Psychological, Social, and Clinical Perspectives on Digital Addiction and Digital Diseases

Özgün Arda Kuş
https://orcid.org/0000-0002-1487-3772
Uskudar University, Turkey

IGI Global
Scientific Publishing
Publishing Tomorrow's Research Today

Vice President of Editorial Melissa Wagner
Director of Acquisitions Mikaela Felty
Director of Book Development Jocelynn Hessler
Production Manager Mike Brehm
Cover Design Jose Rosado

Published in the United States of America by
IGI Global Scientific Publishing
701 East Chocolate Avenue
Hershey, PA, 17033, USA
Tel: 717-533-8845 | Fax: 717-533-7115
Website: https://www.igi-global.com E-mail: cust@igi-global.com

Library of Congress Cataloging-in-Publication Data

LCCN: 2026029205 (CIP Data Pending)
ISBN13: 9798260024683
Isbn13Softcover: 9798260024690
EISBN13: 9798260024706
British Cataloguing in Publication Data
A Cataloguing in Publication record for this book is available from the British Library.

Editorial Advisory Board

Table of Contents

Detailed Table of Contents

Cyberbullying is a major psychosocial risk for young adults, linked to adverse mental health outcomes. The study examined loneliness as a mediator between cyberbullying victimization and psychological distress among undergraduates in Northern India. A cross-sectional survey was conducted, and 427 students who reported cyberbullying victimization were included. Cyberbullying was measured using the Cyber-Bullying and Victimization Experiences Questionnaire, loneliness by the UCLA Loneliness Scale and psychological distress by the Kessler Psychological Distress Scale. Mediation analysis showed cyberbullying victimization was significantly associated with both loneliness and psychological distress. Loneliness also significantly predicted psychological distress. Additionally, loneliness partially mediated the relationship between cyberbullying and psychological distress, indicating both direct and indirect effects. These findings underscore loneliness as a key psychosocial mechanism and highlight the need for interventions targeting cyberbullying and social isolation among undergraduates.

The integration of digital technologies has transformed university life, enhancing learning and connectivity while giving rise to excessive internet use (EIU) among students. University students occupy a vulnerable position due to the combined impact of developmental transitions, academic pressures, social expectations, residential environments and pervasive digital access. This chapter, drawing on multidisciplinary research, examines conceptual and measurement challenges, global prevalence trends, and key psychological, social, and behavioural predictors of EIU. The chapter highlights the academic, psychosocial, and spiritual consequences associated with excessive use, emphasising its role as a maladaptive coping mechanism and difficulties in self-regulation rather than merely a behavioural excess. The chapter emphasises structured, multi-level interventions aimed at strengthening digital self-regulation, adaptive coping, and healthy engagement with technology, positioning universities as key settings for promoting digital well-being, resilience, and sustainable student development.

University students are highly vulnerable to psychological problems, often rooted in low self-acceptance during the quarter-life crisis, a condition closely linked to depression and suicidal ideation. This study is a Formative Context Evaluation with two objectives: (1) assessing the urgency of the problem and (2) designing a structured intervention model. A descriptive survey of 25 students from five universities in Semarang revealed concerning findings: 96% reported insecurity, 88% experienced a quarter-life crisis, and 56% reported suicidal ideation related to difficulties in self-acceptance. These results confirm the urgent need for low-stigma mental health interventions. In response, this study proposes Self-Talks, an interactive literature-based peer support model that employs identification, catharsis, and expressive writing to enhance self-acceptance and strengthen social support. Positioned as a non-digital intervention, Self-Talks aims to mitigate the psychological effects of digital pathology through narrative engagement and structured internal dialogue.

The problem of Internet pornography addiction (IPA) has become a subject of significant academic interest as a multifaceted and complex problem. The I-PACE model describes risk factors, emotional and cognitive reactions, and decision-making deficiencies that contribute to recreational use becoming problematic. Neuroimaging has shown reward circuits and frontal-striatal dysregulation, placing IPA in addiction neurobiology. These data would predict stigma, peer normalization, social isolation, and culturally deep-rooted taboos that enhance relationship or self-stigmatization. Many laws criminalize child sexual abuse material (CSAM) without addressing addiction. This legal and cultural approach stresses modest steps to remove institutional frameworks and human predispositions.This multidisciplinary analysis conceptualizes IPA as a reliance on neurobiological, psychological, social, and legal factors. It advocates for culturally tailored, empirically supported interventions that address individual vulnerabilities within specific sociocultural milieus.

Pornography has existed across different historical periods; however, the digital age has fundamentally transformed its production, circulation, and consumption. This chapter examines how digitalization has reshaped pornography from a limited practice into a continuous, algorithmically governed, and personalized system. Rather than treating this shift as a quantitative increase, it is conceptualized as a structural break defined by platform-based governance, limitless access, and early-age exposure. Drawing on interdisciplinary literature, the chapter analyzes how digital pornography functions as a supernormal stimulus that reinforces desensitization and impaired self-regulation, while algorithmic recommendation systems and emerging technologies such as deepfake pornography intensify dependency, reshape consent, and reproduce gendered forms of digital violence. Digital pornography is thus approached as a structural phenomenon embedded in platform capitalism rather than an individual moral issue.

In this era of rapid technological advancement, it is clear that integration with digital devices shapes human behaviour, including consumption habits and eating behaviours. This situation has the potential to pave the way for an increase in addictive tendencies linked to technology use. In this section, the bidirectional link between excessive technology use—specifically online gaming addiction and problematic smartphone use—and emotional eating and food addiction will be examined. In this context, the section will address how digital platforms that are designed to be engaging and encourage connectivity may simultaneously reduce individuals' self-control over eating behaviours and trigger cravings. In examining the relationship between technology use and eating behaviours, the aim is to address common neurobiological foundations and psychological mechanisms such as impulsivity, particularly in the context of addiction. Furthermore, this chapter offers recommendations for future research and practice by exploring the intersections between eating and technology addiction.

In the digital era, social media has become an integral part of everyday life, particularly among adolescents, young adults, and working professionals. While these platforms provide numerous benefits, including social connectivity, entertainment, and access to information, they also pose significant challenges to users' sleep health. This chapter explores the detrimental impact of late-night social media usage on sleep quality and overall well-being. As screen time during nighttime hours becomes increasingly common, users are exposed to blue light emissions, algorithm-driven content, and cognitive stimulation that delay sleep onset and reduce sleep duration. Biologically, the disruption of circadian rhythms and suppression of melatonin caused by prolonged exposure to screens lead to poor sleep architecture and neural fatigue. Psychologically, users report heightened anxiety, mood swings, and depressive symptoms linked to both insufficient sleep and online social comparison.

This chapter presents a comprehensive public health perspective on digital addictions, focusing on problematic behaviors associated with smartphones, social media, online gaming, and other digital platforms. It explores a range of adverse physical, psychological, and social outcomes linked to these behaviors, including sleep disturbances, mental health challenges, and impaired functioning. The chapter reviews key theoretical frameworks such as behavioral addiction models, cognitive-behavioral approaches, and socio-ecological perspectives to clarify mechanisms and risk factors. It also addresses the influence of social determinants, digital environments, and vulnerable populations. Building on these foundations, the chapter outlines evidence-based, community-level prevention and intervention strategies, emphasizing family, school, and healthcare settings. Interdisciplinary collaboration,

Foreword

The most profound consequences of digital technologies are often not found in the devices themselves, but in the ways they shape human thoughts, emotions, relationships, and everyday experiences. Over the past few decades, digital innovations have transformed how people communicate, learn, work, and participate in society. Alongside these unprecedented opportunities, however, new psychological, social, and clinical challenges have emerged that demand increasing scholarly attention.

As digital technologies become deeply embedded in daily life, concerns surrounding digital addiction and digital diseases have expanded far beyond the boundaries of academic inquiry. These issues now intersect with public health, education, family life, and social policy. What was once viewed simply as excessive technology use is now understood as a complex phenomenon shaped by psychological vulnerabilities, social environments, developmental processes, and technological systems that influence human behavior in powerful and often subtle ways.

Psychological, Social, and Clinical Perspectives on Digital Addiction and Digital Diseases brings together a diverse collection of scholarly contributions that examine these challenges from multiple perspectives. Collectively, the chapters demonstrate that digital addiction is not merely an individual struggle but a multidimensional issue with implications for mental health, social functioning, educational outcomes, and societal well-being.

Particular attention is devoted to the psychological and social dimensions of digital technology use. The contributors explore issues such as cyberbullying victimization, loneliness, psychological distress, excessive internet use among university students, and the broader social consequences of digital pathology. These discussions remind us that digital environments are not simply technological spaces; they are also social and psychological environments that influence identity formation, interpersonal relationships, and emotional well-being.

The book also addresses emerging concerns related to digital sexuality and online pornography. Drawing upon psychological, neurocognitive, social, and developmental perspectives, the authors examine how digital sexual content shapes attitudes, behaviors, and developmental processes, particularly among adolescents and young adults. Their analyses contribute to a more nuanced understanding of one of the most rapidly evolving dimensions of contemporary digital culture.

Equally important are the chapters dedicated to the clinical and public health consequences of technology-related behavioral problems. Sleep disturbances associated with screen exposure, challenges to psychological well-being, intervention strategies, treatment approaches, and broader public health implications are examined through evidence-based perspectives. Together, these contributions demonstrate that digital addiction is not solely a clinical concern but a societal issue requiring coordinated responses from healthcare professionals, educators, families, and policymakers.

One of the defining strengths of this work is its interdisciplinary perspective. Contributions from psychology, psychiatry, communication studies, educational sciences, sociology, public health, and related disciplines provide a comprehensive understanding of both the causes and consequences of digital addiction and digital diseases. Such intellectual diversity is essential for addressing challenges that are dynamic, multifaceted, and continuously evolving.

Importantly, the discussions presented here are neither alarmist nor technologically pessimistic. The contributors recognize that digital technologies have become an indispensable part of contemporary life and that meaningful solutions can emerge only through a balanced understanding of both opportunities and risks. Rather than advocating withdrawal from technology, this book encourages greater awareness, healthier patterns of engagement, and more responsible approaches to digital life.

As digital environments continue to shape the future of human experience, understanding their psychological, social, and clinical implications becomes increasingly important. I believe that this book will serve as a valuable resource for researchers, clinicians, educators, students, and policymakers seeking deeper insight into the challenges and opportunities of the digital age.

It is my sincere hope that the knowledge and perspectives shared throughout this work will contribute to the promotion of digital well-being, the development of effective interventions, and the cultivation of healthier relationships between individuals, communities, and the technologies that increasingly shape modern life.

Nevzat Tarhan
Üsküdar University, Turkey

Preface

Perhaps one of the greatest paradoxes of our age is that humanity has never been more connected, yet many individuals have never felt more isolated. We carry entire worlds in our pockets, communicate instantly across continents, and have access to unprecedented amounts of information. Yet alongside these extraordinary advances, rising levels of loneliness, psychological distress, sleep disruption, emotional exhaustion, and social fragmentation have become increasingly visible realities of contemporary life.

Digital technologies have fundamentally transformed the ways people interact with one another, construct their identities, seek information, form relationships, and experience everyday life. What began as a technological revolution has gradually evolved into a profound psychological and social transformation. As digital environments become embedded in nearly every aspect of human existence, understanding their consequences is no longer a matter of technological interest alone; it has become a matter of individual well-being, public health, and social sustainability.

For many years, discussions surrounding digital technologies focused primarily on access, innovation, efficiency, and connectivity. More recently, however, growing attention has been directed toward the unintended consequences of digital life. Questions concerning digital addiction, online victimization, problematic internet use, digital sexuality, sleep disturbances, mental well-being, and technology-related health outcomes have moved to the forefront of both academic inquiry and public debate.

At the same time, it has become increasingly clear that digital addiction cannot be understood solely as a behavioral issue. The consequences of problematic technology use extend far beyond screen time or excessive engagement. They influence emotional development, interpersonal relationships, psychological resilience, academic performance, social participation, and overall quality of life. In this respect, digital addictions and digital diseases represent not merely technological concerns but complex human concerns.

One of the challenges facing contemporary scholarship is that the psychological, social, and clinical consequences of digital technologies are often studied in isolation from one another. Yet human experience is never fragmented in this way. Emotional difficulties affect social relationships; social environments influence mental health; clinical outcomes are shaped by broader cultural and technological contexts. Consequently, meaningful understanding requires an interdisciplinary approach capable of bringing these interconnected dimensions together.

This book was prepared in response to that need. *Psychological, Social, and Clinical Perspectives on Digital Addiction and Digital Diseases* brings together scholars from diverse disciplines who examine the human consequences of digital life through theoretical, empirical, and applied perspectives.

CHAPTER OVERVIEW

The chapters included in this book explore a wide range of contemporary issues, including cyberbullying victimization, loneliness, psychological distress, excessive internet use among university students, digital pathology, online pornography addiction, adolescent vulnerability, sleep disturbances, mental well-being, public health implications, treatment approaches, and policy perspectives. Collectively, these contributions demonstrate that the effects of digital technologies cannot be reduced to a single discipline, a single symptom, or a single explanation.

One of the greatest strengths of this book lies in its multidisciplinary character. Contributions from psychology, psychiatry, communication studies, educational sciences, sociology, public health, and related fields provide a comprehensive understanding of the challenges emerging at the intersection of human behavior and digital environments. Through this diversity of perspectives, the book seeks not only to identify risks but also to explore pathways toward healthier digital lives.

Importantly, this work does not advocate fear of technology nor a return to a pre-digital world. Digital technologies have become integral to modern society and will continue to shape future generations. The challenge before us is not whether technology should be used, but how it can be used in ways that support psychological well-being, social cohesion, and human flourishing.

As digital environments continue to evolve, so too will the opportunities and challenges they create. It is my hope that this book will contribute to ongoing scientific discussions, inspire future interdisciplinary collaborations, and provide meaningful insights for researchers, clinicians, educators, policymakers, and students seeking to better understand the psychological, social, and clinical dimensions of digital addiction and digital diseases.

Finally, I would like to express my sincere gratitude to all authors, reviewers, and members of the editorial team whose dedication and expertise made this book possible. Their contributions have enriched this work and strengthened our collective understanding of one of the defining issues of the digital age.

Özgün Arda Kus
Uskudar University, Turkey

Acknowledgment

The completion of *Technology Addictions and Digital Diseases: Theories and Practices* has been made possible through the valuable contributions, collaboration, and support of many individuals and institutions.

First and foremost, I would like to express my sincere gratitude to all contributing authors for their scholarly efforts, patience, and commitment throughout the editorial and revision processes. Their interdisciplinary perspectives and academic dedication have significantly enriched the quality and scope of this book.

I would also like to thank the reviewers for their valuable feedback and constructive evaluations, which played an important role in strengthening the chapters included in this volume.

My appreciation extends to the editorial and publishing team at IGI Global Scientific Publishing for their professional guidance, continuous support, and coordination throughout the publication process.

This book was developed with the aim of contributing to the growing body of knowledge surrounding technology addictions, digital diseases, and their psychological, behavioral, social, and neurocognitive dimensions in the rapidly evolving digital era. It is my hope that this work will contribute to future research, academic discussions, and interdisciplinary collaborations in this important field.

Finally, I would like to dedicate this work to the memory of my beloved mother, Canan KARAUÇAK, whose love and guidance continue to inspire me; to my wife, Asena Irmak KUŞ, for her endless patience, understanding, and support throughout this journey; and to my cats, who brought comfort and peace during the long writing process.

Özgün Arda Kuş
Üsküdar University, Turkey

Chapter 1

Digital Diseases:
The Hidden Cost of Connectivity

Arun Agrawal
http://orcid.org/0000-0001-7233-6660
Institute of Technology and Management, Gwalior, India

Pramod Kumar
http://orcid.org/0009-0001-0700-4253
Ganga Institute of Technology and Management, Kablan, India

S. Sindhuja
http://orcid.org/0009-0008-7362-6502
Malla Reddy Engineering College for Women, India

K. Shyam Sunder Reddy
MVSR Engineering College, India

Sujatha Somesula
Chaitanya Bharathi Institute of Technology, Pallavolu, India

Srinivasan Nagaraj
Chaitanya Bharathi Institute of Technology, Proddatur, India

Deeapk Gupta
http://orcid.org/0000-0003-3929-1362
Institute of Technology and Management, Gwalior, India

ABSTRACT

Digital technologies have reshaped modern life through constant connectivity, improving communication, learning, and efficiency. However, continuous and excessive digital engagement has also led to emerging health and behavioral conditions known as digital diseases. This chapter explores the hidden costs of hyperconnectivity by examining psychological, cognitive, physical, and social impacts of prolonged technology use. It conceptualizes digital diseases as lifestyle-related conditions driven by digital dependence, technology addiction, and algorithmic design rather than traditional biological causes. The chapter discusses key theoretical foundations, major categories of digital diseases, impacts across different life stages, and challenges in diagnosis. It also highlights prevention, intervention, and

DOI: 10.4018/979-8-2600-2468-3.ch001

policy approaches required to promote digital well-being. The chapter emphasizes the need for balanced, ethical, and responsible technology use to ensure that digital connectivity enhances rather than harms human health.

INTRODUCTION

This chapter discusses how the internet connectivity of everyday life devices has transformed life. The world today is dominated by digital systems in communication, work, learning and in shopping and leisure. In 2024, the average time spent at the screens across the globe was more than seven hours per day, and teenagers spent even more (DataReportal, 2024, cited in Kaya and Gullu Pinar, 2025). Such omnipresent connectivity is what is also known as "*hyperconnectivity*" that collapses time and space and renders information and social interaction easily accessible. Nonetheless, such systems are also dangerous to the physical and mental health, cognitive abilities, and social well-being of people. These threats have been what this chapter calls as digital diseases.

It is not merely an issue of screens. They are both health and behavioral issues that are caused by constant exposure to digital worlds that aim to stimulate the highest level of user interest via the reward systems of the brain. Such issues are not the fault of some personal weaknesses, but instead generated on the platforms that employ strategies such as elimination of stop lights, variable reinforcement, social comparison, and novelty to encourage their users to remain on the platforms and consume their services unhealthily (Kaya and Güllupinar, 2025; Termann, 2025).

The chapter develops a paradigm of comprehending digital disorders. It establishes the main terms, bridges the theories of addiction and cognitive studies, and suggests a model of how digital disorders are created. The chapter lists the digital disorders, examines the causes behind these disorders and their effects on various life groups and solutions to these problems using the technology, policy, ethical, and regulatory approaches. The discussion of the chapter is summarized with case studies and future research directions.

DIGITAL TECHNOLOGY EVOLUTION AND ALWAYS-CONNECTED LIFESTYLES

A transition between room-sized mainframes and pocket-sized supercomputers was a sixty-year process, but less than fifteen years were needed to perform a transformation between a targeted access and an always-available, everywhere-available connections. Task-specific use was facilitated in the 1990s through email, desktop computing and dial-up internet; the interaction between the users and the technology was functional only (Celebic & Rendulic, 2011). The ubiquity of broadband, Wi-Fi, and 3G/4G/5G mobile networks, the tremendous reduction in the prices of smartphones, have swept away these boundaries (George et al., 2023). This has been done through social media platforms, streaming services, mobile games, and cloud-based office applications which establish a digital domain where social interaction, information, commerce, and entertainment merge. Modern digital infrastructure is not a tool that is easily accessible, but is present everywhere in social life, and has been integrated into homes, schools, health care facilities, transport networks, and street environments (Samala et al., 2024). This structural entrapment renders disconnection amidst the individuals both logistically challenging and socially excessively expensive hence establishing the structural preconditions of the dissemination of digital illnesses.

FROM CONVENIENCE TO COMPULSION: THE SHIFT TO DIGITAL DEPENDENCE

The first reasoning that has resulted in the mass use of digital technologies was mainly practical: the population was using these devices due to fact that they saved time, saved their efforts and increased the area of their application (Costa et al., 2023). This instrumental association is limited to itself; as soon as one has done the job, the instrument is put aside. The transition of using it to reliance, even addiction, is not merely making the use more expansive, but rather a fundamental alteration of the interaction between the users and the technology, this phenomenon is mainly motivated by well thought decisions. The notification, reminder, and variable-ratio rewarding schemes are made to cause compulsive checking behaviors (Kim & Park, 2025), turning intentional interactions into automatic and emotion-controlled interactions. Such dependence is not only excessive but also distressing or dysfunctional in the absence of digital resources, which is also typical of withdrawal responses seen in substance use disorder (Goncalves et al., 2023). This change should be understood since the target of intervention is not screen time, but rather the inherent qualities of digital spaces that usurp volitional control.

Digital Diseases as a Multidisciplinary Public Health Concern

The expanding evidence base in digital health works across a wide range of fields, which include psychiatry, cognitive neuroscience, public health, sociology, organisational behaviour, human-computer interaction, but each of these has communicated with insufficient fluency to produce integrated models. Symptom clusters have been described and proposed as diagnostic criteria using psychology (Moreno et al., 2022); neuroscience has clarified the dopaminergic mechanisms (Termann, 2025); public health has embarked on mapping prevalence at the population level (Iyamu et al., 2022); and technologies that cause greater harm in particular have been analysed through critical technology studies (Kaya and Güllupinar, 2025). The required and what this chapter offers in the explanatory and policy relevant model is the framework that is going to bring these disciplinary efforts together to come up with a complete and coherent explanatory model.

There are three unique contributions to this chapter. First, it theorizes digital diseases as a societal health issue that is established by interplay of algorithmic design, organisational pressures, and cultural practices- not the failure of a behaviour. Second, it combines the insights of the artificial intelligence, attention economy theory, and persuasive digital design to conceptualize the structural processes by which algorithm-based systems can create compulsive consumption patterns and objective health consequences. Third, it offers a life-stage overview of digital disease risk and how children, working adults, and older adults have different but interacting patterns of digital vulnerability. These works collectively build the field, providing a multi-level method of analysis and treatment of digital diseases in hyper-connected societies.

DIGITAL DISEASE FORMATION FRAMEWORK

One of the major contributions of this chapter is the Digital Disease Formation Framework (DDFF), which acts as the roadmap towards the understanding of the digital diseases. It states that, digital diseases are the result of interaction of four forces. The first is platform architecture, which encompasses such design characteristics as reinforcement loops, the removal of stopping cues, algorithmic nudging, and personalised content that optimise engagement at the cost of the user. Second, there are the mechanisms of attention economy where human attention is viewed as a commodity and platforms are optimised to extract it. Third, life-cycle and situational stressors, including vulnerability to developmental changes in children, workers to be always available and caregiving responsibilities, and older adults to lack digital literacy. Fourth, personal psychology and neurobiology, such as individual capacity to self-regulate, react to rewards, mental health, and social environment.

The DDFF is not an earlier model but aims at structural causes of the problem instead of individualizing it in the self-control of the person. It also emphasizes feedback mechanisms in which the outcomes of the digital disease, such as the anxiety or sleep disturbance, predispositions to additional compulsive consumption. Awareness of these loops assists in the design of interventions which do not rely upon the individual attempting to reverse harms and anticipating that they will somehow be able to withstand the systemic leverage points.

CONCEPTUAL FRAMEWORK OF DIGITAL DISEASES

It is obligatory to provide definitional and conceptual parameters before studying digital diseases on the empirical and theoretical level. The conceptual clarity is of particular significance in a discipline where terms like digital addiction, internet disorder, screen addiction, technostress, and digital dependency are subjected to different and even conflicting definitions in literature of different disciplines.

Definition and Scope

Digital diseases refer to disorders which damage physical, mental, cognitive, or social well-being as a result of prolonged, excessive, or forced usage of digital technologies. There are four significant portions of this definition. To begin with, sustained and excessive use exceeds the recommended screen time; it is the use of digital devices when it replaces the significant offline activities, impairs functioning, or behaviors that seem to be out of control (Smits et al., 2022). Second, structurally coerced use is occurring in a setting that requires or reinforces perpetual connectivity, i.e. the issue is not merely a matter of choice. Third, there are various aspects of health influenced by digital diseases, such as body, mind, thinking, and social interactions, demonstrated in clinical and population studies (Raj et al., 2024; Holt-Lunstad, 2024). Fourth, the concept of digital technologies would encompass smartphones, social media, gaming, wearables, streaming, and immersive devices as the issue is in the manner the platforms interface with the users, rather than the gadgets themselves.

Digital diseases are categorized on two dimensions namely impact domain and the level of compulsion. The domain of impact encompasses such psychological problems as anxiety or depression, cognitive ones such as loss of attention or memory impairment, physical such as eye strain or sleeping disturbance, and social-behavioral such as withdrawal or aggression. The degree of compulsion is a distinction between dependency, a partial loss of control is observed, and addiction, which is characterized by an inability to control and ongoing damage (Gonçalves et al., 2023). The system informs interventions: dependency can be ameliorated by changing habits, whereas addiction is frequently a clinical issue that demands a similar approach as substance use therapy (Andrade, 2025).

Distinguishing Digital Addiction from Digital Dependency

Digital dependency and digital addiction are used interchangeably. Digital dependency refers to the habitual engagement with digital technologies to work, communicate, or emotionally satisfy a person, whereby a person is still capable of controlling or decreasing the use in the event that they are motivated and supported by the situational factors. Digital addiction is worse and does entail control loss. It fits the same criteria as substance or behavioral addictions: the activity takes priority of thought, gives a temporary boost, has to be used more and more, is a source of withdrawal, causes conflicts, and it comes back after trying to quit (Gonçalves et al., 2023). According to neurobiological research, there are alterations in dopamine systems and deactivation of the prefrontal activity, which connects digital addiction to other disorders such as gambling (Andrade, 2025). This chapter considers digital addiction as the extreme point of a scale, beginning with normal use, passing to dependency, and finishing with full-fledged addiction. This distinction is valuable in that the policy and intervention strategies must align with the level of this distinction in which milder cases can be treated with changes in habits, and serious cases can be treated with clinical treatment.

Digital Diseases as a Public Health Challenge

It is significant to frame digital diseases as a public health issue as this will influence the way society reacts. Individual case treatment of digital addiction is needed but not sufficient as it is impossible to treat lung cancer instead of controlling tobacco or acting as an awareness campaign. The top three reasons, which are persuasive design, algorithmic nudging, attention-driven features, and workplace connectivity norms, impact a large number of individuals, and not just those who are at risk. Practical actions on the population level require unified interventions in the control of platforms, organizational policy, clinical practice, education, and community awareness (Iyamu et al., 2022). All ages and social groups are affected by digital diseases albeit disproportionately. They pose health burdens, including increased mental health demands, economic costs due to reduced productivity and employee absenteeism, and social costs (poor relationships and community unity). These compounding effects render digital diseases a priority since it concerns the population as would any other lifestyle illness (Vu et al., 2024). By looking at them in this way, prevention, collective accountability, and system-wide remedies are more likely to be considered than individual behavior or pathology.

THEORETICAL FOUNDATIONS

An intensive theoretical explanation of digital diseases should achieve four tasks: labeling the central constructs, locating digital diseases within established systems of addiction and health, harmonising rival or supplementary theoretical approaches, and explaining the way the synthesised framework develops the current models. It discusses each of these, respectively and based on behavioural addiction theory, cognitive overload and attention fragmentation theory, neuroplasticity and dopaminergic reinforcement research, and the socio-technical systems perspective. None of the theories is adequate; it is the combination of them that makes the account explanatory.

Behavioural Addiction Theory

Explaining serious cases of digital illnesses is possible with the help of behavioural addiction theory, which has initially been developed based on the research of gambling, then applied to the use of internet and technology (Andrade, 2025). It demonstrates that non-substance consumption may also develop addictive brain processes similar to drug addiction: dopamine-stimulated gratification in the mesolimbic circuit, habituation in the basal ganglia, and loss of prefrontal control (Termann, 2025). These mechanisms are used to abuse the digital platforms through the provision of variable-ratio rewards that are unpredictable and highly motivating. As likes, comments, or matches, notifications are not delivered consistently, thus the checking devices become compulsory and not deliberate (Kaya and Gullu pinar, 2025).

The theory does not imply that all heavy users are addicted. It describes the transition of normal usage to dependency and then addiction, and features of the platform that accelerate this. Critics believe that it can excessively pathologise normal behaviour, use substance criteria in the wrong way and ignore social and design contexts (Goncalves et al., 2023). Digital Disease Formation Framework (DDFF) is the solution to such problems as it reveals behavioural mechanisms in a broader structural approach. Nevertheless, behavioural addiction theory will still be fundamental to the explanation of severe digital disease, such as the loss of control, withdrawal and irresistible use regardless of harm.

Cognitive Overload and Attention Fragmentation Theory

The cognitive overload theory is a theory that follows the work of Sweller and scaled into digital environments, elaborating on how the digital environment has an impact on the way one thinks (Alimour and Alrabeei, 2025). The capacity of human working memory is limited and in cases where excessive information is presented at a very fast rate, it leads to poor performance: understanding decreases, mistakes increase, learning becomes slow, and the mind becomes fatigued. The digital systems generate a feeling of overload due to constant notifications, multitasking, unending scrolling, and handling more than one communication channel.

The theory of attention fragmentation contributes to the first one and demonstrates that cognitive efficiency declines due to task-switching. Attention residue is the phenomenon when a certain part of the mind remains on the past task, hindering the fresh ones (Alimour and Alrabeei, 2025). Research indicates that it can take 23 minutes to get over an interruption of one notification, which is why continuous notifications do not allow one to think profoundly (Beeson et al., 2024). This has more than productivity effects: it causes anxiety, impairs memory, and impedes reflective thinking, and damages creativity, emotional control, and moral judgment.

These theories have a weakness in that they assume that digital overload is not a design but a given. They characterize the cognitive effects but not platform features with deliberate intent to form them. This chapter responds to this association by relating cognitive overload and fragmentation of attention to socio-technical and attention economy views and demonstrates the construction of digital systems to generate maximum engagement at the expense of overloading users.

Neuroplasticity and Dopamine-Driven Digital Behaviour

Digital diseases are neuroscientific with a reference to neuroplasticity and dopamine reinforcement (Termann, 2025). The release of dopamine, when users get digital rewards they are not expected to get (such as notifications or in-game victory), marks the brain to continue with the behaviour. Frequent exposure reinforces neural pathways, which makes digital interactions simpler and more predominant and offline activities less appealing. With time, the reward system of the brain is re-adjusted making people dependent on digital stimulation.

The dopamine collapse hypothesis proposed by Termann (2025) states that repeated and extreme digital rewards can reduce the dopamine levels of the baselines, which results in the decrease of pleasure, diminished motivation, and the increase of dependence on digital instruments. This is facilitated by clinical observations that reveal that people pull out of offline life but still become compulsively online.

Neuroplasticity poses a problem to children and adolescents too. Their prefrontal cortex, which controls themselves and plans, has not fully developed until the mid-twenties (Pardhan et al., 2022). Early exposure to high reward digital worlds can change reward sensitization and self-regulation that persists into adulthood.

Socio-Technical Systems Perspective

The socio-technical systems school of thought, as an organisation theory and technology studies, is of use in explaining digital diseases as a result of user-technology, user-workplace, user-culture, and user-economic incentive, interaction (Wuersch et al., 2023). Such an opinion goes beyond individualistic explanations that postulate personal weakness as the cause of digital ills.

Digital diseases are not simply accidental and not so much psychological. They are the result of systems that maximise enjoyment: the platforms capitalise on additional screen time, the workplaces insist on full-time availability, cultural norms are rewarding productivity and connectivity and regulation frequently does not ensure safe design (Eke and Stahl, 2024). All these pressures have rendered excessive use of digital becoming predictable as opposed to random.

The socio-technical approach demonstrates that the solutions should be aimed at several levels. Behavior change by individuals is insufficient when work places and platform design promotes excessive use. Similarly, platform redesign will not be expanded without organisational and regulatory assistance. To mitigate the risk of digital disease, coordinated interventions are required at the behaviour, organisational policy, technology design and regulation levels. The chapter is based on this multi-level approach to policy recommendations.

Integration and Synthesis: Why No Single Theory Suffices

All four theoretical frameworks analyzed above reflect a significant aspect of digital diseases, although each of them possesses some characteristic limitations as well. Behavioural addiction theory is more clinically deep, however, it is liable to over-pathologization and does not value structural determinants. Cognitive overload theory sheds light on the cognition processes but assumes that the information environment is fixed. Neuroplasticity studies provide biological support at the cost of determinism and underestimation of social modifiability. The socio-technical approach offers structural examination, yet might not emphasize individual difference in vulnerability. The DDFF formulated in this chapter incorporates these frameworks by giving each a role in a multi-level causal model: neurobiological mechanisms (dopaminergic reinforcement, neuroplasticity) are those that describe how repeated engagement gives that engagement the characteristics of habitual and then compulsive use; the cognitive overload and attention fragmentation mechanisms are those that describe the cognitive costs accrued in the process; the behavioural addiction criteria are those that provide the clinical threshold markers in the severe end of the spectrum; the socio-technical systems perspective are those that describe the structural

TYPOLOGY OF DIGITAL DISEASES

The four-category typology of digital diseases is based on the multi-level framework mentioned above. It presents the interventions by organizing the main areas of impact, system-level-based reinforcement mechanisms and observable outcomes to determine how disorders in one category may affect the others. The typology is theoretically based on a unique study on behavioral addiction, cognitive load, neuroplasticity, and socio-technical studies, but it is not an official system of diagnosis. It is a research and policy instrument, with new integrative constructs being evidently pointed at, instead of a confirmed clinical typology.

Psychological Digital Disorders

The psychological digital disorders mainly impact the emotional well-being and the mental health. One of the most typical examples can be digital anxiety, which is a consequence of the need to remain always connected in several digital mediums. This hypervigilance is strengthened by notifications and alerts and triggers the stress-response system, which negatively affects physical health in the long term (Barbieri et al., 2024). The use of social media is associated with depressive-related symptoms, particularly passive scrolling, which enhances negative emotions, reduces life satisfaction, and exacerbates depression (Moreno et al., 2022). Social comparison only increases these effects because algorithms give precedence to emotionally charged and aspirational content.

Another vital psychological process is the Fear of missing out (FoMO). It is anxiety that is generated by a thought that people are enjoying themselves better than you and leads to compulsive uses of the platform (Jaworska, 2025). One way that FoMO is influenced is through the platform features such as the real-time post activity indicators, disappearing posts, and social metrics. This culminates into checking at late hours, stress and withdrawal in offline relationships. In qualitative studies, FoMO appears to be socially, informational, and professionally different, and how certain design aspects introduce psychological digital disorders. Clinical assessment and intervention require an understanding of these mechanisms.

Cognitive Digital Disorders

Because of constant exposure to digital stimulation that is rapid and multi-source, cognitive digital disorders influence both attention, memory and executive functioning. One of the processes is attentional fragmentation, in which multitasking, notifications, and faster task-switching progressively decrease attention capacity. Prolonged screen use, in addition to leading to visual fatigue, also reduces cognitive functioning, which leads to more errors and less ability to solve problems (Beeson et al., 2024). As negatively captured in the cross-category feedback model of the DDFF, physical and cognitive effects reinforce.

Another process is memory externalisation. Increasing the use of smartphones and apps as a source of information decreases the internal memory consolidation in the brain that may impact long-term memory, reasoning, and the formation of coherent autobiographical stories that enable self-control and identity (Alimour and Alrabeei, 2025). Although, digital tools can enhance the cognitive capacity, excessive dependence can decrease the role of intrinsic memory, an issue that requires long-term research.

Such disorders are of particular concern in schools and work places. Even when students do not consider themselves affected, digitally multitasking during lessons demonstrates a lowered level of comprehension and retention (Timotheou et al., 2023). Exposed professionals commit fewer errors, are less creative, and fail in complicated work, which influences productivity and career performance (Beeson et al., 2024).

Physical Digital Disorders

Physical digital disorders are the most quantifiable one, but people tend to excuse them as a few ergonomic concerns instead of a matter of health. Digital eye strain, which is characterized by dry eyes, blurred vision, headache, and fatigue, is a condition that occurs in 50-90 percent of heavy screen users depending on the measures used (Kaur et al., 2022). The longer the digital task duration the more symptoms deteriorate and productivity decreases, which is associated with physical disorder having the economic and organisational consequences (Beeson et al., 2024). Such effects are influenced not just by the screen time but also by a lack of such design features as the break reminders, blue-light filters, or usage timers.

The most researched physical digital disorder is sleep disruption. Exposure to screen in the evening lowers melatonin, disrupts circadian rhythms, and reduces the quality of sleep (Barbieri et al., 2024). Persistent sleep deprivation elevates cortisol, compromises prefrontal activity, is emotionally reactive, and undermines immunity. This forms a feedback loop: the lack of sleep reduces the levels of self-control, and a person checks his device compulsively, which, in turn, affects sleep negatively an example of the DDFF feedback phenomenon.

Other physical digital disorders are musculoskeletal issues due to excessive sitting like neck, back, and repetitive strain injuries and psychological health issues that relate physical and psychological conditions.

Social and Behavioural Digital Disorders

Digital disorders of social and behavioural nature have implications on relationships, community participation, and social norms. It is typical of social withdrawal, in which the use of the online environment substitutes in-person communication. Such online interactions do not provide emotion, non-verbal communication, and long-term attention in the face-to-face relations; social skills cannot develop with time (Marinucci et al., 2022). This leads to a vicious cycle where face to face interaction becomes more difficult than computer generated interaction.

These forms of digital social disorganisation are behavioural in nature and include online aggression, trolling and cyberbullying. They are conditioned by the characteristics of the platforms, which emphasise the content with a high level of emotional stimulation to increase the engagement and anonymity, which decreases the social responsibility (Holt-Lunstad, 2024). The victims, particularly adolescents, have depression, anxiety, suicidal intentions, and avoidance of school (Pardhan et al., 2022). It is also damaging to perpetrators as they become desensitized to empathy and normalise hostile communication that can be carried over to the real world.

These problems demonstrate that social digital disorders revolve upon platform design and algorithms. Their ethical and regulatory solution should not focus on behaviour but on the characteristics that facilitate and increase digital social harm.

Integrative Table: Comparative Overview of Digital Disease Typology

Table 1 provides a structured comparative overview of the four disorder categories, organised according to the analytical dimensions of the DDFF. The system-level reinforcement mechanisms identified in the rightmost column correspond directly to the platform design features—stopping-cue removal, reinforcement loops, algorithmic nudging—discussed throughout this chapter.

Table 1. Comparative Overview of Digital Disease Typology (synthesised from the theoretical frameworks detailed in the Theoretical Foundations section; see cited sources for primary empirical evidence).

Disorder Category	Primary Impact Domain	Key Clinical Features	Dominant Psychological/ Neurobiological Drivers	Platform-Level Reinforcement Mechanisms	Representative Evidence
Psychological Disorders	Emotional well-being and mental health	Anxiety, depressive symptoms, FoMO, emotional fatigue, mood dysregulation	Variable-ratio reinforcement, social comparison, dopaminergic reward, hypervigilance habituation	Algorithmic content ranking by emotional salience, social comparison metrics, real-time activity indicators, ephemeral content	Moreno et al. (2022); Jaworska (2025); Barbieri et al. (2024)
Cognitive Disorders	Attention, memory, and executive function	Attentional fragmentation, multitasking fatigue, reduced comprehension, memory externalisation, decision-making impairment	Attention residue, cognitive overload, prefrontal inhibitory competition, habituation of deep-focus capacity	Continuous notifications, infinite scrolling, multitask-enabling interfaces, novelty prioritisation algorithms	Alimour & Alrabeei (2025); Beeson et al. (2024); Timotheou et al. (2023)
Physical Disorders	Physiological health and somatic symptoms	Digital eye strain, circadian disruption, sleep disorders, musculoskeletal pathology, psychosomatic symptoms	Blue-light melatonin suppression, sedentary posture, HPA axis activation from chronic stress, attentional strain	Absence of stopping cues, always-on connectivity design, engagement-maximising defaults, no mandatory break architecture	Kaur et al. (2022); Beeson et al. (2024); Barbieri et al. (2024)
Social & Behavioural Disorders	Social relationships, community conduct, and empathy	Social withdrawal, reduced empathy, online aggression, cyberbullying, relationship deterioration, community disengagement	Disinhibition from anonymity, social skill atrophy from offline avoidance, outrage amplification algorithms, reduced accountability	Engagement-driven content moderation prioritising conflict, anonymity affordances, low platform accountability standards	Marinucci et al. (2022); Holt-Lunstad (2024); Pardhan et al. (2022)

Cross-Category Feedback Mechanisms

The four categories of disorders are not stand-alone silos; they are the nodes of a mutually-reinforcing system. The psyche suffers psychological distress due to anxiety or depressive symptoms which interfere with the prefrontal inhibitory control ability needed to withstand compulsive checking- aggravating the cognitive disorders. Emotional exhaustion is increased by cognitive overload and attentional fragmentation, which increases psychological disorder. Sleep disturbance as a result of physical disturbance diminishes the prefrontal control and emotional stability-enhancing psychological disorders as well as cognitive ones. The lack of social withdrawal decreases the offline social support, which is found to act as a protective factor to digital overuse- enhancing the attractiveness of online social interaction. These cross-category feedback processes imply that interventions that focus on one category and ignore the rest are likely to be producing partial and temporary effects. The system of interactions should be considered within the framework of a comprehensive prevention and treatment model and not the parts of it. This is among the major practical implications of the DDFF.

TECHNOLOGY ADDICTION AS A CORE DRIVER OF DIGITAL DISEASE

Technology addiction, which is the clinical extreme of the dependency-to-addiction continuum outlined above, is a fundamental source of the digital disease development, both to the individuals who attain clinical threshold and to the overall population of dependent users whose risk profile is heightened by the same structural means. The two most common and the most well-reported ones are smartphone and social media addiction, and gaming disorder, both of which are inherently informed by the influence of the AI-based concept of personalisation and persuasive design.

Smartphone and Social Media Addiction

The problem of Smartphones being the primary cause of digital disease is that they will have social connection, information, entertainment, gaming, and commerce all in one device that is kept with the user most of the day. The habit has also moved towards checking instead of accomplishing meant tasks, now involving constant checking where individuals check their phones automatically due to boredom, anxiety, or not knowing what to do socially (AL-Zoubi, 2023). Compulsive use happens when individuals use it regardless of their intentions to quit or because its use has a negative impact on sleep, relationships, or activities at work (Goncalves et al., 2023).

The smartphone addiction brought by social media is driven by social rewards: likes, followers, engagement statistics, real-time comparison, and variable, unpredictable feedback in the form of the slot-machine reinforcement (Kaya and Gullupinar, 2025). These groups are particularly susceptible to adolescents and young adults because peer approval and identity building are crucial at that age (Moreno et al.,

2022). Other emotional harms such as anxiety, depression, body image problems, and FoMO are partially designed into platforms, as they also benefit through social comparison and relentless emotional gratification.

Smartphones therefore become the channel and accelerator of digital illnesses, and connect the device design, the platform architecture, and the human psychology in foreseeable habitual patterns of compulsive usage and destructiveness.

Gaming Disorder

Gaming disorder, a formally recognised condition in the World Health Organization in ICD-11 and a topic of current debate regarding the scope of its diagnosis in DSM-5, is an excellent example of technology addiction with the most robust evidence base to support it. Imataka et al. (2024) discuss the neurobiological, psychological, and social aspects of the gaming disorder, and state that the structural aspects of modern games, which include perennial virtual worlds with endless development cycles, social requirements to fellow players, achievement systems, which provide graduated rewards, and the lack of natural narrative endgames, constitute a qualitatively different engagement environment compared to the previous forms of entertainment. The combination of micro-transaction economies and loot-box mechanics adds the extra dimension of financial reinforcement of variable-ratio reward to bring the behavioural architecture of addiction into the economic sector. Gaming disorder is an issue that is particularly high among adolescent males, but the gender disparity is smaller in mobile games, and it has consequences regarding preventive and therapeutic measures.

AI-Driven Personalisation and Persuasive Design as Structural Addiction Drivers

The most clinically investigated types of digital disease include smartphone and social media addiction, as well as gaming disorder, however, they should be regarded in the larger structural framework of the DDFF. The device is not the main point but using AI-based personalisation and convincing design to make the most of engagement. The AI systems track user preference, emotional stimulation, social sensitivities and timing vulnerability, and provide content that appeals to keep the users more engaged (Gujar, 2024). This acts as an individualised operant conditioning, maximizing reinforcement by providing real time feedback of behaviour.

Elements of the platform like endless scrolling, video auto play, adjustable notification time and social comparison indicators are all strategic decisions. They eliminate natural checkpoints, replace decision-making with algorithmic sequencing, use uncertainty to gain rewards, and publicize social performance, with all these measures to support engagement (Kaya & Güllupinar, 2025).

These mechanisms which are design-driven are significant in terms of public health and regulation. Structural solutions such as a requirement to stop cues, a limit on default notification, and the limitation of variable rate reward systems to the underage group are needed to achieve effective responses, as opposed to individual behaviour change.

THE HIDDEN COSTS OF CONTINUOUS CONNECTIVITY

Technology providers and a large part of the business culture put continuous connectivity forward as an opportunity-enabling condition that makes productivity. The experimental evidence has a more complicated narrative: the covert expenses of unrelenting digital involvement - expenses which are systematically understated as they are dispersed among people, distributed over time and are hard to be assigned to particular digital exposure - are substantial and increasing.

Productivity and Cognitive Performance Degradation

The connection of digital connectivity and productivity in the workplace, in a counter-intuitive way, tends to be not only negative but also negative in relation to knowledge workers whose output relies on a persistent focus and extensive cognitive processing. Beeson et al. (2024) show that direct effects of excessive use of digital screens such as digital eye strain alone, are capable of cause direct productivity losses, without any further effects of digital diseases. The effect on productivity is increased when attentional fragmentation due to constant exposure to notification is introduced. This process does not only entail the amount of time wasted to digital disruption per se, but the overall loss of attentional resources due to continuous task-switching, which diminishes the quality of cognitive performance even when work is supposedly not interrupted by digital interruptions. Empirical research on professional email behaviour has uniformly revealed that the perceived ability to receive a prompt reply, which is due not to individual preference but to organisational culture in most instances, causes significant cognitive inaccessibility to complex tasks with most severe effect on work that involves creative and associative thinking.

Educational Consequences

The effects of unremitting connectivity in learning institutions appear in the forms of loss of quality learning, less understanding, and gradual loss of ability to engage in academic pursuit. Timotheou et al. (2023) report a paradox between the adoption of digital technology in the education sector, which may actually increase access and engagement and learning results when used in a considered manner, and the cognitive impact of habitual multitasking across educational apps and social or entertainment applications. The social media behavior of passive and quick content consumption seems to create attentional rhythm that is not well adapted to deep academic study, implying that the cognitive impacts of digital illness is not limited to the situations where digital technology is directly applied to influence attentional capacity more broadly.

Relationship Deterioration and Social Fabric

Social costs of continuous connectivity are the least quantifiable but possibly the most significant. Marinucci et al. (2022) illustrate that online social bonds, although capable of fulfilling some of the cognitive and emotional roles of face-to-face ties, do not systematically do so, and are missing other functions (especially the physiological co-regulation benefits (synchronised cortisol rhythms, oxytocin release, nervous system regulation through physical proximity) that typify face-to-face social bonding and which seem to be required to support long-term mental and physical health. The large-scale review of the social connection and health outcomes conducted by Holt-Lunstad (2024) makes social isolation and loneliness two of the risk factors, equally hazardous to mortality, as smoking, obesity, and physical inactivity. To this degree to which digital social interaction replaces face-to-face contact, being a replacement and not an addition as continuous connectivity and platform architecture are incentivising, it is becoming a public health burden of morbidity and mortality due to loneliness, but not as such.

Economic and Healthcare System Burden

Digital diseases have a high cost to the economy and involve a variety of sectors. On the individual level, fewer occupational performance, greater absenteeism because of digital illness-related mental and bodily malady, and access to healthcare because of illnesses such as apprehension issues, depression, sleeping issues, and musculoskeletal illnesses are considerable personal expenses. At the organisational level, the attentional fragmentation, burnout, and digital overload can be directly related to the loss of productivity and high human resource costs. On the societal level, Vu et al. (2024) estimate that the healthcare sector burden of the conditions related to digital disease-related issues, including mental health services, sleep medicine, occupational health, and musculoskeletal medicine, constitutes already a significant and increasing demand that the current systems were not aimed to fulfil. Preventive spending on digital literacy education, organisational policy revision, and platform requirement control would probably produce the complete health economic returns that are orders of magnitude greater than their expenditure, yet the longitudinal proof base to back such cost-benefit estimates is not well developed yet.

DIGITAL DISEASES ACROSS THE LIFE COURSE

A systemic analysis of the differences in digital disease risk with developmental stages and social roles is one of the unique contributions of this chapter: it provides the development of specific vulnerability patterns and suggests specific priorities of intervention. Digital illnesses do not take an equal toll on all users; they are facilitated by the developmental neurobiology, social surroundings, job position and by situated digital surroundings that prevail at each stage of life.

Children and Adolescents: Developmental Vulnerability

There are two reasons why children and adolescents are the most susceptible to digital diseases. First, their prefrontal cortex, the impulse controller, planner, and self-controller, does not become fully developed until the mid-to-late twenties. This complicates their ability to withstand persuasive features of platform. Second, exposure to highly rewarding digital endeavours at an early age may have long-term consequences in brain reward system and attention with an impact on lifelong development. Research indicates that childhood device usage is associated to the impaired attentional capacity, language, and executive function, whose impact depends on age and daily screen time (Clemente-Suárez et al., 2024).

Teenagers are particularly susceptible to social media. Social and emotional development is disrupted because of upward social comparison, cyberbullying, the use of late-night devices caused by FoMO, and substitution of face-to-face communication (Pardhan et al., 2022). These risks are increased on platforms via social approval ratings, peer notifications and comparison tools, which capitalize on developmental sensitivities. These social determinants reveal the necessity of community-based health intervention and design policies to safeguard the psychological and mental growth of minors with the help of sites where they spend most of their time.

Working Professionals: Organisational and Occupational Dimensions

Unique disease risks are unique to working professionals since they occur due to the interaction of platform features and workplace norms as opposed to platform design. The anticipation to stay online and be reachable and responsive 24/7 is causing incessant stress and mental strain, as well as work-life boundaries (Bossen and Bertelsen, 2024). The conditions are some of the reasons contributing to burnout, anxiety, sleep issues, and the gradual loss of personal time, particularly knowledge workers and high-demand relational positions.

This chapter presents clinical case studies that demonstrate the effects of pressure on occupational factors that restrict the individual behaviour change. Efforts by employees to diminish the digital availability can be penalized at the employment level, and self-regulation is not enough to safeguard health.

This structural limitation emphasises that organisational policies, including email-free hours, explicit meeting principles and official disconnection rights, are interventions that should be considered. This is also necessary in the form of regulatory frameworks, such as the right-to-disconnect laws in France, Ireland and other nations. Systemic solutions are the major path to lessening the threat of digital disease in the work setting, not individual behavioural change.

Older Adults: Digital Inclusion and Novel Vulnerabilities

The digital disease status of the older adult is unique, with equal positive and negative impacts of digital activity. Technology provides them with healthcare access, socialization with relatives physically far away, cognitive engagement and chances of civic engagement. The studies indicate that the adoption of digital technologies can lessen the feeling of isolation and enhance healthcare outcomes (Zaman et al., 2022).

Nevertheless, elderly people are also exposed to certain risk of digital diseases. Poor digital literacy levels make individuals susceptible to misinformation, internet fraud and exploitation. The age-related changes in sensory and cognitive factors make it physically demanding to use a screen, and technological change may lead to anxiety and digital exclusion.

Social equity is also digitally diseased of the elderly. Socio-economic inequality defines access and literacy, better-equipped older adults have opportunities to gain without risk management, whereas low-income earners have to endure marginalization of vital digital services and also fall prey to scammers.

Prevention programmes should thus focus on overuse and underuse and the strategies to be addressed should be dependent on literacy, access and the socio-economic situation. The rights and needs of older adults should be addressed through protection measures, which would allow balancing digital inclusion with physical, cognitive, and social risks.

Socio-Economic and Gender Dimensions

Digital diseases do not impact all individuals in equal measure, as they are based on exposure and vulnerability, by gender and socio-economic factors. It is linked to a higher prevalence of social media anxiety, FoMO, body image concerns, and cyberbullying, whereas men have a higher level of gaming disorder and technology social withdrawal (Jaworska, 2025; Imataka et al., 2024). Those trends are indicative of the interaction between platform design and social norms: appearance-based social media is destructive to the users whose social identity is pegged on their looks, and competitive gaming places the environment favors individuals in need of offline social replacements.

Risk is also determined by the socio-economic variations. Knowledge-intensive workers with higher-SES are exposed to more occupational digital stress, whereas lower-SES workers are more exposed to exploitation, fake news, and poor-quality digital conditions (Upadhyaya, 2024). It is therefore clear that risk profiles are context-dependent as opposed to using a simple gradient implying that interventions are supposed to be specific to particular susceptibilities. To deal with digital disease fairly, it is necessary to acknowledge the interplay of gender, socio-economic status, and platform design, in respect of how they impact exposure, harm, and possible protective measures.

THE ROLE OF DATA, AI, AND ALGORITHMS IN DIGITAL DISEASE GENERATION

The study of AI, data, and algorithms systems does not fall on the periphery of an account of digital diseases; it is central to it. The processes that platform architecture drives the creation of digital disease reinforcement loops, algorithmic nudging, the removal of stopping-cue, personalised vulnerability exploitation are mostly brought to bear on AI systems that are trained on massive behavioural data. It is critical to the practice of clinical medicine and the response of regulation to understand these mechanisms in adequate specificity.

The Attention Economy: Structural Logic

The attention economy is the economic model where user attention is the main commodity that is monetised by platform businesses, which mainly sell advertising exposure. Kaya and Güllu pinan (2025) follow the history of the attention economy, starting with the early broadcast media and progressing to the modern-day algorithmic platforms, and the major shift was the advent of real time behavioural tracking and algorithmic selection of content, which allowed the platforms to shift their focus on approximating the audience preferences and instead focus on continuously refining individualised models of attentional vulnerabilities and reward sensitivities of each particular user. The attention economy logic has a misalignment in structural incentives: the revenue of the platform is maximized by maximising the time spent by users on the platform, whether this time spent is beneficial to user well-being or not. The single-handy design decisions that lead to less interaction, such as required break notifications, easy notification preferences, clear explanations of the algorithm, etc. are economically punished according to the attention economy model, which results in systematic market failure that cannot be remedied by the market forces alone.

Reinforcement Loops, Stopping-Cue Removal, and Algorithmic Nudging

Platform AI maintains digital disease by using three major mechanisms, which are reinforcement loops, stopping-cue removal, and algorithmic nudging. Reinforcement loops are possible when the interaction between users creates data that narrows down individualized models which then provide content that is more likely to attract the user resulting in a self-driven cycle. This procedure has been becoming more focused on the neurobiological vulnerability of the individual user.

Stopping-cue removal is the elimination of natural pauses, i.e. the end of a video, page, or chapter, by mechanisms like infinite scrolling and auto play. Such cues tend to enable users to have control over the timing when to quit using a platform and thus when they are taken away, they relocate power to the system and make users more compulsive.

The algorithmic nudging is based on tools of notification, content recommendations, urgency, and social activity indicators to re-engage. These nudges capitalize on the capture of attention, disruption of the continuous process of cognition and override of stated user preferences to receive more notifications to keep users constantly active (Kim and Park, 2025). These mechanisms jointly work together to strengthen use, diminish self-regulation, and accelerate the development of digital disease.

Ethical Accountability and the Case for Structural Regulation

Ethics of AI-based engagement maximisation is a serious issue. The fact that platforms optimise their experience based on personalised psychological models is not typically known by users, and thus their usage is not fully informed and is definitely not voluntary. Formal rights are provided by data protection models such as GDPR, yet, in reality, users do not have high transparency and control (Eke and Stahl, 2024). The confidentiality of the algorithms, technical obscurity, and default-behavioural configurations that promote information sharing and alerts systematically subvert autonomy.

The moral case of structural regulation resembles other areas in which the information asymmetry and behavioural design generates market failure. Consumers need not be food scientists to demand safe food, drivers do not need engineering skills to demand safety in the traffic, and patients do not need pharmacology education to have confidence in medicines. In the same way, the regulation of digital platforms, obligatory stopping cues, default notifications, prohibiting variable-ratio rewards to underage individuals, and obligatory transparency of algorithms preserve the health of the population and autonomy of the individuals, instead of leaving it to the discretion of the individual user or to self-regulation. These organizational solutions solve the ethical vacuum that opaque, engagement-maximising AI has generated.

DIAGNOSIS AND ASSESSMENT APPROACHES

The digital diseases are a disease whose diagnosis criteria lack full validation with international agreement, the comorbidity with well-established mental health diseases, the heterogeneity of expression among age groups and cultures, and the rapid changes in the digital environments that provoke the conditions under observation, present a set of challenges to their diagnosis. These are not imaginary problems but can be overcome; they require methodological pluralism and further investment in standardisation research, not cynicism on the clinical reality of digital diseases.

Clinical and Psychological Assessment Tools

The clinical assessment tools that are presently available in digital diseases are standardised self-report measures. Internet Addiction Test (IAT) The test was first created by Young; it has been modified by several other researchers multiple times, but its factor structure and cut-off scores differ across different studies and populations (Moreno et al., 2022). The Social Media Addiction Scale, Gaming Disorder Scale and gaming-specific measures offer more specific evaluation in subcategories of digital diseases. Structured diagnostic interviews: The most diagnostically rigorous assessments of severe presentations are structured diagnostic interviews which primarily probabilistically probe the six criteria of behavioural addictions (salience, mood modification, tolerance, withdrawal, conflict, and relapse). The cognitive dimensions of the digital disease can be quantified using cognitive assessment, that is, standardised attention, working memory and executive function and present objective indicators, which are complementary to self-report. The condition of digital addicts assessment tools is discussed by Patel et al. (2025), and the most promising options to prioritize clinical and research practice are exposed; it is stated that the tools require cross-cultural validation and the norms of a specific age range.

Digital Behaviour Metrics and Analytics

The analytical technologies in screen-time, the algorithms that are now the part of the big smartphone operating systems, generate objective behavioural data, which can be used as the secondary source and corroborate the self-report. The data present granular insights into engagement patterns, which is often under-reported by self-report data, such as daily screen time by app, number of unlocks, distributions of session lengths, and time-of-day patterns of use, to give a more detailed view of engagement patterns that is not as evident when it comes to self-reported metrics (Ukabuiro and Agomah, 2025). Passive mobile sensing methods, where a device gathers behavioural or physiological and contextual data in the form of a smartphone sensor, present a prospect of ecological momentary perception of digital disease behaviour in naturalistic environments, where complicated matters of utilization patterns and instantaneous implications on mood, attention, and physiological condition are captured. Subsidiary physiological data capture by wearable gadgets tracking sleep quality, heart rate variability, or physical activity can be operationalised to mirror the physical and autonomic effects of the digital overuse (Khedrabi et al., 2022).

Standardisation Challenges and Diagnostic Boundaries

Digital diseases are not very easy to diagnose since the same behaviour signifies different things to diverse individuals. An excessive mode of smart phone use, excessive gaming or a high rate of frequent use of social media can be detrimental to certain people but healthy or even necessary to others. It is not about the number of hours a person spends on the Internet every day; rather, the question is whether it makes people's lives worse, makes them stressed, or makes them less capable of self-control. Digital diseases regularly come along with other conditions such as depression, anxiety, ADHD or autism. The relationship between them is not always apparent or how they affect one another. An adequate assessment examines mental health history, development and a comparison of the onset of the symptoms against the use of the digital. The majority of types of digital diseases lack official international diagnostic rules, save gaming disorder of ICD-11. This complicates the comparison of research. Instead of monitoring screen time, doctors and researchers have to pay close attention to behaviour and its implications. The objective is to specify whether digital use is addictive, harmful or typical.

PREVENTION AND INTERVENTION STRATEGIES

Effective response to digital diseases should go at the same time and at the same time across several levels of response, as: 1) the determinants of digital disease are in turn themselves multi-level; and 2) as the DDFF reveals, digital disease determinants exist at multiple levels simultaneously. Individual behaviour change tactics though important are not enough in the instance when the structural design aspects of platform and organisational norms are systematic in derailing the self-regulation ability it builds on. The next section will structure evidence-based intervention landscape in terms of the level of intervention, clarifying where the key leverage points of various types of digital disease are.

Individual-Level: Digital Literacy, Self-Regulation, and Therapeutic Approaches

Individual prevention of digital diseases is primarily implemented through digital literacy education (Aydinlare et al., 2024). It does not just show people that excessive screen time is dangerous. It informs the users about the mechanisms that build compulsive use found on platforms, describes individual use patterns, and provides practical skills to use to establish boundaries. This changes the knowledge of symptoms such as you use your phone too much to mechanisms such as how variable rewards and elimination of stop points make use difficult to control. Forming this knowledge makes people feel in control and lessen self-blame. The most efficient treatment in severe cases that qualify as cases of addictions is Cognitive Behavioural Therapy modified to suit digital overuse (Tao et al., 2023). It focuses on the thinking styles and emotional processions as well as habits that perpetuate compulsive usage. The practice of digital detox and mindful technologies, such as taking break periods and rethinking and reconsidering usage, can also aid the development of self-control. These methods are most effective when applied in parallel with formal therapy, but not as substituents to contribute to the long-term process of coping with the digital engagement (Kolhe & Naik, 2025).

Organisational-Level Interventions

Overall, organisational interventions are especially crucial in the case of digital diseases among working adults, where the norm of always-on connectivity takes the primary structural form and digital mindfulness training as a part of occupational health programmes, and behavioural leadership that models healthy digital behaviour. Bossen and Bertelsen (2024) record the complexity of the operation of establishing this kind of policies in organisations where the digital availability has already become part of the competitive culture and that the individual behaviour change in this case is both psychologically expensive and career threatening. A sound organisational intervention thus involves policy commitment on the top and individual support, and ideally, in a regulatory environment, which sets minimum standards (as in right-to-disconnect law), which minimises the competitive drawback on organisations who opt to adopt protective norms.

Platform Design Interventions: Ethical Design as Prevention

Interventions at the design of platforms have the highest potential impact dependent on the amount of investment since they promote the cycle of intervention on the level of the entire population and do not need one-on-one interactions. Specific design changes can be conceptualised in terms of ethical design frameworks, which emphasize the well-being of users, as well as engagement metrics: mandatory usage summaries that will give the user an accurate feedback regarding their engagement patterning; default notification controls that will not be as restrictive to default but instead ensure the user opts-in to high-frequency content-selection; intermittent breaks through pause breaks in the content streams; and consistency in the explanation of the algorithm because this will allow the user to know what is guiding the selection of content to them, and get the opportunity to adjust it (E The data on the effectiveness of certain changes regularly introduced via platforms are evidence-based since their proprietary character, and the financial motive of companies not to share results that potentially could underpin regulatory guidelines. Another research policy of relevance is therefore the access of independent research to platform data and algorithm systems.

TECHNOLOGICAL SOLUTIONS TO DIGITAL DISEASES

The paradox that implementing technology to solve harms caused by technology is there but not fatal, examples of effective interventions that protect the population against health harm often struggle despite or against the same types of products or infrastructure that cause the harm (seatbelts in cars, filtration systems to contaminated water supplies, nicotine replacement therapies). Whether a system of technological solutions is or is not responding to the major determinants of digital disease and is not only responsive to them in their superficial form-at least it is not responding to them at all as well as it ought to be responding to upholding the well-being of its users, or whether it is offering commercially convenient substitutes to structural changes and is responding to them in that way.

AI-Based Monitoring and Early Warning Systems

As a potential early intervention tool, AI-based surveillance systems that are used to compute behaviour patterns in the identification of an emerging digital disease risk are promising especially in populations with potentially low self-awareness of their developing patterns of digital overuse or insufficient access to formal assessment procedures (MacIntyre et al., 2023). Models of machine learning, trained on the data of digital behaviour, screen time patterns, notification response latencies, distribution of usage time, application switching patterns, etc. can pick up the signature of compulsive use more and more accurately and this may lead to early intervention before the clinical threshold is breached. The main challenges in translation have to do with making the alert systems base their reports on actionable guidance instead of causing anxiety by just providing raw information; calibrating sensitivity and specificity to reduce false alarm and missed case; and assuring that the consequences of constant behaviour tracking are taken into consideration with regards to the data privacy concerns.

Wearables, Digital Health Platforms, and Integrated Monitoring

Wearable gadgets tracking physiologic correlates of digital disease, including sleep quality, long-term physical activity as a marker of autonomic stress load, can act as a complementary data stream to behavioural indicators of digital overuse and can determine the physical effects of digital overuse that may not be visibly linked by the user to a particular digital behaviour (Khedraki et al., 2022). Online health applications that combine behavioural, physiological, and self-report measures have the ability to create individualised health profiles and intervention and tailor them to specific patterns and risk factors. Online CBT is especially suitable in digital disease treatment, as it offers scalable administrative assistance to patients with anxiety, depression, and behavioural conditions without the physical presence at a mental provision centre, an important access factor in many populations, and hence therapeutic potential of internet-based CBT offered on the basis of digital platforms is highly applicable. The principles of ethical design concerning the areas of entertainment and social media can also be applied to the sphere of digital health platforms: user benefit should be the central concern, data use should be straightforward and agreeable, and the design should not be based on exploiting the vulnerabilities to achieve engagement metrics.

Limitations, Risks, and Ethical Constraints

Certain limitations and threats are significant in technological solutions of digital diseases. The usage of monitoring systems to gather detailed background behavioural and physiological statistics also brings in underlying privacy issues; the same data to determine the risk of digital diseases can also be employed on the practice of activities that are not favourable to the interests of the user such as commercial profiling, insurance risk, as well as, surveillance by employers. Non-nominal but informed consent to data collection has to be actual and not nominal with the users having any meaningful insight into the use of their data and meaningful ability to make the decisions that the consent signifies. One can also be concerned that the technological solutions to digital disease are offered as screenshot control apps, the use of digital health services, AI-based monitoring services by the technology providers as a way of responsibility shifting: the offering of individual-level tooling becomes an alternative to structural design change, and the causal processes of engagement maximisation are set in stone. The platform design regulation and organisational policy interventions aimed at attaining structural causes of digital disease should not substitute the technological solutions.

POLICY, ETHICS, AND REGULATORY PERSPECTIVES

The policy reaction to the digital illnesses remains immature across the world, however, there are various regulatory measures, ethical codes, and general health awareness that offer hints regarding the avenues in which the influence of efficient policy will probably evolve. The conceptualization of digital disease in terms of a shared public health issue (as opposed to a behavioural issue by individuals) carries significant significance in relation to the form and rightfulness of regulatory intervention.

Emerging Regulatory Frameworks

A number of jurisdictions have also started to create regulatory responses to digital harm that give evidence-of-concept to more robust structures. The Digital Services Act by the European Union imposes transparency and accountability requirements on big platforms, including that they should provide systemic risk assessments about the possible harms to users including harms to their mental health or that they should offer effective content moderation solutions. The Online Safety Act in the UK gives regulatory duties the duty of such online harms that are targeted at children, and there may be age-appropriate services which are given the responsibility of design.

Right-to-disconnect laws, passed in France and Ireland among others, provide a legal safeguard on the entitlement of workers to turn off digital work communication during off-contracted time hours which directly considers the occupational aspect of digital disease by limiting the organisational culture of always-on presence. Although important, these regulatory developments are still partial and fragmented between jurisdictions; a more holistic regulatory framework would cover platform design criteria, algorithmic transparency, restrictions on data use to support engagement maximisation and minimum conditions on user well-being features across digital services (Eke and Stahl, 2024).

Mental Health Rights and Data Privacy

The digital disease encroachment upon the mental health rights and data privacy develops a special ethical sphere that demands legal and ethical frameworks development. The people who are engaged in digital interactions have a fair assumption that mental vulnerabilities that are actively being modelled and exploited by the AI systems to engage the users on their side will not be utilized to work against the interests of the users. The modern regulation does not really offer much protection in practice; GDPR and similar data protection systems make the processing of sensitive health data without explicit consent unlawful, yet predictions made by the engagement of AI systems about psychological vulnerability are not considered health data even when they are practically identical. Such a regulatory loophole would improve the extent to which digital platform users are safeguarded in the maintenance of their mental health rights, in the event of sealing this regulatory loophole by expanding the protections afforded to health data to include algorithmically derived psychological profile types (Eke and Stahl, 2024).

Ethical Design Frameworks and Industry Responsibility

The frameworks of ethical designs put forth by researchers, civil society groups, and by some technology firms, which invest in responsible innovation, define the way operationalisation of user well-being can be realised as one of the design criteria. The designer of the system is already required by the Humane Technology framework, the design principles of the Centre for Humane Technology, and the ACM Code of Ethics to think through the systemic implications of design decisions related to human well-being. These principles must be translated into particular design considerations, such as mandatory stopping signals, limitations on default notification, the ban on dark patterns to control user behaviour contrary to the declared preferences and it needs a regulatory power and acceptance by the industry. These beliefs about the inevitability of ethical design and the essential conflict between the two are not supported by as strong evidence as one might want to think, and platforms that create real user trust and user well-being can maintain a more sustained engagement than platforms that take advantage of the short-term neurobiological weaknesses at the expense of user health and platform confidence.

CASE STUDIES AND PRACTICAL APPLICATIONS

The case studies as presented below demonstrate the processes of digital disease and the results of evidence-based responses in both clinical, educational, and workplace settings. They will be structured to render observable the DDFF explanatory pathways, i.e. platform architecture and contextual pressure to individual health outcome and to show the effectiveness of the multi-level intervention strategies. They are to be interpreted as the examples of reported trends, with reference to published clinical and organisational studies as opposed to the reports of separate patients.

Clinical Case: Adolescent Social Media Addiction and CBT

A 16-year-old female adolescent patient who submitted to a clinical psychology service complaining of anxiety, poor mood, and sleep disturbance stated that she was spending between eight and ten hours each day on various platforms on the social media, mostly on Instagram and Tik Tok. Cognitive evaluation showed that there was much attentional fragmentation; standardised mood assessment evaluation portrayed moderate-to-severe depressive symptoms. A complete clinical formulation revealed the following mechanisms consistent with DDFF algorithmic content selection which differential selected appearance-comparison content, developmental even-number vulnerability to social evaluation, variable-ratio reinforcement by intermittent positive social feedback (likes, comments) that compelled continued compulsive checking notwithstanding negative affect overall, night-time device use that disturbed sleep quality, creating daytime fatigue and emotional reactive state which prone-positioned turn to social comparison content; and late withdrawal in offline peer relationships, the loss of protective social support. The digital adaptation of an eight-session CBT programme, encompassed with structured reduction of screen-time and family-level device use policies yielded great reductions in anxiety and depressive symptoms, a high quality of sleep, and better academic performance at three-month follow-up (Tao et al., 2023). The case demonstrates the cross-category feedback processes (psychological disorder nourishing cognitive disorder nourishing physical disorder) and the usefulness of integrative individual-level clinical intervention and organisational (family system) policy change.

Workplace Case: Professional Burnout and Organisational Intervention

It is a case of a professional services organisation that noted increasing levels of employee burnout, stress-related and anxiety-related sick time, and a poorer quality of performance that resulted in a digital environment assessment that identified unrelenting always-on connectivity norms as the main contributing factor. Employees were checking work email in the evening and weekends, answering and replying to email an hour before going to bed and telling them that they could not think of anything other than work over their time off. A set of organisational intervention measures that included a clear after-hours digital communication policy (no response is expected during working-day hours that are not billed), two-hour block of not responding to emails during the working day that should facilitate deep work as well as manager-style cultural norm modelling were introduced to a business unit. The gap in theoretical understanding between the cognitive overload experienced by the organisation membership in terms of fragmented attention, high error levels, lowering creativity, and the socio-technical systems perspective that attributes the causal agent to the organisational expectations, as opposed to the individual failure of resilience, was clearly reflected in the programme messages. Evaluation after 12 months showed statistically significant decreases in the scores of self-reported stress and burnout, the quality of performance with complex tasks, and no or minor effect on the aspects of client service, which confirmed that the so-called productivity-connectivity trade-off was mostly a myth posited by the pre-intervention culture (Bossen & Bertelsen, 2024).

Educational Case: Digital Literacy Programme for Secondary Students

A digital literacy intervention program offered by a secondary school was found to greatly result in gains to student metacognitive awareness of their digital use habits, as well as the quality of self-regulation behaviour after a ten-week program on the mechanisms of platform engagement design, the cognitive impact of multitasking and attentional fragmentation, and practical skills in digital boundary-setting (Aydinlar et al., 2024). This is at least part of the reason why the programme was so effective, as the framing mechanism was on the mechanism level (the students felt compelled to use their platforms), and only those who realised what aspects of the platform gave them that feeling (because they could individualise) did such area of behaviour change. The intervention group, but not the controls, showed academic performance advantages in subjects that demand a sustained concentration, which is comparable to the attentional advantages of decreased multitasking. Digital environment discussion in the family also received an improvement in the programme which implies systemic spill over effects on the individual student.

FUTURE RESEARCH DIRECTIONS AND EMERGING RISKS

The digital disease terrain does not remain the same; this is due to the technological development trajectory that is still producing new contexts of engagement, new exposure pathways, and new vulnerabilities. The prospective analysis based on mechanisms found in the DDFF and applied to the technical directions most likely to enhance those mechanisms is needed to prepare healthcare systems, research communities, regulators, and the public to new technological threats of disease.

The Metaverse and Immersive Digital Environments

The creation of complete immersive virtual and mixed reality worlds, also known as the Metaverse, is a qualitative intensification of digital disease threat, as immersive worlds remove the natural environmental prompts that already serve as natural barriers to digital activity. The real world is also present in the visual and proprioceptive sense in a screen-based digital world, offering competing factors that will disrupt digital interaction. These competing cues are inhibited or removed in the case of fully immersive virtual reality; the user is entirely in the virtual space. there is no spatial-temporal reference to assist in volitional disengagement. The demons of immersive environments such as novel conditions of digital dissociation, confusion among identities between virtual and real individual, extreme time blindness, and amplified social substitution, must have immediate prospective examination and regulation forecasting, before such surroundings attain the levels of mass usage that would render retroactive regulation as challenging as possible.

AI Companions and Emotional Dependency

The emergence of advanced AI companion systems such as conversational AI which aims to offer emotional support, companionship, and relational interaction have created a new digital disease pathway that cannot be easily categorized or implemented within current systems. This is unlike social media, which facilitates communication between two human beings, and AI companions offer what can look like an attractive alternative to the human relationship—a potential that is exacerbated by the ability of such sources to recreate and react to individual emotional vulnerabilities with the accuracy that cannot be replicated by human relationships. The clinical promise of AI companionship to the socially isolated population such as older adults and those with social anxiety as well as the danger of human functioning is concrete and the social skills and relationship investments in real-world relationships become gradually inactive due to emotional reliance on AI relationships. The development of evidence-based guidelines on the application of AI companion systems as therapeutic or recreational is also a priority area of research and the emergence of AI companionship dependency as a specific category of digital disease have to be monitored.

Research Priorities

The DDFF originated within the framework of this chapter gives rise to a particular range of research priorities that will fill in the most important gaps in the evidence base at the moment. There is a dire need of longitudinal studies of the developmental effects of early digital exposure on neurobiological, cognitive, psychological, and social outcomes; the evidence base of digital disease mechanisms is predominantly cross-sectional and thus cannot answer the most relevant causal questions of relevance to prevention and policy. The research on the digital disease risk profiles and effective intervention choices requires cross-cultural comparative study that would help to establish the scope of how these profiles and the effective interventions could be different based on the cultural setting that can be defined in terms of social norms regarding connectivity, regulatory settings, and platform use habits. Access to platform-level data to independent researchers is required to allow testing on the mechanism of particular algorithms that are being demonstrated in the DDFF since without access to proprietary platform data the causal importance of particular features of the design in triggering outcome of digital disease cannot be tested in a highly rigorous manner. And there is a necessity of interdisciplinary research involving the practices of public health, clinical psychology, organisational science, computational social science and human-computer interaction researchers to create and test the multi-level intervention models, the DDFF implies.

CONCLUSION AND IMPLICATIONS

The chapter introduces an all-inclusive and combined definition of digital diseases, which has three monumental developments to the previous methods. To start with, it acknowledges the actual reasons behind digital diseases not being in personal vulnerabilities like lack of self-control, but the very nature of the digital space as structured and governed by profit, the fixation on attention as a business model, and work cultures where constant connectivity is required. This is a change in the responsibility of the blame on persons, to the analysis of the systems that promote overindulgence in digital activities.

Second, the chapter presents a multi-level predictive model Digital Disease Formation Framework (DDFF) which characterizes the formation of digital diseases. The model relates the design of platforms, the ways thematic systems induce attention, the pressures of life stages, and the personal neurobiological differences to certain health outcomes. It also makes particular attention to feedback loops, which are digital-related health issues (disrupted sleep or anxiety) that grow dependence on digital use, making the situation even worse as time goes on.

Third, the chapter gives a life-stage orientation whereby the risk varies among children, professionals in their careers, and the elderly. This will enable the prevention and intervention strategies to be addressed to the distinctive vulnerabilities of each group.

Another valuable contribution of the chapter is also that it combines various approaches in theory, such as behavioural addiction theory, cognitive overload theory, neuroplasticity research, and socio-technical systems theory. It claims that not one of them can best describe digital diseases but their combination in the DDFF have better explanatory and practical utility. The digital disease classification into psychological, cognitive, physical, and social-behavioural groups provide a good way of research and intervention.

Lastly, the major policy and practical implications are pointed out in the chapter. It demands that technology companies embrace wellbeing conscious design, organisations to consider the issue of digital exposure as a health problem, and policymakers to put in place a regulation to embrace transparency and safer platform architecture. All in all, it is prevention-focused, system-based giving attention to the protection of the population.

REFERENCES

AL-Zoubi., A. (2023, May). Digital technology and changes in media consumption: a case study of smartphone and app usage. In *International Conference on Business and Technology* (pp. 433-444). Cham: Springer Nature Switzerland.

Alimour, S. A., & Alrabeei, M. (2025). Redefining psychopathology in the context of digital overload: Emerging disorders in the age of information saturation. *Frontiers in Digital Health, 7*, 1693287. DOI: 10.3389/fdgth.2025.1693287 PMID: 41312176

Andrade, A. L. M. (Ed.). (2025). *Digital addictions: An interdisciplinary approach to behavioral addictions and digital media.* Springer Nature. DOI: 10.1007/978-3-031-87986-9

Aydınlar, A., Mavi, A., Kütükçü, E., Kırımlı, E. E., Alış, D., Akın, A., & Altıntaş, L. (2024). Awareness and level of digital literacy among students receiving health-based education. *BMC Medical Education, 24*(1), 38. DOI: 10.1186/s12909-024-05025-w PMID: 38191385

Barbieri, V., Piccoliori, G., Engl, A., & Wiedermann, C. J. (2024). Impact of digital media, school problems, and lifestyle factors on youth psychosomatic health: A cross-sectional survey. *Children (Basel, Switzerland), 11*(7), 795. DOI: 10.3390/children11070795 PMID: 39062244

Beeson, D., Wolffsohn, J. S., Baigum, T., Qureshi, T., Gohil, S., Wahid, R., & Sheppard, A. L. (2024). Digital eye strain symptoms worsen during prolonged digital tasks, associated with a reduction in productivity. *Computers in Human Behavior Reports, 16*, 100489. DOI: 10.1016/j.chbr.2024.100489

Bossen, C., & Bertelsen, P. S. (2024). Digital health care and data work: Who are the data professionals? *The HIM Journal, 53*(3), 243–251. DOI: 10.1177/18333583231183083 PMID: 37491822

Celebic, G., & Rendulic, D. (2011). Basic concepts of information and communication technology. *Handbook [Electronic resourse].—URL:* http://www. itdesk. info/ handbook_basic_ ict_concepts. pdf *(дата обращения: 19.05. 2018).*

Clemente-Suárez, V. J., Beltrán-Velasco, A. I., Herrero-Roldán, S., Rodriguez-Besteiro, S., Martínez-Guardado, I., Martín-Rodríguez, A., & Tornero-Aguilera, J. F. (2024). Digital device usage and childhood cognitive development: Exploring effects on cognitive abilities. *Children (Basel, Switzerland), 11*(11), 1299. DOI: 10.3390/children11111299 PMID: 39594874

Costa, F., Frecassetti, S., Rossini, M., & Portioli-Staudacher, A. (2023). Industry 4.0 digital technologies enhancing sustainability: Applications and barriers from the agricultural industry in an emerging economy. *Journal of Cleaner Production, 408*, 137208. DOI: 10.1016/j.jclepro.2023.137208

Eke, D., & Stahl, B. (2024). Ethics in the governance of data and digital technology: An analysis of European data regulations and policies. *Digital Society : Ethics, Socio-Legal and Governance of Digital Technology, 3*(1), 11. DOI: 10.1007/s44206-024-00101-6

George, A. S., George, A. H., & Baskar, T. (2023). The death of analog: Assessing the Impacts of ubiquitous mobile technology. *Partners Universal Innovative Research Publication, 1*(2), 15–33.

Gonçalves, L., Nardi, A., & King, A. (2023). Digital dependence in the past decade: A systematic review. *Journal of Addiction Research and Adolescent Behaviour, 6*(1), 1–18. DOI: 10.31579/2688-7517/059

Gujar, V. (2024). New age marketing: AI personalization strategies in digital world. *International Advanced Research Journal in Science. Engineering and Technology, 11*(3), 288–296.

Holt-Lunstad, J. (2024). Social connection as a critical factor for mental and physical health: Evidence, trends, challenges, and future implications. *World Psychiatry; Official Journal of the World Psychiatric Association (WPA), 23*(3), 312–332. DOI: 10.1002/wps.21224 PMID: 39279411

Imataka, G., Izumi, S., Miyamoto, Y., & Maehashi, A. (2024). Gaming disorders: Navigating the fine line between entertainment and addiction—Gaming history, health risks, social consequences, and pathways to prevention. *Journal of Clinical Medicine, 13*(17), 5122. DOI: 10.3390/jcm13175122 PMID: 39274335

Iyamu, I., Gómez-Ramírez, O., Xu, A. X., Chang, H. J., Watt, S., Mckee, G., & Gilbert, M. (2022). Challenges in the development of digital public health interventions and mapped solutions: Findings from a scoping review. *Digital Health, 8*, 20552076221102255. DOI: 10.1177/20552076221102255 PMID: 35656283

Jaworska, D. (2025). Many faces of FoMO: A qualitative in-depth investigation of context-specific experiences, emotions, and coping strategies. *PLoS One, 20*(9), e0330978. DOI: 10.1371/journal.pone.0330978 PMID: 40892849

Kaur, K., Gurnani, B., Nayak, S., Deori, N., Kaur, S., Jethani, J., & Mishra, D. (2022). Digital eye strain: A comprehensive review. *Ophthalmology and Therapy, 11*(5), 1655–1680. DOI: 10.1007/s40123-022-00540-9 PMID: 35809192

Kaya, F. K., & Güllüpinar, F. (2025). The evolution of attention economy in the age of digital capitalism. *Journal of Consumer & Consumption Research, 17*(1).

Khedraki, R., Srivastava, A. V., & Bhavnani, S. P. (2022). Framework for digital health phenotypes in heart failure. *Heart Failure Clinics, 18*(2), 223–244. DOI: 10.1016/j.hfc.2021.12.003 PMID: 35341537

Kim, J., & Park, S. (2025). Empowering individual preferences in mobile notifications. *IEEE Access : Practical Innovations, Open Solutions*.

Kolhe, D., & Naik, A. R. (2025). Digital detox as a means to enhance eudaimonic well-being. *Frontiers in Human Dynamics, 7*, 1572587. DOI: 10.3389/fhumd.2025.1572587

MacIntyre, C. R., Chen, X., Kunasekaran, M., Quigley, A., Lim, S., Stone, H., & Gurdasani, D. (2023). Artificial intelligence in public health. *The Journal of International Medical Research, 51*(3), 03000605231159335. DOI: 10.1177/03000605231159335 PMID: 36967669

Marinucci, M., Pancani, L., Aureli, N., & Riva, P. (2022). Online social connections as surrogates of face-to-face interactions. *Computers in Human Behavior, 128*, 107102. DOI: 10.1016/j.chb.2021.107102

Moreno, M., Riddle, K., Jenkins, M. C., Singh, A. P., Zhao, Q., & Eickhoff, J. (2022). Measuring problematic internet use. *JMIR Public Health and Surveillance, 8*(1), e27719. DOI: 10.2196/27719 PMID: 34081596

Pardhan, S., Parkin, J., Trott, M., & Driscoll, R. (2022). Risks of digital screen time in children and adolescents. *The Journal of School Health, 92*(8), 765–773. DOI: 10.1111/josh.13170 PMID: 35253225

Patel, D. G., Kshatri, A. H. S., Kommuru, S., & Javvaji, C. K. (2025). A narrative review of digital addiction and health. *Cureus, 17*(12). PMID: 41625856

Raj, G., Sharma, A. K., & Arora, Y. (2024). Analyzing the effect of digital technology on mental health. In *Strategies for E-Commerce Data Security* (pp. 54–82). IGI Global. DOI: 10.4018/979-8-3693-6557-1.ch003

Samala, A. D., Rawas, S., Criollo-C, S., Fortuna, A., Feng, X., Prasetya, F., & Hidayat, R. (2024). Social media in education. *Asian Journal of University Education, 20*(3), 524–539. DOI: 10.24191/ajue.v20i3.27869

Smits, M., Kim, C. M., Van Goor, H., & Ludden, G. D. (2022). From digital health to digital well-being. *Journal of Medical Internet Research, 24*(4), e33787. DOI: 10.2196/33787 PMID: 35377328

Tao, T. J., Lim, T. K., Yeung, E. T. F., Liu, H., Shris, P. B., Ma, L. K. Y., & Hou, W. K. (2023). Internet-based cognitive behavioral therapy. npj. *Digital Medicine*, *6*(1), 80. PMID: 37117458

Termann, S. (2025). The dopamine collapse hypothesis. *SSRN.*

Timotheou, S., Miliou, O., Dimitriadis, Y., Sobrino, S. V., Giannoutsou, N., Cachia, R., & Ioannou, A. (2023). Impacts of digital technologies on education. *Education and Information Technologies*, *28*(6), 6695–6726. DOI: 10.1007/s10639-022-11431-8 PMID: 36465416

Ukabuiro, I. K., & Agomah, S. A. (2025). A digital persuasive system to mitigate health risks. *European Journal of Innovative Studies and Sustainability*, *1*(3), 28–45. DOI: 10.59324/ejiss.2025.1(3).04

Upadhyaya, H. (2024). *Digital education and economic transformation*. Meadow Publication.

Vu, H., François, K. K., Hung, N. X., Trung, N. V., & Hieu, N. L. (2024). Potential of digital health solutions. In *Digitalization of Medicine in LMICs* (pp. 51–68). Springer.

Wuersch, L., Neher, A., & Peter, M. K. (2023). Digital internal communication. *International Journal of Management Reviews*, *25*(3), 614–639. DOI: 10.1111/ijmr.12323

Zaman, S. B., Khan, R. K., Evans, R. G., Thrift, A. G., Maddison, R., & Islam, S. M. S. (2022). ICT adoption for older adults. *JMIR Aging*, *5*(1), e25251. DOI: 10.2196/25251 PMID: 34994695

ADDITIONAL READING

Betoncu, O., & Ozdamli, F. (2019). The disease of 21st century: Digital disease. *TEM Journal*, *8*(2), 598–603. DOI: 10.18421/TEM82-37

Chung, S., & Lee, H. K. (2023). Public health approach to problems related to excessive and addictive use of the internet and digital media. *Current Addiction Reports*, *10*(1), 69–76. DOI: 10.1007/s40429-022-00458-z PMID: 36589709

Ejaz, S., & Khaliq, H. M. H. (2025). Mental health in the age of hyperconnectivity: A crisis hidden in plain sight. *Pakistan Journal of Medicine and Dentistry, 14(3), 01–03.*

Martins, G. D. G., Caricati, V. V., Barbugli, B. C., da Silva Ribeiro, C. M., Lobato, F. B. H., Scatena, A., & Andrade, A. L. M. (2021). The biopsychosocial impact of abusive use of digital media. In *Drugs and human behavior: Biopsychosocial aspects of psychotropic substances use* (pp. 459–468). Springer International Publishing. DOI: 10.1007/978-3-030-62855-0_33

Sandua, D. (2024). The double sides of technology: Internet addiction and its impact on today's society.

Turel, O., Qahri-Saremi, H., & Vaghefi, I. (2021). Dark sides of digitalization. *International Journal of Electronic Commerce*, *25*(2), 127–135. DOI: 10.1080/10864415.2021.1887694

Vaghela, P. S. (2016, March). Digital addiction: an epidemic of digital world—an article on digital addiction among generation D. In *National Conference on Managing Business Through Digital Marketing in the Globalized Era.*

Wadhwa, M. (2021). Digital mental health initiatives in India (No. 60). ICT India Working Paper.

Xue, Y., Zhang, Y., Bai, M., Dong, H., Feng, J., & Jia, F. Y. (2026). The hidden costs of screen time: altered brain network efficiency in children with autism spectrum disorder. BMC Psychiatry.

KEY TERMS AND DEFINITIONS

Digital Diseases: Health problems caused by too much use of digital devices, affecting the body and mind.

Digital Dependency: When a person becomes used to digital devices and finds it difficult to stay without them.

Digital Addiction: When a person cannot control their digital device use even when it causes harm to their health or daily life.

Screen Time: The amount of time a person spends using devices like phones, computers, or tablets.

Attention Economy: A system where apps and websites try to keep users engaged for a long time to capture their attention.

Mental Health: A person's emotional and psychological well-being, including how they think, feel, and handle stress.

Digital Well-being: The healthy and balanced use of digital technology without harming physical or mental health.

Chapter 2
Cyberbullying Victimization and Psychological Distress:
Mediating Role of Loneliness

Rashmi Sharma
Lovely Professional University, India

Jyoti Gupta
http://orcid.org/0000-0002-5864-4998
Lovely Professional University, India

ABSTRACT

Cyberbullying is a major psychosocial risk for young adults, linked to adverse mental health outcomes. The study examined loneliness as a mediator between cyberbullying victimization and psychological distress among undergraduates in Northern India. A cross-sectional survey was conducted, and 427 students who reported cyberbullying victimization were included. Cyberbullying was measured using the Cyber-Bullying and Victimization Experiences Questionnaire, loneliness by the UCLA Loneliness Scale and psychological distress by the Kessler Psychological Distress Scale. Mediation analysis showed cyberbullying victimization was significantly associated with both loneliness and psychological distress. Loneliness also significantly predicted psychological distress. Additionally, loneliness partially mediated the relationship between cyberbullying and psychological distress, indicating both direct and indirect effects. These findings underscore loneliness as a key psychosocial mechanism and highlight the need for interventions targeting cyberbullying and social isolation among undergraduates.

DOI: 10.4018/979-8-2600-2468-3.ch002

INTRODUCTION

Cyberbullying refers to the deliberate and repeated use of digital technologies to harass, threaten, humiliate, or socially exclude individuals through online platforms such as social networking sites, instant messaging applications, gaming environments, and digital forums. Unlike traditional forms of bullying, cyberbullying is characterized by its capacity for anonymity, wide audience reach, and permanence, allowing harmful content to be disseminated rapidly and remain accessible over time. These features intensify the victim's experience by eliminating safe spaces, as digital harassment can occur continuously and intrude into private settings. Cyberbullying often involves behaviors such as online harassment, spreading rumors, public shaming, impersonation, and social exclusion, all of which undermine an individual's sense of dignity, belonging, and security. Conceptually, cyberbullying is not merely an extension of offline aggression but represents a distinct psychosocial stressor rooted in the dynamics of digital communication, where power imbalances are amplified through technological affordances. The global proliferation of internet access and social media use has transformed cyberbullying into a worldwide phenomenon affecting individuals across cultures, age groups, and social contexts. Importantly, cyberbullying operates within social and relational frameworks, as it frequently targets interpersonal connections and social identity, thereby increasing vulnerability to emotional distress, social withdrawal, and psychological harm. As digital interactions become increasingly embedded in everyday life, understanding cyberbullying as a complex, socially mediated form of aggression is essential for explaining its profound and lasting impact on mental health and well-being.

THEORETICAL FRAMEWORK:

Theory of Planned Behaviour (Barlett et al., 2021)

The theory suggests that human behaviour is determined by intention and encompasses three belief-based concepts: the attitude toward the behaviour, subjective norms, and perceived behavioural control over performing the behaviour. The theory examined how comments of a hypothetical Facebook bullying influence users." cyberbullying-specific norms and their confidence in their ability to intervene among pure cyberbullies, pure cyber victims, and cyberbully victims (Leung et al., 2018).

Figure 1. Theory of Panned Behaviour (Barlett et al., 2021)

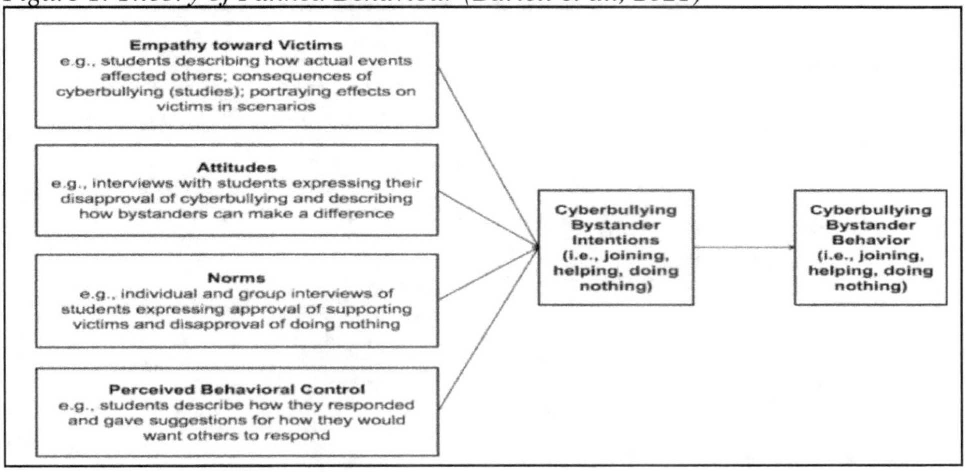

Operationalization of the Barlett Gentile Cyberbullying Model (BGCM)

Figure 1 clearly explained the operationalisation of "The Barlett Gentile Cyberbullying Model (BGCM)". The models begin with the fundamental idea that the early cyber aggressive events serve as the base learning experience where the perpetrator (a) thinks that masculinity is irrelevant in online bullying and (b) thinks he/she is an anonymous. Positive reinforcement for cyber-aggressive behavior, such as peer praise, attention, effective retaliation, and the absence of repercussions, increases the likelihood that the behavior will recur. These recurring behaviors become stronger with time and automatize the fundamental structures that underpin them. Drawing on social cognitive theory proposed by Albert Bandura (1986), these learned experiences and reinforcement mechanisms shape attitudes, which in turn predict cyberbullying perpetration behaviour.

Figure 2. "The Barlett Gentile Cyberbullying Model (BGCM)" (Barlett et al., 2021)

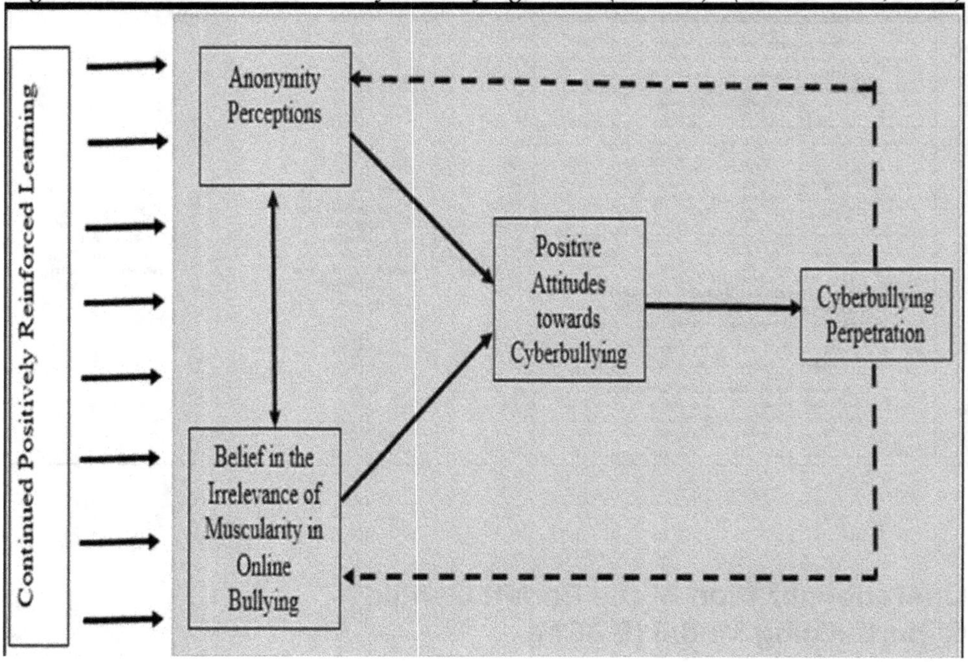

The following figure 2 represents the development of cyberbullying perpetration as per the BGCM model over the period of time.

Figure 3. "The development of the BGCM with continued experiences over time" (Barlett et al., 2021)

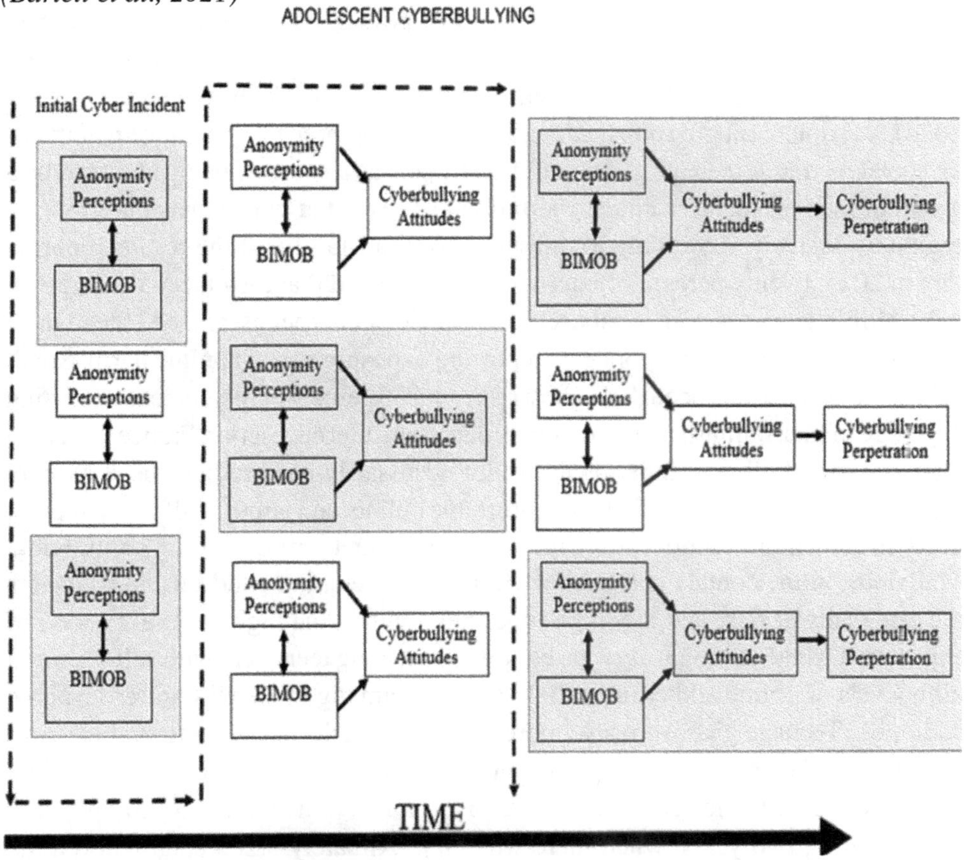

The perception of being anonymous predicts cyberbullying attitude (Barlett, 2015), BIMOB predicts the attitude of cyberbully (Barlett et al., 2017) and Doane et al., (2014) reported that cyberbullying attitude predicts cyberbullying behaviour. Furthermore, the complete model has been validated by longitudinal studies and documented that cyberbullying attitude mediated the relationship between "Wave 1, BIMOB and Wave 3 cyberbullying perpetration" (Barlett et al., 2017). Barlett et al., (2019) conducted four-wave longitudinal research with a three-month gap between waves among the young adults and found that the cyberbullying behaviour continued to strengthen with the cyberbullying knowledge. Therefore, the previous researches suggested that "The Barlett Gentile Cyberbullying Model (BGCM)" was found to be empirically robust.

Prevalence of Cyberbullying

Cyberbullying has become a relatively new type of bullying (Hinduja and Patchin, 2008; Kowalski et al., 2012). Research and media both have turned their attention to the growing concern of cyberbullying. In the recent BBC coverage report (BBC, 2024), an adolescent girl took her own life after being bullied by the group of males on social media. A teenage girl committed suicide as a result of being harassed by a group of men on social media. Cyberbullying does not affect a particular group or region exclusively. According to the survey of Statista (2024) the results reported that in 2023, twenty percent of internet users indicated that they faced the threat of cyberbullying, harassment, or abuse. South African internet users faced the highest risk, with 36 percent of respondents reporting exposure to such online harm. South African internet users faced the highest risk, with 36 percent of respondents reporting exposure to such online harm. In contrast, one in ten internet users in France indicated a risk of cyberbullying. Individuals do not necessarily need to have been a direct victim of online bullying to feel uncomfortable online, and almost half of all internet users in Singapore reported they were worried about exposure to cyberbullying. Malicious online contact is a risk for all internet users, but children and teenagers are especially at risk, and the more time spent online, the higher the likelihood of exposure. Cyberbullying was twice as common among teenagers with self-reported high levels of online addiction in 2023 as it was among those with lower levels of addiction. Teenage girls were also more likely than their male counterparts to have encountered dangerous content on the internet. About 3,092 complaints of criminal harassment over the internet were made to Canadian police in 2023. Compared to the preceding two years, when there were approximately 3,203 such reports, the figure is marginally higher. According to surveys conducted in the UK in 2016 and 2023, as reported by Statista (2025) girls between the ages of seven and ten are increasingly engaging in threatening or distressing online behavior. In 2023, 25% of respondents said they had been the victim of cyberbullying, up from 13% in 2016. Additionally, the percentage of unwanted online contact rose from 16 percent in 2016 to 30 percent in 2023. According to a March 2024 survey results reported in Statista (2024) One in ten Canadian internet users claimed having been the victim of cyberbullying, and other ten percent said they had seen cyberbullying. Pala et al., (2021) reported that 65.3% of teenagers in Turkey experienced cyberbullying. According to the findings of research, cyberbullying is a serious issue that has the potential to affect a large segment of society of the population.

Cyberbullying-Victimization and Loneliness

Loneliness is defined as subjectively perceived social isolation (Hawkley and Cacioppo, 2010) is regarded as a sign of social relationship difficulties (Heinrich and Gullone, 2006), and is defined as the discrepancy between one's desired and existing relationships (Perlman, 1982). Sahin (2012) and Talan et al., (2021) documented that cyberbullying is correlated with loneliness. Loneliness found to predict cyberbullying victimisation (Brewer and Kerslake, 2015). The feeling of loneliness tends to magnify the impact of cyberbullying, whereas resilience and self-control can act as protective factors. Knowledge of these dynamics is essential to the creation of successful interventions to help adolescents deal with cyberbullying situations. The role of encapsulated bullying experience on risk and protective factors for cyberbullying. The more adolescents suffer from loneliness, the more likely they are victims of cyberbullying that subsequently exacerbates the feelings of being alone and feeling deported (Madsen et al., 2024). A meta-analysis of 19 cross-sectional studies from 2007 to 2020 was carried out by Kwan et al., (2020), who discovered that cyberbullying may have a variety of behavioral and psychological impacts. One of the several detrimental effects is loneliness. Samsudin et al., (2024) examined Malaysian adolescents. Their research assessed the impact of cyberbullying on loneliness and well-being. The findings revealed that psychological distress mediated the relationship between cyberbullying victimisation and increased feelings of loneliness, underscoring the emotional toll of such experiences.

Cyberbullying-victimization and Psychological Distress

Cyberbullying-victimization has been persistently correlated to an increased risk of depression, according to research (Reed et al., 2016; Marciano et al., 2020). This correlation consistently reported across various age groups including young adolescents (Hellfeldt et al., 2020), adolescents (Fahy et al., 2016), college students (Watts et al., 2017; Jenaro et al., 2021) younger adults (Balakrishnan, 2018), and adults (Jenaro et al., 2018). According to Samsudin et al., (2023), cyberbullying was more common among young adults who were experiencing high levels of psychological distress. Victims of cyberbullying are more likely to have depressive symptoms and suicide thoughts, and these negative consequences last longer. Therefore, more effective techniques are needed to address cyberbullying and related mental health issues, such as raising knowledge of the subtleties of online harassment among adolescents and young adults (Maurya et al., 2022). Grimland et al., (2025) found that the relationship between combined bullying victimization and suicide attempt was shown to be moderated by emotional symptoms. Reviewing the literature revealed that there is dearth of cross-sectional studies examining the relationship between cyberbullying victimisation and psychological distress with loneliness as a mediator. The existing literature emphasizes the alarming increase in cyberbullying and the harmful consequences it has on its victims, which include a variety of psychological problems like stress, anxiety, despair, low self-esteem, mistrust, negative self-concept, and suicidal thoughts. This concerning pattern emphasizes the urgent need to look into these phenomena, especially among the most susceptible groups of college students. Furthermore, examining the psychosocial factors associated with different bullying roles is crucial for informing the development and implementation of effective prevention and intervention programs within school settings. Additionally in India, very few studies were found on impact of cyberbullying but no study was found which analysed the mediating role of loneliness in the relationship between cyberbullying victimization and psychological distress. Therefore, this study aims to fill this gap by examining the mediating role of loneliness in the relationship between cyberbullying victimisation and psychological distress. The aim of the current study was to explore the mediating role of loneliness in the relationship between cyberbullying and psychological distress among undergraduate victim students. According to the literature, the present study put forward the hypothesis that loneliness will significantly mediate the relationship between cyberbullying victimisation and psychological distress among undergraduate victim students.

RESEARCH, ANALYSIS, FINDINGS

Sample

The current study included the sample from Northern India, 955 students in all have taken part in the survey. After removing outliers (N=8), 947 responses remained for examination. Of them, N=422 said they had been the victim of cyberbullying, while N=525 said they had never been. Therefore, only the 422 students who reported experiencing cyberbullying were included in the data analysis. In the sample, 31.27% of participants were BA students, 12.08% were BBA students, 20.14% were B. Com students, 11.37% were BCA students, 25.11% were B. Tech (CSE) students, and 53.79% of participants were female. 7.3% of the population was under the age of 17, 35.07% was between the ages of 18 and 19, 27.72% was between the ages of 20 and 21, 14.21% was between the ages of 22 and 23, and 15.63% was over the age of 24. The graphical representation of data w.r.t academic program and age is given in figure 4 and 5.

Figure 4. Distribution of cyberbullying victim students w.r.t academic program

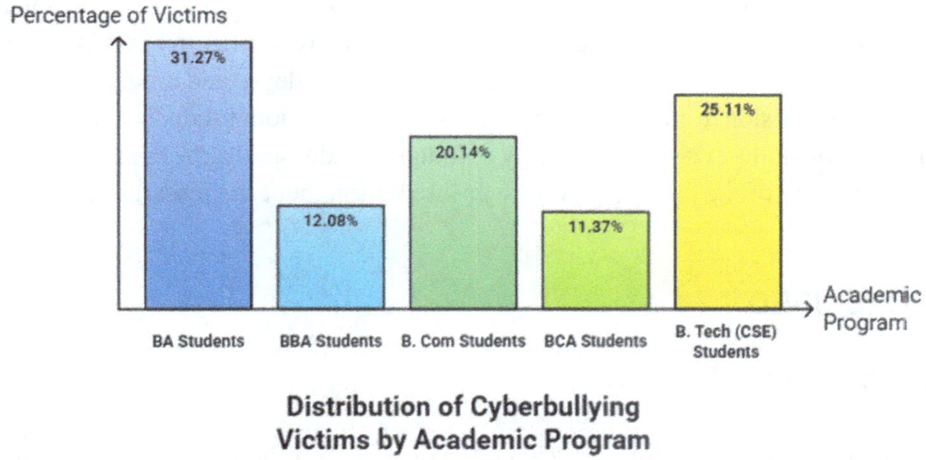

Figure 5. Distribution of cyberbullying victim students w.r.t Age

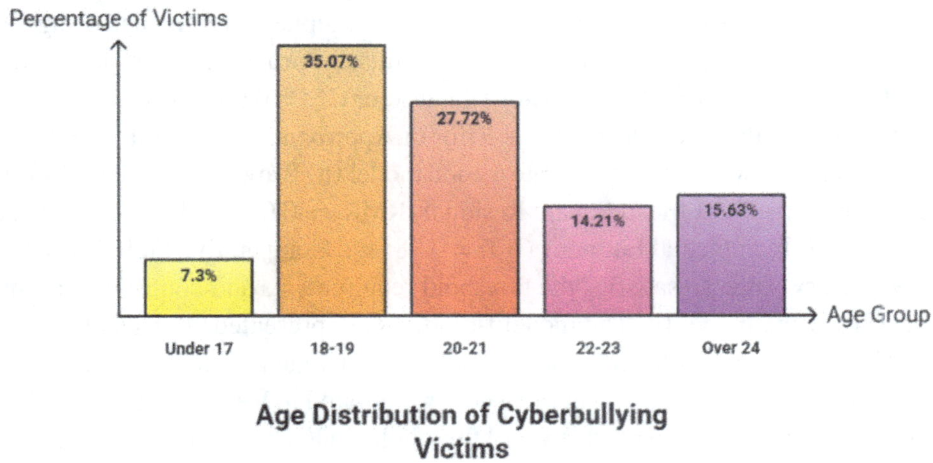

Questionnaire and sample

The present study used self-administered questionnaires. Each scale was adapted and validated on Indian population of university students in order to ensure the cultural relevance. The researcher personally visited the colleges and universities and obtained permission from the respective heads of the institutions to conduct the survey. Participation in the survey was entirely voluntary. Additionally, the confidentiality and anonymity of the participants were ensured throughout the research process.

TOOLS USED

Psychological distress

The psychological distress among undergraduate cyberbullying victim students was measured using "The Kessler Psychological Distress Scale (K10)" (Kessler et al., 2003). Ten items on the scale assess the presence of anxiety and depression symptoms during the previous month, with responses ranging from 1 (never) to 5 (often) (e.g., "How often have you felt desperate?"). The scale was validated on the Indian Population of higher education students. The scale was validated on the Indian population. Construct validity was established using confirmatory factor analysis (CFA) using the SPSS AMOS-23 version, Cronbach's alpha was computed using the IBM SPSS-23 version. According to the CFA results, the proposed model provided a good fit to the data, with a Goodness-of-fit index, or GFI = 0.96, suggesting a good fit. Statistics for the Root Mean Square Error of Approximation (RMSEA) = 0.06, which is satisfactory, also demonstrate a good model fit (Browne & Cudeck, 1993). Furthermore, the Root Mean Square Residual (RMR) = 0.03; Tucker-Lewis Index (TLI) = 0.97; Incremental Fit Index (IFI) = 0.98; and Comparative Fit Index (CFI) = 0.98. Every value so satisfies the threshold requirements and contributes to the validation of the model fit. The model fit indices are presented. The reliability of each dimension and whole scale was computed with Cronbach's α. The dimensions of restlessness, depression, and nervousness were found to have Cronbach's alphas of 0.87, 0.88, and 0.88, respectively and for whole scale Cronbach's α came out to be 0.92 and composite reliability was found to be 0.90. The scale was found to be reliable and valid to be used on the Indian population of higher education.

Cyberbullying Victimisation

Antoniadou and Kokkinos (2016) developed the "Cyber-Bullying and Victimization Experiences Questionnaire Greek (CBVEQ-G)" to measure cyberbullying victimization. It consists of two scales: cyberbullying (CB) and cyber victimization (CV), each with 12 items. Both scales can be used independently by the researcher. Cyber-Bullying and Victimization Experiences Questionnaire-Greek (CBVEQ-G) scores were calculated as follows: 1 = Never, 2 = 1-2 times, 3 = Some times, 4 = Many times, and 5 = Every day. Sadeeq and Kumar (2021) validated the scale on the Indian population of students enrolled in higher education. Following the validation procedure, 11 items were retained from the cyber victimization (CV) scale, and item number 11 from the original scale was eliminated. Therefore, the cyber victimization (CV) scale comprised 11 items. The internal consistency of the scale was computed with Cronbach's α, along with it the composite reliability was also computed. The composite reliability was 0.90, and the construct reliability was also 0.90.

Loneliness

The University of California, Los Angeles Loneliness Scale (UCLA-LS) version 3 by Russell, 1996) was used for examining loneliness. Participants respond to each item on a 1–4 scale, from "never" to "always." The scale has a possible total score ranging from 20 to 80 points, with higher scores indicating greater loneliness. The scale was validated on the Indian Population of higher education students. According to the CFA results, the proposed model provided a good fit to the data, with a Goodness-of-fit index, or GFI = 0.96, suggesting a good fit. Statistics for the Root Mean Square Error of Approximation (RMSEA) = 0.04, which is satisfactory, also demonstrate a good model fit (Browne & Cudeck, 1993). Furthermore, the Root Mean Square Residual (RMR) = 0.04; Tucker-Lewis Index (TLI) = 0.96; Incremental Fit Index (IFI) = 0.97; and Comparative Fit Index (CFI) = 0.97. Every value so satisfies the threshold requirements and contributes to the validation of the model fit. The model fit indices are presented. The reliability of each dimension and whole scale was computed with Cronbach's α. The Cronbach's α for the dimensions "Isolation" = 0.84, "Relational Connectedness" = 0.85, "Social Connectedness" = 0.79, "Social Compatibility" = 0.84, and for "Social Exclusion" =0.83 and for whole scale it came out to be 0.80 and composite reliability was 0.85. Consequently, the scale was found to be reliable and valid to be used on the Indian population of higher education.

Box 1. AVE, Composite Reliability and Construct Reliability

Variable	AVE	Composite Reliability (CR)	Construct Reliability (α)
Cyberbullying Victimization	0.55	0.90	0.90
Loneliness	0.65	0.85	0.80
Psychological Distress	0.69	0.90	0.92

Statistical Analysis

Descriptive analysis was made to depict the demographic characteristics. Mediation analysis was conducted using the bootstrapping procedure in Smart PLS to examine whether loneliness mediates the relationship between cyberbullying victimization and psychological distress.

Results

In order to study the mediating role of loneliness in the relationship between cyberbullying and psychological distress among undergraduate victim students, data was using Smart Pls. the results have been reported in the following table 1.

Table 1. Path coefficients for mediation model (Cyberbullying Victimization, Loneliness, and Psychological Distress)

Path	Standardized Coefficient (β)	t-Statistic	p-Value
Cyberbullying → Loneliness **(path a)**	0.236	5.798**	0.00
Cyberbullying → Psychological Distress **(direct path c)**	0.345	7.699**	0.00
Loneliness → Psychological Distress **(path b)**	0.363	10.068**	0.00
Cyberbullying → Loneliness→ Psychological Distress	0.0857	5.358**	0.00

**significant at 0.01 level of confidence

It is clear from the table 1 that the paths viz. Cyberbullying -> Loneliness, t=5.798, p<0.001, Cyberbullying-> Psychological Distress, t=7.699, p<0.01, and for Loneliness -> Psychological Distress, t=10.068, p<0.001 are found to be significant at 0.01 level of confidence. Additionally, the path Cyberbullying → Loneliness→ Psychological Distress t= 5.358, p<0.01 was also found to be significant. Meaning thereby that all paths are statistically significant and cyberbullying significantly predicting loneliness and psychological distress and loneliness significantly predicts psychological distress. This is indicative of the fact that there is both direct and indirect paths from cyberbullying to psychological distress.

Figure 6. Mediation model showing the relationship between Cyberbullying Victimization, Loneliness, and Psychological Distress)

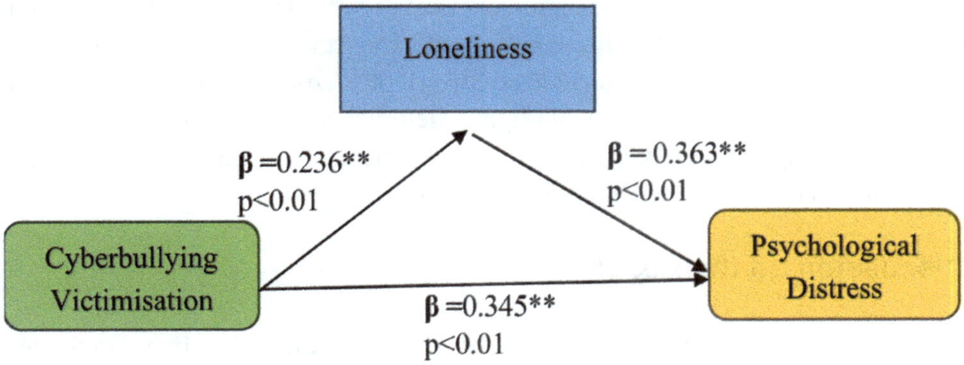

Calculation of Indirect Effects (axb)

From Table 1,
Path a (**Cyberbullying → Loneliness**) = 0.236
Path b (**Loneliness → Psychological Distress**) = 0.363
a x b = 0.236 x 0.363 = 0.0857
Total Effect= Direct Effect + Indirect Effect
Total Effect= 0.345 + 0.0857 = 0.4307

The direct path from cyberbullying to loneliness was found to be significant ($\beta = 0.236$, $t = 5.798$, $p < 0.001$), indicating that higher levels of cyberbullying increase loneliness among undergraduate victim students. Similarly, the path from Loneliness to psychological distress with $\beta = 0.363$, $t=10.068$, $p<0.001$ was also found to be significant, which indicated that higher levels of loneliness were associated with greater psychological distress among the undergraduate victim students. Furthermore, the direct effect of cyberbullying on psychological distress while controlling for loneliness remained significant ($\beta = 0.345$, $t = 7.699$, $p < 0.001$), which indicates a partial mediation. The indirect effect (Cyberbullying→Loneliness→ Psychological Distress) was estimated at 0.0857 (i.e., 0.236 × 0.363), supporting the presence of mediation. The total effect of cyberbullying victimization on psychological distress is positive and statistically significant ($\beta = 0.4307$, $p < 0.001$). This means that higher levels of cyberbullying victimization are associated with substantially higher levels of psychological distress among individuals. Specifically, a one–standard deviation increase in cyberbullying victimization leads to a 0.431 standard deviation increase in psychological distress when both the direct effect and the indirect effect through loneliness are considered together. This indicates a moderately strong overall impact, suggesting that cyberbullying victimization is an important risk factor for psychological distress. The bootstrapped indirect effect of cyberbullying victimization on psychological distress via loneliness was significant at the 95% confidence level, as the confidence interval did not include zero ($\beta = 0.0857, p < 0.01$), indicating partial mediation. This implies that cyberbullying victimization increases psychological distress not only directly, but also indirectly by increasing feelings of loneliness, which in turn exacerbate psychological distress.

Discussion on the Results

The present study aimed to examine the mediating role of loneliness in the relationship between cyberbullying victimization and psychological distress among undergraduate students. The findings provide robust empirical evidence that cyberbullying victimization significantly predicts psychological distress both directly and indirectly through loneliness, indicating partial mediation. These results underscore the complex psychosocial mechanisms through which cyberbullying affects mental health and highlight loneliness as a critical emotional pathway linking online victimization to adverse psychological outcomes. In the context of the increasing digitalization of social interactions among young adults, these findings carry important theoretical, empirical, and practical implications. The direct relationship between cyberbullying victimization and psychological distress observed in this study aligns with a substantial body of prior research demonstrating the detrimental mental health consequences of cyberbullying. Victims of cyberbullying often experience elevated levels of anxiety, depression, stress, and emotional exhaustion, which may persist over extended periods (Reed et al., 2016; Marciano et al., 2020). The present findings corroborate earlier evidence across diverse populations, including adolescents (Hellfeldt et al., 2020), college students (Watts et al., 2017; Jenaro et al., 2021), and young adults (Balakrishnan, 2018), suggesting that cyberbullying victimization constitutes a pervasive psychosocial stressor irrespective of developmental stage. Unlike traditional bullying, cyberbullying possesses unique characteristics—such as anonymity, permanence, and wide audience reach—that intensify victims' psychological vulnerability. The anonymity afforded by digital platforms can embolden perpetrators and leave victims feeling powerless, while the public and enduring nature of online harassment exacerbates shame, humiliation, and fear of social judgment (Hinduja & Patchin, 2015). These factors may explain why cyberbullying exhibits a strong and direct association with psychological distress even after accounting for loneliness. From a stress–diathesis perspective, cyberbullying can be conceptualized as a chronic stressor that overwhelms coping resources, thereby precipitating emotional dysregulation and psychological distress.

Repeated exposure to online harassment may lead victims to internalize negative self-perceptions, heighten rumination, and develop maladaptive cognitive schemas, all of which contribute to depressive and anxiety symptoms (Kowalski et al., 2014). The present findings support this framework by demonstrating that cyberbullying victimization independently predicts psychological distress among undergraduate students.

The significant association between cyberbullying victimization and loneliness observed in this study is consistent with prior empirical evidence indicating that victims of online harassment are more likely to experience social withdrawal and perceived social isolation (Sahin, 2012; Brewer & Kerslake, 2015; Talan et al., 2021). Loneliness, defined as the subjective discrepancy between desired and actual social relationships (Perlman & Peplau, 1982), is particularly salient in the context of cyberbullying, which often targets social identity, peer relationships, and online reputation. Cyberbullying victimization may foster loneliness through several mechanisms. First, victims may withdraw from online and offline social interactions to avoid further harassment, thereby reducing opportunities for social support and connection. Second, public forms of cyberbullying—such as spreading rumors or posting humiliating content—can damage peer relationships and lead to social exclusion, reinforcing feelings of rejection and isolation. Third, the fear of being judged or blamed may prevent victims from disclosing their experiences, further intensifying loneliness. The findings of the present study resonate with the social pain hypothesis, which posits that social exclusion and rejection activate neural and emotional processes similar to physical pain, leading to heightened distress and vulnerability. In this context, cyberbullying functions as a form of social rejection that undermines individuals' sense of belonging, thereby increasing loneliness. Given that undergraduate students are at a developmental stage characterized by heightened sensitivity to peer acceptance and social integration, the impact of cyberbullying on loneliness may be particularly pronounced (Arnett, 2000). The strong positive association between loneliness and psychological distress found in this study is well supported by extensive literature documenting loneliness as a significant risk factor for mental health problems. Loneliness has been linked to depression, anxiety, stress, low self-esteem, and suicidal ideation across age groups and cultural contexts (Hawkley & Cacioppo, 2010; Heinrich & Gullone, 2006). The present findings reinforce the notion that loneliness is not merely an emotional state but a potent psychosocial determinant of psychological well-being. Loneliness may contribute to psychological distress by fostering maladaptive cognitive processes such as negative self-evaluation, hopelessness, and perceived lack of control (Cacioppo et al., 2006). Additionally, lonely individuals often exhibit heightened vigilance for social threats, which may amplify stress responses and exacerbate emotional dysregulation (Qualter et al., 2015). In the context of cyberbullying victimization, loneliness may intensify the psychological impact of online harassment by depriving victims of protective social resources and emotional validation. The findings are consistent with Kwan et al., (2020) meta-analysis, which identified loneliness as one of the key psychological consequences of cyberbullying victimization. Similarly, Samsudin et al., (2024) reported that psychological distress mediated the relationship between cyberbullying victimization and loneliness among adolescents, highlighting the reciprocal and reinforcing nature of these constructs. Together, these findings suggest that loneliness and psychological distress may operate in a feedback loop, wherein cyberbullying initiates a cycle of social withdrawal and emotional suffering. One of the most significant contributions of the present study is the empirical demonstration that loneliness partially mediates the relationship between cyberbullying victimization and psychological distress. This finding indicates that cyberbullying affects mental health both directly and indirectly by increasing feelings of loneliness. The partial mediation suggests that loneliness is an important, but not exclusive, pathway through which cyberbullying influences psychological distress. This result is consistent with previous studies that have identified loneliness as a mediator in the relationship between bullying experiences and mental health outcomes (Baker & Bugay, 2011; Varela et al., 2022). Baker and Bugay (2011) found that loneliness mediated the relationship between peer victimization and psychological symptoms, while Varela et al., (2022) demonstrated that fear of loneliness partially explained the association between cyberbullying victimization and depressive symptoms. The present study extends this literature by focusing specifically on undergraduate students in the Indian context, thereby addressing a notable gap in the existing research. The findings of the present study are particularly significant within the Indian socio-cultural context, where discussions of mental health and cyberbullying remain stigmatized. Indian undergraduate students often face intense academic pressure, familial expectations, and social scrutiny, which may compound the psychological impact of cyberbullying (Deb et al., 2015). Additionally, collectivistic cultural norms place a strong emphasis on social connectedness and group belonging, making experiences of social exclusion and loneliness especially distressing. The relatively high prevalence of cyberbullying victimization observed in this study echoes global trends reported by Statista (2024) and other international surveys, highlighting cyberbullying as a growing public health concern. Given the rapid expansion of internet access and social media use in India, the risk of cyberbullying is likely to increase, underscoring the urgency of addressing its psychosocial consequences.

Implications of the Study

The findings of this study have important implications for prevention and intervention efforts. First, interventions aimed at reducing psychological distress among cyberbullying victims should not focus solely on stopping the bullying behavior but also address its emotional and social consequences, particularly loneliness. Programs that foster social support, peer connectedness, and resilience may help mitigate the adverse mental health effects of cyberbullying.

Second, universities and colleges should implement comprehensive cyberbullying prevention programs that include mental health screening, counseling services, and awareness campaigns. Encouraging help-seeking behavior and reducing stigma around mental health may empower victims to seek support and reduce feelings of isolation. Third, digital literacy programs that educate students about safe online practices and coping strategies may enhance perceived control and resilience, thereby reducing vulnerability to distress.

Limitations of the study

Despite its strengths, the present study has several limitations that should be acknowledged. The cross-sectional design precludes causal inferences, and longitudinal studies are needed to examine the temporal dynamics of cyberbullying, loneliness, and psychological distress. Additionally, reliance on self-report measures may introduce response bias.

FUTURE RESEARCH DIRECTIONS

- Future research could incorporate qualitative methods or multi-informant approaches to gain a more nuanced understanding of victims' experiences.
- Future studies should also explore additional mediators and moderators, such as self-esteem, coping strategies, resilience, and social support, to further elucidate the mechanisms underlying the cyberbullying–mental health relationship. Examining these processes across diverse cultural contexts and age groups would enhance the generalizability of findings.

CONCLUSION

In conclusion, the present study provides compelling evidence that loneliness partially mediates the relationship between cyberbullying victimization and psychological distress among undergraduate students. Cyberbullying emerges as a significant risk factor for mental health problems, operating both directly and indirectly through increased feelings of loneliness. These findings highlight the importance of addressing the social and emotional dimensions of cyberbullying in prevention and intervention efforts. By fostering social connectedness and providing targeted mental health support, educational institutions can play a crucial role in mitigating the harmful consequences of cyberbullying and promoting psychological well-being among young adults.

REFERENCES

Antoniadou, N., Kokkinos, C. M., & Markos, A. (2016). Development, construct validation and measurement invariance of the Greek Cyber-Bullying/Victimization Experiences Questionnaire (CBVEQ-G). *Computers in Human Behavior*, *55*, 380–390. DOI: 10.1016/j.chb.2016.08.032

Arnett, J. J. (2000). Emerging adulthood: A theory of development from the late teens through the twenties. *The American Psychologist*, *55*(5), 469–480. DOI: 10.1037/0003-066X.55.5.469 PMID: 10842426

Baker, Ö. E., & Bugay, A. (2011). Cyberbullying and loneliness: The mediating role of psychological symptoms. *Procedia: Social and Behavioral Sciences*, *30*, 276–280. DOI: 10.1016/j.sbspro.2011.10.253

Baker, O. E., & Bugay, A. (2011). Peer victimization and depressive symptoms: The mediation role of loneliness. *Procedia: Social and Behavioral Sciences*, *30*, 1303–1307. DOI: 10.1016/j.sbspro.2011.10.253

Balakrishnan, V. (2018). Actions, emotional reactions and cyberbullying—From the lens of bullies, victims, bully-victims and bystanders among Malaysian young adults. *Telematics and Informatics*, *35*(4), 1190–1200. DOI: 10.1016/j.tele.2018.02.002

Bandura, A. (1986). *Social foundations of thought and action: A social cognitive theory*. Prentice-Hall.

Barlett, C. P. (2015). Anonymously hurting others online: The effect of anonymity on cyberbullying frequency. *Psychology of Popular Media Culture*, *4*(2), 70–79. DOI: 10.1037/a0034335

Barlett, C. P. (2017). From theory to practice: Cyberbullying theory and its application to intervention. *Computers in Human Behavior*, *72*, 269–275. DOI: 10.1016/j.chb.2017.02.060

Barlett, C. P., Bennardi, C., Williams, S., & Zlupko, T. (2021). Theoretically predicting cyberbullying perpetration in youth with the BGCM: Unique challenges and promising research opportunities. *Frontiers in Psychology*, *12*, 708277. DOI: 10.3389/fpsyg.2021.708277 PMID: 34659022

Barlett, C. P., Kowalewski, D. A., Kramer, S. S., & Helmstetter, K. M. (2019). Testing the relationship between media violence exposure and cyberbullying perpetration. *Psychology of Popular Media Culture*, *8*(3), 280–286. DOI: 10.1037/ppm0000179

Brewer, G., & Kerslake, J. (2015). Cyberbullying, self-esteem, empathy and loneliness. *Computers in Human Behavior, 48*, 255–260. DOI: 10.1016/j.chb.2015.01.073

Browne, M. W., & Cudeck, R. (1993). Alternative ways of assessing model fit. In Bollen, K. A., & Long, J. S. (Eds.), *Testing structural equation models* (pp. 136–162). Sage Publications.

Cacioppo, J. T., Hawkley, L. C., Ernst, J. M., Burleson, M., Berntson, G. G., Nouriani, B., & Spiegel, D. (2006). Loneliness within a nomological net: An evolutionary perspective. *Journal of Research in Personality, 40*(6), 1054–1085. DOI: 10.1016/j.jrp.2005.11.007

Deb, S., Strodl, E., & Sun, J. (2015). Academic stress, parental pressure, anxiety and mental health among Indian high school students. *International Journal of Psychology and Behavioral Sciences, 5*(1), 26–34.

Doane, A. N., Pearson, M. R., & Kelley, M. L. (2014). Predictors of cyberbullying perpetration among college students: An application of the theory of reasoned action. *Computers in Human Behavior, 36*, 154–162. DOI: 10.1016/j.chb.2014.03.051

Fahy, A. E., Stansfeld, S. A., Smuk, M., Smith, N. R., Cummins, S., & Clark, C. (2016). Longitudinal associations between cyberbullying involvement and adolescent mental health. *The Journal of Adolescent Health : Official Publication of the Society for Adolescent Medicine, 59*(5), 502–509. DOI: 10.1016/j.jadohealth.2016.06.006 PMID: 27528471

Grimland, M., Mori, Y., Lesinskiene, S., Li, L., Ong, S. H., Praharaj, S. K., Wiguna, T., Zamani, Z., Heinonen, E., Gilbert, S., Brunstein Klomek, A., & Sourander, A.EACMHS Study Group. (2025). Cyberbullying victimization and suicide attempt among adolescents: A cross-national comparison. *International Journal of Environmental Research and Public Health, 22*(3), 385. DOI: 10.3390/ijerph22030385 PMID: 40238440

Hawkley, L. C., & Cacioppo, J. T. (2010). Loneliness matters: A theoretical and empirical review. *Current Directions in Psychological Science, 19*(2), 70–74. PMID: 20652462

Heinrich, L. M., & Gullone, E. (2006). The clinical significance of loneliness: A literature review. *Clinical Psychology Review, 26*(6), 695–718. DOI: 10.1016/j.cpr.2006.04.002 PMID: 16952717

Hellfeldt, K., López-Romero, L., & Andershed, H. (2020). Cyberbullying and psychological well-being in young adolescence: The potential protective mediation effects of social support from family, friends, and teachers. *International Journal of Environmental Research and Public Health, 17*(1), 45. DOI: 10.3390/ijerph17010045 PMID: 31861641

Hinduja, S., & Patchin, J. W. (2008). Cyberbullying: An exploratory analysis of factors related to offending and victimization. *Deviant Behavior, 29*(2), 129–156. DOI: 10.1080/01639620701457816

Hinduja, S., & Patchin, J. W. (2015). *Bullying beyond the schoolyard: Preventing and responding to cyberbullying* (2nd ed.). Sage.

Jenaro, C., Flores, N., & Frías, C. P. (2018). Systematic review of empirical studies on cyberbullying in adults: What we know and what we should investigate. *Aggression and Violent Behavior, 38*, 113–122. DOI: 10.1016/j.avb.2017.12.003

Jenaro, C., Flores, N., & Frías, C. P. (2021). Anxiety and depression in cyberbullied college students: A retrospective study. *Journal of Interpersonal Violence, 36*(1–2), 579–602. DOI: 10.1177/0886260517730030 PMID: 29294905

Kessler, R. C., Barker, P. R., Colpe, L. J., Epstein, J. F., Gfroerer, J. C., Hiripi, E., Howes, M. J., Normand, S.-L. T., Manderscheid, R. W., Walters, E. E., & Zaslavsky, A. M. (2003). Screening for serious mental illness in the general population. *Archives of General Psychiatry, 60*(2), 184–189. DOI: 10.1001/archpsyc.60.2.184 PMID: 12578436

Kowalski, R. M., Giumetti, G. W., Schroeder, A. N., & Lattanner, M. R. (2014). Bullying in the digital age: A critical review and meta-analysis of cyberbullying research among youth. *Psychological Bulletin, 140*(4), 1073–1137. DOI: 10.1037/a0035618 PMID: 24512111

Kowalski, R. M., Limber, S. P., & Agatston, P. W. (2012). *Cyberbullying: Bullying in the digital age* (2nd ed.). Wiley-Blackwell.

Kwan, I., Dickson, K., Richardson, M., MacDowall, W., Burchett, H., & Stansfield, C. (2020). Cyberbullying and mental health: A systematic review. *The Journal of Adolescent Health : Official Publication of the Society for Adolescent Medicine, 66*(3), 231–242.

Leung, A. N. M., Wong, N., & Farver, J. M. (2018). Cyberbullying in Hong Kong Chinese students: Life satisfaction, and the moderating role of friendship qualities on cyberbullying victimisation and perpetration. *Personality and Individual Differences, 133*, 7–12. DOI: 10.1016/j.paid.2017.07.016

Madsen, K. R., Damsgaard, M. T., Petersen, K. J., Qualter, P., & Holstein, B. E. (2024). Bullying at school, cyberbullying, and loneliness: National representative study of adolescents in Denmark. *International Journal of Environmental Research and Public Health*, *21*(4), 414. DOI: 10.3390/ijerph21040414 PMID: 38673326

Marciano, L., Schulz, P. J., & Camerini, A.-L. (2020). Cyberbullying perpetration and victimization in youth: A meta-analysis of longitudinal studies. *Journal of Computer-Mediated Communication*, *25*(2), 163–181. DOI: 10.1093/jcmc/zmz031

Maurya, C., Muhammad, T., Dhillon, P., & Maurya, P. (2022). The effects of cyberbullying victimization on depression and suicidal ideation among adolescents and young adults: A three- year cohort study from India. *BMC Psychiatry*, *22*(1), 599. Advance online publication. DOI: 10.1186/s12888-022-04238-x PMID: 36085004

Pala, S. Ç., Ünsal, A., Emiral, G. Ö., & Demirtaş, Z.. (2021). Cyberbullying and multidimensional perceived social support among high school students in Turkey. *Journal of Istanbul Faculty of Medicine*, *84*(1), 104–112. DOI: 10.26650/IUITFD.2019.0106

Perlman, D., & Peplau, L. A. (1982). Theoretical approaches to loneliness. In Peplau, L. A., & Perlman, D. (Eds.), *Loneliness: A sourcebook of current theory, research and therapy* (pp. 123–134). Wiley-Interscience.

Qualter, P., Vanhalst, J., Harris, R., Van Roekel, E., Lodder, G., Bangee, M., Maes, M., & Verhagen, M. (2015). Loneliness across the life span. *Perspectives on Psychological Science : A Journal of the Association for Psychological Science*, *10*(2), 250–264. DOI: 10.1177/1745691615568999 PMID: 25910393

Reed, K. P., Cooper, R. L., Nugent, W. R., & Russell, K. (2016). Cyberbullying: A literature review of its relationship to adolescent depression and current intervention strategies. *Journal of Human Behavior in the Social Environment*, *26*(1), 37–45. DOI: 10.1080/10911359.2015.1059165

Russell, D. W. (1996). UCLA Loneliness Scale (Version 3): Reliability, validity, and factor structure. *Journal of Personality Assessment*, *66*(1), 20–40. DOI: 10.1207/s15327752jpa6601_2 PMID: 8576833

Sadeeq, M., & Kumar, V. (2021). Inferring social relationships: Interrelated impact of personological factors and cyber bullying [Doctoral dissertation, Lovely Professional University]. Shodhganga. https://shodhganga.inflibnet.ac.in/handle/10603/123456

Sahin, M. (2012). The relationship between the cyberbullying/cybervictimization and loneliness among adolescents. *Children and Youth Services Review*, *34*(4), 834–837. DOI: 10.1016/j.childyouth.2012.01.010

Samsudin, E. Z., Yaacob, S. S., Wee, C. X., Ruzlin, A. N. M., Azzani, M., Jamil, A. T., & Mohamad, M. (2023). Prevalence of cyberbullying victimisation and its association with family dysfunction, health behaviour and psychological distress among young adults in urban Selangor, Malaysia: A cross-sectional study. *BMJ Open, 13*(11), e072801. DOI: 10.1136/bmjopen-2023-072801 PMID: 37967999

Samsudin, S.. (2024). Cyberbullying victimization, loneliness and well-being among adolescents. *Children and Youth Services Review, 148*, 106896.

Statista. (2024). Canada: experiences with cyberbullying, 2024. Statista. https://www.statista.com/statistics/1498106/canada-experienced-witnessed-cyberbullying/

Statista. (2024). *Cyberbullying – Statistics & facts*. https://www.statista.com/topics/1809/cyber-bullying/

Statista. (2025). *UK girls on upsetting online experiences 2016–2023*. https://www.statista.com/statistics/1448496/uk-girls-on-upsetting-online-experiences/

Talan, M. İ., Bostan, G., & Öztürk, Y. (2021). Investigation of the relationship between high school students' cyberbullying and cyber victimization situations and their perceptions of loneliness. *Journal of Research in Education and Society, 8*(2), 378–398. DOI: 10.51725/etad.905167

Varela, J. J., Hernández, C., Ramos Miranda, R., Barlett, C. P., & Rodríguez-Rivas, M. E. (2022). Victims of cyberbullying: Feeling loneliness and depression among youth and adult Chileans during the pandemic. *International Journal of Environmental Research and Public Health, 19*(10), 5886. DOI: 10.3390/ijerph19105886 PMID: 35627423

Watts, L. K., Wagner, J., Velasquez, B., & Behrens, P. I. (2017). Cyberbullying in higher education: A literature review. *Computers in Human Behavior, 69*, 268–274. DOI: 10.1016/j.chb.2016.12.038

Zalaquett, C. P., & Chatters, S. J. (2014). Cyberbullying in College. *SAGE Open, 4*(1), 215824401452672. DOI: 10.1177/2158244014526721

Zhang, D., Huebner, E. S., & Tian, L. (2020). Longitudinal associations among neuroticism, depression, and cyberbullying in early adolescents. *Computers in Human Behavior, 112*, 106475. DOI: 10.1016/j.chb.2020.106475

ADDITIONAL READING

Amadori, A., Prestera, G., Sangiuliano Intra, F., Taverna, L., Primi, C., & Brighi, A. (2025). Exploring the relationship between peer loneliness, problematic videogame use, and cyberbullying victimisation in adolescence. *Journal of Child and Adolescent Mental Health, 36*(3), 385–401. DOI: 10.2989/17280583.2025.2477126 PMID: 40528354

Ansa Razzaq, , & Ameer Hamza, Dr. Arooj Zahra RizviMuhammad Mohsin Javed Aslam. (2025). Cyberbullying, loneliness and use of social media among college students. *Contemporary Journal of Social Science Review, 3*(4), 158–166. DOI: 10.63878/cjssr.v3i4.1729

González-Abaurrea, E., González-Cabrera, J., Ortega-Barón, J., Escortell, R., & Machimbarrena, J. M. (2026). Bidirectional relationships between peer victimization, loneliness and solitude in adolescence: A systematic review. *Adolescent Research Review, 11*(1), 195–247. DOI: 10.1007/s40894-025-00266-2

Lee, J., Choo, H., Zhang, Y., Cheung, H. S., Zhang, Q., & Ang, R. P. (2026). Cyberbullying victimization and mental health symptoms among children and adolescents: A meta-analysis of longitudinal studies. *Trauma, Violence & Abuse, 27*(2), 391–406. DOI: 10.1177/15248380241313051 PMID: 39828926

Li, Y., Liu, Y., Knoll, M., & Obsuth, I. (2026). Mechanisms linking cyberbullying victimisation to internalising problems in youth: A systematic review and meta-analytic structural equation modelling. *Clinical Psychology Review, 123*, 102672. DOI: 10.1016/j.cpr.2025.102672 PMID: 41330069

Nagata, J. M., Zamora, G., Wong, J. H., Al-Shoaibi, A. A. A., Ganson, K. T., Testa, A., He, J., Lavender, J. M., & Baker, F. C. (2025). Cyberbullying victimisation was associated with greater manic symptoms in early adolescence: A prospective cohort study. *Acta Paediatrica (Oslo, Norway), 114*(8), 1904–1909. DOI: 10.1111/apa.70051 PMID: 40038058

Przepiorka, A., Talik, E., & Blachnio, A. (2025). A Psychological Perspective on the Complex Interplay Between Loneliness and Cyberbullying. In Nelson, T. (Ed.), *The Handbook of Loneliness*. Springer., DOI: 10.1007/978-3-032-02959-1

Vishwakarma, B., Kumari, P., & Kumar Vishwakarma, A. (2025). Predictive role of cyberbullying and victimization on general psychological distress among PhD students. *Indian Journal of Extension Education, 61*(3), 14–18. DOI: 10.48165/IJEE.2025.61303

Xiao, X., Jiang, Z.-L., Lei, Q., Wang, S.-J., Li, S.-X., & Gong, Q.-H. (2025). Loneliness and nervousness mediated the longitudinal association between sleep disorders and cyberbullying victimization in school-aged adolescents. *Frontiers in Psychiatry*, *16*, 1640989. DOI: 10.3389/fpsyt.2025.1640989 PMID: 41367939

Yang, W., Ning, L., Miao, Q., Xu, F., Li, K., Chen, X., & Lu, H. (2025). The mediating roles of anxiety, loneliness, stress, and depression in the relationship between cyberbullying and non-suicidal self-injury: Propensity score matching and causal mediation analysis. *BMC Psychiatry*, *25*(1), 539. DOI: 10.1186/s12888-025-06943-9 PMID: 40420016

KEY TERMS AND DEFINITIONS

Cyberbullying: Cyberbullying was conceptually defined as willful and repeated harm inflicted through the medium of electronic text (Hinduja and Patchin, 2006). In the present study, the cyberbullying was studied with respect to only cyberbullying victimisation. Cyberbullying victimisation was conceptually as the experience of being intentionally harmed, harassed, or threatened by others through digital platforms such as social media, messaging apps, or online forums. In the present study cyberbullying victimisation was operationally defined as experience of insult, abuse, threat, reputation defamation, and masquerading in past 90 days with five-point frequency scale, cyberbullying victimization experiences questionnaire (CBVEQ)-G (Antoniadou et. al., 2016).

Loneliness: Loneliness was conceptually defined as a subjective, distressing feeling that arises when a person's social relationships are perceived to be deficient either in quantity or quality (Perlman & Peplau, 1982). In the present study the loneliness among the cyberbullying victim undergraduate students was operationally defined as measure one's subjective feelings of loneliness as well as feelings of social isolation which was measured through isolation, relational connectedness, social connectedness, social compatibility and social exclusionon 4- point scale, The University of California, Los Angeles Loneliness Scale (UCLA-LS) (Russell, 1996).

Psychological Distress: Psychological Distress was conceptually defined as feelings of anxiety, depression, and irritability, often triggered by experiences such as trauma, loss, or significant life changes. In the present study, psychological distress was operationally defined as a state of mental discomfort characterized by symptoms of depression, nervousness, and restlessness among cyberbullying victim undergraduate students during the last 30 days, the responses were measured on 5-point scale, Kessler Psychological Distress Scale (K-10) (Kessler et al., 2003).

Undergraduate students: Undergraduate students were those enrolled in higher education programs that lead to a bachelor's degree.

Chapter 3
Campus as a Crucible: Understanding and Addressing Excessive Internet Use Among University Students

P. C. Ashfak Ahamed
http://orcid.org/0009-0008-3743-778X
Indian Institute of Technology, Roorkee, India

Zeba Asgari Jinwala
http://orcid.org/0009-0008-6454-7976
Indian Institute of Technology, Roorkee, India

ABSTRACT

The integration of digital technologies has transformed university life, enhancing learning and connectivity while giving rise to excessive internet use (EIU) among students. University students occupy a vulnerable position due to the combined impact of developmental transitions, academic pressures, social expectations, residential environments and pervasive digital access. This chapter, drawing on multidisciplinary research, examines conceptual and measurement challenges, global prevalence trends, and key psychological, social, and behavioural predictors of EIU. The chapter highlights the academic, psychosocial, and spiritual consequences associated with excessive use, emphasising its role as a maladaptive coping mechanism and difficulties in self-regulation rather than merely a behavioural excess. The chapter emphasises structured, multi-level interventions aimed at strengthening digital self-regulation, adaptive coping, and healthy engagement with technology, positioning universities as key settings for promoting digital well-being, resilience, and sustainable student development.

DOI: 10.4018/979-8-2600-2468-3.ch003

1. INTRODUCTION

At two o'clock in the morning, the university hostel corridor is hushed, the occasional vibration of a phone on a shared study desk. Inside one room, a student lies awake on his bed, eyes fixed on the soft glow of a screen. Lecture slides are open in one tab, a social media feed scrolls endlessly in another, and a streaming platform waits in the background, ready to play the next episode. He tells himself he will stop in five minutes—after one more post, one more video, one more message. When he finally checks the time again, the darkness outside is beginning to fade toward dawn. Sleep has slipped away, unease has grown, and the academic day ahead already feels overwhelming. This quiet moment, repeated in hostels across university campuses, captures the often-invisible struggle with excessive internet use (EIU) among students.

Universities have always been crucibles—intense environments where intellectual growth, identity formation, ambition, anxiety, freedom, and vulnerability coexist. Traditionally, this crucible was bounded by physical spaces: classrooms where ideas were debated, libraries where concentration was cultivated, hostels where friendships were forged, and cafeterias where informal social life thrived. In the contemporary era, however, the crucible has expanded far beyond brick-and-mortar boundaries. It now extends into screens carried in students' pockets, backpacks, and hostel rooms. Smartphones glow late into the night in hostels; laptops remain open long after lectures end. Social media feeds, streaming platforms, gaming worlds, and academic portals blur into a single, continuous digital stream that rarely shuts off.

The widespread integration of the internet into university settings has profoundly shaped students' learning processes, communication patterns, and social experiences. Online databases provide rapid access to knowledge, learning management systems structure academic life, and messaging applications help sustain friendships across cities and continents, often offering comfort and a sense of continuity for students living away from home for the first time. At the same time, this pervasive digital presence has given rise to a more troubling pattern. Excessive internet use has emerged as one of the most complex psychosocial challenges on modern campuses, not defined simply by the number of hours spent online but by how, why, and with what consequences students engage with the digital world (Carbonell et al., 2018). Within the university campus—a vibrant ecosystem of learning, discovery, and personal growth—students navigate critical developmental transitions while remaining constantly connected. In this high-risk environment, the boundary between adaptive engagement and maladaptive overuse becomes increasingly blurred, as tools initially adopted for efficiency, connection, or academic support can gradually transform into primary means of emotional regulation, avoidance, or escape.

This chapter conceptualises the university campus as a crucible in which EIU is not only shaped and reinforced but can also be meaningfully challenged, moving beyond explanations that locate the problem solely in individual weakness or poor self-control. Rather than blaming students, it places EIU within a wider developmental, institutional, and cultural context, where academic pressure, transitional life stages, and constant digital availability intersect to influence behaviour.

The chapter therefore pursues two closely connected aims: first, to develop a clear and multidisciplinary understanding of EIU as a digital disease emerging within university settings, exploring how it develops, how it manifests in everyday student life, and what psychological, academic, and social consequences it produces; and second, to translate this understanding into practical, evidence-informed guidance for assessment, prevention, and intervention that can be implemented by counsellors, teachers, administrators, and policy makers. Ultimately, it argues that universities, as spaces of growth and transformation, carry both a responsibility and a unique opportunity to support students in cultivating healthier and more intentional relationships with technology, so that within the pressures of academic life and digital temptation, thoughtful institutional and clinical responses can promote resilience, self-regulation, and well-being rather than burnout and dependence.

2. THEORETICAL FRAMEWORK

Conceptual Foundations and Measurement Challenges

One of the most persistent challenges in the study of EIU lies in how the phenomenon is defined and measured. At the heart of this debate is the absence of a unified definition, resulting in a fragmented academic landscape characterised by competing terms such as Internet Addiction, Problematic Internet Use, Pathological Internet Use, and Internet Use Disorder. Although often used interchangeably, these terms reflect differing theoretical assumptions rather than mere semantic variation. Some scholars conceptualise EIU as a behavioural addiction analogous to substance use disorders, marked by salience, tolerance, withdrawal, loss of control, and functional impairment, while others adopt a more cautious view, framing it as a maladaptive coping strategy, an impulse-control difficulty, or a manifestation of underlying psychosocial distress (Spada, 2014; Kardefelt-Winther, 2014; Anderson et al., 2017; Dahl & Bergmark, 2020; Brand et al., 2022; Tunney & Rooney, 2023). Systematic reviews consistently highlight the lack of consensus in terminology, assessment tools, and diagnostic thresholds, demonstrating how definitional ambiguity continues to hinder theoretical coherence and reliable measurement (Brand et al., 2022). Within this context, EIU may be broadly defined as excessive or poorly controlled preoccupations, urges, or behaviours related to internet and mobile, tablet or computer use that lead to significant distress or impairment in functioning, representing more than heavy usage and instead reflecting a pattern of behaviour that meaningfully disrupts daily life and psychological well-being (Carbonell et al., 2018).

Measurement practices further compound these challenges. While Young's Internet Addiction Test (IAT) remains the most frequently used instrument in campus-based studies, researchers also rely on tools such as Young's Diagnostic Questionnaire (YDQ), the Problematic Internet Use Questionnaire (PIUQ), Assessment of Internet and Computer Game Addiction Scale (AICA-S), Compulsive Internet Use Scale (CIUS), Chen's Internet Addiction Scale, and a range of domain-specific scales targeting social media use, online gaming, or smartphone dependence (Spada, 2014; Kuss & Lopez-Fernandez, 2016; Anderson et al., 2017; Dahl & Bergmark, 2020). These instruments differ substantially in their conceptual focus, scoring systems, reliability, cultural adaptability, and threshold criteria. As a result, reported prevalence rates of excessive or problematic internet use vary dramatically. Such variability is driven not only by contextual differences but also by inconsistent measurement frameworks (Dahl & Bergmark, 2020).

For university populations, these psychometric issues raise critical questions. It remains unclear whether categorical cut-offs meaningfully capture the complexity of students' digital behaviour, or whether dimensional approaches that assess severity along a continuum offer greater clinical and ecological validity. Moreover, self-report instruments are vulnerable to recall bias, social desirability, and limited insight, particularly in environments where heavy internet use is socially normative (Kardefelt-Winther, 2014; Anderson et al., 2017; Dahl & Bergmark, 2020).

In response to these limitations, emerging digital phenotyping methods have been proposed as complementary tools. Passive data sources—such as smartphone telemetry, screen-time metrics, and app usage logs—offer the potential for objective, fine-grained indicators of digital behaviour (Brand et al., 2022). However, their application introduces significant ethical concerns related to privacy, informed consent, surveillance, and data security, especially within educational institutions. Without careful governance, such approaches risk undermining trust and autonomy in campus communities.

Taken together, the evidence points toward the need for a more integrated and standardised framework. A mixed-method measurement strategy—combining validated psychometric instruments, contextual clinical assessment, and ethically governed digital phenotyping—may offer the most nuanced and developmentally sensitive approach to understanding EIU among university students. Achieving greater conceptual clarity and methodological coherence is essential if the field is to move beyond fragmented findings toward effective prevention and intervention.

3. EPIDEMIOLOGY

Global Prevalence in Campus Contexts

A comprehensive synthesis of global epidemiological evidence clearly demonstrates that EIU constitutes a significant and widespread public health concern within university populations worldwide.

Available large-scale epidemiological studies indicate that EIU occurs across populations worldwide, though prevalence varies by age group and context. Among adults, prevalence rates remain relatively low, typically ranging from 0.7% to 1.0%. In contrast, adolescent samples demonstrate greater variability, with estimates ranging from 1.0% to 9.0% in European studies, 1.0% to 12.0% in Middle Eastern populations, and 2.0% to 18.0% in Asian samples. The highest rates are consistently observed among university students, where prevalence estimates range broadly from 6.0% to 35.0%, suggesting heightened vulnerability during emerging adulthood and within academically demanding, digitally intensive environments (Carbonell et al., 2018; Spada, 2014; Dahl & Bergmark, 2020).

Although individual studies report highly divergent prevalence figures—ranging from 4–7% in some contexts to more than 50% in others—this variation largely reflects methodological differences, including inconsistencies in terminology, assessment instruments, sampling procedures, and diagnostic cut-off criteria, rather than genuine epidemiological disparities. When these methodological sources of heterogeneity are accounted for, a more stable global pattern becomes evident: approximately 20% to 30% of university students demonstrate excessive or potentially problematic internet use at any given time, indicating that nearly one in four students experiences some degree of risk or functional impairment (Carbonell et al., 2018; Dahl & Bergmark, 2020).

Across regions, striking epidemiological regularities are observed. Higher prevalence is consistently associated with younger undergraduates, students residing in hostels or dormitories, and those experiencing academic pressure, poor sleep quality, loneliness, reduced self-control, and psychological distress (Dahl & Bergmark, 2020). Meta-analytic evidence further confirms a strong bidirectional relationship between psychological distress—particularly anxiety, depression, and stress—and EIU, suggesting a reinforcing cycle of vulnerability within campus environments (Carbonell et al., 2018).

Taken together, the epidemiological literature positions EIU as neither culturally isolated nor methodologically trivial, but as a global developmental risk embedded in contemporary university life. This level of prevalence firmly establishes EIU as a core campus mental health and public health issue, underscoring the urgent need for systematic screening, targeted prevention, and institution-wide responses within higher education settings.

4. PREDICTIVE FACTORS

EIU among university students is clearly not a random or isolated behaviour, nor can it be explained solely as a by-product of increased technological availability. Rather, it emerges from a complex convergence of psychological vulnerability, maladaptive coping strategies, usage patterns, and lifestyle disruptions, all of which are further shaped and intensified by broader contextual influences such as age, gender, academic demands, cultural expectations, and large-scale societal events, including the COVID-19 pandemic. Within university settings, these interacting dynamics become particularly evident during key transitional and high-stress periods, such as the first year of campus entry, examination cycles, academic probation, placement-related uncertainty, or extended periods of hostel confinement, when students often experience heightened emotional distress, social disconnection, and disruptions to their daily routines.

Adopting a developmental and psychosocial perspective enables a more nuanced understanding of why some students are particularly vulnerable to EIU, while others are not. Students differ in their capacity to regulate emotions, manage stress, maintain sleep–wake routines, and seek adaptive forms of social support. Those experiencing psychological distress, ineffective coping styles, poor sleep hygiene, or intense academic and social pressures are more likely to turn to the Internet as a readily available means of escape, emotional regulation, or avoidance (Kardefelt-Winther, 2014; Montag & Walla, 2016; Anderson et al., 2017; Tokunaga, 2017; Dahl & Bergmark, 2020; Brand et al., 2022; Jin & Jiang, 2025). Over time, this reliance may solidify into habitual or compulsive patterns of use, further undermining academic engagement, interpersonal relationships, and overall well-being.

These insights carry important implications for prevention and intervention within campus settings. Effective responses must move beyond simplistic recommendations that encourage students merely to "reduce screen time." Instead, they should address the underlying psychological needs, developmental challenges, and lifestyle contexts that drive excessive use in the first place (Montag & Walla, 2016). Universities, as critical sites for early identification and support, are uniquely positioned to recognise students at risk, integrate mental health services within academic ecosystems, and cultivate campus environments that promote emotional resilience, social connectedness, healthy routines, and intentional, balanced engagement with digital technologies.

Psychological and Emotional Predictors

Among all identified predictors, psychological distress emerges as the most robust and consistently supported risk factor for EIU. Large-scale evidence demonstrates that symptoms of depression, anxiety, and stress (Kardefelt-Winther, 2014; Kuss & Lopez-Fernandez, 2016; Montag & Walla, 2016; Anderson et al., 2017; Tokunaga, 2017; Brand et al., 2022; Tunney & Rooney, 2023; Jin & Jiang, 2025) show strong positive associations with excessive internet engagement. On campuses, this pattern is often observed during high-pressure academic phases. For example, a student experiencing persistent anxiety about internal assessments or competitive examinations may begin spending excessive hours scrolling through social media or binge-watching content late into the night as a way to temporarily disengage from academic worry. Similarly, students facing depressive symptoms—such as low motivation, hopelessness, or reduced pleasure in offline activities—may retreat into online spaces that offer immediate stimulation or distraction with minimal effort (Brand et al., 2022; Tunney & Rooney, 2023).

The underlying mechanism is relatively consistent: psychological distress increases reliance on the Internet for mood regulation, emotional escape, and avoidance of offline stressors (Montag & Walla, 2016; Brand et al., 2022). Over time, this reliance can become habitual and compulsive, creating a self-reinforcing cycle in which distress fuels excessive use, excessive use disrupts academic performance, sleep, and relationships, and these disruptions further intensify distress (Tokunaga, 2017). Within this triad, stress often shows the strongest association, followed by depression and anxiety, particularly in academically demanding environments such as professional colleges and elite institutions.

Loneliness and Social Disconnection in Campus Life

Loneliness represents one of the most powerful and consistently identified predictors of EIU among university students, particularly those navigating unfamiliar social and cultural environments. Paradoxically, many students report feeling profoundly disconnected from others, despite being constantly surrounded by peers in hostels, classrooms, libraries, and common areas. This experience is especially pronounced among students living in residential campuses, international or out-of-state students, first-generation learners, and those who struggle with language fluency, social confidence, or cultural adjustment (Tokunaga, 2017; Dahl & Bergmark, 2020). In such contexts, online platforms often begin to function as substitutes for face-to-face interaction, offering low-risk avenues for connection without the immediate social demands of offline engagement (Ding et al., 2023).

In the Indian context, this vulnerability is especially salient within premier central-funded institutions such as the Indian Institutes of Technology (IITs), Indian Institutes of Management (IIMs), Indian Institutes of Information Technology (IIITs), and Central Universities. These institutions draw students from across the vast linguistic, cultural, regional, and socio-economic diversity of the Indian subcontinent through highly competitive, all-India level entrance examinations. While this national selection process ensures academic excellence and diversity, it also necessitates an abrupt transition to fully residential campuses, often located far from students' home states and cultural milieus. For many students, entry into such campuses involves simultaneous adjustments to unfamiliar languages of everyday communication, regional food practices, hostel routines, social norms, and distinct campus subcultures that differ markedly from their prior lived experiences.

During the initial months on campus, this sudden cultural and ecological shift frequently triggers adjustment-related stress and a growing sense of social isolation (Ding et al., 2023). Students may struggle to participate in informal conversations due to accent or language differences, feel disconnected during shared meals because hostel food does not align with familiar dietary habits, or experience uncertainty in navigating peer interactions shaped by region-specific humour, values, or social expectations. For instance, a student from a rural or linguistically homogeneous background may struggle to follow rapid, mixed-language conversations in hostels, while another may avoid common dining spaces due to discomfort with unfamiliar food. These challenges are often compounded by intense academic pressure, competitive evaluation systems, and high personal expectations, leaving limited psychological space to process cultural dislocation or seek social support.

Over time, such cumulative experiences can foster a sense of emotional alienation and perceived social exclusion, even within densely populated residential campuses. Although students are physically embedded in vibrant academic communities, they may experience a subjective sense of invisibility or a sense of not belonging. In this context, the Internet becomes a readily accessible and emotionally safer coping medium (Brand et al., 2022). Through social media platforms, regional language content, online gaming communities, or streaming services, students can reconnect with familiar cultural symbols, languages, and identities. For example, a student may spend hours watching content in their native language, engaging in online multiplayer games with peers from similar backgrounds, or maintaining virtual connections with friends and family back home. While such online engagement may initially serve an adaptive function by providing comfort and continuity, prolonged reliance can gradually evolve into EIU, reinforcing withdrawal from offline campus life and further impeding cultural and social adjustment.

In everyday campus terms, a student who feels excluded from peer groups, hesitant to speak up in tutorials, or uncomfortable participating in group projects may increasingly retreat into online spaces where interaction feels more controllable and less threatening. Although these digital environments may initially offer a sense of belonging and validation, over time, they often reduce motivation for real-world engagement, leading to diminished participation in campus activities, student clubs, cultural events, or informal peer gatherings. Clinically, this pattern illustrates how EIU may temporarily mask feelings of loneliness while simultaneously deepening social disengagement, creating a cyclical process that sustains both isolation and problematic digital behaviour (Tokunaga, 2017).

Negative Affect, Emotion Dysregulation, and Maladaptive Coping

Beyond diagnosable distress, studies consistently identify negative affectivity, poor emotion regulation, and maladaptive coping styles as key predictors of EIU (Kardefelt-Winther, 2014; Kuss & Lopez-Fernandez, 2016; Anderson et al., 2017; Brand et al., 2022; Tunney & Rooney, 2023; Jin & Jiang, 2025). Many students struggle not with a single major stressor but with a steady accumulation of minor frustrations—academic setbacks, interpersonal conflicts, homesickness, or uncertainty about the future. When students lack effective skills to tolerate and regulate these emotions, they often turn to immediate digital relief, such as compulsive scrolling, consuming short-form videos, or engaging in prolonged gaming sessions.

On campuses, this is frequently observed during late-night hours, when students report feeling "restless," "empty," or "unable to sleep," and default to their phones or laptops rather than engaging in reflective or restorative coping strategies. Over time, reliance on digital distraction undermines the development of adaptive emotional regulation skills, increasing vulnerability to excessive use.

Cognitive and Personality-Related Contributors

Cognitive factors play a crucial role in sustaining EIU. Many at-risk students hold maladaptive Internet-related beliefs, such as overvaluing online relationships, perceiving online spaces as safer or more controllable than offline interactions, or fearing negative evaluation in real-world social settings (Tokunaga, 2017; Brand et al., 2022; Tunney & Rooney, 2023). For example, a student with social anxiety may feel confident interacting in online discussion forums or gaming platforms but experience significant distress during classroom presentations or group work. These cognitions often mediate the relationship between psychological distress and EIU, reinforcing avoidance of offline challenges.

Personality-related factors further shape vulnerability. Impulsivity and low self-control—manifesting as difficulty delaying gratification, sustaining attention, or inhibiting urges—are consistently associated with loss of control over Internet use (Brand et al., 2014; Brand et al., 2022; Tunney & Rooney, 2023; Jin & Jiang, 2025). Such traits are particularly salient in late adolescence and early adulthood, when self-regulatory capacities are still developing. In contrast, conscientiousness emerges as a protective factor, with organised, goal-directed students being better able to regulate their online behaviour despite high academic demands.

Behavioural Patterns and Lifestyle Disruptions

From a behavioural perspective, time spent online remains one of the most stable predictors of EIU, especially when Internet engagement is non-academic, unstructured, and driven by avoidance rather than purpose. Certain online activities—such as gaming, social media use, and escapist browsing—are consistently associated with a higher risk, whereas academic or task-focused use is associated with a comparatively lower risk (Kuss & Lopez-Fernandez, 2016; Montag & Walla, 2016; Tunney & Rooney, 2023).

Lifestyle factors further compound vulnerability. Poor sleep quality stands out as both a predictor and a consequence of EIU. Many students report disrupted sleep due to late-night screen exposure, which in turn impairs concentration, mood, and stress tolerance, leading to increased reliance on the Internet the following day.

5. MECHANISMS AND NEUROCOGNITIVE CORRELATES

The current literature on EIU among university students is dominated by epidemiological, psychological, and behavioural research, with relatively limited direct investigation of neurobiological or neuroimaging correlates. Despite this limitation, a coherent set of cognitive, psychological, motivational, and neurocognitive mechanisms consistently emerges across studies. These mechanisms allow EIU to be conceptualised not merely as excessive screen exposure but as a maladaptive self-regulation process, shaped by emotional distress, cognitive vulnerabilities, and impaired executive control.

Cognitive Mechanisms: Distorted Thinking and Impulse Control

At the cognitive level, maladaptive Internet-related cognitions represent one of the most consistently identified mechanisms underlying EIU. Research has shown that students with EIU tend to hold distorted beliefs such as overestimating the emotional benefits of Internet use, perceiving online interactions as safer or more rewarding than offline relationships, and believing that digital engagement is essential for stress relief or social acceptance (Kuss & Lopez-Fernandez, 2016; Tokunaga, 2017; Tunney & Rooney, 2023). These cognitions bias decision-making in favour of online activities and reduce motivation to engage with real-world challenges.

On campus, this may be observed in students who repeatedly avoid classroom participation, group discussions, or hostel socialisation, while believing that online gaming communities, social media platforms, or streaming services are their primary sources of comfort or belonging. Over time, such cognitions become self-reinforcing, strengthening avoidance learning and narrowing behavioural repertoires.

Students with EIU consistently demonstrate higher impulsivity scores, indicating impairments in inhibitory control, attentional regulation, and the ability to delay gratification (Brand et al., 2014; Tunney & Rooney, 2023; Jin & Jiang, 2025). In practical terms, this manifests as difficulty disengaging from devices despite academic deadlines, inability to limit "just a few more minutes" of scrolling or gaming, and repeated failure to adhere to self-imposed usage limits. These patterns point to weakened executive control systems that normally regulate goal-directed behaviour.

Psychological Mechanisms: Coping Dysfunction and Self-Regulatory Failure

From a psychological perspective, dysfunctional coping strategies play a pivotal role in the development and maintenance of EIU. Evidence indicates that students with EIU rely disproportionately on avoidance-based coping, using the Internet to escape academic stress, interpersonal discomfort, homesickness, or feelings of inadequacy (Anderson et al., 2017; Tunney & Rooney, 2023). While such coping may offer immediate emotional relief, it prevents active problem-solving and emotional processing, thereby sustaining distress.

In campus life, this mechanism is frequently observed during examination periods, placement uncertainty, or early semesters of adjustment, when students retreat into prolonged online activity rather than seeking peer support, faculty guidance, or structured routines. Over time, Internet use becomes an automatic coping response to stress cues, rather than a conscious choice.

A related psychological mechanism is impaired self-efficacy. Studies consistently report lower confidence in one's ability to regulate Internet use among students with EIU (Anderson et al., 2017). This diminished sense of control contributes to helplessness, resignation, and further loss of behavioural regulation. For instance, students may express beliefs such as "I cannot concentrate without my phone" or "I have no control over my screen time," which undermine attempts at change and reinforce dependency.

Expectancy and Motivational Mechanisms

Another important cognitive–motivational pathway involves outcome expectancies. Students with EIU tend to hold high positive expectancies regarding Internet use—believing it will reliably reduce stress, boredom, loneliness, or negative mood—alongside low refusal self-efficacy, or reduced confidence in their ability to resist online engagement (Kuss & Lopez-Fernandez, 2016; Anderson et al., 2017; Brand et al., 2022; Jin & Jiang, 2025). These expectancies strongly predict continued and excessive use, even in the face of negative academic or health consequences.

On campus, this may appear as a student repeatedly turning to online content late at night to "relax," despite knowing it will disrupt sleep and impair next-day functioning. The anticipated emotional payoff outweighs delayed or abstract costs, biasing choice toward immediate digital rewards.

Neurocognitive Correlates: Executive Control and Reward Sensitivity

Although direct neuroimaging evidence remains limited in student populations, converging findings point to neurocognitive patterns similar to other behavioural addictions. EIU is associated with impairments in executive functions, particularly inhibitory control, sustained attention, and decision-making (Brand et al., 2014; Tunney & Rooney, 2023; Jin & Jiang, 2025). These deficits reflect reduced top-down regulation, making it difficult to interrupt ongoing online behaviour once initiated.

At the same time, students with EIU demonstrate heightened reward sensitivity to digital cues such as notifications, social feedback, gaming achievements, or novel content. Repeated exposure strengthens stimulus–reward associations, gradually shifting Internet use from goal-directed activity to habitual and compulsive behaviour. This process aligns with integrative addiction models such as the I-PACE (Interaction of Person-Affect-Cognition-Execution) framework, which describes how personal vulnerabilities, affective states, cognitive biases, and executive dysfunction interact to sustain addictive behaviours.

6. NAVIGATING THE CONSEQUENCES

Academic Fallout

EIU among university students has been consistently linked to significant academic consequences that extend far beyond simple time management issues. Research across diverse educational contexts demonstrates that EIU disrupts core academic processes, including attention, learning efficiency, motivation, self-regulation, and engagement, ultimately undermining both short-term academic performance and long-term educational trajectories (Kuss & Lopez-Fernandez, 2016; Tunney & Rooney, 2023). In residential university environments, these effects are particularly pronounced due to unrestricted Internet access, academic pressure, and reduced external monitoring.

One of the most concrete and consistently documented academic consequences of EIU is a decline in academic performance, most commonly reflected in lower Cumulative Grade Point Average (CGPA). Empirical studies have consistently demonstrated a significant association between EIU and reduced academic performance, indicating that excessive online engagement directly interferes with academic achievement (Anderson et al., 2017; Ding et al., 2023). In practical campus terms, this is evident in students who initially perform well but gradually experience declining grades as late-night Internet use, online gaming, or continuous social media engagement encroach upon their study time and cognitive resources. Even when students remain enrolled and attend classes, their academic output often deteriorates due to reduced concentration and ineffective learning strategies.

Closely related to objective performance decline is impairment in academic satisfaction and perceived competence. Studies have shown that students with higher levels of EIU report lower satisfaction with their academic performance, reflecting diminished confidence in their academic abilities (Ding et al., 2023). On campus, such students often express feelings of underachievement despite investing long hours "studying," which are frequently fragmented by digital distractions. This mismatch between effort and outcome contributes to frustration, self-doubt, and further disengagement from academic tasks.

Beyond grades alone, EIU exerts a broader impact on overall academic functioning and progress. Research indicates that EIU can inhibit academic progress, undermine scholastic competence, disrupt career planning, and reduce participation in extracurricular and co-curricular activities (Anderson et al., 2017). In university settings, this may manifest as students repeatedly missing internal assessments, failing to meet course requirements on time, or postponing important academic milestones such as internships, projects, or thesis work. Over time, such disruptions can delay graduation and weaken students' preparedness for future academic or professional roles.

EIU also contributes to deterioration in study habits and academic self-regulation, which are essential for success in higher education. Students with EIU exhibit procrastination, irregular study schedules, and last-minute preparation for examinations. In residential hostels, this pattern is frequently reinforced by peer norms of late-night online activity, easy availability of high-speed Internet, and absence of structured routines. As a result, students may spend nights browsing, gaming, or streaming content, only to attempt academic work under conditions of fatigue and heightened stress, leading to suboptimal performance.

From a cognitive perspective, EIU leads to attentional fragmentation and increased cognitive load, impairing students' ability to engage in sustained, effortful learning. Continuous exposure to rapid digital stimulation—such as notifications, scrolling feeds, and gaming rewards—conditions attentional systems toward novelty and immediacy. Consequently, students find it increasingly difficult to focus during lectures, read lengthy academic texts, or engage in complex problem-solving. In classroom settings, this is often observed as students multitasking on laptops or smartphones, switching repeatedly between academic content and non-academic digital activities, thereby compromising the consolidation of learning and conceptual understanding.

EIU is also associated with reduced class attendance and diminished academic engagement. Students with high levels of EIU are more likely to skip lectures, arrive late, or attend classes while mentally disengaged due to late-night Internet use or digital preoccupation. Faculty members frequently report reduced participation, minimal involvement in discussions, and a reliance on recorded lectures or online summaries, rather than actively engaging in the classroom. Over time, this disengagement weakens students' academic identity, limits meaningful interaction with faculty, and reduces access to mentorship and academic guidance.

Sleep disruption represents a critical indirect pathway through which EIU impairs academic functioning. Late-night Internet use is associated with reduced sleep duration, delayed sleep onset, and increased daytime sleepiness (Montag & Walla, 2016; Kuss & Lopez-Fernandez, 2016). Sleep deprivation, in turn, negatively affects attention, memory consolidation, executive functioning, and emotional regulation—all of which are vital for academic success. On residential campuses, this cycle is often normalised, with students collectively engaging in late-night online activities during examinations or project deadlines, leading to cumulative academic impairment across the semester.

Rather than alleviating academic stress, EIU often exacerbates academic pressure and burnout. Poor performance, missed deadlines, and disengagement generate guilt, anxiety, and a sense of academic inadequacy, which may further intensify avoidance-based Internet use. This self-reinforcing cycle increases vulnerability to academic burnout, reduced motivation, and, in more severe cases, academic probation, delayed graduation, or risk of dropout. Research highlights concerns regarding study completion, emphasising the need for timely intervention to ensure fulfilment of academic requirements and successful graduation among students with EIU.

Psychosocial Consequences

A growing body of research indicates that EIU among university students is associated with significant and far-reaching psychosocial consequences that encompass psychological health, academic performance, social relationships, and overall quality of life. Importantly, these consequences are not simply the result of excessive time spent online; rather, they reflect fundamental disruptions in emotional regulation, coping processes, interpersonal engagement, and self-regulatory capacity, particularly within the demanding and transitional context of university life.

Psychological and Mental Health Consequences

One of the most consistently documented psychosocial consequences of EIU is elevated psychological distress, particularly symptoms of depression, anxiety, and chronic stress. Multiple studies demonstrate that students with EIU show significantly higher levels of depressive and anxious symptomatology compared to their non-addicted peers, with some research indicating very strong correlations between EIU and depression and anxiety (Kardefelt-Winther, 2014; Kuss & Lopez-Fernandez, 2016; Tunney & Rooney, 2023). Evidence further suggests that students with moderate to severe depression are several times more likely to exhibit pathological Internet use, highlighting a potent and clinically meaningful association.

On campus, this often manifests as students reporting persistent low mood, emotional exhaustion, irritability, or heightened anxiety, while simultaneously spending long hours online late into the night. Although online activity may initially provide distraction or emotional relief, over time, students frequently report worsening mood, increased restlessness, and a sense of being "stuck" in unproductive routines. This creates a bidirectional cycle in which psychological distress drives EIU, and excessive use further exacerbates emotional difficulties by impairing sleep, academic functioning, and self-esteem.

General psychological distress, increased impulsivity, reduced self-esteem and emotional dysregulation also emerge as prominent psychosocial consequences (Kuss & Lopez-Fernandez, 2016; Tunney & Rooney, 2023). Studies consistently show that moderate to heavy Internet users experience higher perceived stress levels. In academic settings, this is particularly evident during examination periods, project deadlines, or placement seasons, when students may rely heavily on digital platforms to escape pressure. Rather than reducing stress, prolonged online engagement often intensifies feelings of overwhelm, emotional instability, and burnout.

Social and Interpersonal Consequences

Among the most profound psychosocial consequences of EIU are social isolation and impaired interpersonal functioning. Although digital platforms offer avenues for communication, excessive or compulsive use is associated with reduced face-to-face interaction, withdrawal from social activities, and weakened real-world relationships (Kuss & Lopez-Fernandez, 2016; Montag & Walla, 2016; Tunney & Rooney, 2023; Ding et al., 2023). Students often report feeling lonely and disconnected despite being surrounded by peers in hostels, classrooms, and common areas.

In campus settings, this may be observed in students retreating to their hostel rooms, skipping social gatherings, avoiding group discussions, or disengaging from clubs and student organisations, while remaining highly active online. Over time, online interactions begin to replace, rather than supplement, offline relationships, leading to discomfort in real-world social situations and the erosion of social skills.

EIU is also linked to relationship strain and social conflict. Excessive online engagement can reduce emotional availability, disrupt shared responsibilities, and contribute to misunderstandings with peers, roommates, and family members (Kardefelt-Winther, 2014; Tunney & Rooney, 2023). On campus, this may manifest as conflicts over shared hostel spaces, complaints during group projects about lack of participation, or strained friendships due to perceived withdrawal or inattentiveness. These relational difficulties further reduce social support, reinforcing reliance on the Internet as a compensatory coping mechanism.

During emerging adulthood—a critical period for identity development—excessive reliance on online environments may also interfere with identity exploration and role formation. Students may increasingly derive self-worth from online validation, gaming achievements, or curated digital identities, rather than from real-world accomplishments and relationships. On campus, this can translate into reduced initiative, avoidance of leadership roles, and uncertainty about future academic or career goals.

Quality of Life Reduction and Integrated Psychosocial Impact

Taken together, the evidence suggests that EIU leads to a cascade of interconnected psychological and social consequences. These include psychological distress, impaired academic confidence, social withdrawal, maladaptive coping, sleep disruption, and reduced quality of life. Rather than enhancing well-being or connectedness, EIU often narrows students' lived experiences and limits meaningful engagement with campus life.

Spiritual Consequences

Excessive engagement with digital platforms increasingly diverts young individuals from deeper existential reflection and spiritual growth, replacing inward awareness with continuous external stimulation and validation. A central spiritual consequence identified is the erosion of reflective and contemplative capacity. Constant connectivity, rapid content consumption, and the pursuit of online gratification leave little psychological space for silence, self-reflection, or existential questioning.

Practices traditionally associated with spiritual development—such as introspection, mindfulness, prayer, or value-based living—are gradually displaced by habitual scrolling, algorithm-driven engagement, and compulsive checking behaviours. Over time, this weakens young individuals' ability to connect with deeper aspects of self and purpose, fostering a fragmented inner life.

The review also underscores concerns related to identity and moral relativism in the digital realm. Online environments often encourage the construction of curated identities driven by likes, visibility, and approval rather than authenticity. From a spiritual perspective, this can result in an externalised sense of self-worth, where personal value is increasingly measured by digital metrics rather than intrinsic meaning or ethical grounding. It is noted that such dynamics contribute to superficiality and materialistic orientation, undermining stable moral frameworks and long-held spiritual values.

Another important spiritual implication discussed is the commodification of spirituality and morality in online spaces. Digital platforms frequently present spiritual ideas as consumable content—short videos, motivational quotes, or trend-based practices—detached from discipline, ethical responsibility, or lived transformation. This fragmented exposure risks reducing spirituality to momentary emotional uplift rather than a sustained process of moral development, self-restraint, and meaning-centred living. Such patterns may weaken ethical sensitivity and blur moral boundaries, particularly among youth navigating identity formation.

Furthermore, EIU is linked with disconnection from real-life relationships and communities. As online engagement replaces face-to-face interaction, opportunities for empathy, service, shared rituals, and communal meaning-making diminish. This social-spiritual disconnection reinforces isolation and reduces exposure to value-based guidance provided through family, cultural traditions, and community practices.

It conceptualises the spiritual consequences as a gradual shift away from depth toward immediacy, from meaning toward gratification, and from inner coherence toward externally driven identity. These spiritual disruptions do not necessarily manifest as overt crises but emerge as a quiet weakening of reflection, ethical clarity, and purpose. It also argues that addressing EIU therefore requires not only psychological and behavioural interventions but also efforts to restore balance, intentionality, and value-oriented engagement with life, enabling youth to reconnect with meaning, ethics, and spiritual well-being in an increasingly digital world.

7. INTERVENTIONS AND PREVENTION STRATEGIES

Consequently, effective interventions must address the psychological, social, academic, and lifestyle contexts that maintain excessive use. The literature strongly supports multi-level, campus-embedded strategies that combine individual interventions with preventive, institutional approaches.

Individual-Level Psychological Interventions

Cognitive–Behavioural Therapy

Cognitive–behavioural therapy (CBT) approaches are among the most empirically supported interventions for EIU. These interventions target maladaptive cognitions and avoidance-based coping patterns that maintain excessive use. In CBT for EIU, treatment typically begins with identifying and challenging distorted beliefs that maintain excessive online behaviour, such as the assumption that relaxation or optimal performance is only possible through late-night Internet use (Spada, 2014; Kuss & Lopez-Fernandez, 2016; Brand et al., 2022; Jin & Jiang, 2025). For instance, a first-year engineering student presenting to the campus counselling centre reported staying awake until 3 a.m., gaming as a way to "escape academic pressure", and believed that gaming was the only effective method to unwind. Through CBT sessions, the student was guided to examine these beliefs and recognise how late-night gaming was functioning as an avoidance strategy rather than a genuine stress regulator.

Parallel to cognitive restructuring, the intervention focused on developing alternative coping strategies for managing stress, boredom, and loneliness, including brief physical activity, structured peer interaction, and offline relaxation techniques (Tokunaga, 2017). To translate insight into behaviour change, the therapist introduced behavioural scheduling, helping the student plan a structured evening routine that included time-limited gaming, predefined study blocks, and device-free wind-down periods. This graded reduction of unstructured Internet use allowed the student to regain a sense of control without abrupt deprivation. Throughout the process, emphasis was placed on strengthening goal-directed behaviour and self-monitoring, with the student tracking sleep patterns, gaming duration, and academic productivity. Over time, this integrated approach led to improved sleep quality, increased academic engagement, and a marked reduction in reliance on gaming as an emotional escape, illustrating how CBT techniques can be effectively applied within real campus contexts.

Emotion Regulation and Coping Skills Training

Emotion regulation and coping skills training play a central role in interventions for EIU, particularly given the strong association between EIU and emotional dysregulation. Many students with EIU rely predominantly on avoidance-based coping, using online engagement to escape feelings of loneliness, stress, or emotional discomfort rather than addressing these experiences directly (Kuss & Lopez-Fernandez, 2016; Tokunaga, 2017; Brand et al., 2022). For example, a postgraduate student residing on a residential campus presented with excessive social media use, which functioned as a primary means of coping with persistent loneliness and social disconnection. Counselling sessions initially focused on enhancing emotional awareness, helping the student identify specific emotional triggers—such as feelings of isolation during evenings or after academic work—that preceded prolonged online use. Building on this insight, the intervention incorporated campus-based stress-management and relaxation strategies, including regular participation in guided yoga sessions offered by the university wellness or counselling centre, which helped regulate physiological arousal and promote mind–body awareness. In parallel, the student was introduced to neurofeedback sessions offered through the campus mental health service, which enable real-time awareness and modulation of attentional and emotional states. These techniques improved the student's tolerance of emotional discomfort and reduced the immediate urge to seek digital distraction.

Simultaneously, the counsellor focused on developing adaptive coping and help-seeking behaviours, encouraging the student to gradually replace avoidance with interpersonal coping. This involved structured exposure to offline social engagement, such as joining interest-based campus groups and participating in low-pressure peer activities. Over time, as the student's emotional literacy, distress tolerance, and real-world social connections strengthened, reliance on social media as the primary coping mechanism decreased, illustrating the effectiveness of integrating emotion-focused interventions with campus-based resources.

Motivational Interviewing

Motivational Interviewing (MI) represents a particularly effective intervention approach for EIU among university students, especially in cases marked by ambivalence toward change. Many students do not initially conceptualise their Internet use as problematic, even when experiencing academic decline, sleep disturbance, or emotional distress, because online engagement continues to serve important functions such as stress relief, emotional comfort, or social connection. MI addresses this ambivalence through a collaborative, client-centred process that emphasises empathy, autonomy, and evocation rather than confrontation or prescriptive advice. By validating the functional role that Internet use currently plays in students' lives, counsellors create a non-judgmental space in which students can reflect on the costs and benefits of their behaviour. This approach allows students to gradually recognise discrepancies between their current digital habits and broader personal goals—such as academic success, physical well-being, career success and meaningful relationships—thereby enhancing intrinsic motivation and readiness for change within the campus context (Spada, 2014; Kuss & Lopez-Fernandez, 2016).

In practice, MI techniques are readily applicable within university wellness or counselling settings. For example, a postgraduate student presenting with persistent fatigue and reduced academic focus reported late-night Internet use as a primary means of unwinding after stressful academic days. Through open-ended questioning and reflective listening, the counsellor explored both the perceived benefits of online engagement and the student's growing concern about its consequences, highlighting the student's ambivalence without judgment. As the discussion progressed, the counsellor facilitated the development of discrepancy by inviting the student to consider how current Internet use aligned with long-term academic and health goals. Affirmations were used to reinforce the student's emerging insight and prior strengths in self-management, while self-efficacy was supported through collaborative goal setting rather than directive instruction. The student chose to experiment with a modest, self-directed change—reducing screen use by thirty minutes before bedtime on weekdays—which led to noticeable improvements in sleep and concentration. This experiential success naturally increased change talk and readiness for further intervention, illustrating how MI functions as a gateway that enhances engagement with subsequent therapeutic approaches, such as cognitive–behavioural strategies, emotion regulation training, and lifestyle modification, within campus mental health systems.

Academic-Integrated Interventions

Study skills and self-regulation programs constitute a critical intervention pathway for addressing EIU, given its strong association with procrastination, disorganised study routines, and poor academic self-regulation. In university settings, excessive late-night Internet use often disrupts students' ability to plan, prioritise, and sustain focused academic effort. For instance, an undergraduate student who repeatedly missed assignment deadlines reported prolonged late-night browsing, which resulted in daytime fatigue and reduced concentration. A coordinated intervention involving the academic advisor, faculty mentor, and campus counselling services was initiated to address both behavioural and academic difficulties. The student was supported in developing a structured weekly study schedule that clearly delineated academic work periods, planned Internet breaks, and device-free study sessions in the library. Time-management and prioritisation strategies were introduced to help the student break assignments into manageable tasks, while explicit guidance was provided on reducing digital multitasking during lectures and independent study.

Faculty advisors played a key role by monitoring academic progress, reinforcing realistic academic goals, and providing regular feedback, thereby strengthening the student's academic self-efficacy and sense of accountability. In addition, the student was encouraged to enrol in a credit-based life skills or soft skills course offered by the university, which addressed topics such as self-regulation, digital well-being, stress management, and responsible technology use. Embedding these skills within the formal curriculum not only normalised discussions around EIU but also equipped students with transferable competencies for academic and personal functioning. Over time, the combined support from faculty advisors and structured skills training, improved the student's study habits, reduced unregulated Internet use, and enhanced overall academic engagement, highlighting the value of integrated, institutionally supported self-regulation programs in preventing the academic consequences of EIU.

Social and Interpersonal Interventions

Reducing loneliness and enhancing a sense of campus belonging is a critical preventive strategy for EIU, as social disconnection is among the strongest predictors of excessive online engagement. This need is particularly acute during transitional periods such as the first year of admission, when students are adjusting to new academic demands, residential living, and unfamiliar social environments. For example, a student from a different linguistic region experienced significant difficulty adjusting to hostel life and informal peer interactions, leading to increased reliance on online content in their native language as a means of comfort and familiarity. To address this, the university implemented a multi-layered integration approach that included peer-mentorship support, pairing students with senior peers who shared similar transitional experiences and could offer guidance on navigating campus life. The student was also encouraged to participate in structured orientation and transition programs, which provided safe, facilitated spaces to build connections during the early months of campus residence.

In parallel, involvement in student clubs, interest-based groups, and culturally inclusive community activities helped the student reconnect with offline social networks and develop a sense of belonging within the campus culture. Collaborative learning environments within classrooms further supported social integration by fostering peer interaction around shared academic goals. Over time, as the student's sense of inclusion and social confidence strengthened, reliance on online coping decreased, illustrating how institutionally supported belonging initiatives can effectively reduce EIU driven by loneliness.

Preventive Psychoeducation and Digital Well-Being Programs

Preventive psychoeducation and digital well-being programs represent a crucial first line of defence against EIU, as systematic reviews consistently emphasise the value of early, preventive interventions over reactive treatment alone. Such programs aim to normalise open discussions about digital habits, mental health, and self-regulation, helping students recognise early warning signs before significant impairment develops (Kuss & Lopez-Fernandez, 2016; Brand et al., 2022).

Within university settings, psychoeducation focuses on enhancing students' understanding of the continuum between healthy and problematic Internet use, clarifying the psychological, academic, and psychosocial consequences of excessive online engagement. By promoting intentional and goal-directed technology use, these initiatives encourage students to reflect on how digital behaviours align with academic responsibilities, sleep routines, and overall well-being (Kuss & Lopez-Fernandez, 2016; Jin & Jiang, 2025).

Equally important is the emphasis on reducing stigma around help-seeking, reinforcing the message that seeking support for digital-related difficulties is a proactive and adaptive step rather than a sign of failure. In practice, many universities have successfully implemented these principles by integrating digital well-being modules into first-year foundation or orientation courses, where topics such as time management, stress regulation, sleep hygiene, and responsible technology use are embedded within an academic success framework. This curricular integration ensures broad reach, reinforces healthy norms early in the student lifecycle, and equips students with practical skills to maintain balanced digital engagement throughout their university years.

Institutional and Policy-Level Strategies

Universities play a crucial role in shaping students' digital environments, and the effective prevention of EIU requires institutional commitment, rather than relying solely on individual responsibility. A coordinated, system-level approach is essential, integrating mental health services with academic support structures so that students experiencing digital-related difficulties are identified and supported early (Jin & Jiang, 2025).

Central to this approach is the training of faculty members, academic advisors, and hostel or residential staff to recognise early warning signs such as sudden academic decline, frequent absenteeism, sleep-related concerns, or marked changes in behaviour and engagement. Establishing clear, accessible referral pathways between academic departments, faculty advisors, and counselling or wellness centres ensures that concerns are addressed promptly and consistently, without placing the burden solely on students to seek help.

At the cultural level, universities can actively promote balanced digital norms, encouraging healthy technology use through institutional messaging, campus policies, and role modelling by staff and faculty. For example, a university wellness centre may collaborate with academic departments to monitor indicators such as repeated deadline extensions or unexplained drops in academic performance, using these signals to initiate early, supportive outreach rather than punitive action. Such proactive, compassionate institutional responses not only reduce stigma but also foster a campus climate in which digital well-being is recognised as a shared responsibility and an integral component of student success.

Tiered Intervention Model for Campuses

A tiered intervention framework is recommended to address EIU in university settings, ensuring that support is matched to the severity and complexity of students' difficulties. At the level of primary prevention, universities focus on promoting digital literacy, healthy technology use, and resilience through orientation programs, first-year experience courses, and campus engagement activities that foster a sense of belonging and balanced routines. Secondary prevention targets students who begin to show early signs of distress or functional impairment, incorporating systematic screening for psychological distress, brief counselling interventions such as motivational interviewing, and targeted academic support to prevent escalation. For students with more severe or persistent impairment, tertiary intervention involves structured psychotherapeutic approaches—such as cognitive–behavioural therapy, emotion regulation training, or integrated behavioural interventions—along with psychiatric referral when clinically indicated and ongoing follow-up to support sustained recovery. This stepped-care model allows universities to intervene early, allocate resources efficiently, and provide individualised support, thereby reducing the risk of chronic impairment and promoting long-term academic and psychosocial well-being.

Faculty Engagement

Faculty members play a pivotal role in shaping students' digital behaviours through both explicit policies and implicit modelling. Classroom practices that encourage intentional, rather than reactive, technology use can significantly buffer the negative academic effects of excessive Internet engagement. When teachers articulate clear expectations—for instance, specifying when laptops or mobile devices are appropriate for learning and when device-free engagement is encouraged—students are better able to regulate their attention without feeling policed or infantilised.

Relational teaching styles further strengthen this impact. Faculty who engage students through discussion, collaborative problem-solving, and real-time feedback reduce reliance on passive, screen-mediated learning. For example, a lecturer who pauses during a session to invite reflection or peer discussion creates natural breaks from digital distraction, reinforcing the value of presence and interaction. Faculty can also model healthy digital boundaries by avoiding excessive late-night communication, normalising realistic response times, and acknowledging the cognitive costs of constant connectivity. Through such everyday practices, teachers contribute to a campus culture where technology is used deliberately as a learning tool rather than an automatic default.

Environmental Design

Beyond curriculum and teaching practices, the physical and social design of campus environments plays a powerful preventive role in shaping digital behaviour. Reimagining campus spaces to support offline engagement allows students to regulate Internet use without coercion or surveillance. Quiet study zones, device-free reading rooms, nature-integrated spaces, and communal lounges designed for conversation and collaboration all provide alternatives to screen-dominated routines.

For instance, a library that designates certain floors as device-free reading areas subtly encourages deep focus, while outdoor seating or green spaces invite informal social interaction away from screens. Hostel common rooms, designed around shared activities—such as board games, music, or group discussions—offer students opportunities for connection that naturally compete with solitary online engagement. These environmental cues communicate institutional values, signalling that student well-being, attention, and connection are priorities embedded in campus life, not merely addressed through counselling services.

Ethical Challenges in Campus Mental Health Practice

Ethical challenges frequently arise in campus mental health practice when counsellors are asked to navigate the complex intersection of student distress, institutional requirements, and diagnostic responsibility. One common dilemma involves requests for medical or psychological certification to support academic accommodations such as re-examinations, deadline extensions, or reduced course loads.

EIU often occupies a diagnostic grey zone: students may experience significant functional impairment in sleep, academic performance, or emotional regulation without clearly meeting formal diagnostic criteria for a mental disorder. For example, a student may seek certification attributing missed examinations to "Internet addiction," while clinical assessment reveals maladaptive coping and disrupted routines rather than a diagnosable psychiatric condition. In such cases, ethical practice requires counsellors to resist pressure to medicalise behaviour for administrative convenience, while still validating the student's distress and functional difficulties. This involves transparent communication with the student, appropriate referral when diagnostic clarification is needed, and careful documentation that focuses on observed impairments in functioning—such as sleep disruption, academic disengagement, or stress-related difficulties—rather than inferred or exaggerated diagnoses.

Equally important is the ethical responsibility to avoid moral panic and stigmatisation in responding to EIU. Labelling students prematurely as "addicted" can unintentionally reinforce feelings of helplessness, shame, and reduced self-efficacy, particularly in developmental contexts where identity and autonomy are still evolving. Ethical frameworks, therefore, emphasise capacity-building, developmental sensitivity, and shared responsibility, framing EIU as a maladaptive but reversible coping pattern shaped by academic pressure, social transition, and institutional digital environments. By focusing on skill development, support systems, and environmental modification—rather than blame or pathologisation—campus mental health professionals uphold ethical practice while fostering empowerment and recovery.

8. CHALLENGES

Despite increasing recognition of the importance of digital well-being initiatives on university campuses, implementing effective programs remains complex. Students' reliance on digital technologies is deeply embedded in both academic and personal domains, as demonstrated by studies in which attempts at short-term digital disconnection resulted in low adherence and withdrawal-like discomfort. These challenges are intensified by structural features of modern higher education, including mandatory online submissions, digital research practices, continuous academic communication, and social expectations of constant availability. Consequently, restrictive or punitive approaches to technology use are neither practical nor sustainable within contemporary university environments.

9. FUTURE RESEARCH DIRECTIONS

Although research on EIU among university students has expanded, several important gaps remain.

First, longitudinal studies are required to clarify causal relationships between psychological distress and EIU. Most existing evidence is cross-sectional, limiting understanding of whether distress precedes excessive use or whether digital over-engagement exacerbates vulnerability. Prospective research across key academic transitions—such as entry into university, examination periods, and career-related stress phases—would provide stronger causal insight.

Second, greater conceptual clarity is needed to distinguish generalised EIU from domain-specific problematic behaviours, including gaming disorder, social media overuse, and smartphone dependence. Future studies should examine whether these represent distinct clinical conditions or variations of shared self-regulation difficulties.

Third, emerging approaches such as digital phenotyping require careful ethical and empirical evaluation. While passive usage data may offer opportunities for objective assessment, issues of privacy, feasibility, and student acceptability must be systematically examined before institutional implementation.

Fourth, intervention-focused research in campus settings remains limited. Randomised controlled trials evaluating stepped-care models, integrated academic–counselling approaches, and campus-wide digital well-being programs are necessary to establish evidence-based prevention frameworks.

Finally, future scholarship should integrate neurocognitive, psychosocial, and broader developmental dimensions into unified explanatory models. A multidisciplinary research agenda will better capture the complexity of students' experiences within increasingly immersive digital ecosystems.

10. CONCLUSION

EIU among university students should not be understood as a moral failing or simply an individual pathology. Rather, it represents a predictable response to developmental vulnerability, academic pressure, social transition, and digitally saturated environments. In this sense, EIU reflects not only individual coping difficulties but also the broader structures within which students learn and live.

Universities, as crucibles of intellectual and personal growth, hold both the responsibility and the opportunity to shape healthier digital cultures. Moving away from control-based models—such as blanket bans or punitive monitoring—toward approaches that emphasise conscious, intentional engagement with technology allows students to develop agency rather than dependence. When campuses integrate digital well-being into curricula, model healthy norms through faculty practices, and design environments that invite presence and connection, students are supported in reclaiming their attention, strengthening relationships, and using technology as a purposeful tool rather than a psychological refuge. Such a shift not only mitigates the risks of EIU but also fosters deeper learning, resilience, and well-being across the university community.

REFERENCES

Anderson, E. L., Steen, E., & Stavropoulos, V. (2017). Internet use and problematic Internet use: A systematic review of longitudinal research trends in adolescence and emergent adulthood. *International Journal of Adolescence and Youth, 22*(4), 430–454. DOI: 10.1080/02673843.2016.1227716

Brand, M., Potenza, M. N., & Stark, R. (2022). Theoretical models of types of problematic usage of the Internet: When theorists meet therapists. *Current Opinion in Behavioral Sciences, 45*, 101119. DOI: 10.1016/j.cobeha.2022.101119

Brand, M., Young, K. S., & Laier, C. (2014). Prefrontal control and Internet addiction: A theoretical model and review of neuropsychological and neuroimaging findings. *Frontiers in Human Neuroscience, 8*, 375. Advance online publication. DOI: 10.3389/fnhum.2014.00375 PMID: 24904393

Carbonell, X., Chamarro, A., Oberst, U., Rodrigo, B., & Prades, M. (2018). Problematic use of the Internet and smartphones in university students: 2006–2017. *International Journal of Environmental Research and Public Health, 15*(3), 475. DOI: 10.3390/ijerph15030475 PMID: 29518050

Dahl, D., & Bergmark, K. H. (2020). Problematic internet use: A scoping review – Longitudinal research on a contemporary social problem, 2006–2017. *Nordisk Alkohol- & Narkotikatidskrift : NAT, 37*(6), 497–525. DOI: 10.1177/1455072520941997 PMID: 35308651

Ding, H., Cao, B., & Sun, Q. (2023). The association between problematic internet use and social anxiety within adolescents and young adults: A systematic review and meta-analysis. *Frontiers in Public Health, 11*, 1275723. DOI: 10.3389/fpubh.2023.1275723 PMID: 37841708

Jin, Y., & Jiang, S. (2025). Theoretical perspectives on adolescent internet addiction: A comprehensive literature review. *Health & Social Care in the Community, 2025*(1), 4875332. Advance online publication. DOI: 10.1155/hsc/4875332

Kardefelt-Winther, D. (2014). A conceptual and methodological critique of internet addiction research: Towards a model of compensatory internet use. *Computers in Human Behavior, 31*, 351–354. DOI: 10.1016/j.chb.2013.10.059

Kuss, D. J., & Lopez-Fernandez, O. (2016). Internet addiction and problematic Internet use: A systematic review of clinical research. *World Journal of Psychiatry, 6*(1), 143–176. DOI: 10.5498/wjp.v6.i1.143 PMID: 27014605

Montag, C., & Walla, P. (2016). Carpe diem instead of losing your social mind: Beyond digital addiction and why we all suffer from digital overuse. *Cogent Psychology*, *3*(1), 1157281. DOI: 10.1080/23311908.2016.1157281

Spada, M. M. (2014). An overview of problematic Internet use. *Addictive Behaviors*, *39*(1), 3–6. DOI: 10.1016/j.addbeh.2013.09.007 PMID: 24126206

Tokunaga, R. S. (2017). A meta-analysis of the relationships between psychosocial problems and internet habits: Synthesizing internet addiction, problematic internet use, and deficient self-regulation research. *Communication Monographs*, *84*(4), 423–446. DOI: 10.1080/03637751.2017.1332419

Tunney, C., & Rooney, B. (2023). Using theoretical models of problematic internet use to inform psychological formulation: A systematic scoping review. *Clinical Child Psychology and Psychiatry*, *28*(2), 810–830. DOI: 10.1177/13591045221104569 PMID: 36916053

ADDITIONAL READING

Carli, V., Durkee, T., Wasserman, D., Hadlaczky, G., Despalins, R., Kramarz, E., Wasserman, C., Sarchiapone, M., Hoven, C. W., Brunner, R., & Kaess, M. (2013). The association between pathological internet use and comorbid psychopathology: A systematic review. *Psychopathology*, *46*(1), 1–13. DOI: 10.1159/000337971 PMID: 22854219

Cimino, S., & Cerniglia, L. (2018). A longitudinal study for the empirical validation of an etiopathogenetic model of internet addiction in adolescence based on early emotion regulation. *BioMed Research International*, *4038541*, 1–8. Advance online publication. DOI: 10.1155/2018/4038541 PMID: 29707569

Dong, G., & Potenza, M. N. (2014). A cognitive-behavioral model of Internet gaming disorder: Theoretical underpinnings and clinical implications. *Journal of Psychiatric Research*, *58*, 7–11. DOI: 10.1016/j.jpsychires.2014.07.005 PMID: 25062755

Ho, R. C., Zhang, M. W. B., Tsang, T. Y., Toh, A. H., Pan, F., Lu, Y., Cheng, C., Yip, P. S., Lam, L. T., Lai, C.-M., Watanabe, H., & Mak, K.-K. (2014). The association between internet addiction and psychiatric co-morbidity: A meta-analysis. *BMC Psychiatry*, *14*(1), 183. DOI: 10.1186/1471-244X-14-183 PMID: 24947851

Jin, Y., & Jiang, S. (2025). Theoretical perspectives on adolescent internet addiction: A comprehensive literature review. *Health & Social Care in the Community*, *2025*(1), 4875332. Advance online publication. DOI: 10.1155/hsc/4875332

Laconi, S., Rodgers, R. F., & Chabrol, H. (2014). The measurement of Internet addiction: A critical review of existing scales and their psychometric properties. *Computers in Human Behavior, 41*, 190–202. DOI: 10.1016/j.chb.2014.09.026

Przybylski, A. K., Weinstein, N., & Murayama, K. (2017). Internet gaming disorder: Investigating the clinical relevance of a new phenomenon. *The American Journal of Psychiatry, 174*(3), 230–236. DOI: 10.1176/appi.ajp.2016.16020224 PMID: 27809571

Weinstein, A., Feder, L. C., Rosenberg, K. P., & Dannon, P. (2014). Internet addiction disorder: Overview and controversies. In Rosenberg, K. P., & Feder, L. C. (Eds.), *Behavioral addictions* (pp. 99–117). Academic Press. DOI: 10.1016/B978-0-12-407724-9.00005-7

KEY TERMS AND DEFINITIONS

Academic-Integrated Intervention: Collaborative support involving counsellors, faculty, and academic advisors to address excessive internet use through the academic curriculum.

Behavioural Addiction: A non-substance-related addictive pattern involving frequent engagement in rewarding behaviours despite harmful consequences in personal and professional life.

Campus Belongingness: A student's sense of inclusion and social connection within the university community acts as a protective factor against excessive internet use.

Digital Escape Mechanism: The use of an online ecosystem to temporarily avoid real-life stressors, emotional discomfort, or interpersonal pressures.

Digital Literacy: The knowledge and skills required to use technology responsibly, critically and intentionally.

Digital Phenotyping: The use of passive digital data to objectively assess behavioural patterns related to mental health and technology use.

Digital Well-Being: Balanced, intentional, and healthy engagement with technology that supports psychological well-being, productivity, and meaningful life participation.

Excessive Internet Use (EIU): A pattern of excessive or poorly controlled Internet-related behaviours that result in significant psychological distress, functional impairment, or disruption in academic, social, or personal life.

Chapter 4
Literature-Based Peer Support to Enhance Self-Acceptance Among University Students:
Addressing Digital Pathology in Semarang

Ika Rizki Refima Putri
http://orcid.org/0009-0005-7228-7578
Universitas Negeri Semarang, Indonesia

ABSTRACT

University students are highly vulnerable to psychological problems, often rooted in low self-acceptance during the quarter-life crisis, a condition closely linked to depression and suicidal ideation. This study is a Formative Context Evaluation with two objectives: (1) assessing the urgency of the problem and (2) designing a structured intervention model. A descriptive survey of 25 students from five universities in Semarang revealed concerning findings: 96% reported insecurity, 88% experienced a quarter-life crisis, and 56% reported suicidal ideation related to difficulties in self-acceptance. These results confirm the urgent need for low-stigma mental health interventions. In response, this study proposes Self-Talks, an interactive literature-based peer support model that employs identification, catharsis, and expressive writing to enhance self-acceptance and strengthen social support. Positioned as a non-digital intervention, Self-Talks aims to mitigate the psychological effects of digital pathology through narrative engagement and structured internal dialogue.

DOI: 10.4018/979-8-2600-2468-3.ch004

INTRODUCTION

The contemporary world is currently situated within a golden era of digitalization, in which information technology no longer functions merely as a supporting instrument but has evolved into a primary environment where identity is constructed, negotiated, and validated. Digital platforms now play a central role in shaping self-perception, social comparison, and individual aspirations. However, alongside these advancements, digital transformation has produced significant pathological consequences that pose serious risks to mental health.

Patterns of addictive device use have been empirically shown to increase the risk of anxiety disorders and suicidal ideation by up to twofold among early adult populations. University students, whose identities are heavily mediated by digital platforms, are particularly vulnerable to the erosion of self-acceptance due to continuous exposure to unrealistic and idealized standards of success, productivity, physical appearance, and life trajectories (Xiao et al., 2025). In digital spaces, success is often portrayed as linear, accelerated, and flawless, leaving little room for failure, delay, or personal struggle.

A needs assessment conducted in the city of Semarang indicates that academic pressure combined with uncertainty about future careers and life directions manifests as an acute identity crisis among university students. This phenomenon aligns with what is commonly referred to as the quarter-life crisis, a developmental phase characterized by emotional instability, self-doubt, fear of failure, and confusion regarding personal and professional identity. Although awareness of mental health issues among university students has increased in recent years, a substantial gap persists in the availability of interventions that are both humanistic in orientation and low in social stigma.

Existing mental health services within academic institutions often remain underutilized due to cultural stigma, fear of judgment, and concerns regarding confidentiality. Consequently, many students experiencing psychological distress choose to internalize their struggles rather than seek formal help. This gap underscores the urgent need for alternative intervention models that are accessible, culturally sensitive, and capable of addressing emotional distress without reinforcing stigmatization.

This chapter aims to empirically validate the urgency of mental health challenges faced by university students in Semarang through data-driven analysis and to propose an innovative intervention model entitled "Self-Talks." By harnessing the therapeutic potential of literature and structured internal dialogue, the Self-Talks model is designed to mediate the process of narrative repair, defined as an intentional effort to reclaim authorship over personal life narratives that have become fragmented due to persistent digital comparison and performance pressure (Gualano et al., 2017; Zhai et al., 2025). Through this approach, students are encouraged to reinterpret their experiences, reconstruct self-meaning, and cultivate a healthier sense of self-acceptance within an increasingly digitized social environment.

THEORETICAL BACKGROUND

Media Ecology and Digital Identity Distortion

From the perspective of media ecology, media are not merely channels of information but environments that fundamentally shape human perception, cognition, and behavior. In the contemporary digital landscape, social media platforms function as immersive ecosystems that continuously stimulate social comparison processes. For university students who are situated in the developmental phase of emerging adulthood or the quarter-life crisis, this environment significantly disrupts identity formation.

Digital platforms routinely present filtered, curated, and excessively positive representations of life, success, and personal achievement. As a result, students are exposed to distorted benchmarks that redefine success as immediate, flawless, and hyper-visible. Empirical studies demonstrate that adolescents and young adults who exhibit addictive patterns of digital device use face a twofold increase in the risk of suicidal ideation, suicide attempts, and symptoms of anxiety and depression. University students, whose daily academic and social experiences are deeply intertwined with digital platforms, represent a particularly vulnerable population within this context.

Students experiencing quarter-life crisis frequently turn to digital media as a coping mechanism to escape academic pressure, social anxiety, or uncertainty about the future. However, this form of avoidance paradoxically generates a negative feedback loop. Rather than alleviating distress, compulsive digital engagement intensifies feelings of inadequacy and self-comparison. Over time, these dynamic shifts the primary risk factors for suicidality away from academic difficulties and toward addictive digital behavior as a maladaptive coping strategy. This maladaptive reliance not only exacerbates psychological distress but also stabilizes a chronic crisis of self-acceptance.

Consequently, the core contributor to suicidal risk is no longer limited to external stressors such as grades or workload, but increasingly rooted in internalized narratives of failure reinforced by digital comparison. Breaking this cycle of addiction through explicitly non-digital interventions therefore emerges as a primary clinical and preventive priority (Zhu et al., 2024).

Quarter-Life Crisis, Fear of Missing Out, and Self-Acceptance

Quarter-life crisis is commonly characterized by pervasive fear of career failure, social inadequacy, and existential uncertainty. In the digital era, this developmental crisis is significantly intensified by continuous exposure to social media. One of the central psychological mechanisms underlying this intensification is Fear of Missing Out (FoMO), a pervasive anxiety that others are experiencing rewarding events from which one is absent. FoMO has been shown to strongly predict compulsive social media engagement, particularly among university students (Weill Cornell Medicine, 2025).

At the conceptual core of quarter-life crisis among students lies low self-acceptance. Self-acceptance refers to an individual's capacity to acknowledge and embrace both strengths and limitations while maintaining a stable sense of self-worth. Digital platforms such as Instagram, TikTok, and LinkedIn amplify upward social comparison, wherein individuals compare themselves to others perceived as more successful, attractive, or accomplished. This form of comparison has been empirically linked to significant declines in self-esteem and body esteem (Gerber, 2018; Mabonga, 2024).

When self-acceptance deteriorates, students become increasingly vulnerable to maladaptive cognitive patterns, including perfectionism, self-criticism, and hopelessness. Research consistently identifies failure in self-acceptance as a pathological pathway toward suicidality, positioning self-acceptance as a central target for mental health intervention.

Pathology of Social Comparison Among University Students

In-depth empirical assessment conducted among university students in the city of Semarang reveals that, despite increasing awareness of mental health issues, the capacity for self-acceptance remains critically low. This deficiency extends beyond superficial dissatisfaction and constitutes a foundational driver of severe depression and suicidal ideation.

Within this context, the integration of self-talk mechanisms or internal dialogue, with literature therapy (bibliotherapy) offers a novel therapeutic paradigm. Rather than focusing solely on symptom reduction, this integrated approach aims to restore narrative identity, enabling students to reinterpret personal experiences through meaning-making processes facilitated by literary engagement.

The pathological impact of digital social comparison manifests not only at the emotional level but also at the cognitive level, where students internalize rigid success narratives that delegitimize personal struggle and non-linear life trajectories. Bibliotherapy, when combined with structured self-talk, provides an alternative symbolic framework that challenges these dominant digital narratives and replaces them with more adaptive, humanistic interpretations of selfhood.

This paradigm shift reframes mental health intervention as a restorative process, emphasizing identity reconstruction rather than mere psychological stabilization. Through narrative engagement, students are guided to reclaim interpretive authority over their experiences, thereby fostering resilience and sustainable self-acceptance.

MAIN FOCUS OF THE CHAPTER

Issues, Controversies, and Problems

Mental health issues have become a central and increasingly visible topic of discussion, particularly among university students. This population is consistently identified in the literature as being more psychologically vulnerable than the general population. The combination of academic demands, daily life pressures, inadequate time management, and difficulties in meeting academic obligations frequently results in significant psychological stress.

Mental disorders that remain unaddressed during this critical developmental period are closely associated with declining academic achievement and impaired psychosocial functioning. In the Indonesian context, these challenges are further exacerbated by limited social support systems and, in some cases, dysfunctional family environments. This situation is reinforced by findings from The Indonesia National Adolescent Mental Health Survey (I-NAMHS) conducted in collaboration with Universitas Gadjah Mada, which reported that 2.45 million adolescents in Indonesia experienced mental health disorders in 2022.

These psychological conditions often function as precursors to the emergence of quarter-life crisis, a developmental phenomenon characterized by fear, confusion, and uncertainty regarding future life trajectories, career prospects, and social relationships. Quarter-life crisis is most commonly experienced between the ages of 18 and 30 and is driven by both internal and external factors. Internally, students experience anxiety, self-doubt, and a lack of commitment to long-term life goals, particularly in relation to post-graduation careers. Externally, sociocultural pressures intensify these internal conflicts.

Within Asian cultural contexts, quarter-life crisis assumes an amplified dimension due to strong sociocultural expectations surrounding success, family honor, and conformity. Empirical studies indicate that perfectionism discrepancy, defined as the gap between personal expectations and lived reality, serves as a significant predictor of psychological distress and suicidality among university students. This discrepancy is further magnified by digital environments that normalize exceptional achievement while obscuring struggle and failure.

To adequately understand quarter-life crisis in the contemporary era, it is necessary to shift analytical focus away from total screen time toward addictive and compulsive patterns of digital behavior. Emerging research consistently demonstrates that negative mental health outcomes are not primarily associated with the quantity of time spent on digital devices, but rather with compulsive usage patterns characterized by loss of control, emotional dependence, and avoidance coping.

This paradigm shift offers a critical explanation for the heightened risk of suicidality among university students. Compulsive digital engagement functions as a maladaptive coping mechanism that temporarily alleviates distress while simultaneously reinforcing feelings of inadequacy and failure. Mortier et al. (2018) emphasize that such behavioral patterns significantly elevate vulnerability to suicidal thoughts and behaviors among first-year university students.

At the core of both quarter-life crisis and broader mental health disturbances lies low self-acceptance. Self-acceptance is defined as an individual's capacity to maintain satisfaction with personal qualities, acknowledge limitations, and engage in continuous self-development. When self-acceptance is compromised, individuals tend to experience persistent dissatisfaction with themselves, which can precipitate depressive symptoms and, in severe cases, suicidal ideation.

This relationship is strongly supported by empirical evidence. Studies consistently demonstrate that low self-esteem is negatively correlated with suicidal ideation, while regression analyses confirm that self-acceptance exerts a significant protective effect against suicidal thoughts (Rector et al., 1996; Wilcox et al., 2004). Consequently, self-acceptance emerges as a central psychological construct and a critical target for intervention.

Low self-acceptance is directly connected to Fear of Missing Out (FoMO), a global psychological phenomenon that exerts a powerful influence on university students. FoMO operates as a psychological antecedent shaping social comparison dynamic in digital environments (Błachnio et al., 2024). In an effort to alleviate FoMO, individuals are compelled to engage compulsively with social media platforms, leading to problematic social media use and increased risk of digital addiction (Servidio et al., 2024; Li et al., 2025).

Within digital contexts, social comparison is predominantly characterized by upward social comparison, in which individuals compare themselves to others perceived as more successful, attractive, or accomplished. Platforms such as Instagram and TikTok, which prioritize highly curated and idealized content, actively promote upward comparison processes. Extensive empirical evidence demonstrates that such exposure significantly undermines self-esteem and psychological well-being (Sabet et al., 2019; Hulme, 2018; Wang et al., 2024).

The interrelationship between quarter-life crisis and digital pathology is clearly reflected in empirical findings derived from a descriptive needs analysis involving 25 university students in the city of Semarang, drawn from both public and private higher education institutions, including Universitas Negeri Semarang, Universitas Islam Negeri Walisongo, Universitas Dian Nuswantoro, Universitas Diponegoro, and Universitas PGRI Semarang. This study employed a Program Development Research Design, with a sample size of N = 25. The methodological justification for this sample size rests on the study's positioning as a Formative Context Evaluation rather than a statistical generalization study. The sample size was deemed sufficient based on the achievement of insight saturation, prioritizing depth of understanding over numerical representativeness for the purpose of intervention design.

Table 1.

Psychological Indicator	Percentage	Clinical Implications
Feeling of insecurity	96%	Chronic barriers to self-acceptance
Suicidal ideation	56%	Direct correlation with failure of self-acceptance
Currently experiencing quarter life crisis	88%	Urgent need for life direction and meaning
Need for media or tools to facilitate self-acceptance and coping	60%	Demand for structured psychological support

Analysis of these data indicates that strong academic performance does not guarantee psychological stability. On the contrary, academic demands often constitute an additional stressor, exacerbating time management difficulties and emotional exhaustion, which in turn worsen mental health outcomes. In sociocultural contexts such as Indonesia, where strong emphasis is placed on family honor, achievement, and social conformity, students frequently experience intense pressure to meet rigid standards of success. When lived realities fail to align with these expectations, students may enter a destructive cycle of self-rejection and internalized failure.

The data above shows that 88% of student respondents are in the quarter-life crisis phase. Notably, although the majority of respondents reported caring about themselves, 96% acknowledged experiencing insecurity related to academic achievement, physical appearance, or career progression. Most critically, 56% of respondents reported having experienced suicidal ideation due to difficulties in accepting themselves. These findings underscore the urgent need for innovative and structured psychological support mechanisms aimed at fostering self-acceptance among university students.

The 96% prevalence of insecurity is consistently associated with the psychological consequences of continuous digital social comparison. Self-acceptance becomes increasingly unattainable when persistent upward social comparison systematically positions individual limitations as definitive failures. Consequently, the quarter-life crisis, rooted in chronic self-dissatisfaction, transforms into a sustained psychological condition under constant digital pressure, thereby exacerbating feelings of inferiority and contributing to digital burnout.

Qualitative data further reveal that one of the primary triggers of insecurity among students is exposure to peers' achievements on digital platforms such as LinkedIn and Instagram. Several respondents reported feeling left behind in terms of career progression despite being in early semesters, illustrating a distortion of temporal perception driven by digital comparison. These findings demonstrate that effective interventions must penetrate emotional and narrative layers of experience rather than merely offering cognitive or informational guidance. Students require spaces that allow for emotional processing, meaning-making, and identity reconstruction.

Given the high prevalence of digital pathology, there is a critical need for explicitly non-digital mental health interventions that align with the Good Health and Well-being objective of the Sustainable Development Goals (SDGs). In response to this urgency, structured and contextually appropriate psychological support strategies are required. The Self-Talks program which is conceptualized as an interactive discussion space utilizing literature therapy is positioned as a digital detox intervention designed to counteract internet addiction and digital burnout. Literature therapy (bibliotherapy), functioning as *dulce et utile*, both entertaining and educational, offers an alternative medium for structured emotional and cognitive processing.

The primary objective of this reformulation is to analyze how literature therapy functions as a narrative repair mechanism, enabling the reconstruction of identities distorted by digital pressure. Through this process, students are supported in enhancing self-acceptance and mitigating associated mental health risks.

Based on an in-depth needs analysis and the methodological relevance of literature therapy, this study focuses on two primary objectives: (1) to empirically identify the urgency of mental health issues and low levels of self-acceptance among university students in Semarang City, and (2) to design an innovative interactive support group model grounded in literary therapy as a digital detox intervention targeted at the student population.

SOLUTIONS AND RECOMMENDATIONS

The Theoretical Foundations of Literature Therapy and Internal Dialectical Mechanisms

Literature therapy, globally recognized as bibliotherapy, is defined as the guided and intentional use of reading materials to assist individuals in resolving psychological difficulties or adapting to developmental transitions. Etymologically, the term combines *biblion* (book) and *therapeia* (healing), reflecting a long-standing historical tradition in which literary engagement has been employed to soothe emotional distress and restore psychological balance (Akbar et al., 2025). Literature, by providing coherent narrative structures, enables individuals to process adverse or traumatic experiences and integrate them into an evolving and meaningful self-narrative (Luo et al., 2025).

Empirical evidence suggests that literary texts possess the capacity to shape character development and psychological resilience. Through engagement with literary narratives, individuals are able to analogize their personal experiences with the struggles, conflicts, and transformations of fictional characters. This process facilitates catharsis, emotional release, and ultimately self-acceptance. The therapeutic framework of bibliotherapy is grounded in three core stages of bibliotherapy: (1) Identification, during the identification stage, participants establish emotional and cognitive connections between themselves and literary characters or themes, (2) Catharsis, allows for the release of suppressed emotions and the processing of internal conflicts. Third, the insight stage enables participants to achieve self-recognition, a deeper understanding of personal motivations, emotional responses, and behavioral patterns, and (3) Insight, defined as the attainment of self-recognition, namely a deeper understanding of one's own motives and emotions which is essential for facilitating self-acceptance.

Self-talk refers to the internal dialogue that occurs consciously or unconsciously within an individual's mind. According to dialogical self theory, the self is composed of multiple internal voices representing different identity positions. Within therapeutic contexts, self-talk functions not merely as internal speech, but as a cognitive strategy through which individuals interpret emotions, regulate beliefs, and provide guidance or reinforcement to themselves.

When maladaptive, self-talk may reinforce negative self-evaluations, perfectionism, and hopelessness. Conversely, structured and positive self-talk serves as a powerful mechanism for emotional regulation, cognitive restructuring, and resilience building. In therapeutic settings, self-talk enables individuals to challenge irrational beliefs, replace self-critical narratives with adaptive interpretations, and foster psychological flexibility.

The integration of self-talk into literature therapy gives rise to an interactive discussion space referred to as "Self-Talks". Within this model, literary texts function as external stimuli that activate internal dialectical processes. When university students engage with literary narratives depicting personal struggle, identity conflict, or resilience, their internal dialogues are naturally triggered, prompting reflection and meaning-making.

The Self-Talks model positions literature as a mirror through which participants recognize their own experiences. Internal dialogue then operates to map similarities between textual narratives and personal life stories. This integration transforms passive reading into an active therapeutic process characterized by reflection, emotional processing, and narrative reconstruction.

Conceptualization of the "Self-Talks" Intervention Model

Based on the urgency identified through empirical needs analysis, this study proposes an innovative interactive peer-support intervention grounded in literature therapy, branded as "Self-Talks". The program is explicitly designed as a non-digital intervention that functions as a digital detox strategy to restore mental well-being among university students. In its implementation, the Self-Talks program adapts literary elements as methodological tools. The intervention consists of two primary components: Literary Dialogue and Creative Writing (Literary Creation).

Literary Dialogue

The Literary Dialogue component is designed to cultivate self-acceptance through the mechanisms of identification and catharsis. Activities within this component include the reading of poetry, viewing video recitations of poems, reading short stories, and watching dramatic performances that explicitly address themes of self-acceptance, identity struggle, and personal growth. Discussions are guided by facilitators using reflective prompts that encourage participants to analyze internal conflicts experienced by literary characters and connect these conflicts to their own lived experiences. This guided dialogue fosters collective catharsis and normalizes emotional vulnerability within a supportive group environment.

Through repeated engagement in Literary Dialogue sessions, students are expected to develop a deeper conceptual and emotional understanding of self-acceptance. This understanding then serves as the foundation for subsequent expressive activities.

Creative Writing (Literary Creation)

Following the insights gained through Literary Dialogue, participants are guided to produce their own literary works as a form of self-expression and narrative re-authoring. This creative process allows students to confront personal limitations, reconcile with perceived shortcomings, and articulate aspirations for future self-development (Ackerman, 2017).

Creative writing within the Self-Talks model aligns with the principles of expressive writing, which has been empirically shown to enhance self-awareness, reduce rumination, and facilitate cognitive reorganization (Baikie, et. al., 2005; Przybylski, et. al., 2013). According to Pennebaker's theory (1986), writing about emotionally charged experiences enables individuals to restructure internal narratives and reduce maladaptive emotional processing. By engaging in expressive literary creation, students reclaim narrative authorship, regaining control over life stories that have been fragmented by persistent digital comparison and external validation pressures (Elhai et al., 2020).

Psychological Stages of Change in Literature Therapy

The effectiveness of bibliotherapy in enhancing self-acceptance is grounded in a systematic three-stage process. These stages function as a cognitive bridge that enables university students to transition from self-rejection toward the development of a healthy and integrated sense of identity.

Stage 1: Identification and Projection

The first psychological stage in literature therapy is identification, a process through which participants recognize aspects of themselves within literary narratives. Identification occurs when readers perceive emotional, cognitive, or experiential parallels between their own lives and the characters, conflicts, or themes presented in literary texts. This stage is particularly crucial for university students experiencing quarter-life crisis, as it provides a safe symbolic space for self-recognition without direct self-disclosure.

During identification, literary texts function as projective mirrors that allow students to externalize internal struggles such as insecurity, fear of failure, identity confusion, and self-doubt. By observing these struggles embodied in fictional characters, participants are able to acknowledge their own emotional states indirectly, reducing psychological defensiveness and stigma.

From a psychological perspective, identification facilitates empathic engagement and emotional resonance. Students begin to realize that their experiences are neither isolated nor abnormal, which contributes to the normalization of distress. This recognition marks the initial disruption of self-blame narratives and initiates the process of self-acceptance.

Stage 2: Emotional Catharsis

The second stage, catharsis, involves the release of suppressed emotions that emerge during engagement with literary narratives. As students encounter stories that resonate with their personal struggles, emotions such as sadness, anger, grief, or disappointment are activated and expressed within a controlled and supportive environment.

Catharsis serves a critical psychological function by alleviating emotional tension and enabling emotional clarity. In the context of the Self-Talks intervention, catharsis is facilitated through guided discussion, reflective questioning, and collective dialogue. These activities encourage participants to articulate feelings that may have previously been internalized or silenced.

Empirical literature consistently demonstrates that emotional suppression is associated with heightened psychological distress and increased vulnerability to depressive symptoms. By contrast, emotional expression through narrative engagement promotes psychological relief and enhances emotional regulation. In group-based settings, shared cathartic experiences further strengthen interpersonal connectedness and reduce feelings of isolation.

Stage 3: Insight and Integration

The final stage of psychological change in literature therapy is integration, wherein insights gained through narrative engagement are internalized and translated into everyday attitudes and behaviors. Integration signifies the consolidation of self-acceptance as a stable psychological orientation rather than a temporary emotional state.

During this stage, students demonstrate increased tolerance for personal limitations, reduced dependence on external validation, and enhanced emotional resilience. Internal self-talk becomes more supportive and constructive, enabling individuals to navigate academic and social challenges with greater psychological flexibility.

Integration is further reinforced through creative writing activities, which allow participants to articulate newly constructed self-narratives. By authoring personal texts such as poems and short narratives students symbolically affirm their capacity for self-definition and agency.

The Strategic Function of Self-Talk as a Catalyst in Literary Therapy

Within the Self-Talks intervention model, internal dialogue strategies are not merely regarded as byproducts of the reading process, but rather as the primary mechanisms driving behavioral change. Self-talk functions as a mediating process that translates literary symbols into operational cognitive instructions.

Message Filtering and Rationalization

Within the Self-Talks framework, self-talk functions as a cognitive filtering system that selectively screens and restructures negative messages generated by irrational or maladaptive thought patterns. When university students are exposed to literary narratives that embody values of resilience, perseverance, and self-compassion, self-talk facilitates the internalization of these values by actively disputing irrational beliefs.

For example, absolutist internal narratives such as "I must be perfect in everything" are cognitively challenged and replaced with more adaptive and realistic self-statements. This rationalization process plays a critical role in addressing social anxiety and depressive symptoms, as individuals are systematically trained to counter destructive self-criticism using arguments grounded in logic, evidence, and contextual realism.

Through repeated engagement, self-talk enables students to dismantle rigid cognitive distortions and reconstruct healthier belief systems that support psychological well-being and self-acceptance.

Emotional Regulation and Self-Soothing Mechanisms

Constructive internal dialogue also functions as a powerful self-soothing tool in the face of emotional turbulence. By habituating positive self-talk, students activate neural soothing systems associated with feelings of safety, calmness, and emotional containment.

In particular, the use of distanced self-talk, referring to oneself using one's own name or third-person pronouns has been empirically shown to enhance self-regulatory capacity by creating psychological distance from intense emotional experiences. This distancing mechanism allows students to appraise stressful situations as challenges rather than threats, a critical cognitive shift that significantly strengthens mental resilience. Such emotional regulation processes enable students to manage distress without avoidance or emotional suppression, fostering greater emotional stability and adaptive coping.

Enhancement of Academic Self-Efficacy and Productivity

The integration of Self-Talks within literary therapy demonstrates a positive correlation with increased academic self-efficacy, defined as students' belief in their ability to successfully complete academic tasks and overcome learning challenges. Students with higher levels of academic self-efficacy tend to exhibit greater persistence, increased willingness to take intellectual risks, and more effective learning strategies.

Literary therapy provides behavioral and cognitive role models through characters who successfully navigate academic obstacles and personal adversity. Self-talk enables students to borrow the narrative voice of these successful characters and incorporate it into their own cognitive repertoire. As a result, students internalize narratives of competence and perseverance as part of their self-concept.

This internalization process directly enhances academic productivity, as students are no longer trapped in cycles of anxiety, self-doubt, and avoidance that previously undermined performance. Instead, they develop adaptive internal scripts that support sustained motivation, focus, and goal-directed behavior.

Narrative Repair Theory and the Restoration of Disrupted Identity

Human identity is fundamentally narrative in nature, meaning that individuals understand themselves through stories constructed about their past, present, and imagined future. However, traumatic experiences, chronic social pressure, or negative social labeling can lead to identity disruption, in which personal narratives become fragmented, rigid, or self-devaluing.

Deconstruction of Master Narratives

University students are frequently trapped within rigid master narratives, such as "an exemplary student must never fail" or "a graduate must immediately secure employment in a prestigious company." When students fail to meet these socially imposed standards, their sense of identity may collapse, leading to feelings of shame, inadequacy, and existential distress.

Literature therapy enables students to deconstruct these master narratives by exposing them to alternative life stories that demonstrate multiple pathways toward a meaningful and fulfilling life. Through narrative comparison and reflection, students are encouraged to release unrealistic expectations and reconstruct more authentic and flexible self-narratives. This process allows individuals to renegotiate identity on their own terms rather than conforming to externally imposed ideals of success.

Re-authoring: Reclaiming the Pen of One's Life

The process of re-authoring, or rewriting one's life story, lies at the core of narrative recovery. Within the Creative Writing component of the Self-Talks program, students are positioned as active authors of their own lives, rather than passive characters shaped solely by circumstance.

By externalizing problems, treating difficulties as entities separate from one's core identity, students are able to perceive themselves as agents capable of altering the direction of their narratives. Journaling and literary creation provide a private reflective space that functions as a psychological lifeline, particularly for emotions that are difficult to articulate verbally. This narrative distance empowers students to reinterpret adversity without self-condemnation.

Neurobiology of Empathy and Cognitive Simulation in Literary Reading

Research in neurocognitive poetics has demonstrated that engagement with fictional literature activates complex neural networks within the brain. These findings provide a biological foundation for the effectiveness of literature therapy in reshaping students' cognitive and emotional patterns.

Mirror Neuron System and Affective Empathy

Mirror neurons are neural cells that activate both when an individual performs an action and when they observe the same action performed by others. In literary reading, mirror neuron activation enables embodied simulation, allowing readers to internally replicate the emotional states, intentions, and struggles of fictional characters.

This mechanism explains why reading fiction has been empirically linked to increased empathy and enhanced Theory of Mind (ToM), the ability to understand the mental states of others. These capacities are essential for healthy social relationships and emotional intelligence within university environments.

Cognitive Benefits of Poetry and Prose

Different literary genres elicit distinct neurological responses. Fictional prose tends to activate the Default Mode Network (DMN), which supports self-reflection, imagination, and hypothetical simulation, making it particularly effective for stress reduction and emotional regulation.

In contrast, poetry often contains ambiguity, metaphor, and unconventional structure, which compel the brain to engage in continuous cognitive reappraisal. This heightened mental activity enhances cognitive flexibility and increases students' tolerance for uncertainty, an essential skill for navigating real-life ambiguity and future-related anxiety.

Table 2.

Brain Region	Therapeutic Function	Implications for Students
Left Inferior Orbitofrontal Cortex (OFC)	Emotional and reward processing	Improved mood and self-satisfaction
Bilateral Insula	Somatic awareness and empathy	Strengthened mind–body integration
Dorsomedial Prefrontal Cortex	Social cognition and emotional understanding	Enhanced interpersonal communication
Limbic System	Regulation of basic emotional responses	Reduced anxiety and fear intensity

University Students in the Digital Era: Pathology and Restoration

As digital natives, university students face unique psychological pressures resulting from excessive technological exposure. The digital era has generated new forms of distress that require targeted mental literacy interventions.

Digital Dementia and Cognitive Consequences

Overreliance on digital devices for information storage and navigation has given rise to the phenomenon of digital dementia, characterized by reduced attention span, weakened memory capacity, and impaired concentration without digital assistance. Additionally, behaviors such as doomscrolling and Zoom fatigue contribute to cognitive fragmentation and emotional exhaustion, significantly undermining psychological well-being (Prasad et al., 2025).

Social Comparison and Social Media Addiction

Social media platforms create environments that continuously promote upward social comparison, in which students compare their complex lived realities to the curated highlight reels of others. This process drastically diminishes self-esteem and reinforces feelings of inadequacy. Social media addiction is often rooted in unmet needs for validation and belonging. Ironically, algorithm-driven validation frequently intensifies loneliness and depressive symptoms when expected recognition is not achieved.

Table 3.

Digital Pathology	Mechanism of Harm	Restorative Role of Literature Therapy
Infobesity	Attention fragmentation and cognitive overload	Encourages deep focus and reflective engagement
FOMO (Fear of Missing Out)	Social anxiety and negative comparison	Cultivates internal fulfillment through aesthetic appreciation
Digital Sickness/ Digital Fatigue	Sleep disruption and reduced cognitive empathy	Restores authentic emotional connection

Literature Therapy as a Digital Detox Strategy

In response to the digital crisis, bibliotherapy functions as an effective digital detox strategy (Hossain et al., 2025). Reading physical books or engaging with immersive narratives demands sustained cognitive involvement, far exceeding the shallow engagement typical of social media consumption.

Through deep narrative engagement, students are trained to reclaim control over their attention and restore neural connectivity in brain regions responsible for imagination, empathy, and meaning-making.

The Indonesian Student Context: Stigma, Loneliness, and Suicide Risk

The mental health conditions of Indonesian university students, particularly in metropolitan academic centers such as Semarang, require urgent attention. Despite high academic achievement, emotional distress among students remains alarmingly prevalent.

Prevalence of Mental Disorders and Barriers to Help-Seeking

Data indicate that Indonesian students experience mild to severe depressive and anxiety symptoms. However, social stigma remains the primary barrier to treatment. Many students suppress psychological distress due to fear of appearing weak or bringing shame upon their families. Limited utilization of university counseling services further exacerbates this crisis.

Loneliness and Suicidal Ideation

Low social support and high levels of loneliness are strong predictors of suicidal ideation among university students. Students who feel emotionally or socially isolated tend to develop maladaptive self-perceptions.

Within this context, the Self-Talks group-based intervention offers a preventive solution by fostering positive social connectedness. Through shared narratives and collective reflection, students realize that they are not alone, significantly reducing suicide risk.

Implementation of the Self-Talks Program Based on Literary Therapy

The potential efficacy of the Self-Talks model lies in its capacity to provide narrative restoration through the humanities, offering a robust alternative to counter identity fragmentation induced by digital pressure. Expressive writing plays a significant role in reducing maladaptive rumination, while the program simultaneously addresses mental health stigma and provides a low-barrier, non-digital intervention pathway to mitigate internet addiction.

This approach is further supported by empirical data indicating that approximately 60% of university students express a preference for such alternative intervention mechanisms. To ensure systematic and sustainable impact, the Self-Talks program should be implemented through a structured five-stage strategy, as outlined below.

Enabling Stage: The initial enabling stage involves an in-depth analysis of the university environment and the identification of the specific needs of students in Semarang. This stage includes the mapping of mental health data, patterns of psychological distress, and digital behavior trends among the target population. The objective is to establish a contextual foundation that ensures the program is grounded in the actual ecological and sociocultural conditions of the campus community.

Strengthening Stage: The strengthening stage focuses on the collection of empirical data through questionnaires and in-depth interviews to validate the identified issues, such as the prevalence of quarter-life crisis and barriers to self-acceptance. This stage ensures that the designed intervention is evidence-based and directly aligned with students' lived experiences, rather than relying on assumed or generalized psychological conditions.

Protection Stage: The protection stage involves the development of a safe and confidential interactive discussion format for Self-Talks sessions. At this stage, clear group norms and ethical guidelines are established to guarantee emotional safety, confidentiality, and mutual respect among participants. This protective framework is essential for fostering trust and encouraging open narrative expression without fear of judgment or exposure.

Supporting Stage: The supporting stage consists of the regular implementation of Literary Dialogue and Creative Writing sessions, typically scheduled on weekends to provide a form of healthy mental recreation outside academic obligations. These sessions function as structured yet flexible spaces for reflective reading, guided discussion, and expressive literary creation, reinforcing positive self-talk and emotional regulation through sustained engagement.

Maintenance Stage: The final maintenance stage involves continuous monitoring and evaluation to assess the program's impact on enhancing self-acceptance and reducing levels of emotional distress among students. Ongoing assessment enables iterative refinement of the program and ensures its long-term effectiveness, adaptability, and relevance within the evolving mental health landscape of higher education.

Integrating the Bio-Psycho-Social-Digital Model for Student Well-Being

Future mental health support for university students must adopt a more comprehensive and integrative framework, namely the bio-psycho-social-digital model. This model recognizes that human well-being is shaped simultaneously by biological, psychological, social, and digital factors, all of which interact dynamically rather than functioning in isolation.

Biological Dimension and Cognitive Restoration

From a biological perspective, interventions should prioritize the restoration of neurocognitive health that has been disrupted by excessive screen exposure. Literary therapy functions as a form of cognitive training that strengthens neural circuits responsible for sustained attention, working memory, and executive control.

In addition, the use of recovery-oriented narratives in digital formats, often categorized as Digital Health Interventions (DHIs), has been shown to be effective in enhancing individuals' self-efficacy in achieving personal health goals. When implemented thoughtfully, such digital narratives can complement offline literary engagement by reinforcing motivation and self-regulatory capacity.

Psychological Dimension and Narrative Repair

Psychologically, the primary focus lies in narrative repair and the reinforcement of individual agency. Narrative coaching training that incorporates creative tools such as serious games and narrative-based board games can assist students in reconstructing more positive, coherent, and future-oriented identities.

Through these narrative processes, students are encouraged to perceive themselves as the protagonists of their own life journeys, a literary metaphor that is particularly empowering within the context of mental health recovery. This reframing supports the development of hope, self-direction, and psychological resilience, which are essential for long-term well-being.

Social and Digital Dimensions: Building Healthy Virtual Communities

From a social standpoint, technology should be leveraged to reduce social isolation rather than exacerbate it. Digitally enabled peer support programs have been empirically demonstrated to significantly decrease levels of loneliness and depressive symptoms among university students.

Online communities offer a unique space in which students can share vulnerability and emotional experiences without fear of immediate physical stigma. However, such interactions must remain within healthy digital boundaries to prevent adverse effects associated with excessive screen use and negative social comparison. When properly moderated, digital communities can foster authentic connection, mutual support, and collective resilience.

Implications for Stakeholders in Higher Education

The findings of this comprehensive analysis provide strategic recommendations for multiple stakeholders within the higher education system, as outlined below.

The Role of Counselors and Educators

University counselors are encouraged to integrate narrative-based and self-talk techniques into their professional practice, given their demonstrated cognitive effectiveness and cultural sensitivity. Educators may incorporate bibliotherapy approaches into the curriculum, particularly within character development modules or professional ethics courses.

Such integrative practices foster essential character strengths, including empathy, self-awareness, and interpersonal communication, at an early stage before psychological challenges escalate into more severe clinical pathologies. By embedding preventive mental health strategies within academic learning environments, universities can promote holistic student development beyond purely academic outcomes.

The Role of Academic Librarians

Academic librarians should no longer be viewed solely as custodians of books, but as strategic partners in supporting students' digital well-being. Librarians are well positioned to curate collections of therapeutic and reflective literature and to collaborate with counseling services in facilitating guided reading groups and literary discussion forums.

Enhancing librarians' competencies in bibliotherapy and narrative facilitation is a critical prerequisite for the successful implementation of such initiatives within university settings. Through active engagement, libraries can evolve into inclusive spaces that support mental restoration and intellectual reflection.

Institutional Policy and the Creation of Safe Spaces

Higher education institutions must invest in the creation of counter-spaces protected environments in which students can engage in self-reflection and identity exploration without the pressures of public visibility or social media performance metrics.

In addition, the development of digital suicidality notification systems can facilitate early detection and rapid response to students who express extreme psychological distress in online environments. Such systems, when implemented ethically and responsibly, can serve as a crucial component of campus-wide mental health surveillance and crisis prevention strategies.

FUTURE RESEARCH DIRECTIONS

Randomized Controlled Trial (RCTs)

Given that the present study constitutes a formative context evaluation with a limited sample size (N = 25), future research should advance toward the product evaluation (efficacy) phase. Subsequent studies are strongly recommended to move beyond formative evaluation and conduct empirical validation through Randomized Controlled Trial (RCT) designs involving larger samples and well-defined control groups.

Such trials are essential for testing the causal impact of the Self-Talks model on reducing symptoms of digital addiction, Fear of Missing Out (FoMO), and enhancing self-acceptance over the long term. To ensure the highest level of academic rigor, future research should employ internationally validated measurement instruments.

This step is crucial to establishing causal evidence regarding whether the Self-Talks model is genuinely effective in increasing self-acceptance scores and reducing suicidal ideation when compared to control conditions.

Technology Integration and E-Bibliotherapy

Future studies may explore the development of dedicated digital platforms or applications for the Self-Talks model in order to enhance accessibility and scalability. Research should examine the viability of e-bibliotherapy or digital Self-Talks applications as intervention tools capable of reaching students in remote or underserved regions. In-depth comparative research is also needed to assess the relative effectiveness of face-to-face (offline) interventions versus digital (online) formats in mitigating digital stress and social isolation among university students.

The Use of Objective Digital Metrics

Rather than relying solely on self-report measures, future research is encouraged to incorporate more objective digital behavioral metrics, such as analyses of device usage patterns, application-switching frequency, and total duration of social media exposure. The development of internationally validated digital well-being measurement instruments would yield more precise and reliable outcomes in detecting and monitoring digital-related psychopathologies.

Narrative Repair Analysis Using Natural Language Processing (NLP)

Technology-driven research utilizing Natural Language Processing (NLP) techniques may be employed to analyze emotional shifts within students' expressive writing during the Creative Writing phase of the intervention. Computational analysis of students' textual outputs can be used to objectively measure sentiment change and emotional tone across intervention stages. Such approaches would provide more sensitive and quantifiable insights into the narrative identity repair process, thereby strengthening methodological innovation in literary therapy research.

Cross-Cultural Perspectives and Master Narratives

Future research should investigate how Asian cultural factors, such as family honor values and mental health stigma, interact with social media pressures in shaping students' identity development. Studies may focus on how counter-stories within literary therapy function to deconstruct rigid master narratives and socially imposed standards of success in the digital era.

Longitudinal Studies on the Sustainability of Effects

It is essential to conduct longitudinal follow-up studies, for example at 6–12 months post-intervention, to evaluate whether improvements in self-acceptance achieved through literary therapy are sustained or transient. Longitudinal research may also examine whether the intervention is effective in preventing the recurrence of depressive symptoms associated with future exposure to social media stressors.

CONCLUSION

Self-acceptance is not an innate or static trait, but rather a narrative achievement facilitated by supportive intrapersonal and interpersonal environments. The Self-Talks model, which integrates the cognitive precision of internal dialogue with the emotional depth of literary therapy, offers a robust framework through which university students can engage in meaningful identity work. Through the stages of identification, catharsis, and insight attainment, students are enabled to reclaim the authorship of their lives and rewrite their personal narratives using the language of resilience and agency.

Amid the cognitive fragmentation and social pressures characteristic of the digital era, low-tech solutions such as deep reading and structured internal dialogue remain among the most fundamental and evidence-based methods for restoring our shared humanity. The successful implementation of this program within the Semarang context provides a replicable roadmap for higher education institutions globally as they confront the escalating mental health crisis among future leaders.

Identity restoration through literature and self-talk is not merely an act of individual healing, but a form of cognitive resistance against increasingly impersonal societal demands. By integrating biological, psychological, social, and digital dimensions, educational ecosystems can be cultivated that enable students not only to survive academically, but also to flourish personally as whole, resilient, and self-directed individuals.

REFERENCES

Ackerman, C. E. (2017). *Writing therapy: Using a pen and paper to enhance personal growth.* PositivePsychology.com. https://positivepsychology.com/writing-therapy/

Akbar, Z., & Alamsyah, R. (2025). The impact of social media usage on student mental health: A study of social comparison and FOMO. *International Journal of Educational Studies*, *8*(1), 12–24.

Baikie, K. A., & Wilhelm, K. (2005). Emotional and physical health benefits of expressive writing. *Advances in Psychiatric Treatment*, *11*(5), 338–346. DOI: 10.1192/apt.11.5.338

Błachnio, A., Przepiórka, A., & Gorbaniuk, O. (2024). Relationship between fear of missing out and adolescents' mental health. *Annals of Agricultural and Environmental Medicine : AAEM*, *31*(2), 266–271.

Elhai, J. D., Yang, H., & Montag, C. (2020). Fear of missing out (FoMO): Symptom associations with depression, anxiety, and problematic smartphone use. *Addictive Behaviors Reports*, *11*, 100262.

Gerber, J. P. (2018). Social comparison on social media: A meta-analysis. *Social Psychology (Göttingen).*

Gualano, M. R., Bert, F., Martorana, M., Voglino, G., Andriolo, V., Thomas, R., Gramaglia, C., Zeppegno, P., & Siliquini, R. (2017). The long-term effects of bibliotherapy in depression treatment: Series of case reports. *BioMed Research International*, *2017*, 4306473.

Hossain, M. S., & Islam, M. S. (2025). Digital detox for young hearts: Bibliotherapy within a bio-psycho-social model embedding AETCOM in medical humanities for digital-age challenges.

Hulme, K. (2018). *The effects of social media on self-esteem and emotional well-being* [Graduate Research Paper, University of Northern Iowa]. UNI ScholarWorks. https://scholarworks.uni.edu/grp/589/

Indonesia, C. N. N. (2022). *Studi: Sebanyak 2,45 juta remaja Indonesia kena gangguan jiwa* [Study: As many as 2.45 million Indonesian teenagers have mental disorders]. https://www.cnnindonesia.com/gaya-hidup/20221212142530-255-886337/studi-245-juta-remaja-indonesia-kena-gangguan-jiwa

Karyanta, N. A. (2012). *Terapi puisi: Dasar-dasar penggunaan puisi sebagai modalitas dalam psikoterapi* [Poetry therapy: Basics of using poetry as a modality in psychotherapy]. Universitas Sebelas Maret.

Kübler-Ross, E. (1969). *On death and dying*. Macmillan.

Li, Y., & Wang, X. (2025). The relationship between fear of missing out and problematic social media use: A moderated mediation model. *Scientific Reports, 15*, 2468.

Luo, T., Wang, M., & Wu, L. (2025). Fear of missing out and problematic social media use: A moderated mediation model of social comparison and self-control. *International Journal of Mental Health and Addiction, 23*(1).

Mabonga, B. (2024). *Impact of social media use (Instagram) on body image and self-esteem: The role of social comparison and FOMO* [Tesis Master, Bournemouth University]. Bournemouth University Institutional Repository. https://eprints.bournemouth.ac.id/40501/

Merdeka.com. (2022). *Mahasiswa Unhas bunuh diri karena tugas, Dekan: Tidak ada hubungannya* [Unhas student commits suicide due to assignments, Dean: No connection]. https://www.merdeka.com/peristiwa/mahasiswa-unhas-gantung-diri-diduga-karena-tugas-kuliah-dekan-tidak-ada-hubungannya.html

Mortier, P., Auerbach, R. P., Alonso, J., Bantjes, J., Benjet, C., Cuijpers, P., Ebert, D. D., Green, J. G., Hasking, P., Nock, M. K., O'Neill, S., Pinder-Amaker, S., Sampson, N. A., Vilagut, G., Zaslavsky, A. M., Bruffaerts, R., Kessler, R. C., Boyes, M., Kiekens, G., & Vives, M.WHO WMH-ICS Collaborators. (2018). Suicidal thoughts and behaviors among first-year college students: Results from the WMH-ICS project. *Journal of the American Academy of Child and Adolescent Psychiatry, 57*(4), 263–273. DOI: 10.1016/j.jaac.2018.01.018 PMID: 29588052

Prasad, S., & Kumar, R. (2025). *From detection to detox: A hybrid model of machine learning and bibliotherapy in digital dementia care*. ResearchGate.

Przybylski, A. K., Murayama, K., DeHaan, C. R., & Gladwell, V. (2013). Motivational, emotional, and behavioral correlates of fear of missing out. *Computers in Human Behavior, 29*(4), 1841–1848. DOI: 10.1016/j.chb.2013.02.014

Rector, N. A., & Roger, D. (1996). Cognitive style and symptom presentation in depression. *Journal of Affective Disorders, 39*(2), 79–87.

Sabet, A. G., & Gountas, S. (2019). Social comparison on Instagram and its relationship with self-esteem. *The International Journal of Health, Wellness & Society, 9*(3), 33–47.

Servidio, R., Soraci, P., Griffiths, M. D., Boca, S., & Demetrovics, Z. (2024). Fear of missing out and problematic social media use: A serial mediation model of social comparison and self-esteem. *Addictive Behaviors Reports, 19*, 100536. DOI: 10.1016/j.abrep.2024.100536 PMID: 38495391

Wang, J., & Zhao, Y. (2024). Social comparison on social media and its influence on subjective well-being: A systematic review. *International Journal of Environmental Research and Public Health, 21*(3), 345. PMID: 38541344

Weill Cornell Medicine. (2025). *Study finds addictive screen use, not total screen time, linked to youth suicide risk.* https://news.weill.cornell.edu/news/2025/06/study-finds-addictive-screen-use-not-total-screen-time-linked-to-youth-suicide-risk

Wilcox, H. C., & Wyman, P. A. (2004). Self-esteem, perceived social support, and suicidal ideation and behavior among African American public housing residents. *Archives of Suicide Research : Official Journal of the International Academy for Suicide Research, 8*(3), 239–252. PMID: 16081390

Xiao, Y., Meng, Y., Brown, T. T., Keyes, K. M., & Mann, J. J. (2025). Addictive use of social media and mobile phones, but not total time, kopingis associated with future suicidal behavior. *International Journal of Environmental Research and Public Health, 22*(1), 57. PMID: 39857510

Zhai, B., & Fang, G. (2025). The relationship between social media use intensity and life satisfaction: A moderated mediation model. *Frontiers in Psychology, 16*, 1463671.

Zhu, L., & Lan, J. (2024). The Influence of Negative Emotion and Self-Acceptance on Suicidal Ideation of Disabled College Students: The Mediating Effect of Hopelessness. *Iranian Journal of Public Health, 53*(12), 2759–2767. DOI: 10.18502/ijph.v53i12.17319 PMID: 39759216

ADDITIONAL READING

Bernard, M. E. (Ed.). (2013). *The Strength of Self-Acceptance: Theory, Practice and Research.* Springer. DOI: 10.1007/978-1-4614-6806-6

Brown, B. (2010). *The Gifts of Imperfection: Let Go of Who You Think You're Supposed to Be and Embrace Who You Are.* Hazelden Publishing.

Burns, D. D. (1999). *Feeling Good: The New Mood Therapy.* Avon Books.

Hari, J. (2018). *Lost Connections: Uncovering the Real Causes of Depression – and the Unexpected Solutions*. Bloomsbury Publishing.

Neff, K. (2011). *Self-Compassion: The Proven Power of Being Kind to Yourself.* William Morrow.

Robbins, A., & Wilner, A. (2001). *Quarterlife Crisis: The Unique Challenges of Life in Your Twenties*. TarcherPerigee.

Rubin, R. J. (1978). *Using Bibliotherapy: A Guide to Theory and Practice*. Oryx Press.

Turkle, S. (2011). *Alone Together: Why We Expect More from Technology and Less from Each Other*. Basic Books.

Turkle, S. (2015). *Reclaiming Conversation: The Power of Talk in a Digital Age*. Penguin Press.

van der Kolk, B. (2014). *The Body Keeps the Score: Brain, Mind, and Body in the Healing of Trauma*. Viking.

KEY TERMS AND DEFINITIONS

Digital Detox: A voluntary period of reduced digital device use aimed at restoring cognitive focus and reducing mental overload.

Expressive Writing: A writing technique focused on articulating deep emotions and personal experiences to facilitate cognitive reorganization.

Narrative Repair: The process of reconstructing disrupted identity through coherent and empowering life narratives.

Quarter Life Crisis: A phase of emotional uncertainty and identity crisis experienced during early adulthood (ages 18–30).

Self-Acceptance: The ability to acknowledge and embrace both strengths and limitations while maintaining self-worth.

Self-Talk: Internal dialogue, conscious or unconscious, that shapes self-perception, evaluation, and behavior.

Upward Social Comparison: The tendency to compare oneself with others perceived as superior, often resulting in insecurity.

Chapter 5
Online Pornography Addiction:
Psychological, Neurocognitive, Social, and Legal Perspectives

Geetika Saxena
http://orcid.org/0000-0003-1420-8243
JECRC University, Rajasthan, India

Ruchika Dwivedi
JECRC University, Rajasthan, India

Richa Saxena
Gurukul Kangri University, Haridwar, India

ABSTRACT

The problem of Internet pornography addiction (IPA) has become a subject of significant academic interest as a multifaceted and complex problem. The I-PACE model describes risk factors, emotional and cognitive reactions, and decision-making deficiencies that contribute to recreational use becoming problematic. Neuroimaging has shown reward circuits and frontal-striatal dysregulation, placing IPA in addiction neurobiology. These data would predict stigma, peer normalization, social isolation, and culturally deep-rooted taboos that enhance relationship or self-stigmatization. Many laws criminalize child sexual abuse material (CSAM) without addressing addiction. This legal and cultural approach stresses modest steps to remove institutional frameworks and human predispositions.This multidisciplinary analysis conceptualizes IPA as a reliance on neurobiological, psychological, social, and legal factors. It advocates for culturally tailored, empirically supported interventions that address individual vulnerabilities within specific sociocultural milieus.

DOI: 10.4018/979-8-2600-2468-3.ch005

INTRODUCTION

Online pornography addiction is growing as a major public health issue and is considered to be a complex issue of sexual behavior, irresponsibility, and compulsive use of pornographic sexual material despite apparent negative effects. The ever-expanding accessibility of the Online coupled with the development of smartphone technology has enabled access to sexually suggestive content to be affordable, difficult to control, and tailored to intentions (Dinçer et al., 2025). The online availability of pornographic content has made it a normal part of life, rather than something luxurious. Such accessibility has increased the number of consumers and has integrated pornography into modern sexual culture (Duffy et al., 2016; Grubbs and Kraus, 2021; Lewczuk et al., 2024). In the past, viewing pornographic material was a conscious act that could have social consequences, today it is so easy to access with different devices from anywhere and anytime, with a high degree of anonymity and impunity, that the emergence and manifestation of online sexual addictive behavior are changing. (Singh, 2024) The inclusion of compulsive sexual behavior disorder (CSBD) within the International Classification of Diseases 11th Revision (ICD-11) is another step towards recognizing this behavioral disorder as one that needs clinical intervention. The International Classification of Diseases, Eleventh Revision (ICD-11) does classify the disorder within a group of disorders under the name 'compulsive sexual behavior disorder (CSBD)'; even if the Diagnostic and Statistical Manual of Mental Disorders, Fifth Edition (DSM-5) has not classified pornography addiction as a disorder, it raises several questions regarding whether it belongs to the same category as CSBD or whether it is a variation of hypersexual disorder, among other possibilities. (Kraus & Sweeney, 2019). This official designation has spurred interdisciplinary studies on the neurobiological foundations, psychological processes, social impacts, and legal consequences of pornography addiction. (Love et al., 2015; Ince et al., 2026).

The prevalence of Online pornography addiction is also rising among younger age groups, partly due to especially early exposure to pornography in developmental windows of opportunity and the embedding of pornography watching within the digital lives of adolescents and young people (Grant et al., 2025). The high number of Online pornography use depends on the approach and criteria used to define it, but 3-6% of adults meet the clinical criteria, with more men than women reporting pornography addiction. In community samples, 10% or more of younger adults use it. 2020 (Kowalewska et al. 2020). In addition to epidemiology, Indian and other non-Western studies indicate that the severity of addiction is greatly increased by young age, single marital status, and restricted legitimate sexual gratification, thus making the interaction of cultural, social, and individual factors in the expression of this addiction an important one. (Jaiswal et al., 2025)

People who struggle with compulsive sexual behavior often find that they are unable to fulfil their own promises to themselves, have constant and intrusive thoughts and urges about sex, and feel a strong sense of losing control of their sexual desires. The psychological burden of the condition is high, with patients with CSBD and PPU having a significantly higher number of comorbid depressions, anxiety, attention-deficit/hyperactivity disorder (ADHD), and obsessive-compulsive symptoms than control populations.(Marchetti, 2023) In addition to psychiatric comorbidities, Online pornography addiction has been shown to interfere with basic psychosocial functioning, such as relationship dissatisfaction, sexual dysfunction, low self-esteem, social isolation, occupational dysfunction, and, in severe cases, suicidal ideation (Grant et al., 2025;Odlaug et al., 2013). The neurocognitive processes that underlie Online pornography addiction are a fundamental field of current addiction study. Several neuroimaging studies have identified neural hyperreactivity to sexual cues in the ventral striatum, nucleus accumbens, and orbitofrontal cortex (OFC), which are key brain regions associated with reward processing and motivation and emotional salience attribution, among individuals with pornography addiction (Brand et al., 2016). This increased cue reactivity is thought to represent a type of incentive sensitization, in which sexual cues increasingly acquire increased motivational salience and automatically attract attention and elicit strong "wanting" responses even when the individual is aware that it would be counterproductive. At the same time, studies reveal the key deficits in other executive functions like inhibitory control, decision-making, impulse control, and working memory that occur when dealing with cues related to addiction (Robinson & Berridge, 2025).The tripartite relationship among the impulsive system (facilitating automatic, reward-driven behaviors), the reflective system (allowing conscious, deliberate processes and inhibitory control), and the interoceptive system (enabling the subjective experience of craving) provides a comprehensive understanding of how dysregulation in these neural systems sustains compulsive sexual behavior(Christensen et al., 2024).

The impact of online pornography addiction on our social interactions goes beyond the personal psychological harm to sexual relationships, attitudes towards gender, and societal norms. The findings support Online pornography addiction use as being linked to diminished relationship quality, decreased sexual satisfaction in relationships, increased infidelity, and increased rates of relationship dissolution (Ince et al., 2026). Among the most troubling are the correlations found between pornography consumption and unrealistic sexual expectations, lowered levels of empathy for sexual partners, acceptance of sexual coercion and aggression, and the reinforcement of gender stereotypes of women as objects for men's sexual gratification (Harun et al., 2025). Finally, Online pornography addiction use is often comorbid with other addictive behaviors, such as substance use, risky sexual behaviors, gambling, and compulsive shopping, highlighting the necessity of integrated and comprehensive conceptualizations of addictive behaviours as decontrols. (Wdowiak et al., 2025) Moreover, adolescents and individuals with autism spectrum disorder (ASD), ADHD, prior trauma histories, and sexual and gender minorities are at an increased risk of Online pornography addiction use and may be more sensitive to intervention approaches that need to be adapted to their cultural and developmental backgrounds (Ince et al., 2026). Online pornography addiction can sometimes instigate or enable criminal behavior, which in turn leads to actions that elicit legal responses, such as obtaining or distributing illicit materials (Kraus & Sweeney, 2019; Gola et al., 2022). The clinical and social importance of differentiating between non-addictive and addictive usage patterns is enhanced when the nature of non-addictive use patterns shifts towards patterns of law violation, such as the sharing of non-consensual content or access to prohibited content. Consequently, such behavior can often lead to legal implications ranging from CSAM possession, sexual violence, rape, domestic violence (e.g., strangulation), non-consensual image sharing, and harassment as a result of desensitization, escalation to explicit content, and aggression (Tomei et al., 2021; Wright et al., 2025). There is a lack of coherence in terms of legislative and regulatory responses to Online pornography addiction, which are inadequate to address the complex nature of the addiction while considering the principles of freedom of speech, protecting children, criminal law, and public health concerns. While certain jurisdictions have established laws making the creation and dissemination of specific forms of pornography illegal (e.g., minors in pornography or non-consensual deepfake pornography), the vast majority of legislation fails to address the clinical problem of addiction in any way. The problem, in essence, is trying to find a balance between safeguarding the welfare of minors against exposure to damaging sexual content while respecting the privacy of adults, ensuring their autonomy, protecting performers' rights, preventing exploitation within the pornography industry, and developing regulatory frameworks capable of adapting to innovations in technology like artificial pornography. Therefore, this chapter address a comprehensive synthesis within the areas of psychology, neurocognition, social science, and law is presented to highlight the complex facets of online pornography addiction. It is possible to gain a deeper understanding of this increasingly prevalent disorder through the integration of results obtained from neuroimaging studies, clinical investigations, epidemiology, and the legal field.

PORNOGRAPHY ADDICTION: DEFINITIONAL AMBIGUITY AND PHENOTYPES

"Pornography addiction" refers to the broader term in historical usage, indicating an uncontrollable habit of indulging in porn irrespective of how it is consumed (De

Alarcón et al., 2019). Scholars and therapists use varying terms, such as "pornography addiction," "online pornography addiction," "addictive pornography use" (PPU), "compulsive sexual behavior disorder" (CSBD), and "pornography-watching disorder" (PWD), interchangeably without specifying what each means (Dinçer et al., 2025; Kraus & Sweeney, 2019). Such inconsistencies highlight the ambiguity on whether the disorders are addictions, compulsions, impulse-control problems, or simply cases of moral discrepancies. Online pornography addiction, popularly known as "cybersex addiction," gained traction in the 2000s. Online pornography addiction takes note of unique qualities of the Online, including accessibility, affordability, and anonymity (the "triple A" theory) that might enhance inappropriate habits (De Alarcón et al., 2019).

Addictive pornography consumption is the most common behavioural expression (Gola et al., 2022) and denotes a lack of control over online pornography consumption—characterized by an inability to regulate frequency, duration, or content—alongside functional impairment in personal, occupational, social, or relational spheres (Chen et al., 2022).

Compulsive sexual behavior disorder is an impulse-control disease, not an addiction (Gola et al., 2022). The CSBD (ICD-11) defines a persistent loss of control of sexual impulses in a period of 6 months or longer, which involves pornography, masturbation, commercial sex, and partnered sex (Ince et al., 2026).

Pornography-Watching Disorder (PWD) is a disorder that is assessed using DSM-5 substance use criteria, which deals with impaired control, salience, mood modulation, interpersonal conflict, tolerance, and persistence despite negative outcomes (Erdosz et al., 2025).

PSYCHOLOGICAL FRAMEWORKS

The I-Pace Model

The Interaction of Person-Affect-Cognition-Execution (I-PACE) model can be applied to the online pornography addiction (Brand et al., 2016) and other behavioural addictions including gaming disorder (e.g., Deleuze et al., 2015; Sariaysk et al., 2015; Paulus et al., 2018), compulsive sexual behavior disorder, including addictive pornography use (e.g., Carnes and Love, 2017; Wery et al., 2018). The model suggests that predisposing factors (neurobiological and psychological vulnerabilities), the affect/cognitive response to situational triggers, and diminished executive functioning (Brand et al. 2016) interact together to create specific online -use disorders. These components interact dynamically and the conditioning processes intensify the links in an addictions cycle. The I-PACE model suggests a holistic explanation, stating that individual predispositions of vulnerability and previous learning experiences make individuals recidivist in their engagement with particular online addiction to seek gratification or relief (Brand et al., 2016; Brand et al., 2019). With repeated exposure, the affective and cognitive responses are biased—they become more craving and cue responsive, and the ability to respond flexibly is weakened as a result of reduced executive control. This inter-relaxation leads to a gradual progression from voluntary behavior to compulsive consumption, with online pornography consumption situated along the continuum of addictive behaviors.

Predisposing variables are those that make a person central traits, which can be comparatively constant with time (Brand et al., 2016). High trait sexual motivation could result in an increased tendency of highly motivated people to develop hypersexual behavior or pornography-use disorder (Stark et al., 2022). This model of particular online-use disorders contains psychopathology elements (e.g., depression, social anxiety) and dysfunctional personality traits, among other variables (e.g., stress vulnerability), as the variables that signify predispositions. In addition to these more global factors of vulnerability, studies suggested that people are particularly more vulnerable to becoming addicted to using some types of applications or sites. Indicatively, the intense interest in gaming or sexual promiscuity in general can be, in part, the reason behind the people using certain applications/sites (e.g., gaming or pornography-viewing, respectively) to receive gratification and enjoyment. The predisposing variables do not necessarily influence the course of a particular Online-use disorder but are correlated with some online -use expectancies and dysfunctional coping styles. Online-use expectancies and coping have been regarded as personal core cognitions and could be a critical moderating or mediating variable. The last element of the model is the utilization of the first-choice application/site that leads to the experience of the gratification and positive reinforcement (Everitt & Robbins, 2016).The positive (and somewhat negative) reinforcement of the dysfunctional coping style, anticipations regarding the application of particular online applications/sites, and certain fundamental attributes, especially psychopathological ones and the particular preferences, is brought about through gratification. More biopsychological considerations, which can predispose people to the onset of a mental disorder in general or an addictive behavior in particular, include negative early childhood experiences, including early trauma, emotional or physical abuse, and social isolation. Negative experiences during childhood life have also been associated with some types of online use disorders (Dalbudak et al., 2014). The insecure attachment style is linked to early negative experiences in childhood life that result in the development of an online use disorder, such as online pornography use (Kor et al., 2014). This association agrees with the assumption that online use disorders are linked to negative experiences in early life. The development of a negative and addictive behavior only comes from the interaction of the predisposing variables in people and the specifications that specific situations bring in, one of the major ideas of the inner circle of the I-PACE model. The interrelations lead to gratification and compensation experiences, which are linked to a specific behavior. Online pornography addiction within the concept of Person-Affect-Cognition-Execution can be best explained as the result of the dynamic interactions between situational triggers and reinforcement learning (Brand et al., 2016; Brand et al., 2019). Continuous exposure to pornography gives a short-lived satisfaction and relief of the negative effect, solidifying the expectation that porn makes me feel better, which slowly turns pornography into a maladaptive coping mechanism (Laier et al., 2013; Bibi et al., 2022). Over time, these expectations become generalized, prompting individuals to turn to pornography as a means of coping with stress, boredom, or rejection. This behaviour is linked to the correlation of online pornography addiction with depression, anxiety, and diminished self-esteem resulting from maladaptive coping mechanisms (Bibi et al., 2022). As expectation for rewards and coping mechanisms develop, more exposure to internal stimuli (e.g., loneliness) or exterior stimuli (e.g., sexual images) intensifies desire and cue reactivity, culminating in skewed decision-making favouring pornography consumption (Wegmann et al., 2025).Therefore, Online pornography addiction shows up as an obsession with losing control, which is caused by executive dysfunction, reward dysregulation, unhealthy coping, and biased cognitive-affective responses (Brand et al., 2019).

Attachment and emotion regulation in online pornography addiction

One of the key theories explaining the phenomenon of pornography addiction is the interaction between attachment and deficits in emotion regulation (Wizła & Lewczuk, 2024). According to the presented theoretical framework, deficits in emotion regulation lead to an increased effect of attachment insecurity (attachment anxiety and attachment avoidance) on the development of pornography addiction online. Emotional dysregulation, together with loneliness, appears as a reliable predictor of pornography abuse regardless of age and stress levels (Cardoso et al., 2022; Kató et al., 2024). The proposed mechanism includes using pornography to cope with various emotional issues. According to the Emotional Escape Mechanism, emotional dysregulation facilitates pornography addiction use disorder. In qualitative studies, when men were asked about their reasons for pornography addiction, they stated that it helped them to cope with negative feelings and emotions (Hanseder & Dantas, 2023). Insecure people who have troubles in controlling and managing their emotions find pornography as an easy-to-access solution to their problems (Shafly et al., 2025).

NEUROCOGNITIVE FRAMEWORK

According to this Neurocognitive model, the imbalance in the fronto-striatal network, especially the ventral striatum, amygdala, and dorsolateral prefrontal cortex, leads to the onset of addiction via increased sensitivity to cues and craving, followed by the recruitment of dorsal striatum-related processes as the behavior becomes more automatic. (Brand et al., 2019).

Dopaminergic system and reward processing in pornography addiction

The neural biology underlying addiction to online pornography relies heavily on the disturbance in the dopaminergic reward pathway, which exhibits common principles with addictions to drugs. (Love et al., 2015) The mesolimbic dopaminergic pathway, emanating from the ventral tegmental area (VTA) and converging into the nucleus accumbens (NAc), seems to play an important role in the formation and perpetuation of pornography consumption. (Peng et al., 2025) The neurobiological changes involved in pornography addiction include neuroplasticity of the dopaminergic reward pathway. The repeated exposure to sexually stimulating stimuli leads to the enhanced incentive salience linked to the cues associated with pornography, which results from the overactivity of the ventral striatum (responsible for reward processing), dorsal anterior cingulate cortex (involving conflict monitoring and attention), and anterior orbitofrontal cortex (assigning value to rewards). During the process of learning, the reward pathway becomes highly responsive to cues, thus enabling the arousal of powerful motivational responses. Notably, studies involving extinction training demonstrate that the aforementioned behavior can persist even when there is no anticipated reward present, indicating the pathological nature of the neuroplastic adaptation process (Wojciechowski et al., 2025).

Neuroimaging studies have revealed that men receiving therapy for their pornography usage display heightened activation in the ventral striatum when presented with erotic reward prediction cues, with the elevated activation showing positive correlations with the severity of pornography usage, the duration of pornography viewing, and the frequency of masturbation. (Gola et al., 2017) Importantly, the increased striatal response to the erotic stimuli is juxtaposed by a reduced response to monetary rewards, which further implies selective sensitization of the reward system in relation to specific stimuli instead of general reward hypersensitivity. The observed trend corroborates the incentive sensitization theory, which stipulates that addiction is characterized by increased "wanting" of an addicted object without "liking" it.

The orbitofrontal cortex (OFC) can also be considered another important part of the reward system involving dopamine that exhibits dysfunctions in pornography addiction cases. According to Golec et al., when looking at cue reactivity among patients who suffer from compulsive sexual behavior disorder, there is increased anticipatory response in the ventral striatum and anterior OFC triggered by erotic cue stimuli. It is noteworthy that OFC functioning depends on reward probability, as individuals affected by compulsive sexual behaviors exhibit abnormal probability processing. In addition, erotic reward cues activate further OFC sections than those recruited by monetary rewards. (Golec et al., 2021)

Brian structure alteration and functions

Studies utilizing neuroimaging techniques have uncovered consistent alterations in the structural integrity of the brain among people addicted to pornographic material and those with compulsive sexual behavior disorder by pointing out regions associated with reward mechanisms, executive functioning, and emotion regulation. (Görts et al., 2023) The study of the cortical surface area and thickness among people with compulsive sexual behavior disorder showed a significant reduction in the cortical surface area of the right posterior cingulate cortex among patients compared to the healthy group, along with a negative correlation between the degree of symptoms and surface areas.

White matter integrity is yet another vital structural factor affected by the use of porn in unhealthy ways. (Draps et al., 2021) A study employing diffusion sensor imaging in people with compulsive sexual behavior disorder compared to those without the condition revealed marked decreases in fractional anisotropy, which is an index of white matter microstructure, within a number of important fiber tracts such as the superior corona radiata, internal capsule, cerebellar tracts, and the occipital gyri. It is worth mentioning that all of these regions of white matter tracts are involved in other addictive conditions, meaning that there exist anatomical similarities between substance abuse and pornography addiction. The deterioration of white matter connectivity between reward pathways, areas responsible for executive functioning, and emotion-related brain regions may underlie the lack of inhibition in porn addiction.

Altered gray matter volumes represent further evidence for remodelling associated with pornography addiction. (Draps et al., 2020) The comparison between neuroimaging conducted on patients with compulsive sexual behavior disorder, gambling disorder, and alcohol use disorder has shown similarities in terms of having a lower gray matter volume in the orbitofrontal cortex. The highest amount of gray matter decrease has been observed in gambling disorder and alcohol use disorder, followed by lesser yet still significant reductions in compulsive sexual behaviours disorder. It is possible that the reduced volume of gray matter in the brain region (orbitofrontal cortex) could cause poor decision-making and increased sensitivity to rewarding stimuli in those who suffer from pornography addiction.

The amygdala is an essential brain area that plays a critical role in emotion processing and reward processing and shows morphological and functional alterations in pornography addiction. (Schmidt et al., 2017) In studies conducted by comparing individuals with pornographic addiction against normal controls, elevated gray matter volume was identified in the left amygdala, while lower resting-state functional connectivity was revealed between the amygdala and bilateral dorsolateral prefrontal cortex in individuals with online addiction disorder. The high gray matter volume of the amygdala was due to heightened emotional sensitivity toward sex, while the low functional connectivity might be related to suboptimal prefrontal control over this heightened emotional sensitivity. Consequently, the amygdala of individuals with pornographic addiction appeared to have enhanced limbic reactivity to sexual stimuli but weak prefrontal modulation of such reactivity. (Schmidt et al., 2017) More recently, recurrent quantification analysis was applied to examine the bilateral differences in subdivisions of the amygdala between individuals with pornographic addiction and healthy subjects. Such bilateral differences showed negative correlations with depression, anxiety, and impulsivity (the factors that caused the disorder). (Adamus et al., 2025)

There is a significant alteration in the functioning and anatomy of the prefrontal cortex in cases of addiction to pornography, indicating deficient executive control. (Brand et al., 2014) In studies of neuropsychology and neuroimaging, it has been found that functions of the prefrontal cortex, including executive control processes, are compromised in subjects suffering from Online addiction, and the deficiency of control processes becomes more pronounced during encounters with the cue of the Online, which represents their preferred object of addiction. These cues interfere with working memory and decision-making abilities, similar to what is seen in other behavioural and substance addictions.

Dysregulation of Autonomic Nervous System

Apart from dopaminergic changes and structural abnormalities, new findings indicate the dysregulation of the autonomic nervous system (ANS) in pornography addiction, characterized by imbalances between the sympathetic and parasympathetic nervous systems. (Stark et al., 2022) During acute stress induction before and during sexually stimulating media viewing, there is an exaggerated cortisol response, which has been shown to have a positive correlation with neural responses to sexual stimuli in the reward pathway, especially within the nucleus accumbens and dorsal anterior cingulate cortex. Sensitivity to the effects of stress and the length of addiction to pornography affect the way in which cortisol affects activation of the reward pathways, suggesting that the dysregulation of the ANS caused by stress can be both an activator and amplifier of porn cue reactivity. Dysregulation of autonomic processes has been found among individuals addicted to pornography, just as it has been reported in other behavioral addictions. Levels of resting-state catecholamines were found to be lower, accompanied by high levels of anxiety, suggesting a state of imbalance between the sympathetic and parasympathetic systems.

Thus, owing to the long-lasting activity of the sympathetic nervous system, the level of physiological arousal becomes increased at the time of presentation of the stimulus, thus making it difficult for the parasympathetic system to achieve the recovery process and leading to a violation of the homeostasis process. In this connection, the effect of an imbalance between the processes of stress and its regulation on the functioning of the autonomic nervous system regarding the development of pornography addiction plays a vital role. Under circumstances where anticipation and consumption of pornographic materials occur, the increase in the production of cortisol makes the process of activating the dopaminergic reward system more likely, thus positively affecting the stimulation of sexual desire and addiction (Stark et al., 2022; Sič et al., 2025).

SOCIAL STRUCTURAL AND CULTURAL EMBEDDEDNESS

Online pornography addiction is not only considered an individual psychopathology but also a process based in the structural and cultural system. A critical analysis of the use of online pornography shows that such practices

fall under the scope of behavioural addiction, impulse-control problems, and compulsive behavior, as well as risk and protective factors associated with these phenomena. Sociology recognizes that norms, culture expectations, interaction with others, and processes of stigma inside the organization are critical for the emergence and perpetuation of norms of online pornographic addiction consumer practices. With the advent of smartphones and streaming applications, there has been a major change in the pornography consumption habits of young people that have made it common to watch porn regularly as a means to sexual arousal and a way to relieve tension. This phenomenon is now widespread enough for the normalization of casual sexuality while, simultaneously, damaging the usual behavioral control mechanisms that were introduced by family, peers, and communities. (Dinçer et al., 2025) In today's digital world, it is challenging to influence conventional behavioural control instruments like parents, peers, and social surveillance because of unique characteristics of the digital world such as algorithms and privacy.

Differential Gender Socialization and Conformity

Gender is a significant factor in the process of Online pornography use and has different social pathways. Research has identified key sex and gender differences in behavioral dyscontrol in addictive behaviors (Fattore & Melis, 2016). Peer pressure is greater for males in consuming pornographic material on a regular basis, whereas female consumption of pornographic material leads to a sense of social shame or social disapproval because of its cultural acceptance among peer groups. Culture – specifically the construction of masculinity – appears to have a significant role in patterns of pornography use, as this relationship is moderated by gender in several countries and is highly significant for sexually objectifying attitudes (Willis et al., 2022). Conformity pressures related to the construction of masculinity (and social status) form the basis of the peer effect involved in these gendered patterns. In the past 20 years, researchers have found that pornography users tended to be mostly boys and men, sensation-seekers, and boys and men with poor or troubled relationships with their families. (Peter & Valkenburg, 2016) This is a pressure of conformity that applies to men and shapes a series of norms that are conducive to the proliferation of pornography among men, while also creating shame and internalized stigma for women. Different cultural and gender differences in pornography use patterns highlight that secretiveness is connected to both reduced sexual satisfaction and higher feelings of shame, but that this relationship could be two-way, with those who hide reflecting both the potential costs of the relationship and the potential sources of shame and dissatisfaction.

Dysfunctional Relationships

The dysfunctional family interactions, which resulted in isolation and made individuals turn to pornography to regulate their emotions (Lochner et al., 2024), showed a moderate positive correlation between the functioning of the family and Online use. However, the level of the quality of the family interactions was lower for Online pornography users compared to those who did not use pornographic material online. In fact, there is a two-way relationship between pornography use and family functioning, where more frequent pornography use was related to poorer family functioning. Nevertheless, the negative impacts of pornography use may outweigh the benefits.Pornography can provide some form of short-term escape from negative emotions. But most of the time, such situations may lead to more instability and emotional detachment, among other forms of dysfunctional coping. Negative emotional states and Online pornography addiction have a complicated relationship because, at some point, social support may serve as a buffer. Depression, anxiety, self-esteem and loneliness are all important predisposing factors to online pornography use, and the presence of craving and coping are important serial mediators that perpetuate and intensify online pornography addiction . (Hanseder & Dantas, 2023).

Moral Incongruence, Shame and Religious Stigmatisation

However, the problem with Online pornography addiction use is not necessarily the act of use itself, but rather the attitudes consumers have about the repugnant and immoral nature of such use. Individual religious shame-proneness is significantly related to moral disapproval on the basis of individual religious beliefs and these moral disapprovals subsequently predict pornography use symptoms. These mechanisms of moral/psychological suffering are unique to these types of consumption. The severe moral codes of religion forbid the use of pornography, and this causes the users to feel strongly guilty and struggling with their conscience, which leads to alienation from the community and family. The research conducted among religious adolescents indicate the existence of a relationship between disapproval of pornographic content and sexual guilt in all three spheres of behavior, and disapproval was found to be the highest among religious adolescents. (Kaplan et al., 2025)

It is intriguing that religiosity was associated with lower shame despite controlling for disapproval, indicating that moral commitment and inner distress may have a complex interplay. Shame-based psychopathology is especially vulnerable because of the connection between religious trauma and religious identity with sexual conduct. The partners of those individuals who struggle with sexual addiction and compulsive sexual behavior have pointed out that most religious communities failed to provide validation and safety once they disclosed their loved ones' addiction or behavior (Aghamiri et al., 2024). They have expressed significant spiritual transformation experiences, such as changing their beliefs, fearing judgment from others regarding their religion, the pastor's pressure to forgive and forget the abuse inflicted upon them, and blaming God for being a silent accomplice. These community reactions add more shame and social exclusion to their victims and their intimate partners. This moral schema further perpetuates the process of self-stigmatization, which is characterized by the internalization of negative beliefs and stereotypical perceptions about oneself. Narrative analysis of self-help groups on the Internet, which focus on the etiology of online pornography usage, reveals the dialectical relationship between available resources, material circumstances, and feelings of vulnerability, which are articulated in order to achieve escape and validation. Abstinence, which is articulated through a discourse of recovery/relapse, constitutes an important issue that leads to distress.

Sexual minorities and Intersecting Stressors

The sexual minority individual is subject to various stressors that impact their route toward developing an internet pornography addiction (Lewczuk et al., 2023). Sexual stigmatization, sexual discrimination, and stress from hiding one's sexuality have been found to be significantly correlated with CSBD and internet pornography abuse. Experiences of discrimination due to sexual orientation and engagement in sexualized drug use are associated with higher compulsive sexual behavior symptom severity. Internalized sexual stigma particularly relates to greater online pornography use severity.

In particular, the effect of social support is strongly protective among sexual minorities. (Jennings et al., 2024) LGBQ-affirming clinical guidelines for compulsive sexual behavior disorder stress that the delineation needs to be made between the sociocultural variables in the clients' environment and their symptoms, since current issues revolve around the erroneous conflation of these variables leading to misdiagnosis. The concept of minority stress theory offers an empirical rationale explaining how the stigmatization of LGBQ individuals leads to the emergence of online pornographic addiction.

Cultural Variation and the Construction of Online Use

The definition and conceptualization of Online pornography use is very different from sub-culture to sub-culture and across geographical regions, and the identification of 'pathology' is therefore culturally dependent. In conservative cultures like China, if sexual attitudes are negative (disapproval of nonmarital or casual sex) but sexual behaviors are positive (online sexual activity), then the incongruence between sexual attitudes and behaviors further enhances the perception of Online pornography use (Chen et al. 2023). The earlier studies shows that the cultural attitudes towards sexuality have a strong impact on the understanding and experience of sexuality that is manifested in excessive or Online social media use, but that the exact mechanisms of these influences differ depending on the cultural context (Chen et al. 2023). Family climate, attachment patterns, social support, self-esteem, resilience, peer pressure, emotion regulation, fear of missing out, and cognitive factors are key factors that affect excessive or Online use of social media, with cultural factors influencing the exact nature of these effects. Cultural differences are evident in the discussions about pornography exposure, with the "turn blind eye" approach fitting boys' pornography use and sweeping prohibition and denial fitting the replies given to girls' potential exposure. Exposure to pornography in the context of families and social environment with youths' online behavior is increasingly recognized, and culturally sensitive intervention design is necessary; the "turn blind eye" approach fits boys' pornography use, while sweeping prohibition and denial fit the replies given to potential exposure of girls' pornography. Boys said they watched pornography a lot but at the same time had feelings of guilt because of the conflict between modernity and traditional values, whereas girls said they weren't engaged but admitted their peers were watching pornography. In these patterns, cultural and religious taboos have implications for consumption patterns and the psychological effects that are felt.

LEGAL FRAMEWORKS

Online pornography addiction is becoming an acknowledged behavioural disorder with compulsive use, tolerance, withdrawal, and lack of self-control, which is similar to the effect of substance-related addictions (Paquette et al., 2025). Despite the fact that consumption of adult pornographic content is not a criminal offence in most jurisdictions, the compulsive use of it has been found as a risk factor towards the escalation into criminal activities, specifically, the purchase, distribution, or creation of child sexual abuse material (CSAM), grooming, or other such activities. Difference is of paramount importance: although addiction is a clinical and social issue, its further development in the illicit content leads to legal actions. Addictive pornographic consumption has been linked to paraphilias and hypersexual behavior, and is strongly related to CSAM offending (Seto, 2015).

The deterrence-dominant and rehabilitation-integrated models are opposing philosophies of dealing with online pornography addiction (OPA) in the criminal justice system. The U.S. federal system has deterrence-dominant models that are based on the rational choice theory and impose severe penalties, registries, and surveillance to intimidate and curb recidivism by instilling cost-benefit awareness (Morgan and Klein, 2024). Nevertheless, online pornography addiction is counterproductive due to its compulsiveness, which is promoted by affective stimuli such as anxiety, cognitive distortions, and feedback cycles, because lack of insight (Grade I denial caused by psychosis-like states) does not allow thinking rationally, and punishment is ineffective in the transition into escalation to online pornography addiction offences (Brand et al., 2019).

Included in rehabilitation-based models are the underlying pathologies, which include addiction, paraphilias, and emotional dysregulation treated through forced therapy, psychological testing, and relapse prevention based on the assumption that the offender is reformable through clinical intervention (Morgan and Klein, 2024). This is consistent with the treatment focus of MHCA 2017 as well as the discretion in sentencing of behavioral offenses under IT Act and stricter liability of POCSO (Information Technology Act, 2000; Protection of Children from Sexual Offences Act, 2012). Nordic rehabilitation focuses lowers recidivism better than U.S. punitiveness in compulsive crimes, and the integration of forensic psychology is required to balance the issue of accountability and evidence-based change.

Global Legal Frameworks and International Consensus

There is extensive worldwide consensus regarding the illegality of CSAM, as demonstrated by legal frameworks such as the United Nations Convention on the Rights of the Child and its Optional Protocol, the Lanzarote Convention, and EU Directive 2011/93/EU. All these laws are in total agreement that the manufacture, distribution, and possession of CSAM is illegal, considering the content to be an expression of abuse and not freedom of speech. However, there is a notable absence of consistency in the definition of CSAM in most countries and the law surrounding it.Countries such as Tanzania and the Philippines have updated their legislation in terms of identifying CSAM, convicting perpetrators of grooming, and applying victim-centered laws (Ardhanariswari et al., 2026). Nevertheless, advancements in technology, in particular, the use of AI-produced imagery and deepfakes, bring challenges in defining virtual CSAM. While some countries ban the creation of artificial photographs, others limit the definition to real images of children only.

All legal systems around the world give precedence to regulations that target harmful content, as opposed to those that criminalize addiction or compulsive consumption. The international laws and conventions support this principle by emphasizing prohibitions against harmful content, rather than the behavioural disorders associated with the act. There emerges a clear doctrinal distinction between the two – the crime in question here is participation in the production or distribution of online pornography addiction and exploitative content, rather than addiction or compulsive behavior. Global laws place emphasis on regulating content, rather than criminalizing addiction. Universal prohibitions against CSAM have been established under international conventions. Some examples of approaches to jurisdiction are as follows:

1. In India, it is criminalized through the Information Technology Act (art. 67B) and POCSO (art. 15), and possession has been accepted by the courts as punishable. Metadata, browser history and morphed CSAM detection, and juvenile offender profiling are areas of focus in forensics.
2. The USA has very serious CSAM laws (18 U.S.C. 2252) and obscenity requirements (Miller v. California, 1973). Forensic software (FTK and EnCase) recovers deleted caches, and addiction has been identified as a risk factor leading to recidivism—compulsive pornography users presently show up to fourfold higher recidivism rates.

3. The EU unifies protections against revenge porn and deep fakes through the Digital Services Act (2024) and Directive 2011/93. At Europol, hashing databases (ICSE) and deep-fake detection are conducted using forensic AI.
4. The harmful content is regulated by the Online Safety Act (2023) in the UK and the prosecutions by the Coroners Act in the case of CSAM. Forensic imaging is used by the National Crime Agency to match grooming behavior.
5. CSAM is criminalized by Criminal Code Div. 474 in Australia, and federal police detect it through Tor-network forensics to reveal concealed distribution.
6. China implements prohibitions with the help of the Cybersecurity Law and anti-vice movements based on the analysis of traffic controlled by the state.
7. The state of the Middle East (e.g., UAE) imposes a ban based on Federal Law No. 5/2012, and forensic attention is paid to the tracing of imports/distribution

FUTURE RESEARCH DIRECTIONS

Despite advancements in psychology, neuroscience, laws, and regulation of online pornographic addiction, the current state of research in the field of pornography is fragmented rather than integrated. The gap between these areas leads to an "integration paradox" when the development of effective methods for dealing with the problem becomes difficult due to the presence of highly sophisticated knowledge in all these areas. First of all, the lack of agreement regarding definitions and diagnoses can be considered a serious drawback. Different approaches to defining CSBD, hypersexual disorder, and porn addiction make diagnosis and treatment processes vary from one system to another. Also, different treatments for ICD-11 and DSM due to theoretical contradictions exist. The constraints of measurement further intensify this problem. Current evaluation instruments lack cross-cultural validity, depend significantly on self-report metrics, and frequently do not differentiate between high-frequency usage and clinically detrimental behavior. The existence of substantial comorbidities, such as depression, anxiety, and impulse-control disorders, confuses causal interpretation and hinders the diagnosis of basic severity classifications.

Neurobiological research enables us to comprehend how rewards are perceived by individuals and how executive control functions. However, it cannot establish causality because, due to the cross-sectional nature of most research, it is difficult to determine whether brain changes are a cause or consequence of the behavior. Moreover, a neurobiological perspective may cause a reductionist view because it excludes psychological and environmental considerations that affect an individual's actions. The reductionist view, in turn, leads to the development of inaccurate conclusions regarding the culpability of criminals and their risk assessment.

The stigma and guilt that come from having sex create significant barriers to seeking help and intervening. People hide their inappropriate behavior to avoid being judged by society, thus delaying any treatment or worsening their condition. The culture of individuals plays a vital role in determining the nature of their experience and reaction to the problem. However, the methods currently used for diagnosing and treating this disorder primarily target Western society.

While there is a general consensus that online pornography addiction is forbidden, law enforcement agencies find it challenging to manage other types of sexual conduct that happen online. The international efforts to regulate this phenomenon face obstacles in the form of differences in the jurisdiction, implementation, and organization of the rehabilitation process. The deterrence-based model, which involves punishing the offender, fails to address the compulsion that drives the individual to engage in sexual behavior.

Technology is making regulatory issues even more difficult. Technology such as artificial intelligence, deepfake, and algorithmic content recommendations has been introduced, creating new ways for individuals to exploit others and manipulate them. The current laws do not take into consideration the role of technology in encouraging exploitative practices and behavior intensification. This demonstrates the need for having an extensive set of regulations that incorporate technology responsibility.

CONCLUSION

Online pornography addiction is a complex issue that spans across several disciplines such as psychology, neurocognition, social processes, and law. From a clinical standpoint, it entails behaviours similar to other forms of addiction, including compulsiveness, tolerance, withdrawal symptoms, and continued usage despite negative outcomes, all of which resonate with psychological and neurocognitive theories of impulsiveness, reflective control, and interoception. In treatment, research indicates that psychotherapy techniques, including CBT, relapse prevention through mindfulness training, ACT, and EMDR, have been proven to be the most effective means to address the condition, with pharmacotherapy, such as SSRIs and naltrexone, acting as complementary tools. A multimodal therapeutic strategy that emphasizes psychoeducation, cognitive restructuring, and relapse prevention is paramount, especially in cases where other conditions coexist, for instance, depression, anxiety disorders, trauma, and sexual dysfunction. The addition of Compulsive Sexual Behavior Disorder (CSBD) in ICD-11 is an important step from a policy point of view, but at the same time, there are issues associated with its definition that pose problems regarding stigmatization of normal sexuality. There needs to be a fine balance between freedom, sexual wellness, and safeguarding individuals from any kind of harm through legislation, including problems such as verifying someone's age, making the platform liable, and personalizing using technology. Generative AI and deepfake technology bring about novel forms of harm such as identity violation, non-consensual sexualizing of victims, and amplified distribution of AI-generated content depicting intimate images. Victims suffer unique types of trauma, while the offenders receive the advantage of low barriers of entry. The existing legal regime proves to be inadequate as it does not provide for proper criminalization of deep-fake production, victim rights, nor platform liability. In the future, policies need to emphasize the importance of victim-centric approaches, law reforms, mandated AI requirements, and international coordination efforts. Additionally, educational programs should extend to encompass synthetic media awareness, which will allow young people to identify deepfakes and grasp consent violation issues. Policies differ from one country to another, from criminalizing non-consensual production of pornography and deepfake content to developing ineffective policies. Preventive methods involve providing comprehensive sex education, pornography literacy, and digital wellbeing via school curriculum, parental mediation, and community sensitization programs. These preventive efforts have to be integrated into health education that focuses on emotion regulation, stress management, and media literacy skills. However, issues in terms of preparedness for professionals, longitudinal evaluations, and adaptation to fast-changing digital contexts still exist.There is a need for future research to focus on addressing methodological flaws such as a lack of diversity in male heterosexual samples and inadequate experimental design. It would also be necessary to conduct longitudinal, cross-cultural, and multimodal investigations to determine the trajectory of development, risk factors, and biological underpinnings. There is also a need to investigate alternative pathways to addiction such as habitual consumption, trauma, difficulties in forming attachments, and moral incongruity while examining the influence of sexual gratification, quality of relationships, and platform characteristics.

CONFLICT OF INTEREST STATEMENT

The authors declare no competing interests.

REFERENCES

Adamus, S., Bielski, K., Szatkowska, I., Gola, M., & Draps, M. (2025). Exploring the role of the amygdala in Compulsive Sexual Behavior Disorder via a parcellation pipeline based on Recurrence Quantification Analysis. *Journal of Behavioral Addictions, 14*(1), 204–219. DOI: 10.1556/2006.2025.00014 PMID: 40063093

Aghamiri, F. S., Luetz, J. M., & Hills, K. (2024). Why did God let this Happen? Assessing the Spiritual Impacts of Sexual Addiction on Intimate Female Partners: A Qualitative Investigation. *Sexuality & Culture, 28*, 2113–2142. DOI: 10.1007/s12119-024-10221-3

Ardhanariswari, R., Azzahro, F., Fauzan, M., Pamuji, K., & Murniati, T. (2026). Digital Technology as a Tool for Fulfilling Women's Rights: A Legal Analysis of Online Gender-based Violence (OGBV) Within the Framework of SDG 5. *KnE Social Sciences, 11*(1), 213–234. DOI: 10.18502/kss.v11i1.20610

Bibi, K., Fatima, A., Amin, R., & Rowland, D. L. (2022). Understanding Serial Mediators of Problematic Pornography Use in Pakistani Men and Women. *International Journal of Environmental Research and Public Health, 19*(21), 14336. DOI: 10.3390/ijerph192114336 PMID: 36361229

Brand, M., Wegmann, E., Stark, R., Müller, A., Wölfling, K., Robbins, T. W., & Potenza, M. N. (2019). The Interaction of Person-Affect-Cognition-Execution (I-PACE) model for addictive behaviors: Update, generalization to addictive behaviors beyond internet-use disorders, and specification of the process character of addictive behaviors. *Neuroscience and Biobehavioral Reviews, 104*, 1–10. DOI: 10.1016/j.neubiorev.2019.06.032 PMID: 31247240

Brand, M., Young, K. S., & Laier, C. (2014). Prefrontal control and online addiction: A theoretical model and review of neuropsychological and neuroimaging findings. *Frontiers in Human Neuroscience, 8*, 375. DOI: 10.3389/fnhum.2014.00375 PMID: 24904393

Brand, M., Young, K. S., Laier, C., Wölfling, K., & Potenza, M. N. (2016). Integrating psychological and neurobiological considerations regarding the development and maintenance of specific Internet-use disorders: An Interaction of Person-Affect-Cognition-Execution (I-PACE) model. *Neuroscience and Biobehavioral Reviews, 71*, 252–266. DOI: 10.1016/j.neubiorev.2016.08.033 PMID: 27590829

Cardoso, J., Ramos, C., Brito, J., & Almeida, T. C. (2022, April). Predictors of Pornography Use: Difficulties in Emotion Regulation and Loneliness. *Journal of Sexual Medicine, 19*(4), 620–628. DOI: 10.1016/j.jsxm.2022.01.005 PMID: 35165051

Carnes, S., & Love, T. (2017). Separating Models Obscures the Scientific Underpinnings of Sex Addiction as a Disorder. *Archives of Sexual Behavior, 46*(8), 2253–2256. DOI: 10.1007/s10508-017-1072-8 PMID: 28948394

Chen, L., Wang, D., Wang, H., Zhang, Y., & Jiang, X. (2023). Moderating Role of Sexual Attitudes in the Association between Online Sexual Activity and Problematic Pornography Use: Evidence from the Chinese Community and Help-Seeking Men. *International Journal of Sexual Health : Official Journal of the World Association for Sexual Health, 35*(4), 555–572. DOI: 10.1080/19317611.2023.2257688 PMID: 38601807

Christensen, E., Albertella, L., Chamberlain, S. R., Suo, C., Brydevall, M., Grant, J. E., Yücel, M., & Lee, R. S. C. (2024). A comprehensive evaluation of the neurocognitive predictors of problematic alcohol use, eating, pornography, and internet use: A 6-month longitudinal study. *Journal of Behavioral Addictions, 13*(3), 823–840. DOI: 10.1556/2006.2024.00041 PMID: 39141435

Dalbudak, E., Evren, C., Aldemir, S., & Evren, B. (2014). The severity of Internet addiction risk and its relationship with the severity of borderline personality features, childhood traumas, dissociative experiences, depression and anxiety symptoms among Turkish university students. *Psychiatry Research, 219*(3), 577–582. DOI: 10.1016/j.psychres.2014.02.032 PMID: 25023365

de Alarcón, R., de la Iglesia, J. I., Casado, N. M., & Montejo, A. L. (2019). Online Porn Addiction: What We Know and What We Don't-A Systematic Review. *Journal of Clinical Medicine, 8*(1), 91. DOI: 10.3390/jcm8010091 PMID: 30650522

Deleuze, J., Rochat, L., Romo, L., Van der Linden, M., Achab, S., Thorens, G., Khazaal, Y., Zullino, D., Maurage, P., Rothen, S., & Billieux, J. (2015). Prevalence and characteristics of addictive behaviors in a community sample: A latent class analysis. *Addictive Behaviors Reports, 1*, 49–56. DOI: 10.1016/j.abrep.2015.04.001 PMID: 29531979

Dinçer, E. M., Durmuş, H., Demirgül, S. A., Kavla, Y., Kitapçıoğlu, S., Aktürk, İ., Bozdemir, T., Sandıkçı, T., Büyükçorak, M., & Barış, F. Y. (2025). A roadmap to online pornography use: Research, assessment, and treatment. *Addicta : The Turkish Journal on Addictions, 12*(4), 498–514. DOI: 10.5152/ADDICTA.2025.25572

Draps, M., Kowalczyk-Grębska, N., Marchewka, A., Shi, F., & Gola, M. (2021). White matter microstructural and Compulsive Sexual Behaviors Disorder - Diffusion Tensor Imaging study. *Journal of Behavioral Addictions, 10*(1), 55–64. DOI: 10.1556/2006.2021.00002 PMID: 33570504

Draps, M., Sescousse, G., Potenza, M. N., Marchewka, A., Duda, A., Lew-Starowicz, M., Kopera, M., Jakubczyk, A., Wojnar, M., & Gola, M. (2020). Gray Matter Volume Differences in Impulse Control and Addictive Disorders-An Evidence From a Sample of Heterosexual Males. *Journal of Sexual Medicine, 17*(9), 1761–1769. DOI: 10.1016/j.jsxm.2020.05.007 PMID: 32690426

Duffy, A., Dawson, D. L., & das Nair, R. (2016). Pornography Addiction in Adults: A Systematic Review of Definitions and Reported Impact. *Journal of Sexual Medicine, 13*(5), 760–777. DOI: 10.1016/j.jsxm.2016.03.002 PMID: 27114191

Everitt, B. J., & Robbins, T. W. (2016). Drug Addiction: Updating Actions to Habits to Compulsions Ten Years On. *Annual Review of Psychology, 67*(1), 23–50. DOI: 10.1146/annurev-psych-122414-033457 PMID: 26253543

Fattore, L., & Melis, M. (2016). Exploring gender and sex differences in behavioral dyscontrol: From drug addiction to impulse control disorders. *Frontiers in Psychiatry, 7*, 19. DOI: 10.3389/fpsyt.2016.00019 PMID: 26941657

Gola, M., Lewczuk, K., Potenza, M. N., Kingston, D. A., Grubbs, J. B., Stark, R., & Reid, R. C. (2020). What should be included in the criteria for compulsive sexual behavior disorder? *Journal of Behavioral Addictions, 11*(2), 160–165. DOI: 10.1556/2006.2020.00090 PMID: 34329192

Gola, M., Wordecha, M., Sescousse, G., Lew-Starowicz, M., Kossowski, B., Wypych, M., Makeig, S., Potenza, M. N., & Marchewka, A. (2017). Can Pornography be Addictive? An fMRI Study of Men Seeking Treatment for Problematic Pornography Use. *Neuropsychopharmacology : Official Publication of the American College of Neuropsychopharmacology, 42*(10), 2021–2031. DOI: 10.1038/npp.2017.78 PMID: 28409565

Golec, K., Draps, M., Stark, R., Pluta, A., & Gola, M. (2021). Aberrant orbitofrontal cortex reactivity to erotic cues in compulsive sexual behavior disorder. *Journal of Behavioral Addictions, 10*(3), 646–656. Advance online publication. DOI: 10.1556/2006.2021.00051 PMID: 34437297

Görts, P., Savard, J., Görts-Öberg, K., Dhejne, C., Arver, S., Jokinen, J., Ingvar, M., & Abé, C. (2023). Structural brain differences related to compulsive sexual behavior disorder. *Journal of Behavioral Addictions, 12*(1), 278–287. DOI: 10.1556/2006.2023.00008 PMID: 36943775

Grant, J. E., Boutouis, S., Collins, M., & Chamberlain, S. R. (2025). Compulsive sexual behavior disorder: Rates and clinical correlates in a community sample. *Frontiers in Psychiatry, 16*, 1561885. DOI: 10.3389/fpsyt.2025.1561885 PMID: 40475952

Grubbs, J. B., & Kraus, S. W. (2021). Pornography use and psychological science: A call for consideration. *Current Directions in Psychological Science, 30*(1), 68–75. DOI: 10.1177/0963721420979594

Hanseder, S., & Dantas, J. A. R. (2023). Males' Lived Experience with Self-Perceived Pornography Addiction: A Qualitative Study of Problematic Porn Use. *International Journal of Environmental Research and Public Health, 20*(2), 1497. DOI: 10.3390/ijerph20021497 PMID: 36674250

Harun, N. U., Jaafar, A. B., Razak, T. M. T. A., Rahman, N. A. A., & Musah, N. S. M. (2025). A Comprehensive Review of the Psychological, Societal, and Technological Dimensions of Pornography Use and Impact. *International Journal of Research and Innovation in Applied Science, 9*(24), 977–984.

Ince, C., Antons, S., Ashton, S., Borgogna, N. C., Brand, M., Briken, P., Castro-Calvo, J., Chen, L., Coleman, E., Efrati, Y., Fernández, D. P., Fuss, J., Gleason, N., Gola, M., Jennings, T. L., Kowalewska, E., Kraus, S. W., Lewczuk, K., Grubbs, J. B., & Bőthe, B. (2026). Compulsive sexual behavior disorder (CSBD) and problematic pornography use (PPU): A comprehensive, interdisciplinary, and expert-informed narrative review with suggested future directions. *Journal of Behavioral Addictions, 15*(1), 32–98. DOI: 10.1556/2006.2025.00337 PMID: 41879870

Jaiswal, N., Deshpande, S., Gokani, N., Sahore, A., & Gowande, T. (2025). Understanding Pornography Addiction in India: Insights from a Retrospective, Observational Study. *BJPsych Open, 11*(S1, Suppl 1), S46. DOI: 10.1192/bjo.2025.10153

Jennings, T. L., Gleason, N., Pachankis, J. E., Bőthe, B., & Kraus, S. W. (2024). LGBQ-affirming clinical recommendations for compulsive sexual behavior disorder. *Journal of Behavioral Addictions, 13*(2), 413–428. DOI: 10.1556/2006.2024.00012 PMID: 38592797

Kaplan, M., Lazter, Y., Bőthe, B., & Gewirtz Meydan, A. (2025). The Sacred, the Sinful, and the Shamed: The Association Between Compulsive Sexual Behavior, Moral Disapproval, and Sexual Shame Among Jewish Religious Adolescents. *International Journal of Sexual Health : Official Journal of the World Association for Sexual Health*, *37*(3), 486–502. DOI: 10.1080/19317611.2025.2530511 PMID: 40843156

Kató, S., Pintér-Eszenyei, Z. G., Rándo Hurtado, M. A., Csinády, A. K., & Szemán-Nagy, A. (2024). Associations of sexual dysfunction with problematic pornography use and attachment styles: A cross-sectional study of Hungarian-Spanish samples. *European Psychiatry : The Journal of the Association of European Psychiatrists*, *67*(S1, Suppl 1), S49–S50. DOI: 10.1192/j.eurpsy.2024.153

Kor, A., Zilcha-Mano, S., Fogel, Y. A., Mikulincer, M., Reid, R. C., & Potenza, M. N. (2014). Psychometric development of the Problematic Pornography Use Scale. *Addictive Behaviors*, *39*(5), 861–868. DOI: 10.1016/j.addbeh.2014.01.027 PMID: 24583276

Kowalewska, E., Gola, M., Kraus, S. W., & Lew-Starowicz, M. (2020). Spotlight on Compulsive Sexual Behavior Disorder: A Systematic Review of Research on Women. *Neuropsychiatric Disease and Treatment*, *16*, 2025–2043. DOI: 10.2147/NDT.S221540 PMID: 32943868

Kraus, S. W., & Sweeney, P. J. (2019). Hitting the Target: Considerations for Differential Diagnosis When Treating Individuals for Problematic Use of Pornography. *Archives of Sexual Behavior*, *48*(2), 431–435. DOI: 10.1007/s10508-018-1301-9 PMID: 30229519

Kumar, S., & Saxena, G. (2021). Child online pornography: Criminal methods and investigation. In *Combating the exploitation of children in cyberspace: Emerging research and opportunities* (pp. 117–145). IGI Global., DOI: 10.4018/978-1-7998-2360-5.ch006

Laier, C., Schulte, F. P., & Brand, M. (2013). Pornographic picture processing interferes with working memory performance. *Journal of Sex Research*, *50*(7), 642–652. DOI: 10.1080/00224499.2012.716873 PMID: 23167900

Lewczuk, K., Wizła, M., Glica, A., & Dwulit, A. D. (2024). Compulsive Sexual Behavior Disorder and Problematic Pornography Use in Cisgender Sexual Minority Individuals: The Associations with Minority Stress, Social Support, and Sexualized Drug Use. *Journal of Sex Research*, *61*(8), 1246–1260. DOI: 10.1080/00224499.2023.2245399 PMID: 37676791

Lochner, C., van den Berg, G., Chamberlain, S. R., Marincowitz, C., & Coetzee, B. (2024). Family functioning and problematic usage of the internet in youth: A cross-sectional investigation. *Journal of Psychiatric Research, 173*, 239–244. DOI: 10.1016/j.jpsychires.2024.03.038 PMID: 38554619

Love, T., Laier, C., Brand, M., Hatch, L., & Hajela, R. (2015). Neuroscience of Internet Pornography Addiction: A Review and Update. *Behavioral Sciences (Basel, Switzerland), 5*(3), 388–433. DOI: 10.3390/bs5030388 PMID: 26393658

Marchetti, I. (2023). The Structure of Compulsive Sexual Behavior: A Network Analysis Study. *Archives of Sexual Behavior, 52*(3), 1271–1284. DOI: 10.1007/s10508-023-02549-y PMID: 36735169

Morgan, C., & Klein, C. (2024). How online data informs forensic mental health evaluations of sexual behavior: An overview. *Behavioral Sciences & the Law, 42*(3), 186–204. DOI: 10.1002/bsl.2650 PMID: 38459739

Odlaug, B. L., Lust, K., Schreiber, L. R., Christenson, G., Derbyshire, K., Harvanko, A., Golden, D., & Grant, J. E. (2013). Compulsive sexual behavior in young adults. *Annals of Clinical Psychiatry, 25*(3), 193–200. DOI: 10.1177/104012371302500305 PMID: 23926574

Paquette, M. M., Bergeron, S., Bigras, N., Koós, M., Nagy, L., Kraus, S. W., Demetrovics, Z., Potenza, M. N., Ballester-Arnal, R., Batthyány, D., Billieux, J., Briken, P., Burkauskas, J., Cárdenas-López, G., Carvalho, J., Castro-Calvo, J., Chen, L., Ciocca, G., Corazza, O., & Bőthe, B. (2025). Sexual satisfaction across cultures, genders, languages, and sexual orientations: Validation of the Global Measure of Sexual Satisfaction. *Psychology of Sexual Orientation and Gender Diversity*. Advance online publication. DOI: 10.1037/sgd0000774

Paulus, F. W., Ohmann, S., von Gontard, A., & Popow, C. (2018). Internet gaming disorder in children and adolescents: A systematic review. *Developmental Medicine and Child Neurology, 60*(7), 645–659. DOI: 10.1111/dmcn.13754 PMID: 29633243

Peng, Z., Jia, Q., Mao, J., Luo, X., Huang, A., Zheng, H., Jiang, S., Ma, Q., Ma, C., & Yi, Q. (2025). Neurotransmitters crosstalk and regulation in the reward circuit of subjects with behavioral addiction. *Frontiers in Psychiatry, 15*, 1439727. DOI: 10.3389/fpsyt.2024.1439727 PMID: 39876994

Peter, J., & Valkenburg, P. M. (2016). Adolescents and Pornography: A Review of 20 Years of Research. *Journal of Sex Research, 53*(4-5), 509–531. DOI: 10.1080/00224499.2016.1143441 PMID: 27105446

Robinson, T. E., & Berridge, K. C. (2025). The Incentive-Sensitization Theory of Addiction 30 Years On. *Annual Review of Psychology*, *76*(1), 29–58. DOI: 10.1146/annurev-psych-011624-024031 PMID: 39094061

Schmidt, C., Morris, L. S., Kvamme, T. L., Hall, P., Birchard, T., & Voon, V. (2017). Compulsive sexual behavior: Prefrontal and limbic volume and interactions. *Human Brain Mapping*, *38*(3), 1182–1190. DOI: 10.1002/hbm.23447 PMID: 27787929

Seto, M. C. (2015). *Internet sexual offending: Theory, practice, and policy*. American Psychological Association., DOI: 10.1037/14644-000

Shafly, M. S. N., Ahadiah, H. R., Syadza, L., Algristian, H., & Setyorini, D. (2025). Compulsive Sexual Behavior as a Maladaptive Coping Mechanism in Bipolar Affective Disorder: A Case Report. *Sinergi International Journal of Psychology*, *3*(3), 137–147. DOI: 10.61194/psychology.v3i3.785

Singh, R. (2024). Cyber pornography and its control mechanisms: An evaluation. *Research Review*, *9*(12), 73–78.

Stark, R., Markert, C., Kruse, O., Walter, B., Strahler, J., & Klein, S. (2022). Individual cortisol response to acute stress influences neural processing of sexual cues. *Journal of Behavioral Addictions*, *11*(2), 506–519. DOI: 10.1556/2006.2022.00037 PMID: 35895611

Tomei, A., Studer, J., & Gmel, G. (2021). Prosocialness in young males with substance and behavioral addictions. *Journal of Behavioral Addictions*, *10*(2), 327–337. DOI: 10.1556/2006.2021.00035 PMID: 34191744

Wdowiak, K., Maciocha, A., & Wąż, J. (2025). Pornography through the lens of the 21st century and its impact on society. *Journal of Psychiatry & Clinical Psychology/Psychiatria i Psychologia Kliniczna, 25*(2). https://doi.org/DOI: 10.15557/PiPK.2025.0018

Wegmann, E., Antons, S., Schmidt, L. D., Klein, L., Montag, C., Rumpf, H. J., Müller, S. M., & Brand, M. (2025). Feels good, and less bad: Problematic use of the Internet is associated with heightened experiences of both gratification and compensation. *Journal of Behavioral Addictions*, *14*(1), 263–275. DOI: 10.1556/2006.2024.00067 PMID: 39786377

Wéry, A., Deleuze, J., Canale, N., & Billieux, J. (2018). Emotionally laden impulsivity interacts with affect in predicting addictive use of online sexual activity in men. *Comprehensive Psychiatry*, *80*, 192–201. DOI: 10.1016/j.comppsych.2017.10.004 PMID: 29128857

Willis, M., Bridges, A. J., & Sun, C. (2022). Pornography use, gender, and sexual objectification: A multinational study. *Sexuality & Culture, 26*(4), 1298–1313. DOI: 10.1007/s12119-022-09943-z

Wizła, M., & Lewczuk, K. (2024). The Associations Between Attachment Insecurity and Compulsive Sexual Behavior Disorder or Problematic Pornography Use: The Mediating Role of Emotion Regulation Difficulties. *Archives of Sexual Behavior, 53*(9), 3419–3436. DOI: 10.1007/s10508-024-02904-7 PMID: 38898361

Wojciechowski, J., Draps, M., Kublik, E., Dubiejko, P., Wolak, T., & Gola, M. (2025). Enhanced conditioning and disrupted extinction processes in men struggling with compulsive sexual behaviors. *Journal of Behavioral Addictions, 14*(1), 191–203. DOI: 10.1556/2006.2025.00012 PMID: 40014056

Wright, P. J., Tokunaga, R. S., & Herbenick, D. (2025). Pornography Use, Moral Incongruence, Psychological Distress, and Sexual Satisfaction. *Archives of Sexual Behavior, 54*(1), 7–17. DOI: 10.1007/s10508-024-03055-5 PMID: 39718733

ADDITIONAL READING

Bayer, H. M., & Glimcher, P. W. (2005). Midbrain dopamine neurons encode a quantitative reward prediction error signal. *Neuron, 47*(1), 129–141. DOI: 10.1016/j.neuron.2005.05.020 PMID: 15996553

Briken, P., Bőthe, B., Carvalho, J., Coleman, E., Giraldi, A., Kraus, S. W., Lew-Starowicz, M., & Pfaus, J. G. (2024). Assessment and treatment of compulsive sexual behavior disorder: A sexual medicine perspective. *Sexual Medicine Reviews, 12*(3), 355–370. DOI: 10.1093/sxmrev/qeae014 PMID: 38529667

Donevan, M. (2025, March). Exposing pornography's true nature: A conceptual framework. In *Women's Studies International Forum* (Vol. 109, p. 103029). Pergamon. https://doi.org/DOI: 10.1016/j.wsif.2024.103029

Fineberg, N. A., Menchón, J. M., Hall, N., Dell'Osso, B., Brand, M., Potenza, M. N., Chamberlain, S. R., Cirnigliaro, G., Lochner, C., Billieux, J., Demetrovics, Z., Rumpf, H. J., Müller, A., Castro-Calvo, J., Hollander, E., Burkauskas, J., Grünblatt, E., Walitza, S., Corazza, O., & Zohar, J. (2022). Advances in problematic usage of the internet research - A narrative review by experts from the European network for problematic usage of the internet. *Comprehensive Psychiatry, 118*, 152346. DOI: 10.1016/j.comppsych.2022.152346 PMID: 36029549

Fineberg, N. A., Menchón, J. M., Hall, N., Dell'Osso, B., Brand, M., Potenza, M. N., Chamberlain, S. R., Cirnigliaro, G., Lochner, C., Billieux, J., Demetrovics, Z., Rumpf, H. J., Müller, A., Castro-Calvo, J., Hollander, E., Burkauskas, J., Grünblatt, E., Walitza, S., Corazza, O., & Zohar, J. (2022). Advances in problematic usage of the internet research - A narrative review by experts from the European network for problematic usage of the internet. *Comprehensive Psychiatry*, *118*, 152346. DOI: 10.1016/j.comppsych.2022.152346 PMID: 36029549

Lee, K. Y., Chen, C. Y., Chen, J. K., Liu, C. C., Chang, K. C., Fung, X. C. C., Chen, J. S., Kao, Y. C., Potenza, M. N., Pakpour, A. H., & Lin, C. Y. (2023). Exploring mediational roles for self-stigma in associations between types of problematic use of internet and psychological distress in youth with ADHD. *Research in Developmental Disabilities*, *133*, 104410. DOI: 10.1016/j.ridd.2022.104410 PMID: 36603311

Müller, S. M., Antons, S., Wegmann, E., Ioannidis, K., King, D. L., Potenza, M. N., Chamberlain, S. R., & Brand, M. (2023). A systematic review and meta-analysis of risky decision-making in specific domains of problematic use of the internet: Evidence across different decision-making tasks. *Neuroscience and Biobehavioral Reviews*, *152*, 105271. DOI: 10.1016/j.neubiorev.2023.105271 PMID: 37277009

Privara, M., & Bob, P. (2023, August 1). Pornography Consumption and Cognitive-Affective Distress. *The Journal of Nervous and Mental Disease*, *211*(8), 641–646. DOI: 10.1097/NMD.0000000000001669 PMID: 37505898

Sharpe, M., & Mead, D. (2021). Problematic Pornography Use: Legal and Health Policy Considerations. *Current Addiction Reports*, *8*(4), 556–567. DOI: 10.1007/s40429-021-00390-8 PMID: 34518793

Zare-Bidoky, M., Baldacchino, A. M., Demetrovics, Z., Fineberg, N. A., Kamali, M., Khazaal, Y., Potenza, M. N., Stein, D. J., & Ekhtiari, H. (2025). Problematic usage of the internet: Converging and diverging terminologies and constructs. Journal of behavioral addictions, 2006.2025.00085. Advance online publication. https://doi.org/DOI: 10.1556/2006.2025.00085

KEY TERMS AND DEFINITIONS

Child Sexual Abuse Material (CSAM): Child Sexual Abuse Material (CSAM), which is also known legally as child pornography, is defined by the images depicting sexual activity where the child may either have participated or been a part of virtually. The term "Child Sexual Exploitation Material (CSEM)" may be applied to denote all sexual imagery containing images of children except for CSAM (Kumar, S., & Saxena, G. (2021).

Compulsive Sexual Behaviour Disorder (CSBD): The characteristics of QE83 according to the ICD-11 criteria can be listed as follows: (a) loss of control over one's sexual drives or actions, (b) an escalation in the intensity or frequency necessary to derive gratification, (c) persistence regardless of adverse effects on health, relationships, job, and finances, and (d) a functional disturbance for at least a period of six months (Gola et al., 2020).

Compulsive sexual behaviour disorder: is an impulse-control disease, not an addiction (Gola et al., 2022). The CSBD (ICD-11) defines a persistent loss of control of sexual impulses in a period of 6 months or longer, which involves pornography, masturbation, commercial sex, and partnered sex (Ince et al., 2026).

Moral Incongruence: "Moral Incongruence," a form of psychological discomfort, arises when there is an inconsistency between the sexual behaviors of an individual and the moral/ethical values held by that individual. Belief violation rather than dysfunction (professional/personal consequences) forms the basis of distress among people. Particularly common in religious and conservative societies; non-existent in liberal societies (Jaiswal et al., 2025).

Online Pornography Addiction (OPA): Online Pornography Addiction (OPA) is a colloquial word (not a diagnostic category in DSM-5 or ICD-11) that characterizes addiction-like behaviors associated with pornography use via digital platforms. Emphasizes the obsession aspect, tolerance (requires greater stimulation or novelty), withdrawal effects (irritation and anxiety due to limited access), and the continuity of activity despite negative repercussions. Increasingly recognized within academic studies alongside CSBD, although there is controversy concerning the precise definition of the term (Basu & Dalal, 2016).

Online pornography consumption: is the most common behavioral expression (Gola et al., 2022) and denotes a lack of control over online pornography consumption—characterized by an inability to regulate frequency, duration, or content—alongside functional impairment in personal, occupational, social, or relational spheres (Chen et al., 2022).

Pornography-Watching Disorder (PWD): is a disorder that is assessed using DSM-5 substance use criteria, which deals with impaired control, salience, mood modulation, interpersonal conflict, tolerance, and persistence despite negative outcomes (Erdosz et al., 2025).

Chapter 6
The Influence of Online Pornography on Young Learners:
Shaping Minds and Distorting Realities

Ratan Sarkar
http://orcid.org/0009-0008-5480-0165
Tezpur University, India

ABSTRACT

The rapid expansion of digital media has reshaped childhood and adolescence, transforming how young learners access information, form identities, and understand relationships. A critical yet underexplored consequence is minors' increasing exposure to online pornography. This chapter frames online pornography as a technology-mediated developmental challenge within the broader context of technology addiction and digital disorders. Drawing on interdisciplinary research across psychology, neuroscience, education, sociology, and policy studies, it examines exposure pathways, algorithmic drivers, and the cognitive, emotional, behavioral, and socio-cultural impacts on adolescents. The analysis highlights adolescents' heightened vulnerability due to ongoing brain development, limited impulse control, and inadequate educational and parental guidance. Focusing on India, the chapter advocates shifting from censorship-based approaches toward evidence-informed, public health–oriented interventions involving families, schools, policymakers, and digital platforms.

DOI: 10.4018/979-8-2600-2468-3.ch006

1. INTRODUCTION

The rapid expansion of digital technologies has profoundly reshaped the social, cognitive, and emotional environments in which children and adolescents grow and learn (Romer, 2016). Digital devices are no longer peripheral tools but central mediators of everyday experience, influencing how young learners acquire knowledge, construct identities, and engage with peers and wider society. Internet connectivity, mobile technologies, and algorithm-driven platforms have transformed childhood and adolescence into increasingly digitized life stages, characterized by continuous access to information, entertainment, and social interaction (Schmitt & Woolf, 2018; Ng, 2015). While these transformations have opened new educational and communicative possibilities, they have simultaneously introduced novel risks that existing social, educational, and regulatory frameworks are often ill-equipped to address (Turner et al., 2017).

One of the less visible yet deeply consequential outcomes of this digital transformation is the increasing exposure of minor-age learners to online pornographic content (Chatterjee & Kar, 2023). In earlier eras, access to pornography was constrained by physical, legal, and social barriers that, despite their limitations, delayed exposure until adulthood for many individuals (Carnevali et al., 2022). In contrast, contemporary digital environments have dismantled these barriers. Pornographic material is now accessible through personal and often privately used devices, frequently without effective age-verification mechanisms, contextual warnings, or adult mediation (Przybylski & Nash, 2018). The portability, anonymity, and immediacy of digital media have rendered pornography a readily available component of the online ecosystem encountered by young learners, sometimes unintentionally and at increasingly early ages (Byron, 2023).

This shift is not merely a matter of increased availability but reflects a structural transformation in how sexual content is produced, distributed, and consumed. Online pornography operates within platform-based economies driven by attention, engagement, and algorithmic optimization (Daneback & Ross, 2011). Recommendation systems, data-driven personalization, and commercial imperatives amplify exposure by prioritizing content that maximizes user retention, often without regard for developmental appropriateness (Massey et al., 2020). Consequently, young learners may encounter sexually explicit material not solely through deliberate seeking but through algorithmic spillovers, pop-up advertisements, hyperlinks, or peer-mediated sharing. Such exposure situates pornography within the broader architecture of digital capitalism rather than framing it as an isolated or purely individual choice (Healy-Cullen et al., 2021).

The implications of this transformation are particularly significant for children and adolescents, whose cognitive, emotional, and neurological development is still in progress (Marciano et al., 2025). Adolescence represents a critical period for the formation of sexual understanding, moral reasoning, impulse control, and relational norms. When exposure to pornography occurs during this formative stage, it intersects with developmental vulnerabilities, potentially shaping perceptions of intimacy, consent, gender roles, and sexuality in ways that are misaligned with healthy relational development. Unlike formal educational contexts, online pornography offers no pedagogical structure, ethical framing, or emphasis on mutual respect, yet it may function as a de facto source of sexual knowledge for many young learners (Maas et al., 2025).

Despite the magnitude of these concerns, public and academic discourse has often oscillated between moral panic and permissive neglect. Moralistic approaches tend to frame pornography exposure as a problem of individual immorality or parental failure, while libertarian perspectives emphasize personal freedom and technological inevitability (Maes et al., 2024). Both positions obscure the complexity of the issue and divert attention from the systemic forces- technological design, Crabbe, educational gaps, and cultural silence- that shape young people's digital experiences. As a result, responses remain fragmented, reactive, and insufficiently grounded in developmental and educational research (Thorneycroft et al., 2024).

The increasing exposure of minor-age learners to online pornography therefore raises critical concerns for education, mental health, and child development that demand systematic academic inquiry (Maes et al., 2024). Understanding this phenomenon requires moving beyond simplistic binaries of prohibition versus permissiveness and toward an integrative analysis that recognizes online pornography as a technology-mediated developmental challenge. Such an approach must account for the interaction between digital infrastructures, adolescent neurodevelopment, sociocultural norms, and institutional responses (Rojas-Estrada et al., 2024). Situating pornography consumption within the broader framework of technology addiction and digital disorders provides a valuable lens through which to examine its causes, consequences, and potential interventions in a rapidly evolving digital landscape.

1.1 Background and Context

Childhood and adolescence in the twenty-first century are increasingly shaped by digital environments (Bozzola, 2021). Smartphones, tablets, and personal computers provide young learners with unprecedented access to information, entertainment, and social interaction (Schmitt & Woolf, 2018). While digital technologies offer significant educational and developmental opportunities, they also expose children to content that was previously inaccessible or heavily regulated (Robb & Lauricella, 2014). Sexual content, particularly online pornography, has become a routine part of the digital landscape encountered by many adolescents, often unintentionally and at increasingly younger ages (Paulus et al., 2024).

Historically, access to pornographic material was limited by physical, social, and legal barriers. These barriers acted- however imperfectly- as filters that delayed exposure until adulthood (Przybylski & Nash, 2018). In contrast, contemporary digital ecosystems are characterized by constant connectivity, privacy of use, and algorithmic content delivery systems designed to maximize engagement. As a result, pornographic material is no longer confined to intentional searches but may appear through advertisements, pop-ups, hyperlinks, or recommendation algorithms embedded within mainstream platforms (Nesi, 2022). This ubiquity has transformed pornography from a marginal phenomenon into a normalized component of digital media consumption (Rainwater, 1974).

Importantly, the contemporary debate on pornography exposure among minors must move beyond moralistic framings that focus solely on notions of obscenity or individual deviance. Online pornography is fundamentally a technology-mediated phenomenon, shaped by platform architectures, commercial incentives, and algorithmic logics (Thorneycroft et al., 2024). Its widespread availability is not simply a consequence of adolescent curiosity but a structural outcome of digital economies that monetize attention and arousal. Understanding pornography consumption among young learners therefore requires situating it within broader discussions of technology use, digital cultures, and behavioral addictions (Rojas-Estrada et al., 2024).

From an educational and developmental perspective, this context is particularly significant. Adolescence is a critical period of identity formation, sexual development, and cognitive maturation (Coyle et al., 2015). The meanings that young learners attach to intimacy, consent, gender roles, and relationships are shaped during this phase. When pornography becomes a primary or unmediated source of sexual knowledge, it risks distorting these understandings in ways that have long-term consequences for psychological wellbeing and social relationships (Vertongen et al., 2022).

1.2 Problem Statement

Despite growing recognition of technology-related addictions, the exposure of minor-age learners to online pornography remains inadequately addressed within educational and policy frameworks (Crabbe & Flood, 2021). Evidence indicates that adolescents are frequently exposed to such content at early developmental stages, where heightened reward sensitivity and underdeveloped impulse control increase susceptibility to compulsive engagement and distorted sexual learning (Chatterjee & Kar, 2023; Vertongen et al., 2022; Bava et al., 2010). Rather than being incidental, this exposure is amplified by the highly stimulating and reinforcing nature of digital sexual content, which can shape behavioral patterns, emotional responses, and expectations regarding intimacy and relationships (Vertongen et al., 2022).

Critically, this issue is sustained not merely by individual vulnerability but by systemic failures across key social institutions. Persistent taboos within families limit open communication, educational systems often lack comprehensive sexuality education and media literacy, and policy frameworks inadequately regulate everyday access to pornography on mainstream platforms (Dawson et al., 2024; Rojas-Estrada et al., 2024; Flood, 2009). As a result, adolescents are left to navigate complex digital environments without adequate guidance or critical tools. This institutional fragmentation transforms pornography exposure from a peripheral risk into a normalized and enduring developmental challenge, highlighting the limitations of framing the issue as individual behavior rather than as a structurally embedded problem requiring coordinated intervention (Massey et al., 2020; Roberto, 2023).

1.3 Objectives of the Chapter

The objectives of the chapter are as follows

1. To examine the prevalence, causes, and patterns of online pornography use among minor-age students
2. To analyze neuropsychological, behavioral, and socio-cultural impacts of early exposure
3. To explore technological and algorithmic drivers facilitating compulsive use
4. To situate online pornography addiction within the broader framework of technology addictions and digital disorders
5. To propose multi-level intervention strategies

2. REVIEW OF LITERATURE

The expanding body of scholarship on online pornography reflects growing concern regarding its psychological, social, and developmental implications. However, the literature remains marked by conceptual inconsistencies, a disproportionate focus on adult populations, and a strong Western orientation. Addressing these limitations, this review synthesizes research on the conceptualization, prevalence, neuropsychological effects, and socio-cultural consequences of online pornography, while highlighting gaps in the Indian context and the fragmented nature of interdisciplinary inquiry.

2.1 Conceptualizing Online Pornography Use

Online pornography is generally defined as sexually explicit material intended to elicit sexual arousal and disseminated through digital platforms such as websites, social media, streaming services, and mobile applications (Franjic, 2022). Despite this broad definition, the literature emphasizes the need to differentiate between varying forms and intensities of engagement. Scholars commonly distinguish between exposure, use, problematic use, and addiction, each representing qualitatively distinct experiences with different developmental implications (Gonsalves et al., 2015; Sabina et al., 2008).

Exposure typically refers to incidental or unintentional encounters, often arising from pop-up advertisements, algorithmic recommendations, or peer sharing (Flood, 2009). Use denotes intentional but non-problematic consumption, whereas problematic use is characterized by compulsivity, impaired control, and adverse emotional or functional outcomes (Ballester-Arnal et al., 2022). The notion of pornography addiction—though contested—describes persistent, compulsive engagement marked by craving, tolerance, and continued use despite harm (de Alarcón et al., 2019). The absence of consensus on these categories and their diagnostic thresholds contributes to conceptual ambiguity, particularly in adolescent populations whose developmental capacities differ from those of adults (Healy-Cullen et al., 2024).

2.2 Theoretical Perspectives

Understanding adolescents' exposure to online pornography requires a multi-theoretical approach that situates the phenomenon within broader frameworks of media influence, social learning, and digital platform structures. This chapter draws on three complementary perspectives—media effects theory, sexual socialization theory, and platform governance/political economy—to provide a more integrated analytical foundation.

From a media effects perspective, exposure to mediated content is understood to shape attitudes, beliefs, and behaviors through processes such as cultivation, social learning, and cognitive priming (Bandura, 2001; Huesmann, 2007). Pornographic content, characterized by repetitive and often exaggerated representations, may contribute to the normalization of particular sexual scripts and expectations. However, contemporary media effects research also emphasizes that such influences are neither uniform nor deterministic but mediated by individual, social, and contextual factors (Valkenburg & Peter, 2013).

Closely related, sexual socialization theory conceptualizes media as a key agent in shaping individuals' understanding of sexuality, alongside family, peers, and education (Fisher & Barak, 2001). In contexts where open discussions of sexuality are limited, pornography may function as an informal source of sexual knowledge, influencing perceptions of gender roles, consent, and intimacy. Sexual script theory further suggests that repeated exposure to mediated representations can inform internalized expectations about sexual behavior and relationships (Wright, 2011). Importantly, these effects are contingent upon adolescents' interpretive capacities and the availability of alternative sources of information.

Finally, insights from platform governance and digital political economy highlight the structural conditions under which exposure occurs. Digital platforms operate within attention-driven economies that prioritize engagement, personalization, and data extraction (Srnicek, 2017). Algorithmic recommendation systems, autoplay features, and content amplification mechanisms are designed to maximize user retention, often without regard for developmental appropriateness (van Dijck et al., 2018). From this perspective, exposure to online pornography is not merely a function of individual choice but a systemic outcome of platform architectures and commercial incentives. This aligns with broader critiques of surveillance capitalism, where user behavior—including that of minors—is monetized through predictive and engagement-based systems (Zuboff, 2019).

Taken together, these theoretical frameworks enable a more nuanced understanding of online pornography as a technology-mediated, socially embedded, and structurally influenced phenomenon. They move the analysis beyond simplistic causal assumptions, emphasizing the interaction between media content, adolescent development, and digital infrastructures in shaping outcomes.

2.3 Technology Addiction and Digital Disorders

Within the broader framework of behavioral addictions, online pornography is increasingly examined alongside related phenomena such as gaming disorder, social media addiction, and compulsive internet use (Palazzolo, 2023). These frameworks identify shared characteristics, including excessive engagement, diminished control, withdrawal-like symptoms, and functional impairment (Love et al., 2015). Pornography consumption is argued to operate through similar mechanisms, particularly its reliance on immediacy, novelty, and reward-based reinforcement (Blinka et al., 2022).

However, its classification as an addiction remains contested. While certain behavioral addictions, such as gaming disorder, have gained formal diagnostic recognition, compulsive pornography use continues to occupy an ambiguous position, often subsumed under broader constructs such as compulsive sexual behavior or internet addiction (Sancho-Cantus, 2024). Critics warn against the over-pathologization of sexual behavior, whereas proponents emphasize the intensified and technologically mediated nature of online pornography (Love et al., 2015). This debate is especially salient for adolescents, for whom adult diagnostic criteria may be developmentally inappropriate, underscoring the need for age-sensitive conceptual frameworks (Smaniotto et al., 2021).

2.4 Prevalence and Patterns of Use among Adolescents

Empirical evidence consistently demonstrates that a substantial proportion of adolescents encounter online pornography, often at early developmental stages (Bryant, 2009). Global studies indicate that initial exposure frequently occurs during early adolescence and, in some cases, late childhood (Ybarra & Mitchell, 2005). Patterns of engagement vary widely, ranging from occasional, curiosity-driven viewing to more habitual and solitary consumption (Nesi, 2022).

Gender differences are evident, with boys generally reporting higher frequency and more intentional use, while girls tend to report lower engagement but greater emotional discomfort upon exposure (McArthur et al., 2024). However, emerging evidence suggests that these differences may be narrowing as digital access becomes more widespread (Ybarra & Mitchell, 2005). Importantly, many studies emphasize that exposure is often unintentional, challenging assumptions that adolescent pornography use is solely driven by deliberate choice (Field, 2020).

2.5 Neuropsychological Effects of Pornography Consumption

Neuroscientific research offers critical insights into adolescents' heightened vulnerability to online pornography. During adolescence, reward-related neural systems—particularly those associated with dopamine activity—are highly responsive, while executive control functions remain underdeveloped (Adarsh & Sahoo, 2023). Pornographic content, characterized by novelty and high-intensity stimulation, strongly activates these reward pathways, reinforcing repeated engagement (Stark & Klucken, 2017).

Repeated exposure may contribute to desensitization and tolerance, potentially leading individuals to seek increasingly explicit material to maintain arousal. Although most neuroimaging studies focus on adults, scholars argue that these mechanisms may operate more intensely in adolescents due to ongoing brain development (Stark & Klucken, 2017). This raises concerns regarding habit formation, impaired impulse control, and possible long-term alterations in reward processing, particularly when exposure occurs at an early age.

2.6 Psychological and Behavioral Consequences

A substantial body of literature associates problematic pornography use with a range of psychological and behavioral outcomes. Adolescents frequently report emotions such as guilt, shame, anxiety, and confusion, particularly in contexts where sexuality is stigmatized (Bryant, 2009; Peter & Valkenburg, 2016). These emotional responses are often intensified by secrecy and fear of judgment, limiting opportunities for open discussion and guidance (Chatterjee & Kar, 2023).

Behaviorally, excessive consumption has been linked to reduced academic engagement, attention difficulties, and social withdrawal (Schiebener et al., 2015). Some studies also identify associations with compulsive patterns of digital use and reliance on online content for emotional regulation (Vieira & Griffiths, 2024). While causal relationships remain contested, converging evidence suggests that pornography use intersects with broader patterns of psychological vulnerability and digital overuse (Privara & Bob, 2023).

2.7 Socio-cultural and Gender Perspectives

From a socio-cultural standpoint, pornography functions as a significant agent of sexual socialization (Fisher & Barak, 2001). It transmits implicit norms regarding gender, power, and intimacy, often privileging male desire, objectifying women, and marginalizing the role of consent (Allen et al., 1995). In the absence of comprehensive sexuality education, adolescents may rely on pornography as a primary source of sexual knowledge.

Gender-focused research further highlights how repeated exposure can reinforce stereotypical roles and normalize dynamics of dominance and aggression (Li, 2023). However, these effects are not uniform; they are mediated by cultural norms, family communication, and educational contexts (Steyer, 2014). In conservative or patriarchal societies, tensions between publicly endorsed values and privately consumed content may intensify confusion and internal conflict among adolescents (Magis-Weinberg et al., 2021).

2.8 Indian Context: Key Insights and Gaps

In India, research on adolescent pornography consumption remains limited and fragmented (Daneback et al., 2018). Available studies indicate rising exposure driven by rapid digitalization, affordable internet access, and widespread smartphone use (Jiang & Li, 2018). However, cultural taboos surrounding sexuality continue to constrain open dialogue within families and educational institutions (Vinnakota et al., 2021).

The absence of comprehensive sexuality education further increases adolescents' reliance on unregulated online sources for sexual information (Wylie, 2010). At the policy level, regulatory frameworks primarily address extreme forms of sexual exploitation, with insufficient attention to routine access to adult pornography by minors (Green et al., 2020). Weak enforcement and inadequate age-verification mechanisms exacerbate these gaps. Consequently, Indian adolescents navigate a digital environment characterized by high exposure and limited guidance, underscoring the urgent need for context-sensitive research and intervention (Bryant, 2009).

Synthesis of Literature and Research Gap

The literature consistently establishes that adolescent exposure to online pornography is widespread, developmentally significant, and embedded within contemporary digital media ecosystems (Sabina et al., 2008). Interdisciplinary research highlights adolescents' neuropsychological vulnerability to highly stimulating sexual content, with documented links to emotional distress, compulsive behaviors, and distorted understandings of gender, intimacy, and consent (Field, 2020). However, despite this growing body of work, significant conceptual and empirical limitations persist (Massey et al., 2020).

A primary limitation lies in conceptual inconsistency. Studies employ overlapping terms—such as exposure, use, problematic use, and addiction—without clear operational distinctions, while diagnostic frameworks remain contested, particularly for minors (Byun et al., 2008; Yu et al., 2013). These inconsistencies hinder comparability and the development of coherent, developmentally appropriate models (D'Angelo, 2020). Additionally, much of the literature remains disproportionately focused on adult populations or extreme behaviors, with adolescents often treated as a secondary subgroup, thereby overlooking their distinct developmental and psychosocial contexts (Sabina et al., 2008; Maes et al., 2024).

Geographical limitations further constrain the field. Existing research is predominantly Western, reflecting contexts with relatively open sexual discourse and established educational and regulatory frameworks (Mattuck et al., 2005; Simon & Daneback, 2013). In contrast, non-Western contexts—particularly India—remain underrepresented, despite unique conditions shaped by rapid digitalization, cultural conservatism, limited sexuality education, and uneven regulatory enforcement (Adarsh & Sahoo, 2023).

Moreover, the literature is fragmented across disciplinary boundaries. Psychological, neuroscientific, sociological, and educational perspectives often operate in isolation, limiting the development of integrated frameworks capable of capturing pornography consumption as a technology-mediated, developmental, and sociocultural phenomenon (Casale, 2020; Štulhofer et al., 2022). This fragmentation constrains both theoretical advancement and the design of effective interventions (Whitehand, 2022).

Addressing these gaps, there is a clear need for interdisciplinary, context-sensitive scholarship that situates online pornography within the broader ecology of technology addiction and digital disorders affecting young learners (Vertongen et al., 2022). The present chapter responds to this need by adopting an integrative analytical approach to examine the causes, consequences, and responses to adolescent pornography exposure, with particular emphasis on educational and policy implications in the Indian context (Gupta, 2024).

3. METHODOLOGY

3.1 Research Design

This chapter adopts a qualitative, conceptual, review-based design. Due to ethical and practical constraints in studying minors, no primary data were collected. Instead, an interdisciplinary analytical approach integrates perspectives from education, psychology, neuroscience, sociology, and public policy to examine online pornography as a technology-mediated developmental phenomenon.

3.2 Sources of Data

The study draws on secondary sources, including peer-reviewed articles, academic books, and policy reports. Documents from international organizations (e.g., UNESCO, WHO) and Indian legal and policy frameworks were also reviewed to ensure contextual relevance.

3.3 Inclusion and Exclusion Criteria

Literature focusing on adolescents (10–18 years) and online pornography was prioritized. Only scholarly, peer-reviewed, and policy-relevant sources were included; anecdotal and non-academic materials were excluded to ensure rigor.

3.4 Analytical Framework

A thematic synthesis approach was employed to identify key patterns across the literature. Analysis was guided by the technology addiction framework and the ecological systems approach, enabling a multi-level understanding of individual, social, technological, and policy influences.

3.5 Ethical Considerations

The study adopts a non-stigmatizing, child-centered, harm-reduction perspective. Discussions are framed within developmental and educational contexts, ensuring sensitivity and alignment with principles of child wellbeing.

4. FINDINGS AND ANALYSIS

Drawing on the thematic synthesis of interdisciplinary literature, this section presents key findings related to the patterns of exposure, technological drivers, and neuropsychological impacts of online pornography on young learners. Rather than reporting empirical results, the analysis interprets convergent evidence across studies to elucidate how online pornography exposure is initiated, sustained, and potentially transformed into compulsive engagement within adolescent digital environments.

4.1 Patterns and Pathways of Exposure

A consistent finding across the literature is that adolescents' exposure to online pornography often occurs through multiple, overlapping pathways rather than through deliberate and informed choice alone (Sabina et al., 2008). Accidental exposure emerges as a common entry point, particularly for younger adolescents. Pop-up advertisements, misleading hyperlinks, and algorithmic spillovers from otherwise non-sexual content frequently expose minors to explicit material without prior intent (Vertongen et al., 2022). Such encounters are often unanticipated and occur in private digital spaces, limiting opportunities for immediate adult guidance or contextualization (Maas et al., 2025).

Peer-mediated access represents another significant pathway. Adolescents commonly encounter pornographic material through friends, siblings, or peer networks, either via direct sharing or informal recommendations (Weber et al., 2012). Peer contexts not only facilitate access but also play a role in normalizing consumption, framing pornography as a routine or expected aspect of adolescent digital culture (Nesi, 2022). This normalization can reduce perceived risk and discourage critical reflection, particularly when peer approval is a salient developmental concern (Field, 2020).

In addition, curiosity-driven exploration becomes increasingly prominent with age. As adolescents undergo sexual maturation, curiosity about bodies, relationships, and sexual practices motivates intentional searching (Fortenberry, 2013). In the absence of comprehensive sexuality education or open family communication, online pornography often becomes a readily accessible—though unregulated—

source of information (Bryant, 2009). The literature suggests that these pathways are not mutually exclusive; accidental exposure may trigger curiosity, which is then reinforced through peer validation and repeated engagement.

4.2 Technological and Algorithmic Drivers

Findings consistently indicate that exposure patterns are deeply shaped by the technological architecture of digital platforms. Online pornography operates within an engagement-driven digital economy, where platform design prioritizes user retention, repeated visits, and prolonged viewing (Bryant, 2009). Features such as autoplay, infinite scrolling, and instant access reduce friction and facilitate continuous consumption, particularly for users with limited impulse control (Keilty, 2015).

Recommendation algorithms further intensify exposure by personalizing content based on prior viewing behavior (Vertongen et al., 2022). Even minimal interaction can generate increasingly explicit or novel recommendations, contributing to rapid escalation (Elbaum & Panter, 2025). The literature highlights that such algorithmic amplification is largely indifferent to users' age or developmental stage, effectively treating adolescent engagement as equivalent to adult consumption (Uludag, 2023). This design logic transforms pornography exposure from episodic encounters into sustained patterns of use.

Compounding these issues are weak age-verification mechanisms, which often rely on self-declaration rather than robust authentication. Scholars note that existing safeguards function more as symbolic compliance than effective barriers, enabling minors to access adult content with minimal effort (Dombrowski et al., 2007). Together, platform design, algorithmic optimization, and inadequate regulatory enforcement create a digital environment in which exposure is not only likely but structurally facilitated.

4.3 Neuropsychological Impacts on Young Learners

The literature reveals strong convergence around the neuropsychological implications of early and repeated exposure to online pornography. Adolescents exhibit heightened reward sensitivity, with neural systems responsive to novelty and arousal developing earlier than executive control mechanisms (Astuti & Winarti, 2022). Pornographic content, characterized by high-intensity visual stimulation, strongly activates reward pathways, reinforcing viewing behavior and increasing the likelihood of repetition (Astuti & Winarti, 2022).

Repeated exposure may contribute to reduced impulse control, particularly when consumption occurs in private, unsupervised contexts (Kuhn et al., 2013; Maldonado-Devincci et al., 2010; Gibbons et al., 2016). The developing prefrontal cortex, responsible for self-regulation and decision-making, may struggle to moderate engagement with highly stimulating content. As a result, adolescents may experience difficulty limiting use, even when aware of negative emotional or functional consequences.

Over time, these processes can support habit formation, wherein pornography use becomes routinized and integrated into daily digital practices (Grubbs et al., 2017). The literature suggests that such habits may develop without conscious intent, shaped instead by repeated reinforcement and ease of access (Wdowiak et al., 2025; Büsche et al., 2022). While not all exposure leads to problematic outcomes, the findings underscore how neurodevelopmental vulnerability interacts with digital design to heighten the risk of compulsive patterns among young learners.

4.4 Cognitive and Emotional Outcomes

The literature consistently indicates that early and repeated exposure to online pornography can shape adolescents' cognitive schemas related to sexuality, intimacy, and relationships (Vertongen et al., 2022). One prominent outcome is the development of distorted sexual expectations, as pornography often presents exaggerated, unrealistic, and performance-oriented representations of sexual bodies and behaviors. For young learners, particularly those lacking alternative sources of accurate sexual information, these portrayals may be internalized as normative (Massey et al., 2020). Such internalization can lead to misconceptions about physical appearance, sexual readiness, and relational dynamics, potentially influencing expectations in future interpersonal relationships (Maas et al., 2024).

A closely related consequence is the misunderstanding of consent and intimacy. Pornographic content frequently minimizes or omits explicit communication, mutuality, and emotional connection, instead emphasizing dominance, submission, or transactional interactions (Rojas-Estrada et al., 2024). Adolescents exposed to such representations may struggle to distinguish between performative sexual scripts and healthy relational norms (Adarsh & Sahoo, 2023). The literature suggests that this misalignment can impair the development of respectful attitudes toward consent, boundaries, and reciprocal intimacy, particularly when exposure occurs before young learners have developed critical media literacy skills (Vertongen et al., 2022).

Emotionally, exposure to online pornography is often associated with distress and secrecy (Willoughby et al., 2018). Adolescents report feelings of guilt, shame, confusion, and anxiety, especially in cultural contexts where sexuality is stigmatized or rarely discussed openly (Adarsh & Sahoo, 2023). These emotional responses are frequently intensified by the private and hidden nature of consumption, which discourages disclosure and dialogue with parents, teachers, or peers (Schepis et al., 2008; Salimian et al., 2014). The resulting secrecy can limit opportunities for corrective guidance and emotional support, potentially exacerbating internal conflict and psychological strain.

4.5 Educational and Behavioral Consequences

Beyond cognitive and emotional effects, the literature identifies several educational and behavioral consequences associated with problematic pornography use among adolescents (Bryant, 2009). One recurring finding is academic disengagement, manifested in reduced concentration, diminished motivation, and difficulty sustaining attention on academic tasks (Barton et al., 2018). Excessive screen time devoted to pornography consumption—often occurring late at night- may disrupt sleep patterns, further impairing cognitive functioning and classroom engagement (Astuti & Winarti, 2022).

Social withdrawal also emerges as a notable behavioral outcome. As pornography consumption is typically solitary, habitual engagement may reduce time spent in peer interaction and offline social activities (Cardoso et al., 2022). Some studies suggest that adolescents may retreat from real-world relationships due to unrealistic expectations, social anxiety, or diminished interest in non-digital forms of connection. This withdrawal can weaken social skills and reduce opportunities for experiential learning critical to adolescent development (Adarsh & Sahoo, 2023).

Additionally, the literature points to reduced participation in offline activities, including sports, hobbies, and family interactions. As digital consumption becomes more central to daily routines, adolescents may increasingly rely on online content for stimulation and emotional regulation (Odgers et al., 2020; Ophir et al., 2020). This shift not only narrows developmental experiences but also reinforces patterns of digital dependency (Dienlin & Johannes, 2020). While not all adolescents exposed to pornography exhibit these outcomes, the convergence of findings underscores how problematic engagement can intersect with broader patterns of behavioral disengagement and digital overuse (Nesi, 2022).

4.6 Socio-cultural and Gendered Effects

The socio-cultural implications of online pornography exposure among young learners extend beyond individual cognition and behavior, implicating broader structures of gender, power, and cultural meaning-making (Flood, 2009). A recurring finding across the literature is the tendency of mainstream pornographic content to reproduce and normalize patriarchal gender norms, often portraying sexual interactions through hierarchies of dominance and submission (Healy-Cullen et al., 2024). Masculinity is frequently associated with control, aggression, and sexual entitlement, while femininity is framed through passivity, availability, and objectification (Paulus et al., 2024). For adolescents in the formative stages of gender identity development, repeated exposure to such representations can contribute to the internalization of unequal relational scripts that privilege power over reciprocity (Rojas-Estrada et al., 2024).

This internalization is particularly consequential because pornography functions as an informal yet influential agent of sexual socialization. In contexts where open discussion of sexuality is limited, pornographic media may fill an educational void, shaping beliefs about what constitutes "normal" sexual behavior (Landripet & Štulhofer, 2021). Unlike comprehensive sexuality education, pornography rarely emphasizes mutual consent, emotional intimacy, or respect for boundaries (Layden, 2021). Instead, it often presents sexual encounters as performance-driven and detached from relational accountability. The literature suggests that when these portrayals are consumed uncritically, they may distort adolescents' understanding of intimacy and reinforce gendered expectations that persist into adulthood (Rojas-Estrada et al., 2024; Strasburger, 2010).

Closely intertwined with patriarchal scripting is the objectification and normalization of aggression. Many studies highlight how pornographic content reduces bodies - particularly women's bodies - to objects of visual consumption, severed from agency or subjectivity (Vera-Gray et al., 2021). Aggressive acts, coercive dynamics, or unequal power relations are frequently eroticized rather than problematized (Klaassen & Peter, 2014). For young learners, repeated exposure to such content may blur the distinction between consensual desire and coercive behavior, particularly when adolescents lack the critical literacy skills to contextualize what they are viewing (Aznar-Martínez et al., 2024). This normalization is not merely attitudinal but may influence expectations within real-life relationships, shaping how young people interpret desire, refusal, and emotional responsiveness (Yue, 2022).

In non-Western and culturally conservative societies, these effects are further complicated by value dissonance between digital exposure and socio-cultural norms (Daneback et al., 2018). Adolescents may encounter explicit sexual representations online that directly contradict the moral frameworks promoted by families, schools, and religious institutions. Rather than facilitating healthy negotiation of sexual identity, this dissonance often produces silence, secrecy, and internal conflict (Gesser-Edelsburg & Arabia, 2018). The literature suggests that such tensions can intensify feelings of guilt and confusion, reinforcing cycles of private consumption and public denial. In the absence of supportive spaces for dialogue, young learners are left to reconcile contradictory cultural messages independently, increasing vulnerability to misinformation and emotional distress (Ojala, 2022; Coppola & Pihkala, 2023).

Thus, the socio-cultural and gendered effects of online pornography cannot be understood solely at the level of individual choice or preference. They reflect the interaction between digital media systems, entrenched gender ideologies, and cultural silences surrounding sexuality (Attwood, 2005). Recognizing these dynamics is essential for developing educational and policy responses that address not only behavior but also the underlying power structures shaping young learners' sexual socialization (Maes et al., 2024).

4.7 Pornography within the Ecology of Digital Disorders

An important analytical insight emerging from the literature is that online pornography consumption among adolescents is rarely an isolated behavior (Cerniglia & Cimino, 2022). Instead, it operates within a broader ecology of digital disorders, characterized by overlapping and mutually reinforcing patterns of excessive screen use. Studies increasingly document the co-occurrence of problematic pornography use with social media overuse, online gaming addiction, and compulsive internet engagement, suggesting shared underlying mechanisms rather than discrete, unrelated problems (Healy-Cullen et al., 2024).

These digital behaviors are united by common structural features: constant availability, algorithmic reinforcement, rapid reward cycles, and immersive design (Almourad et al., 2020). Social media platforms often expose adolescents to sexualized imagery that normalizes explicit content, while gaming environments encourage prolonged screen time, late-night use, and emotional immersions (Ashata, 2024). Pornography may emerge within this saturated digital context as one among several high-arousal activities that provide immediate gratification and temporary relief from stress, boredom, or emotional discomfort. The convergence of these behaviors amplifies overall screen dependency, making self-regulation increasingly difficult for young learners (Tabish, 2025).

The literature further highlights screen saturation and digital escapism as central dynamics linking pornography to broader digital disorders. Adolescents facing academic pressure, social anxiety, or limited recreational opportunities may turn to digital media as a coping strategy (Field, 2020). Pornography, due to its intensity and privacy, can become a particularly potent form of escapism. Over time, reliance on digital stimulation for emotional regulation may displace offline activities such as physical play, creative pursuits, and face-to-face social interaction (Healy-Cullen et al., 2024). This displacement narrows developmental experiences and weakens protective factors associated with resilience and wellbeing (Chatterjee & Kar, 2023).

Importantly, framing pornography within the ecology of digital disorders shifts the analytical focus from individual pathology to systemic conditions. It underscores how platform design, educational gaps, and socio-cultural stressors interact with adolescent neurodevelopment to produce patterns of overuse (Vertongen et al., 2022). Interventions that target pornography in isolation—through censorship or punitive measures—are therefore unlikely to be effective. Instead, the literature points toward the need for holistic strategies that address overall digital habits, promote media literacy, and strengthen offline engagement opportunities (Astuti & Winarti, 2022).

By situating online pornography within interconnected digital practices, this perspective reinforces the argument that adolescent pornography consumption is best understood as part of a broader technological and developmental landscape (Vertongen et al., 2022). Such an ecological understanding provides a more robust foundation for educational, psychological, and policy interventions aimed at supporting healthy development in a digitally saturated world.

5. DISCUSSION

This chapter set out to examine online pornography exposure among young learners as a technology-mediated developmental issue situated within the broader ecology of digital disorders. The findings reveal that pornography exposure among minors is not an incidental or marginal phenomenon but a structurally facilitated outcome of contemporary digital environments. Interpreting these findings requires moving beyond narrow behavioral explanations to consider developmental vulnerability, socio-cultural power relations, and systemic digital governance failures. This discussion integrates the key insights and situates them within broader theoretical and policy debates.

5.1 Pornography as a Developmental Risk in the Digital Age

A central insight emerging from the analysis is that minors are uniquely vulnerable to the effects of online pornography due to the intersection of neurodevelopmental immaturity and technologically amplified exposure (Sabina et al., 2008). Adolescence is characterized by heightened reward sensitivity, ongoing development of executive control, and an increased drive for novelty and experimentation (Adarsh & Sahoo, 2023). When highly stimulating sexual content is encountered during this developmental window, it can exert a disproportionate influence on learning, habit formation, and emotional regulation (Carnevali et al., 2022).

Unlike adults, young learners lack the cognitive maturity, critical media literacy, and experiential reference points needed to contextualize pornographic representations. As the findings demonstrate, pornography may function as a de facto educator in the absence of structured guidance, shaping sexual expectations, relational norms, and understandings of consent (Bryant, 2009). The developmental risk, therefore, lies not merely in exposure itself but in the timing and context of that exposure-occurring before adolescents have developed the capacity to critically evaluate and regulate their engagement with digital content (Štulhofer, Kohut, & Koletić, 2022).

Viewing pornography through a developmental lens also underscores the inadequacy of individual responsibility narratives (Galatzer-Levy, 2021). Adolescents' interactions with digital media are shaped by platform architectures, peer dynamics, and socio-cultural silences. Framing pornography use as a personal failing or moral weakness obscures these structural determinants and risks further marginalizing young learners rather than supporting their development (Vertongen et al., 2022).

5.2 Rethinking Moral Panic versus Public Health Perspectives

Public discourse on pornography and minors has often been polarized between moral panic and permissive indifference (Flood, 2009). Moral panic approaches tend to portray pornography as an existential threat to social values, advocating blanket bans or punitive controls. While such responses may resonate culturally, the findings of this chapter suggest that censorship-only approaches are inherently limited in digitally networked environments (Bond & Phippen, 2020). Technical workarounds, private device use, and global content distribution render absolute restriction both impractical and ineffective (Bond & Phippen, 2020).

Conversely, libertarian or normalization perspectives downplay potential harms by framing exposure as inevitable or developmentally inconsequential (Zurcher, 2017). This stance neglects substantial evidence pointing to psychological distress, distorted sexual cognition, and behavioral consequences among young learners. The limitations of both extremes highlight the need for a public health–oriented framework that emphasizes prevention, early intervention, and harm reduction (Vertongen et al., 2022).

A public health perspective reframes pornography exposure as a population-level risk shaped by environmental factors rather than individual deviance (Potenza, 2018). It prioritizes evidence-based responses, acknowledges varying degrees of vulnerability, and recognizes that not all exposure leads to harm. Importantly, it shifts the focus from moral judgment to developmental support, aligning interventions with principles of child wellbeing and educational responsibility.

5.3 Implications for Education

The findings have significant implications for educational systems, particularly regarding the urgent need for media literacy and comprehensive sexuality education. Media literacy education equips young learners with the skills to critically analyze digital content, understand algorithmic influences, and distinguish between mediated representations and real-life relationships (Setty, 2022). Without such literacy, adolescents remain vulnerable to internalizing distorted narratives presented by pornography.

Equally critical is the role of comprehensive, age-appropriate sexuality education that addresses not only biological aspects of sex but also consent, respect, emotional intimacy, and healthy relationships (Judge, 2008) (Khemkhaeng et al., 2022). In the absence of formal educational guidance, pornography often fills an informational vacuum, despite its lack of pedagogical intent or ethical framing. Educational institutions therefore have a central role in providing credible, contextualized alternatives that can counteract misinformation and normalize open, respectful discussion.

For contexts such as India, where sexuality education remains contested, the findings underscore the costs of silence (Sharma, 2020). Avoidance does not prevent exposure; it merely ensures that exposure occurs without guidance. Integrating media literacy and sexuality education within school curricula is thus not a cultural imposition but a protective developmental necessity in digitally saturated environments.

5.4 Policy and Platform Accountability

The analysis reveals substantial limitations in existing policy and digital governance frameworks, particularly in their capacity to address the routine exposure of minors to online pornography. Current legal approaches are predominantly oriented toward criminalizing extreme forms of sexual exploitation, such as child sexual abuse material, while largely neglecting the everyday accessibility of adult pornography through mainstream digital platforms (Binford, 2018). This narrow focus reflects a reactive rather than preventive regulatory paradigm, one that fails to engage with the structural conditions enabling widespread exposure. Consequently, age-verification mechanisms remain weak, often relying on self-declaration systems that are easily circumvented, while enforcement practices are inconsistent and fragmented across jurisdictions (Carnevali et al., 2022). This regulatory insufficiency effectively shifts the burden of protection onto families and educational institutions, which are themselves unevenly equipped to manage complex digital risks.

Critically, such policy limitations must be understood within the broader context of global digital governance, where jurisdictional boundaries, platform sovereignty, and the transnational nature of online content complicate enforcement. Regulatory frameworks often lag behind technological innovation, resulting in symbolic compliance rather than substantive protection. Moreover, an overreliance on access-restriction measures risks oversimplifying the problem, as it does not address the underlying dynamics of exposure embedded in platform design and digital consumption patterns.

Beyond state policy, the findings underscore the central role of technology companies as active agents in shaping exposure environments. Platform architectures—driven by algorithmic recommendation systems, engagement-maximizing features, and data-driven personalization—are not neutral but are structurally oriented toward maximizing user retention and profit (Hawdon et al., 2016). These systems frequently amplify sexually explicit or suggestive content due to its high engagement value, thereby increasing the likelihood of adolescent exposure, whether intentional or incidental. The treatment of adolescent users as indistinguishable from adults reflects a critical failure to incorporate child-centered design principles into digital ecosystems.

From a critical perspective, this raises fundamental questions about the political economy of digital platforms. The prioritization of attention extraction and monetization often comes at the expense of developmental appropriateness and user wellbeing. In this sense, adolescent exposure to pornography is not merely a byproduct of individual behavior but a predictable outcome of platform logics that privilege engagement over protection. Ethical digital governance, therefore, requires a shift from reactive moderation to proactive design responsibility. This includes implementing robust age-assurance systems, limiting algorithmic amplification of explicit content, enhancing content labeling and filtering mechanisms, and embedding safety-by-design principles that explicitly account for developmental vulnerabilities (Moreno & Radesky, 2024).

However, calls for increased platform accountability must also be critically balanced with concerns related to privacy, surveillance, and digital rights. More stringent age-verification systems, for instance, may involve biometric data or identity tracking, raising significant ethical and legal questions. Similarly, content moderation at scale presents challenges related to over-censorship, cultural bias, and algorithmic opacity. These tensions highlight that regulatory solutions are not merely technical but inherently political, requiring careful negotiation between child protection, individual freedoms, and corporate interests.

Ultimately, effective responses demand a multi-level and coordinated governance approach. Regulatory reform must move beyond punitive or symbolic measures toward comprehensive frameworks that integrate platform accountability, educational interventions, and public awareness. Schools and families cannot be positioned as primary regulators in an environment shaped by powerful technological infrastructures. Instead, a shared responsibility model is required, wherein states, technology companies, educational systems, and civil society collectively engage in safeguarding young learners. Such an approach acknowledges that no single intervention—whether legal, technological, or educational—can adequately address the complexity of pornography exposure in digitally mediated environments.

6. RECOMMENDATIONS AND INTERVENTION STRATEGIES

The findings highlight that online pornography exposure among young learners is a structurally embedded and multifaceted phenomenon shaped by technological architectures, developmental vulnerabilities, cultural silences, and institutional inadequacies (Maas et al., 2024; Maes et al., 2024). Consequently, isolated or punitive interventions are insufficient. A critical, multi-level, and harm-reduction–oriented approach is required, integrating family, educational, policy, and psychological domains.

6.1 Family-Level Interventions

Family environments play a foundational role in mediating adolescents' digital experiences. Evidence underscores the protective value of open, age-appropriate communication about sexuality and online content (Mullis, 2022). Rather than avoidance or fear-based control, dialogic engagement that normalizes curiosity while addressing consent, relationships, and risks is more effective in reducing secrecy and fostering help-seeking behaviors (Rank, 2023; Allison et al., 2023). Critically, a shift from surveillance-based monitoring to active parental mediation is essential. Excessive control may intensify concealment, whereas collaborative boundary-setting and modeling of responsible digital practices promote self-regulation and critical awareness (Vaterlaus et al., 2015; Steinfeld, 2020; Fardouly et al., 2022). However, such approaches presuppose parental digital literacy, which remains uneven and necessitates broader support mechanisms.

6.2 School and Educational Interventions

Educational institutions are central to addressing informational and developmental gaps. Media literacy education is crucial for enabling adolescents to critically interpret digital content, including the algorithmic and commercial logics underlying pornography (Boyd & Dobrow, 2011; Maas, 2024). Equally important is comprehensive sexuality education, which provides normative frameworks around consent, intimacy, and emotional wellbeing, thereby countering pornography as an informal and often misleading educator (Zen et al., 2024). However, implementation remains constrained by cultural resistance and institutional reluctance. Teacher preparedness is a critical bottleneck; without adequate training and support, educators may avoid or inadequately address these issues (Romero Rodríguez et al., 2024). Institutionalizing teacher training and establishing clear referral systems for psychological support are therefore essential, though often underdeveloped in practice.

6.3 Policy and Regulatory Measures

At the policy level, existing frameworks demonstrate a gap between intent and effectiveness, particularly in addressing routine access to pornography by minors (Steel, 2015). Strengthening age-verification systems is necessary but insufficient if treated as a standalone solution. Broader regulatory approaches must address platform accountability, including algorithmic transparency and child-centered design (Pasquale et al., 2020). Current platform architectures prioritize engagement over wellbeing, effectively normalizing exposure. Regulatory interventions must therefore extend beyond access restriction to encompass systemic design reforms. However, enforcement challenges, global content flows, and privacy concerns complicate implementation, underscoring the need for integrated strategies combining regulation, education, and public awareness.

6.4 Psychological and Preventive Interventions

From a psychological perspective, interventions should prioritize prevention and harm reduction rather than pathologization (Rehm et al., 2004). Early identification of problematic use—manifested in compulsivity, distress, or functional impairment—is critical, yet often hindered by stigma and lack of institutional capacity (Wright, 2018). Expanding school-based mental health services can provide accessible, non-judgmental spaces for adolescents to process experiences and develop adaptive coping strategies (Openshaw, 2011). Importantly, harm-reduction approaches acknowledge the impracticality of eliminating exposure in digitally saturated environments (Lopez-Fernandez, 2020). Instead, emphasis should be placed on resilience-building, emotional regulation, and critical engagement with digital content. Nonetheless, the effectiveness of such interventions depends on sustained institutional support, which remains uneven across contexts.

Overall, these recommendations underscore that meaningful intervention requires systemic, coordinated, and context-sensitive responses rather than fragmented or reactive measures.

7. FUTURE RESEARCH DIRECTIONS

Future research on adolescent exposure to online pornography must adopt longitudinal, interdisciplinary, and culturally sensitive approaches to address significant gaps in current knowledge. Long-term studies are needed to examine how early exposure influences cognitive, emotional, behavioral, and relational development over time, while neurodevelopmental research should further explore how repeated exposure interacts with brain maturation, impulse control, and emotional regulation. There is also a critical need for context-specific research in India and other non-Western societies, where rapid digitalization intersects with cultural taboos and limited sexuality education. Additionally, empirical studies should evaluate the effectiveness of media literacy programs, comprehensive sexuality education, parental mediation, and school-based interventions in promoting healthy development and critical digital awareness. Future research must also investigate the role of algorithmic recommendation systems and platform design in shaping exposure patterns, as well as identify protective factors such as family communication, educational support, and psychological resilience. Ultimately, integrating perspectives from psychology, neuroscience, education, sociology, public health, and digital governance will be essential for developing comprehensive theoretical frameworks and evidence-based interventions to support adolescent wellbeing in digitally mediated environments.

8. LIMITATIONS OF THE STUDY

The present chapter is subject to several methodological limitations arising from its reliance on a qualitative, conceptual, and review-based research design. As the study is grounded entirely in secondary data, it does not incorporate primary empirical evidence, thereby limiting its ability to establish causal relationships or generate context-specific insights into adolescents' lived experiences. The analysis is inherently dependent on the scope, quality, and potential biases of existing literature, which may vary in methodological rigor and conceptual clarity. Furthermore, inconsistencies in key definitions—such as exposure, use, problematic use, and addiction—across studies pose challenges for synthesis and comparative interpretation. Another limitation concerns the predominance of Western-centric research within the reviewed literature, which may constrain the generalizability of findings to the Indian socio-cultural context emphasized in the chapter. Additionally, the absence of direct engagement with participants restricts the ability to capture emerging digital behaviors, nuanced patterns of media interaction, and evolving technological influences. Consequently, while the interdisciplinary review provides valuable theoretical and analytical insights, the findings should be interpreted as indicative rather than empirically definitive.

9. CONCLUSION

This chapter has examined online pornography exposure among young learners by situating it at the intersection of digital technology, adolescent development, and socio-cultural context. The analysis demonstrates that such exposure is not incidental but structurally embedded within contemporary digital ecosystems, facilitated by platform architectures, algorithmic amplification, and inadequate regulatory safeguards. Adolescents encounter pornography through multiple pathways—including accidental exposure, peer mediation, and curiosity-driven exploration—interacting with neurodevelopmental vulnerabilities to shape cognitive, emotional, behavioral, and socio-cultural outcomes related to gender, intimacy, and consent.

A key contribution of this chapter is the reconceptualization of online pornography as a technology-mediated developmental challenge rather than a purely moral or individual issue. This perspective highlights how exposure is shaped by systemic forces—digital economies, educational deficits, cultural silences, and governance gaps—rather than solely by personal choice. Situating pornography within the broader ecology of technology addiction and digital disorders further underscores its entanglement with patterns of screen saturation, digital escapism, and overlapping online behaviors, thereby challenging reductionist and polarized framings of the issue.

The findings also emphasize the limits of fragmented or single-level responses. Effective intervention requires coordinated, multi-sectoral engagement involving families, educational institutions, policymakers, digital platforms, and mental health systems. Approaches grounded in media literacy, comprehensive sexuality education, ethical platform design, and accessible psychological support offer more sustainable pathways than censorship or punitive control alone, though their implementation remains uneven and context-dependent.

At the same time, significant gaps persist in the evidence base. The dominance of Western-centric research, limited longitudinal data, and insufficient attention to non-Western contexts—particularly India—constrain both theoretical generalization and policy relevance. Future research must therefore prioritize context-sensitive, interdisciplinary, and longitudinal approaches to better understand developmental trajectories, protective factors, and the effectiveness of interventions.

Ultimately, in digitally saturated environments where exposure is difficult to eliminate, the challenge lies not in suppressing adolescent curiosity but in equipping young learners with the knowledge, critical capacities, and supportive environments necessary for healthy, informed, and respectful development.

DECLARATIONS

- **Ethical Compliance:** This study follows academic and ethical standards and is based on secondary literature.
- **Consent to Participate/Publication:** Not applicable.

- **Conflict of Interest:** The author declares no conflict of interest.
- **Funding:** No external funding was received.
- **Data Availability:** No primary data were used.
- **Use of AI Tools:** Grammarly and Paperpal (Premium) were used only for language editing and readability improvement.

ACKNOWLEDGEMENTS

The author sincerely acknowledges the contributions of scholars and researchers whose work informed this chapter. The author also expresses gratitude to colleagues and family for their support and encouragement.

REFERENCES

Adarsh, H., & Sahoo, S. (2023). Pornography and its impact on adolescent/teenage sexuality. *Journal of Psychosexual Health*, *5*(1), 35–39. DOI: 10.1177/26318318231153984

Allen, M., Emmers, T., Gebhardt, L., & Giery, M. A. (1995). Exposure to pornography and acceptance of rape myths. *The Journal of Communication*, *45*(1), 5–26. DOI: 10.1111/j.1460-2466.1995.tb00711.x

Allison, K., Dawson, R. M., Messias, D. K. H., Culley, J. M., & Brown, N. (2023). Early adolescent online sexual risks on smartphones and social media: Parental awareness and protective practices. *The Journal of Early Adolescence*, *44*(7), 882–908. DOI: 10.1177/02724316231212560

Almourad, M. B., McAlaney, J., Skinner, T., Pleya, M., & Ali, R. (2020). Defining digital addiction: Key features from the literature. *Psihologija*, *53*(3), 237–253. DOI: 10.2298/PSI191029017A

Ashata, G. P. (2024). Digital dynamics: Investigating the impact of social media on sexual behavior. *IDOSR Journal of Communication and English*, *9*(2), 1–6. DOI: 10.59298/IDOSR/JCE/92.16.202412

Astuti, S. A. T., & Winarti, Y. (2022). A scoping review: The impact of pornography addiction on adolescents. *Muhammadiyah International Public Health and Medicine Proceeding*, *2*(1), 366–381. DOI: 10.61811/miphmp.v1i2.265

Attwood, F. (2005). What do people do with porn? Qualitative research into the consumption, use, and experience of pornography and other sexually explicit media. *Sexuality & Culture*, *9*(2), 65–86. DOI: 10.1007/s12119-005-1008-7

Aznar-Martínez, B., Lorente-De-Sanz, J., López-I-Martín, X., & Castillo-Garayoa, J. A. (2024). Pornography and gender-based violence: Two neglected topics in sexuality education. A systematic review. *Sex Education*, *25*(2), 256–272. DOI: 10.1080/14681811.2024.2316154

Ballester-Arnal, R., García-Barba, M., Castro-Calvo, J., Giménez-García, C., & Gil-Llario, M. D. (2022). Pornography consumption in people of different age groups: An analysis based on gender, contents, and consequences. *Sexuality Research & Social Policy, 20*(2), 766–779. DOI: 10.1007/s13178-022-00720-z

Bandura, A. (2001). Social cognitive theory of mass communication. *Media Psychology, 3*(3), 265–299. DOI: 10.1207/S1532785XMEP0303_03

Barton, B. A., Adams, K. S., Browne, B. L., & Arrastia-Chisholm, M. C. (2018). The effects of social media usage on attention, motivation, and academic performance. *Active Learning in Higher Education, 22*(1), 11–22. DOI: 10.1177/1469787418782817

Bava, S., & Tapert, S. F. (2010). Adolescent brain development and the risk for alcohol and other drug problems. *Neuropsychology Review, 20*(4), 398–413. DOI: 10.1007/s11065-010-9146-6 PMID: 20953990

Binford, W. (2018). Viewing pornography through a children's rights lens. *Sexual Addiction & Compulsivity, 25*(4), 415–444. DOI: 10.1080/10720162.2019.1578311

Blinka, L., Ševčíková, A., Dreier, M., Škařupová, K., & Wölfling, K. (2022). Online sex addiction: A qualitative analysis of symptoms in treatment-seeking men. *Frontiers in Psychiatry, 13*, 907549. DOI: 10.3389/fpsyt.2022.907549 PMID: 35873234

Bond, E., & Phippen, A. (2020). Tackling teen sexting- policing challenges when society and technology outpace legislation. In *Advanced sciences and technologies for security applications* (pp. 157–177). https://doi.org/DOI: 10.1007/978-3-030-50613-1_7

Boyd, M. J., & Dobrow, J. (2011). Media literacy and positive youth development. *Advances in Child Development and Behavior, 41*, 251–271. DOI: 10.1016/B978-0-12-386492-5.00010-5 PMID: 23259195

Bozzola, E. (2021). Media use during childhood and adolescence. *International Journal of Environmental Research and Public Health, 18*(3), 967. DOI: 10.3390/ijerph18030967 PMID: 33499274

Bryant, C. (2009). *Adolescence, pornography and harm* (Trends & Issues in Crime and Criminal Justice No. 368). Australian Institute of Criminology.

Büsche, K., Stark, R., Brand, M., & Antons, S. (2022). Self-regulatory processes in problematic pornography use. *Current Addiction Reports, 9*(4), 344–352. DOI: 10.1007/s40429-022-00447-2

Byron, P. (2023). Porn literacy and young people's digital cultures. *Porn Studies, 11*(1), 32–39. DOI: 10.1080/23268743.2023.2174173

Byun, S., Ruffini, C., Mills, J. E., Douglas, A. C., Niang, M., Stepchenkova, S., Lee, S. K., Loutfi, J., Lee, J., Atallah, M., & Blanton, M. (2008). Internet addiction: Metasynthesis of 1996–2006 quantitative research. *Cyberpsychology & Behavior, 12*(2), 203–207. DOI: 10.1089/cpb.2008.0102 PMID: 19072075

Cardoso, J., Ramos, C., Brito, J., & Almeida, T. C. (2022). Predictors of pornography use: Difficulties in emotion regulation and loneliness. *Journal of Sexual Medicine, 19*(4), 620–628. DOI: 10.1016/j.jsxm.2022.01.005 PMID: 35165051

Carnevali, D., Cavazzana, L., Grimoldi, L., Magnoni, P., Principi, N., Pellai, A., Carnevali, D., Cavazzana, L., Grimoldi, L., Magnoni, P., Principi, N., & Pellai, A. (2022). The use of online pornography among minors: Epidemiological analysis of the phenomenon. *Minerva Pediatrics, 74*(5), 579–585. DOI: 10.23736/S2724-5276.19.05342-8 PMID: 35166482

Casale, S. (2020). Problematic social media use: Conceptualization, assessment and trends in scientific literature. *Addictive Behaviors Reports, 12*, 100281. DOI: 10.1016/j.abrep.2020.100281 PMID: 32426449

Cerniglia, L., & Cimino, S. (2022). Some Considerations about Pornography Watching in Early Adolescence. *International Journal of Environmental Research and Public Health, 19*(17), 108–118. DOI: 10.3390/ijerph191710818 PMID: 36078525

Chatterjee, S., & Kar, S. K. (2023). Teen Pornography: An emerging mental health challenge. *Journal of Psychosexual Health, 5*(1), 30–34. DOI: 10.1177/26318318231154230

Coppola, I., & Pihkala, P. (2023). Complex dynamics of climate emotions among environmentally active Finnish and American young people. *Frontiers in Political Science, 4*, 1063741. Advance online publication. DOI: 10.3389/fpos.2022.1063741

Coyle, K., Anderson, P., & Laris, B. A. (2015). Schools and sexuality education. In *Evidence-based approaches to sexuality education* (1st ed., pp. 23–45). Routledge.

Crabbe, M., & Flood, M. (2021). School-based education to address pornography's influence on young people: A proposed practice framework. *American Journal of Sexuality Education, 16*(1), 1–37. DOI: 10.1080/15546128.2020.1856744

D'Angelo, J. D. (2020). Problematic and addictive technology use. In *Elsevier eBooks* (pp. 347–364). https://doi.org/DOI: 10.1016/B978-0-12-817319-0.00016-5

Daneback, K., & Ross, M. W. (2011). The complexity of internet sexuality. *Advances in Psychosomatic Medicine, 31*, 121–134. DOI: 10.1159/000328920 PMID: 22005208

Daneback, K., Ševčíková, A., & Ježek, S. (2018). Exposure to online sexual materials in adolescence and desensitization to sexual content. *Sexologies, 27*(3), e71–e76. DOI: 10.1016/j.sexol.2018.04.001

Dawson, K., Gabhainn, S. N., Friday, R., & MacNeela, P. (2024). Barriers and recommendations for parent–child conversations about pornography. *Frontiers in Sociology, 9*, 1349549. DOI: 10.3389/fsoc.2024.1349549 PMID: 38726390

De Alarcón, R., De La Iglesia, J. I., Casado, N. M., & Montejo, A. L. (2019). Online porn addiction: What we know and what we don't-A systematic review. *Journal of Clinical Medicine, 8*(1), 91. DOI: 10.3390/jcm8010091 PMID: 30650522

Dienlin, T., & Johannes, N. (2020). The impact of digital technology use on adolescent well-being. *Dialogues in Clinical Neuroscience, 22*(2), 135–142. DOI: 10.31887/DCNS.2020.22.2/tdienlin PMID: 32699513

Dombrowski, S. C., Gischlar, K. L., & Durst, T. (2007). Safeguarding young people from cyber pornography and cyber sexual predation: A major dilemma of the internet. *Child Abuse Review, 16*(3), 153–170. DOI: 10.1002/car.939

Elbaum, S., & Panter, J. (2025). Managing escalation in off-the-shelf large language models. *arXiv (Cornell University)*. https://doi.org//arxiv.2508.01056DOI: 10.48550

Fardouly, J., Magson, N. R., Rapee, R. M., Oar, E. L., Johnco, C. J., Richardson, C., & Freeman, J. (2022). Investigating longitudinal and bidirectional relationships between parental factors and time spent on social media during early adolescence. *New Media & Society, 26*(3), 1610–1626. DOI: 10.1177/14614448221076155

Field, T. (2020). Adolescent pornography: A narrative review. *International Journal of Psychological Research and Reviews, 36*, 36. Advance online publication. DOI: 10.28933/ijprr-2020-03-0505

Fisher, W. A., & Barak, A. (2001). Internet pornography: A social psychological perspective on internet sexuality. *Journal of Sex Research, 38*(4), 312–323. DOI: 10.1080/00224490109552102

Flood, M. (2009). The harms of pornography exposure among children and young people. *Child Abuse Review, 18*(6), 384–400. DOI: 10.1002/car.1092

Fortenberry, J. D. (2013). Sexual development in adolescents. In *Elsevier eBooks* (pp. 171-192). DOI: 10.1016/B978-0-12-387759-8.00007-6

Franjic, S. (2022). A few words about pornography. *International Journal of Social Science and Economics, 2*(1), 7. DOI: 10.22158/ijsse.v2n1p7

Galatzer-Levy, R. M. (2021). Adolescent boys and pornography: Notes on a complex system. *The Psychoanalytic Study of the Child, 74*(1), 191–208. DOI: 10.1080/00797308.2020.1859279

Gesser-Edelsburg, A., & Arabia, M. A. E. (2018). Discourse on exposure to pornography content online between Arab adolescents and parents: Qualitative study on its impact on sexual education and behavior. *Journal of Medical Internet Research, 20*(10), e11667. DOI: 10.2196/11667 PMID: 30305264

Gibbons, F. X., Kingsbury, J. H., Wills, T. A., Finneran, S. D., Cin, S. D., & Gerrard, M. (2016). Impulsivity moderates the effects of movie alcohol portrayals on adolescents' willingness to drink. *Psychology of Addictive Behaviors : Journal of the Society of Psychologists in Addictive Behaviors, 30*(3), 325–334. DOI: 10.1037/adb0000178 PMID: 27099959

Gonsalves, V. M., Hodges, H., & Scalora, M. J. (2015). Exploring the use of online sexually explicit material: What is the relationship to sexual coercion? *Sexual Addiction & Compulsivity, 22*(3), 207–221. DOI: 10.1080/10720162.2015.1039150

Green, L., Lumby, C., McKee, A., & Ólafsson, K. (2020). National contexts for the risk of harm being done to children by access to online sexual content. In Tsaliki, L., & Chronaki, D. (Eds.), *Discourses of anxiety over childhood and youth across cultures* (pp. xx–xx). Palgrave Macmillan., DOI: 10.1007/978-3-030-46436-3_11

Grubbs, J. B., Wilt, J. A., Exline, J. J., Pargament, K. I., & Kraus, S. W. (2017). Moral disapproval and perceived addiction to internet pornography: A longitudinal examination. *Addiction (Abingdon, England), 113*(3), 496–506. DOI: 10.1111/add.14007 PMID: 28833800

Gupta, S. (2024). Child pornography and internet subcultures in India - A legal perspective. *Journal of Law and Sustainable Development, 12*(1), e2997. DOI: 10.55908/sdgs.v12i1.2997

Hawdon, J., Oksanen, A., & Räsänen, P. (2016). Exposure to online hate in four nations: A cross-national consideration. *Deviant Behavior, 38*(3), 254–266 DOI: 10.1080/01639625.2016.1196985

Healy-Cullen, S., Taylor, J. E., Ross, K., & Morison, T. (2021). Youth encounters with internet pornography: A survey of youth, caregiver, and educator perspectives. *Sexuality & Culture, 26*(2), 491–513. DOI: 10.1007/s12119-021-09904-y

Healy-Cullen, S., Taylor, K., & Morison, T. (2024). Youth, pornography, and addiction: A Critical review. *Current Addiction Reports, 11*(2), 265–274. DOI: 10.1007/s40429-024-00549-z

Huesmann, L. R. (2007). The impact of electronic media violence: Scientific theory and research. *The Journal of Adolescent Health : Official Publication of the Society for Adolescent Medicine, 41*(6), S6–S13. DOI: 10.1016/j.jadohealth.2007.09.005 PMID: 18047947

Jiang, Q., & Li, Y. (2018). Factors affecting smartphone dependency among the young in China. *Asian Journal of Communication, 28*(5), 508–525. DOI: 10.1080/01292986.2018.1431296

Judge, A. C. D. E. (2008). *Sex education: Are schools teaching what teens need to know?* NEJM Journal Watch., DOI: 10.1056/WH200804030000006

Keilty, P. (2015). Embodied engagements with online pornography. *The Information Society, 32*(1), 64–73. DOI: 10.1080/01972243.2015.1107162

Khemkhaeng, A. C., Pravat, P. N., Thiha, T., Hayma, T., & Zeya, Z. (2022). Enhancing adolescent well-being: The impact of comprehensive sex education on knowledge, consent, and sexual violence Prevention. *Jurnal Sosial Sains Terapan Dan Riset (Sosateris), 10*(2), 151–161. DOI: 10.35335/gze4k733

Klaassen, M. J. E., & Peter, J. (2014). Gender (In)equality in internet pornography: A content analysis of popular pornographic internet videos. *Journal of Sex Research, 52*(7), 721–735. DOI: 10.1080/00224499.2014.976781 PMID: 25420868

Kuhn, C. M., Wilson, W., & Swartzwelder, S. (2013). Enduring effects of adolescent drug exposure. *Biological Psychiatry, 74*(7), 480–481. DOI: 10.1016/j.biopsych.2013.07.030 PMID: 24034365

Landripet, I., & Štulhofer, A. (2021). Pornography use and sexual satisfaction: The role of sexual socialization. In Maggino, F. (Ed.), *Encyclopedia of quality of life and well-being research.* Springer., DOI: 10.1007/978-3-319-69909-7_4145-2

Layden, M. A. (2021). Pornified: Pornography's connection to long-term damage and violence. In Caffo, E. (Ed.), *Online child sexual exploitation: Treatment and prevention of abuse in a digital world* (pp. 57–74). Springer Nature Switzerland AG., DOI: 10.1007/978-3-030-66654-5_6

Li, W. (2023). Gender stereotyping in media - Bias and discrimination. *Lecture Notes in Education Psychology and Public Media, 29*(1), 237–241. DOI: 10.54254/2753-7048/29/20231518

Lopez-Fernandez, O. (2020). Considering existing classic and contemporary proposals for preventing online addiction problems: Some old recipes for new problems. *Journal of Behavioral Addictions, 9*(4), 903–907. DOI: 10.1556/2006.2020.00084 PMID: 33242026

Love, T., Laier, C., Brand, M., Hatch, L., & Hajela, R. (2015). Neuroscience of internet pornography addiction: A review and update. *Behavioral Sciences (Basel, Switzerland)*, *5*(3), 388–433. DOI: 10.3390/bs5030388 PMID: 26393658

Maas, M. K., Wright, P. J., Rothman, E. F., Nelson, K. M., Weigle, P., & Herbenick, D. (2025). Pornography use during adolescence: The current state of knowledge and recommendations. In Christakis, D. A., & Hale, L. (Eds.), *Handbook of children and screens* (pp. 341–347). Springer., DOI: 10.1007/978-3-031-69362-5_47

Maes, C., Vandenbosch, L., & Wright, P. J. (2024). The impact of online pornography consumption on youth. In Rich, G. J., Kumar, V. K., & Farley, F. H. (Eds.), *Handbook of media psychology: The science and the practice* (pp. 101–111). Springer Nature Switzerland AG., DOI: 10.1007/978-3-031-56537-3_8

Magis-Weinberg, L., Suleiman, A. B., & Dahl, R. E. (2021). Context, development, and digital media: Implications for very young adolescents in LMICs. *Frontiers in Psychology*, *12*, 632713. DOI: 10.3389/fpsyg.2021.632713 PMID: 33967899

Maldonado-Devincci, A. M., Badanich, K. A., & Kirstein, C. L. (2010). Alcohol during adolescence selectively alters immediate and long-term behavior and neurochemistry. *Alcohol (Fayetteville, N.Y.)*, *44*(1), 57–66. DOI: 10.1016/j.alcohol.2009.09.035 PMID: 20113874

Marciano, L., Dubicka, B., Magis-Weinberg, L., Morese, R., Viswanath, K., & Weber, R. (2025). Digital media, cognition, and brain development in adolescence. In Christakis, D. A., & Hale, L. (Eds.), *Handbook of children and screens* (pp. 21–29). Springer., DOI: 10.1007/978-3-031-69362-5_4

Massey, K., Burns, J., & Franz, A. (2020). Young people, sexuality and the age of pornography. *Sexuality & Culture*, *25*(1), 318–336. DOI: 10.1007/s12119-020-09771-z

Mattuck, R., Blanchet, R., & Wait, A. D. (2005). Data representativeness for risk assessment. *Environmental Forensics*, *6*(1), 65–70. DOI: 10.1080/15275920590913886

McArthur, J., Stewart, S., & Al-Hamdani, M. (2024). Vaping frequency in young users: The role of gender and age among regular users. *Substance Use & Misuse*, *59*(12), 1778–1784. DOI: 10.1080/10826084.2024.2374975 PMID: 39028136

Moreno, M. A., & Radesky, J. S. (2024). Benefits and harms of proposed social media legislation. *JAMA Pediatrics*, *178*(9), 857. DOI: 10.1001/jamapediatrics.2024.2380 PMID: 39037793

Mullis, M. D. (2022). Parent-child communication about sex. *The International Encyclopedia of Health Communication*, 1-4. https://doi.org/DOI: 10.1002/9781119678816.iehc0887

Nesi, J. (2022). The facts about pornography use in teens. *Brown University Child and Adolescent Behavior Letter*, *38*(12), 8. DOI: 10.1002/cbl.30677

Ng, W. (2015). Learners in a digital society: Digital practices of young people and their teaching implications. In *New digital technology in education* (pp. 51–71). Springer., DOI: 10.1007/978-3-319-05822-1_3

Odgers, C. L., Schueller, S. M., & Ito, M. (2020). Screen time, social media use, and adolescent development. *Annual Review of Developmental Psychology*, *2*(1), 485–502. DOI: 10.1146/annurev-devpsych-121318-084815

Ojala, M. (2022). How do young people deal with border tensions when making climate-friendly food choices? On the importance of critical emotional awareness for learning for social change. *Climate (Basel)*, *10*(1), 8. DOI: 10.3390/cli10010008

Openshaw, L. L. (2011). School-based support groups for traumatized students. *School Psychology International*, *32*(2), 163–178. DOI: 10.1177/0143034311400830

Ophir, Y., Rosenberg, H., Lipshits-Braziler, Y., & Amichai-Hamburger, Y. (2020). "Digital adolescence": The effects of smartphones and social networking technologies on adolescents' well-being. In N. Van Zalk & C. P. Monks (Eds.), *Online peer engagement in adolescence: Positive and negative aspects of online social interaction* (pp. 122-139). Routledge/Taylor & Francis Group. https://doi.org/DOI: 10.4324/9780429468360-8

Palazzolo, F. (2023). Internet pornography use disorder: In search of a non-pathologizing description of an evolving clinical issue. *Sexual Health & Compulsivity*, *30*(4), 328–341. DOI: 10.1080/26929953.2023.2254785

Pasquale, L., Zippo, P., Curley, C., O'Neill, B., & Mongiello, M. (2020). Digital age of Consent and age verification: Can they protect children? *IEEE Software*, *39*(3), 50–57. DOI: 10.1109/MS.2020.3044872

Paulus, F. W., Nouri, F., Ohmann, S., Möhler, E., & Popow, C. (2024). The impact of internet pornography on children and adolescents: A systematic review. *L'Encéphale*, *50*(6), 649–662. DOI: 10.1016/j.encep.2023.12.004 PMID: 38519310

Peter, J., & Valkenburg, P. M. (2016). Adolescents and pornography: A review of 20 years of research. *Journal of Sex Research*, *53*(4-5), 509–531. DOI: 10.1080/00224499.2016.1143441 PMID: 27105446

Potenza, M. N. (2018). Pornography in the current digital technology environment: An overview of a special issue on pornography. *Sexual Addiction & Compulsivity, 25*(4), 241–247. DOI: 10.1080/10720162.2019.1567411

Privara, M., & Bob, P. (2023). Pornography consumption and cognitive-affective distress. *The Journal of Nervous and Mental Disease, 211*(8), 641–646. DOI: 10.1097/NMD.0000000000001669 PMID: 37505898

Przybylski, A. K., & Nash, V. (2018). Internet filtering and adolescent exposure to online sexual material. *Cyberpsychology, Behavior and Social Networking, 21*(7), 405–410. DOI: 10.1089/cyber.2017.0466 PMID: 29995533

Rainwater, L. (1974). The effects of pornography. In *Deviance and liberty* (pp. 8–25). Routledge., DOI: 10.4324/9780203793343-16

Rank, M. R. (2023). *Talking to children about pornography.* https://doi.org/DOI: 10.4324/9781003189787-10

Rehm, J., Fischer, B., Graham, K., Haydon, E., Mann, R. E., & Room, R. (2004). The importance of environmental modifiers of the relationship between substance use and harm. *Addiction (Abingdon, England), 99*(6), 663–666. DOI: 10.1111/j.1360-0443.2004.00719.x PMID: 15139864

Robb, M. B., & Lauricella, A. R. (2014). Connecting child development and technology: What we know and what it means. In *Technology and digital media in the early years* (1st ed., pp. 16–32). Routledge., DOI: 10.4324/9781315856575-18

Roberto, C. A. (2023). An inconvenient truth: Difficult problems rarely have easy solutions. *The Behavioral and Brain Sciences, 46*, e173. DOI: 10.1017/S0140525X23000882 PMID: 37646295

Rojas-Estrada, E., Vizcaíno-Verdú, A., & Bonilla-Del-Río, M. (2024). Sexual (Mis) information. In *Advances in educational technologies and instructional design book series* (pp. 265-284). https://doi.org/DOI: 10.4018/979-8-3693-2053-2.ch015

Romer, D. (2016). Introduction to the issue "adolescents in the digital age: Effects on health and development.". *Media and Communication, 4*(3), 1–3. DOI: 10.17645/mac.v4i3.658

Romero-Rodríguez, J., Berral-Ortiz, B., Martínez-Domingo, J., & Victoria-Maldonado, J. (2024). Online protection measures to prevent sexting among minors. In *Advances in educational technologies and instructional design book series* (pp. 246-264). https://doi.org/DOI: 10.4018/979-8-3693-2053-2.ch014

Sabina, C., Wolak, J., & Finkelhor, D. (2008). The nature and dynamics of internet pornography exposure for youth. *Cyberpsychology & Behavior, 11*(6), 691–693. DOI: 10.1089/cpb.2007.0179 PMID: 18771400

Salimian, P. K., Chunara, R., & Weitzman, E. R. (2014). Averting the perfect storm: Addressing youth substance use risk from social media use. *Pediatric Annals, 43*(10), 411. DOI: 10.3928/00904481-20140924-08 PMID: 25290130

Sancho-Cantus, D. (2024). Pornography addiction: Conceptual and methodological approaches in the post-pandemic era. Mini-Review. *Global Journal of Addiction & Rehabilitation Medicine, 7*(4). Advance online publication. DOI: 10.19080/GJARM.2024.07.555718

Schepis, T. S., Marlowe, D. B., & Forman, R. F. (2008). The availability and portrayal of stimulants over the internet. *The Journal of Adolescent Health : Official Publication of the Society for Adolescent Medicine, 42*(5), 458–465. DOI: 10.1016/j.jadohealth.2007.11.140 PMID: 18407040

Schiebener, J., Laier, C., & Brand, M. (2015). Getting stuck with pornography? Overuse or neglect of cybersex cues in a multitasking situation is related to symptoms of cybersex addiction. *Journal of Behavioral Addictions, 4*(1), 14–21. DOI: 10.1556/JBA.4.2015.1.5 PMID: 25786495

Schmitt, K. L., & Woolf, K. D. (2018). Cognitive development in digital contexts. *Journal of Children and Media, 1-3*, 1–3. Advance online publication. DOI: 10.1080/17482798.2018.1522116

Setty, E. (2022). Digital media and relationships, sex, and health education in the classroom. *Pastoral Care in Education, 41*(3), 289–305. DOI: 10.1080/02643944.2022.2095418

Sharma, R. (2020). Vital need for sex education in Indian youth and adolescents. *Indian Journal of Pediatrics, 87*(4), 255. DOI: 10.1007/s12098-020-03240-z PMID: 32048223

Simon, L., & Daneback, K. (2013). Adolescents' use of the internet for sex education: A thematic and critical review of the literature. *International Journal of Sexual Health : Official Journal of the World Association for Sexual Health, 25*(4), 305–319. DOI: 10.1080/19317611.2013.823899

Smaniotto, B., Bigot, J. L., & Camps, F. (2021). "Pornography addiction": Elements for discussion of a case report. *Archives of Sexual Behavior, 51*(2), 1375–1381. DOI: 10.1007/s10508-021-02133-2 PMID: 34786657

Srnicek, N. (2017). *Platform capitalism*. Polity Press.

Stark, R., & Klucken, T. (2017). Neuroscientific approaches to (online) pornography addiction. In *Studies in neuroscience, psychology and behavioral economics* (pp. 109-124). https://doi.org/DOI: 10.1007/978-3-319-46276-9_7

Steel, C. M. (2015). Web-based child pornography: The global impact of deterrence efforts and its consumption on mobile platforms. *Child Abuse & Neglect*, *44*, 150–158. DOI: 10.1016/j.chiabu.2014.12.009 PMID: 25605590

Steinfeld, N. (2020). Parental mediation of adolescent Internet use: Combining strategies to promote awareness, autonomy and self-regulation in preparing youth for life on the web. *Education and Information Technologies*, *26*(2), 1897–1920. DOI: 10.1007/s10639-020-10342-w

Steyer, I. (2014). Gender representations in children's media and their influence. *Campus-Wide Information Systems*, *31*(2/3), 171–180. DOI: 10.1108/CWIS-11-2013-0065

Strasburger, V. C. (2010). Sexuality, contraception, and the media. *Pediatrics*, *126*(3), 576–582. DOI: 10.1542/peds.2010-1544 PMID: 20805150

Štulhofer, A., Kohut, T., & Koletić, G. (2022). Pornography use in adolescence and young adulthood. In *Focus on sexuality research* (pp. 385-421). https://doi.org/DOI: 10.1007/978-3-030-84273-4_14

Tabish, S. (2025). From evolution to obsession: Understanding digital addiction among youth in the modern age. *American Journal of Health Research*, *13*(4), 248–258. DOI: 10.11648/j.ajhr.20251304.17

Thorneycroft, R., Smith, E., & Nicholas, L. (2024). Whose concerns? Young adults discussing (their) concerns with pornography. *Sex Education*, *25*(4), 465–480. DOI: 10.1080/14681811.2024.2356635

Turner, K. H., Jolls, T., Hagerman, M. S., O'Byrne, W., Hicks, T., Eisenstock, B., & Pytash, K. E. (2017). Developing digital and media literacies in children and adolescents. *Pediatrics*, *140*(Supplement_2), S122–S126. DOI: 10.1542/peds.2016-1758P PMID: 29093046

Uludag, K. (2023). Personalized video recommendation system and its potential role as a trigger of addiction. *Scientific Studios on Social and Political Psychology*, *29*(2), 44–46. DOI: 10.61727/sssppj/2.2023.44

Valkenburg, P. M., & Peter, J. (2013). The differential susceptibility to media effects model. *The Journal of Communication*, *63*(2), 221–243. DOI: 10.1111/jcom.12024 van Dijck, J., Poell, T., & de Waal, M. (2018). *The platform society: Public values in a connective world.* Oxford University Press. DOI: 10.1093/oso/9780190889760.001.0001

Vaterlaus, J. M., Beckert, T. E., & Bird, C. V. (2015). At a certain age it's not appropriate to monitor one's child. *Emerging Adulthood, 3*(5), 353–358. DOI: 10.1177/2167696815581277

Vera-Gray, F., McGlynn, C., Kureshi, I., & Butterby, K. (2021). Sexual violence as a sexual script in mainstream online pornography. *British Journal of Criminology, 61*(5), 1243–1260. DOI: 10.1093/bjc/azab035

Vertongen, R., Chamberlain, K., & Van Ommen, C. (2022). Pornography and adolescents: Unravelling dominant research assumptions. *Porn Studies, 9*(4), 430–444. DOI: 10.1080/23268743.2022.2114532

Vertongen, R., Van Ommen, C., & Chamberlain, K. (2022). Adolescent dilemmas about viewing pornography and their efforts to resolve them. *Journal of Adolescent Research, 40*(1), 226–254. DOI: 10.1177/07435584221133307

Vieira, C., & Griffiths, M. D. (2024). Problematic pornography use and mental health: A systematic review. *Sexual Health & Compulsivity, 31*(3), 207–247. DOI: 10.1080/26929953.2024.2348624

Vinnakota, D., Arafat, S. M. Y., Kar, S. K., Sivasubramanian, M., Hossain, S. R., Parsa, A. D., & Kabir, R. (2021). Pornography and sexual violence against women in India: A scoping review. *Journal of Psychosexual Health, 3*(3), 216–221. DOI: 10.1177/26318318211023935

Wdowiak, K., Maciocha, A., & Wąż, J. (2025). Pornography through the lens of the 21st century and its impact on society. *Psychiatria I Psychologia Kliniczna, 25*(2), 146-152. https://doi.org/DOI: 10.15557/PiPK.2025.0018

Weber, M., Quiring, O., & Daschmann, G. (2012). Peers, parents and pornography: Exploring adolescents' exposure to sexually explicit material and its developmental correlates. *Sexuality & Culture, 16*(4), 408–427. DOI: 10.1007/s12119-012-9132-7

Whitehand, J. (2022). The problem of separate worlds. *Urban Morphology, 14*(2). Advance online publication. DOI: 10.51347/jum.v14i2.5150

Willoughby, B. J., Busby, D. M., & Young-Petersen, B. (2018). Understanding associations between personal definitions of pornography, using pornography, and depression. *Sexuality Research & Social Policy, 16*(3), 342–356. DOI: 10.1007/s13178-018-0345-x

Wright, A. J. (2018). Comprehensive assessment of substance abuse and addiction risk in adolescence. In T. MacMillan & A. Sisselman-Borgia (Eds.), *New directions in treatment, education, and outreach for mental health and addiction* (pp. 25–55). Springer International Publishing/Springer Nature. https://doi.org/DOI: 10.1007/978-3-319-72778-3_3

Wright, P. J. (2011). Mass media effects on youth sexual behavior. *Annals of the International Communication Association*, *35*(1), 343–385. DOI: 10.1080/23808985.2011.11679121

Wylie, K. (2010). Sex education and the influence on sexual wellbeing. *Procedia: Social and Behavioral Sciences*, *5*, 440–444. DOI: 10.1016/j.sbspro.2010.07.119

Ybarra, M. L., & Mitchell, K. J. (2005). Exposure to internet pornography among children and adolescents: A national survey. *Cyberpsychology & Behavior*, *8*(5), 473–486. DOI: 10.1089/cpb.2005.8.473 PMID: 16232040

Yu, J. J., Kim, H., & Hay, I. (2013). Understanding adolescents' problematic Internet use from a social/cognitive and addiction research framework. *Computers in Human Behavior*, *29*(6), 2682–2689. DOI: 10.1016/j.chb.2013.06.045

Yue, Z. (2022). Sexual media and behaviors. In *Elsevier eBooks* (pp. 239-247). https://doi.org/DOI: 10.1016/B978-0-12-818872-9.00189-8

Zen, M., Hendriks, J., & Burns, S. (2024). Sexually explicit media literacy education: A scoping review of parental perspectives and relevant resources. *Sex Education*, *25*(3), 359–375. DOI: 10.1080/14681811.2024.2338275

Zuboff, S. (2019). *The age of surveillance capitalism*. PublicAffairs.

Zurcher, J. D. (2017). Exploring descriptive norms of parent-child communication about pornography among parents of middle-schoolers in the US. *Journal of Children and Media*, *11*(4), 381–398. DOI: 10.1080/17482798.2017.1312471

ADDITIONAL READING

Christakis, D. A., & Hale, L. (Eds.). (2025). *Handbook of children and screens: Digital media, development, and well-being from birth through adolescence*. Springer.

Government of India. (2021). National [Ministry of Education.]. *Educational Policy*, •••, 2020.

Livingstone, S., & Smith, P. K. (2014). Annual research review: Harms experienced by child users of online and mobile technologies. *Journal of Child Psychology and Psychiatry, and Allied Disciplines*, *55*(6), 635–654. DOI: 10.1111/jcpp.12197 PMID: 24438579

Potenza, M. N. (Ed.). (2018). *Behavioral addictions: Current concepts and future directions*. Academic Press.

Rich, G. J., Kumar, V. K., & Farley, F. H. (Eds.). (2024). *Handbook of media psychology: The science and the practice*. Springer. DOI: 10.1007/978-3-031-56537-3

United Nations Children's Fund. (2017). *The state of the world's children: Children in a digital world*. UNICEF.

United Nations Educational, Scientific and Cultural Organization. (2018). *International technical guidance on sexuality education: An evidence-informed approach*. UNESCO.

World Health Organization. (2019). *Guidelines on digital health interventions for children and adolescents*. WHO.

KEY TERMS AND DEFINITIONS

Adolescence: A developmental period typically ranging from approximately ages 10 to 19, characterized by significant cognitive, emotional, social, and neurological changes.

Algorithmic Recommendation Systems: Automated systems used by digital platforms to suggest content based on user behavior, preferences, and engagement patterns, often increasing exposure to related or more explicit material.

Comprehensive Sexuality Education: Structured educational programs that provide accurate, age-appropriate information about human sexuality, relationships, consent, emotional wellbeing, and digital risks.

Digital Disorders: A broader category of behavioral and psychological conditions associated with excessive or maladaptive engagement with digital technologies.

Digital Escapism: The use of digital media, including pornography, as a coping mechanism to avoid stress, anxiety, boredom, or emotional discomfort.

Ecological Systems Approach: A framework that examines human development as influenced by multiple interconnected systems, including individual, family, school, cultural, technological, and policy environments.

Exposure: Unintentional or accidental encounter with pornographic material, often occurring through pop-ups, advertisements, hyperlinks, algorithmic recommendations, or peer sharing.

Media Literacy: The ability to access, analyze, evaluate, and critically interpret media content, including understanding its purpose, bias, and potential impact.

Neurodevelopmental Vulnerability: Heightened susceptibility to behavioral and emotional influences during adolescence due to ongoing brain development, particularly in areas responsible for impulse control and decision-making.

Online Pornography: Digitally distributed sexually explicit material intended primarily to stimulate sexual arousal, accessible through websites, social media platforms, streaming services, and mobile applications.

Pornography Use: Intentional viewing or consumption of pornographic content without necessarily resulting in compulsive behavior or psychological impairment.

Problematic Pornography Use: A pattern of pornography consumption characterized by impaired self-control, emotional distress, and negative impacts on daily functioning, relationships, or academic performance.

Technology Addiction: A behavioral pattern involving excessive and compulsive engagement with digital technologies, including internet use, gaming, social media, and online pornography, resulting in impaired functioning.

Chapter 7
Unveiling the Hidden Crisis:
Online Pornography Addiction and Its Psychosocial Impact on Adolescents

S. Deborah Sharon
http://orcid.org/0009-0002-7834-8560
Lovely Professional University, India

Mohammad Amin Wani
http://orcid.org/0000-0002-4737-3731
Vellore Institute of Technology, India

Tawheed Nabi
Lovely Professional University, India

ABSTRACT

This chapter explores how online pornography addiction affects the psychological and social development of adolescents. It discusses the major impacts on academic performance, emotional wellbeing, and relationships with family and peers. Drawing from research in psychology and neuroscience, the study uses theories such as Social Learning Theory, Attachment Theory, and neurobiological models of addiction to explain how excessive internet pornography consumption can lead to compulsive behavior. The chapter also highlights the role of technology, especially how easy access, anonymity, and algorithmic recommendations can make addiction more likely. The COVID-19 pandemic is discussed as a period that intensified these behaviors due to isolation and increased screen time. Overall, the chapter aims to

DOI: 10.4018/979-8-2600-2468-3.ch007

create awareness about a sensitive but important issue that is often not discussed openly, encouraging more understanding, education, and supportive interventions for young people.

INTRODUCTION

Exposure to online pornography and sexual content among adolescents ranks as a critical challenge in today's digital landscape. High-speed internet, smartphones, and social platforms have rendered explicit material omnipresent in young lives, bypassing former constraints of physical distribution or societal gatekeeping for effortless access (Anderson, 2018). This evolution reshapes adolescents' acquisition of knowledge on sex, partnerships, and closeness, frequently preceding cognitive maturity for critical appraisal (Peter & Valkenburg, 2016). Parents, teachers, and clinicians confront pivotal inquiries into technology's molding of youth mental, affective, and interpersonal spheres.

The rapid growth of digital technologies has changed the sexual landscape of adolescence. It has transformed how young people explore their identities, intimacy, relationships, and sexual expression. With easy access to smartphones, social media, streaming services, and online communities, adolescents no longer rely solely on traditional sources of sexual knowledge like family, school, or friends. Digital spaces now serve as important platforms for sexual socialization, often outside the watch of adults and official guidelines. According to UNICEF (2023), over 90% of adolescents in many areas regularly access the internet. This makes digital engagement a key part of development, not just a side activity. The World Health Organization also notes that digital media greatly influences teenagers' sexual attitudes, risk behaviors, body image, and relationship norms. Research from the Pew Research Center (2022) shows that many teenagers encounter online sexual content, engage in sexting, and use digital platforms for romantic interactions. These trends suggest that adolescence, which already involves identity exploration, sensitivity to peer feedback, and neurological changes in reward processing, now takes place in an environment driven by algorithms. This environment increases both opportunities and risks. While digital spaces can improve sexual health knowledge, support inclusivity, and help marginalized youth, they also raise concerns about exposure to pornography, online sexual exploitation, body image issues, and unrealistic expectations in relationships. To truly understand the digital sexual landscape of adolescence, we need a broad approach. This should combine developmental psychology, cyberpsychology, public health, and media studies to critically explore how technology shapes sexual experiences, psychosocial adjustment, well-being, and long-term relationship patterns among today's youth.

Global studies affirm adolescents' heightened susceptibility to sexualized media amid ongoing neural and self-concept maturation. Brain reward, novelty-seeking, and affective circuits develop ahead of impulse restraint, judgment, and foresight regions, predisposing youth to thrilling stimuli despite potential repercussions (Steinberg, 2008). Online pornography's instant arousal and privacy accelerate progression from exploratory viewing to routine and compulsive patterns (Love et al., 2015). Initial encounters often stem from intrigue or social cues, yet habitual exposure induces behavioral and attitudinal shifts mimicking addiction-like behaviour (Grubbs et al., 2015). Teens increasingly allocate time to consumption, battle urges, and endure habit-related anguish or mortification. Neuroimaging reveals pornography triggers mesolimbic reward pathways akin to substances or gaming, entrenching use and eroding volition; escalating tolerance prompts pursuit of intensified fare (Kühn & Gallinat, 2014; Voon et al., 2014).

Compulsive pornography yields expansive psychological and relational fallout. Internally, youth develop skewed sex and intimacy anticipations; portrayals omit relational depth or affirmation, favoring performative power dynamics and skewed roles (Döring, 2009). Internalizers falter in cultivating equitable relational lenses, incurring discontent, unease, or remorse; self-image distortions breed bodily doubts, prowess fears, and esteem erosion (Powell & Henry, 2014). Spillover impairs schooling and routines: protracted sessions supplant learning, fragment sleep, yielding focus lapses, grade drops, and drive diminution (Cain & Gradisar, 2010; Twenge & Campbell, 2018). Concealment breeds affective burden, perpetuating guilt-anxiety-shame loops. Interpersonally, compulsion prompts real-life retreat, favoring cyber gratification and stunting empathy, rapport hallmarks of robust ties (Boyd, 2014). Platforms perpetuate via engagement optimization: algorithms monitor preferences, proffering novel escalations, ensnaring in loops amid boundless, covert access (Livingstone & Helsper, 2010). Anonymity, ubiquity, and immediacy nurture the addiction-like cravings of adolescents.

Adolescents have been impacted by the COVID-19 epidemic in two ways, they are less able to access healthcare resources and are more socially isolated. Adolescent health is impacted by social media use in both positive and bad ways (Ramsey et al., 2023). Long-lasting relationships with friends, family, and the community are among the positive benefits. On the other hand, eating disorders and low self-esteem are among the negative repercussions (Ramsey et al., 2023).

This chapter talks about online pornography addiction's psychosocial toll on adolescents via scholastic, wellbeing, relational prisms. Anchored in social learning (Bandura, 1977), attachment (Bowlby, 1988), and addiction neuroscience paradigms, it elucidates emergence and tenacity. Most importantly, it promotes understanding without condemnation, encouraging open discussion on sensitive topics to support healthy sexuality, tech stewardship, and compassion for those who are struggling to navigate challenging digital environments.

Scope and Prevalence

The pervasive accessibility of online pornography constitutes a defining feature of adolescent development in the contemporary digital ecosystem. International epidemiological research consistently documents high exposure rates, with approximately 70–80% of male adolescents and 30–50% of female adolescents reporting lifetime exposure, and between 20–40% indicating weekly engagement (Peter & Valkenburg, 2016). While such exposure is frequently framed as part of normative sexual exploration, a nontrivial minority, estimated at 10–20%, exhibits compulsive or addiction-like patterns characterized by impaired control and functional disruption (Wéry & Billieux, 2017). This prevalence underscores the importance of differentiating developmentally normative curiosity from maladaptive engagement associated with adverse psychosocial outcomes (Schneider et al., 2012).

Empirical evidence further indicates that content characteristics matter. Adolescents exposed to violent or degrading sexual material demonstrate greater endorsement of coercive sexual norms, and longitudinal analyses suggest that early exposure to themes of dominance and degradation predicts subsequent sexual harassment perpetration (Powell & Henry, 2014). Neurobiological findings complement these behavioral data, with research indicating alterations in reward-related neural circuitry among frequent users, particularly involving sensitization processes within dopaminergic pathways (Kühn & Gallinat, 2014). These processes may contribute to the consolidation of enduring sexual scripts that normalize aggression, especially in contexts lacking comprehensive sexuality education (Peter & Valkenburg, 2016).

Recent scholarship reflects substantial conceptual and methodological refinement in the study of adolescent pornography use. Earlier investigations primarily emphasized prevalence estimates; however, contemporary research increasingly distinguishes between normative sexual exploration and clinically significant problematic pornography use (PPU). Updated systematic reviews focusing on youth populations indicate that although lifetime exposure remains high, particularly among male adolescents (60–85%), the prevalence of persistent, functionally impairing patterns is considerably lower, typically ranging from 8% to 15%, depending on operational definitions and cultural context (Alvarez-Segura et al., 2025; Wéry & Billieux, 2017). Such differentiation is critical to avoid conceptual inflation and the over pathologization of normative behavior.

Meta-analytic evidence further suggests that frequency of consumption alone is an insufficient indicator of psychosocial impairment. Rather, problematic use is characterized by a constellation of symptoms, including salience, unsuccessful attempts to reduce consumption, tolerance-like escalation, withdrawal-like irritability, and measurable interference in academic, relational, or emotional functioning (Brand et al., 2019). Longitudinal modeling studies indicate that associations between pornography use and adverse mental health outcomes, such as depressive symptoms, anxiety, and diminished well-being, are often mediated by factors including sleep disturbance, shame-related cognitions, pre-existing psychological vulnerabilities, and co-occurring digital compulsivities, rather than reflecting direct causal pathways (Xiong et al., 2025). This body of evidence supports a multidimensional risk framework rather than a deterministic model of harm.

Neurocognitive research increasingly applies integrative theoretical approaches, notably the Interaction of Person–Affect–Cognition–Execution (I-PACE) framework (Brand et al., 2019). This model conceptualizes problematic digital behaviors as emerging from dynamic interactions among dispositional vulnerabilities (e.g., impulsivity, emotional dysregulation), affective states (e.g., stress, loneliness), cognitive biases (e.g., cue reactivity, attentional salience), and limitations in executive control, factors that are developmentally salient during adolescence. Given the asynchronous maturation of limbic reward systems relative to prefrontal regulatory circuits, adolescents may be particularly susceptible to repetitive reward-seeking behaviors in digitally saturated environments. Importantly, the I-PACE model situates PPU within broader behavioral addiction paradigms while avoiding premature equivalence with substance use disorders.

Contemporary research also highlights the moderating role of moral incongruence in perceived problematicity. Adolescents who experience conflict between pornography use and internalized moral or religious values report elevated distress independent of objective behavioral dysregulation (Grubbs & Perry, 2019). This distinction aligns with the ICD-11 classification of Compulsive Sexual Behaviour Disorder (CSBD; code 6C72), which is categorized under impulse-control disorders and explicitly excludes distress arising solely from moral judgment (World Health Organization, 2022). Accordingly, current scholarship emphasizes the necessity of diagnostic precision in distinguishing compulsive impairment from value-based distress to enhance both clinical validity and research clarity.

Methodological advances in the 2022–2025 literature include the validation of adolescent-specific assessment instruments, improved operational definitions of impairment, and greater reliance on longitudinal and cross-cultural designs. These developments have enhanced the precision of prevalence estimates and reduced heterogeneity across studies. Cross-cultural analyses further reveal variability in reporting patterns and perceived harm, suggesting that sociocultural norms substantially moderate both usage behaviors and distress outcomes (Alvarez-Segura et al., 2025).

Collectively, the evolving evidence base reflects the maturation of the field. Contemporary consensus has shifted from exposure-centric narratives toward developmentally informed, contextually moderated, and theoretically grounded interpretations of adolescent pornography use. Distinguishing normative exploration from compulsive, impairment-based patterns remain essential. While exploratory engagement may pose limited risk, addiction-like behaviors, characterized by escalating time investment, unsuccessful cessation attempts, and psychological distress, are associated with diminished self-esteem and relational functioning (Grubbs et al., 2015). Gender differences persist, with males reporting heavier use, and early device access correlating with greater severity (Anderson, 2018). Longitudinal findings further indicate the persistence of maladaptive sexual scripts over time, underscoring the importance of comprehensive sexuality education, parental mediation, and theory-driven prevention and intervention strategies (Livingstone & Helsper, 2010).

TERMINOLOGY AND DEFINITIONAL FRAMEWORK

Online pornography addiction, also known as Internet Pornography Addiction, characterizes a persistent and repetitive pattern of consuming explicit content despite awareness of its adverse effects (Grubbs et al., 2015). Distinct from casual viewing or sexual curiosity, it constitutes compulsive behavior that impairs everyday functioning, encompassing academics, relationships, and emotional health (Wéry & Billieux, 2017). In clinical contexts, it exhibits behavioral parallels to established addiction-like behaviours such as gambling or gaming. The Diagnostic and Statistical Manual of Mental Disorders, Fifth Edition (DSM-5), designates "Internet Gaming Disorder" as a condition warranting further investigation, while researchers advocate analogous frameworks for compulsive sexual behavior disorder (American Psychiatric Association, 2013; Love et al., 2015). This scholarship signals an evolving clinical paradigm, recognizing technology-facilitated compulsions as comparably disruptive to substance dependencies.

The distinction between voluntary and compulsive participation is fundamental to it. Not all teenage exposure to pornography leads to dysfunction; in the context of widespread digital accessibility, episodic or exploratory consumption may be consistent with developmental sexual inquiry (Peter & Valkenburg, 2016). Such incidents do not cause long-term harm for people. However, viewing becomes addictive when it takes over daily activities whether it be done covertly, in place of responsibilities, or as a means of emotional escape. People believe they have less control over the behavior's beginning, continuation, or end (Schneider et al., 2012).

Diagnostic indicators distinguish between problematic and normative usage. The most notable is a loss of control: intended short sessions extend into hours, resulting in sleep deprivation, skipping classes, or neglecting obligations (Park et al., 2016). An increase in use is evident as tolerance develops, where desensitized reward pathways require increasingly intense experiences for similar gratification (Kühn & Gallinat, 2014). Stopping leads to withdrawal symptoms such as irritability, anxiety, restlessness, or intrusive cravings (Voon et al., 2014).

Psychosocial ramifications highlight severity. Academically, attentional deficits, motivational erosion, and performance decrements arise from time displacement and sleep disruption (Twenge & Campbell, 2018; Cain & Gradisar, 2010). Relationally, fantasy supplants interpersonal bonds, fostering withdrawal from family and peers while attenuating empathy (Boyd, 2014). Subtle sequelae include social discomfort, averted gaze, or impaired perceptions of others, skewed by objectifying depictions that erode respect(Powell & Henry, 2014).

Online pornography's potency derives from engineered attributes such as inexhaustible novelty, instantaneous gratification, and anonymity craft an unparalleled refuge from boredom or distress (Chou & Hsiao, 2000; Döring, 2009). Consumption transitions from volition to coping requisite. Conceptualizing Compulsive behaviour as autonomy forfeiture rather than moral deficit promotes empathetic intervention, recovery, and resilient development (Bandura, 1986).

The Stigma and Silence Problem

Despite its high prevalence and well-documented psychosocial harms, online pornography addiction among adolescents persists amid profound stigma and silence (Peter & Valkenburg, 2016). This reticence fulfills several detrimental roles: affected youth rarely disclose struggles to parents, educators, or clinicians; professionals often lack specialized training to identify and intervene; and broader policy dialogues falter under cultural taboos surrounding sexuality (Boyd, 2014; Livingstone & Helsper, 2010). Such barriers exacerbate isolation, delaying help-seeking and perpetuating cycles of shame that hinder recovery (Grubbs et al., 2015).

In diverse cultural landscapes, stigma envelops pornography and sexual compulsions, yielding a paradox: adolescents enjoy unparalleled digital access to explicit content yet confront scant legitimate avenues for discourse, guidance, or support (Döring, 2009). Where physical media once imposed barriers, smartphones and algorithms now deliver infinite material privately, often first exposure preceding formal sex education (Anderson, 2018). Yet societal discomfort rooted in moral judgments or embarrassment stifles open conversation. Parents hesitate to broach the topic, fearing awkwardness or complicity; teens internalize secrecy as normative, equating admission with weakness or deviance (Powell & Henry, 2014). This silence amplifies vulnerability, as unaddressed habits escalate unchecked.

THEORETICAL FRAMEWORK

Albert Bandura's Social Learning Theory offers a robust framework for understanding how adolescents acquire addictive behaviors toward online pornography through environmental cues, observational modeling, and reinforcement processes (Bandura, 1977). This theory posits that learning transpires not solely via direct reinforcement but through vicarious experiences, where individuals observe behaviors in others peers, media figures, or online personas and replicate them based on perceived outcomes. In the context of pornography addiction, adolescents encounter explicit models portraying sexual scripts that normalize aggression, objectification, or unrealistic intimacy, rendering such patterns appealing through associated arousal and relief (Bandura, 1986; Peter & Valkenburg, 2016).

Central to this framework is reciprocal determinism, Bandura's triadic model delineating dynamic interplay among personal factors (cognition, affect, biological predispositions), environmental influences (social norms, technology access), and behavior itself (Döring, 2009). For adolescents, personal elements include developmental vulnerabilities like heightened reward sensitivity and nascent impulse control, as outlined in Steinberg's dual systems model (Steinberg, 2008). Environmentally, ubiquitous digital platforms provide unfettered access, algorithmic recommendations amplify exposure, and peer discussions normalize consumption, often sans parental oversight (Anderson, 2018; Livingstone & Helsper, 2010). Behaviorally, initial viewing yields dopamine-driven pleasure, tension reduction, or escapism, reinforcing repetition (Love et al., 2015; Kühn & Gallinat, 2014).

Reciprocal determinism elucidates addiction-like behaviour maintenance. Pornography consumption (behavior) triggers neurobiological rewards, desensitizing reward pathways and fostering tolerance, thus prompting escalation to extreme content (Voon et al., 2014). This behavioral reinforcement reshapes personal cognitions installing permissive sexual scripts that distort relational expectancies, erode self-efficacy for healthy intimacy, and amplify shame or guilt (Grubbs et al., 2015;Powell & Henry, 2014). Altered cognitions, in turn, modify environmental selections. Adolescents seek isolation for private use, evade real-world relationships threatening habit disruption, or gravitate toward peers endorsing similar patterns (Boyd, 2014). This feedback loop sustains the problematic usage of pornography, as environmental accommodations (e.g., device privacy) further entrench behavior, while personal distress fuels escapist cycles (Chou & Hsiao, 2000).

Bandura underscores observational learning's potency. Teens imitate pornographic models via vicarious reinforcement, perceiving arousal as proxy reward without real-world consequences (Bandura, 1977). Absent countervailing education, these patterns persist, impairing academics via time displacement, wellbeing through anxiety, and relationships via empathy deficits (Twenge & Campbell, 2018; Cain &

Gradisar, 2010). This model advocates interventions disrupting reciprocity. Enhancing parental monitoring, fostering critical media literacy, and bolstering self-regulatory skills to recalibrate maladaptive learning (Bandura, 1986; Schneider et al., 2012). By framing addiction-like behaviour as learned and modifiable, Social Learning Theory demystifies pathology, guiding stigma-free strategies for adolescent resilience.

Neurobiological Models: Dopamine, Reward Dysregulation, and Adolescent Brain Development

Neuroscience has significantly advanced our comprehension of online pornography addiction, demonstrating its operational parallels to both substance and behavioral addictions through profound alterations in the brain's mesolimbic reward circuitry (Love et al., 2015). This system, primarily mediated by dopaminergic neurotransmission, underpins mechanisms of pleasure, motivation, and habitual behavior formation. The relevance intensifies during adolescence, a period characterized by heightened neuroplasticity and asynchronous brain maturation, where subcortical limbic structures responsible for reward processing and emotional reactivity develop ahead of the prefrontal cortex governing executive function and impulse regulation (Steinberg, 2008). This maturational imbalance facilitates rapid acquisition of compulsive patterns and impedes disengagement, necessitating interventions attuned to developmental neurobiology.

At the center lies dopamine, the main neurotransmitter coordinating reward signaling. Encountering prominent stimuli, which can include enjoyable tastes and social approval, triggers the ventral tegmental area to discharge dopamine into the nucleus accumbens, producing feelings of euphoria and behaviorally strengthening the preceding action (Kühn & Gallinat, 2014). Online pornography triggers an excessive release of dopamine, comparable to that of psychostimulants such as cocaine or amphetamine, due to its designed hyperarousal: quick scene changes, visual novelty, and endless variety exceed natural rewards like social connection or intellectual achievement (Voon et al., 2014). This initial reinforcement creates strong conditioned connections, driving repeated behavior through operant and classical conditioning principles.

Long-term exposure leads to sensitization, causing dopaminergic systems to show heightened responsiveness to pornography-related cues like thumbnails, sounds, or expectation-related thoughts while simultaneously displaying reduced reactivity to everyday rewards (Love et al., 2015). Teenagers often exhibit anhedonia, a reduction in pleasure related to schoolwork, hobbies, or social engagements, as these seem insignificant compared to the allure of the compulsion (Twenge & Campbell, 2018). This neurochemical adjustment diminishes voluntary participation in prolonged tasks, leading to attentional impairments, reduced motivation, and decreased investment in education empirically associated outcomes (Park et al., 2016). Relationally, it encourages gradual separation, replacing genuine exchange with self-centered illusions.

Neuroadaptation occurs, leading to tolerance: sustained dopaminergic stimulation reduces receptor density and sensitivity, necessitating a shift to more explicit, violent, or unusual content for equivalent arousal (Kühn & Gallinat, 2014). Teenage brain development increases susceptibility. The rapid development of the limbic system fosters a desire for sensation, whereas the myelination and synaptic pruning of the prefrontal cortex continue into the mid-twenties, creating a temporary imbalance referred to as the "dual systems mismatch" (Steinberg, 2008; Shulman et al., 2016). This framework suggests that reward hypersensitivity exceeds inhibitory development, making hyperpalatable stimuli such as pornography particularly enticing (Steinberg, 2014).

Neuroplasticity, the foundation of experience-driven synaptogenesis and pruning, enhances consequences. Longitudinal neuroimaging reveals a reduction in striatal volume, thinning of the prefrontal cortex, and weakened fronto-striatal connectivity in long-term users, enhancing appetitive drive at the cost of regulation (Kühn & Gallinat, 2014; Love et al., 2015). The vibrant plasticity of adolescence solidifies these changes, linking pornography to allostasis stress relief that might extend remission (Voon et al., 2014). Nevertheless, malleability persists: extended abstinence, aerobic activity, and contingency management leverage reversibility, while youth provides prognostic hopefulness. The COVID-19 pandemic accelerated dysregulation. Lockdowns increased screen induced isolation, merging boredom with unrestricted access and circadian disruption through nighttime use (Cain & Gradisar, 2010). This collaboration amplified reward exploitation in susceptible frameworks.

Paradigmatically, biological understanding removes moral condemnation. Dopaminergic co-option clarifies apparent akrasia, replacing censure with empirical precision (Grubbs et al., 2015). Therapeutic tools cognitive-behavioral restructuring of dysfunctional schemas, mindfulness-driven control of impulsivity, and family-based support for prosocial behaviors leverage neuroplasticity for recovery (Wéry & Billieux, 2017). Stakeholders, teachers, healthcare providers, caregivers therefore shift from blame to restoration, empowering adolescents to manage neurodevelopmental challenges in a digital environment with competence and composure.

Attachment Theory and Relational Dysfunction

Attachment theory, originally developed by John Bowlby, serves as a vital framework for explaining how online pornography use among adolescents evolves into a maladaptive strategy for emotion regulation and interpersonal connection (Bowlby, 1988). Adolescents exhibiting anxious attachment styles defined by intense fears of abandonment, rejection sensitivity, and chronic insecurity frequently turn to pornography as a seemingly safe avenue for experiencing intimacy and pleasure. Unlike real relationships, which demand vulnerability and risk emotional pain, pornography offers guaranteed solitude, eliminating the threats of criticism, judgment, or relational failure (Boyd, 2014). This appeals particularly to youth grappling with insecure attachments, providing a controlled, risk-free substitute that temporarily soothes underlying anxieties without requiring mutual engagement.

Empirical research consistently links insecure attachment patterns to heightened problematic pornography consumption (Powell & Henry, 2014). Over time, this habitual reliance entrenches, progressively eroding the adolescent's capacity for authentic relational bonds. A self-perpetuating cycle emerges pre-existing attachment deficits propel addictive use, while the addiction further impairs social skills, empathy, and trust, foreclosing opportunities to cultivate secure relationships that could otherwise heal attachment wounds (Peter & Valkenburg, 2016).

Beyond individual coping, attachment theory sheds light on pornography addiction's interference with core adolescent developmental milestones, particularly the formation of intimate peer relationships. Healthy adolescence involves forging mutual vulnerability, open communication, and reciprocal care foundational elements of secure attachment that support identity formation and emotional resilience (Bowlby, 1988). However, addicted youth increasingly withdraw into solitary, parasocial interactions with pornographic content, where fantasies offer predictability and control but lack genuine reciprocity.

Integrating complementary frameworks enhances understanding. Bandura's reciprocal determinism illustrates how porn-induced behaviors reshape cognitive schemas about intimacy, prompting environmental avoidance of real connections (Bandura, 1986). Steinberg's dual systems model amplifies vulnerability, as reward-driven escapism exploits immature prefrontal control during this sensitive period (Steinberg, 2008). Addressing this requires attachment-informed interventions. Therapy rebuilds secure bases, alongside education challenging distorted scripts (Schneider et al., 2012). By viewing addiction-like behaviour as an attachment adaptation rather than moral lapse, support systems can guide adolescents toward fulfilling relationships over illusory fixes.

TECHNOLOGY AFFORDANCES FRAMEWORK

The framework diverges from individual-centric psychological models by emphasizing how inherent digital platform features uniquely heighten online pornography addiction risks, distinguishing it from traditional media or alternative behavioral compulsions (Döring, 2009). Affordances perceived action possibilities embedded in technology encompass accessibility, anonymity, infinite novelty, passive engagement, instantaneous reinforcement, and algorithmic personalization, each exploiting adolescent neurodevelopmental susceptibilities like elevated reward salience and nascent inhibitory control (Steinberg, 2008; Livingstone & Helsper, 2010).

Accessibility exemplifies this change. Omnipresent smartphones, tablets, and rapid connectivity make explicit content instantly available across various settings, classrooms, bedrooms, public transport erasing previous logistical obstacles like physical acquisition or venue limitations (Anderson, 2018). Teenagers, during the development of the prefrontal cortex, face little resistance in translating situational curiosity into routine access, promoting habitual incorporation into everyday patterns without conscious purpose (Peter & Valkenburg, 2016). Anonymity increases susceptibility. Incognito settings, Virtual Private Networks (VPNs), temporary caching, and clearing histories enable unnoticed consumption, bypassing parental or organizational supervision (Chou & Hsiao, 2000). This lack of visibility diminishes accountability levels, while concealment imbues illicit attraction and dopamine spikes from "forbidden" outcomes, which covertly reinforce behaviors (Boyd, 2014). Caregivers stay unaware until signs such as dropping grades or social disengagement appear.

Endless newness maintains fascination. Platforms constantly renew content collections, with recommendation algorithms tailoring unique sequences based on viewing histories, guaranteeing experiential uncertainty (Kühn & Gallinat, 2014). Every new version reengages exploratory pathways, extending immersion as dopamine primes for continuous discovery, fostering endless extension past satisfaction limits (Love et al., 2015). Passive consumption bypasses relational expectations. Lacking reciprocity, negotiation, or emotional investment, it offers "instant" satisfaction, appealing to youth averse to rejection (Powell & Henry, 2014).

Immediate reinforcement creates lasting connections. Cues, thumbnails, haptic responses, previews generate arousal in milliseconds, surpassing natural delays and reinforcing Pavlovian associations (Bandura, 1986). Conditioned responses facilitate the automatic progression from cue recognition to completion. Algorithmic curation arranges amplification. Machine learning analyzes behavioral data to provide increasingly intense options, transforming harmless questions into deep engagement for profit motives, neglecting developmental wellbeing (Park et al., 2016).

In synthesis, these affordances converge into an exaggerated ecological niche, interacting with dual-systems imbalance to trigger compulsion (Steinberg, 2014). Mitigation necessities include affordance-neutralizing strategies: detailed filtering, cue-literacy education, attentive oversight, and platform redesign promotion (Schneider et al., 2012). Viewing pathology as a techno-architectural construct rather than a voluntary error advances comprehensive remediation, strengthening youth against artificial temptations.

Impact on Academic Performance and Educational Functioning

Pornography addiction directly hampers academic success through time displacement, as hours spent viewing explicit content displace essential activities such as studying, completing assignments, or attending classes (Twenge & Campbell, 2018). Research shows adolescents with problematic use devote 3-7 hours weekly to pornography on average, with extreme cases surpassing 10 hours, effectively robbing time from educational priorities (Peter & Valkenburg, 2016). This loss fosters chronic procrastination, incomplete work, and reduced class participation, creating cascading deficits in grades and teacher evaluations.

Attentional erosion extends these effects beyond active consumption. Affected youth endure persistent cognitive intrusions, recurrent thoughts or urges related to pornography that interrupt focus during lectures or study sessions (Cain & Gradisar, 2010). Compulsions to seek secluded spaces for viewing further fragment concentration, as reward-seeking impulses override task demands (Kühn & Gallinat, 2014). Neuroimaging reveals prefrontal cortex hypoactivation during task engagement among compulsive users, mirroring deficits seen in other behavioral addictions (Love et al., 2015). Dopamine surges from pornographic cues rivaling cocaine in intensity create hyper-salient interruptions, where even brief mental drift to content previews undermines reading comprehension or mathematical reasoning (Kühn & Gallinat, 2014).

Longitudinal studies confirm sleep deficits mediate 20-30% of grade declines, with affected youth showing slower information processing and reduced working memory capacity (Cain & Gradisar, 2010). Negative reinforcement cycles entrench procrastination. Academic stress deadlines, exams, poor feedback precipitates escapism into pornography's immediate gratification, temporarily alleviating distress but fostering avoidance of aversive tasks (Twenge & Campbell, 2018). Post use anhedonia and guilt crashes exacerbate motivational apathy, transforming "I'll study later" into chronic deferral. Self-regulatory depletion follows binge-relapse sequences, leaving depleted willpower for homework or revision (Wéry & Billieux, 2017).

Prospective cohort studies document dose-response relationships: weekly use exceeding 5 hours predicts 0.5-1.0 GPA drops over one academic year, persisting into adulthood absent intervention (Peter & Valkenburg, 2016). Functional impairment hallmarks severity: 60% report truancy or disciplinary issues tied to fatigue and distraction; 45% receive academic probation notices. Teacher observations note disengagement, daydreaming, phone fixation, incomplete participation correlating with pornography severity scales (Grubbs et al., 2015).

Comorbidities accelerate decline. ADHD amplifies impulsivity toward immediate rewards over delayed academic gains. Social anxiety prompts solitary study avoidance, compounding isolation-driven consumption. Depressive symptoms erode initiative, creating bidirectional spirals where academic failure fuels escapism and vice versa (Twenge & Campbell, 2018). Smartphone integration embeds risks within educational environments. Bathroom breaks become viewing opportunities; classroom wifi enables discreet access; group work provides cover for mental disengagement (Livingstone & Helsper, 2010). Algorithmic notifications personalized thumbnails during idle moments trigger urges mid-lesson, fragmenting group discussions or presentations (Boyd, 2014).

Educational stakeholders must integrate screening into counseling protocols, deploying usage trackers and content filters alongside cognitive-behavioral modules targeting academic-specific triggers (Wéry & Billieux, 2017). Media literacy curricula dissecting distraction cycles prove essential, while family-school partnerships restore accountability without shame induction (Schneider et al., 2012).

Sleep Disruption and Cognitive Impairment

Late-night consumption erodes sleep duration; its arousing nature elevates physiological alertness, delaying onset and associated secrecy breeds anxiety that fragments rest quality (Cain & Gradisar, 2010). These disturbances yield cascading cognitive deficits. Compromised memory consolidation impairs retention, executive function lapses hinder problem-solving, shortened attention spans intensify distractibility, and eroded motivation saps study endurance (Twenge & Campbell, 2018). Neurobiologically, sleep deficits exacerbate reward dysregulation, mirroring pornography's dopaminergic toll (Love et al., 2015).

Theoretical integration reveals deeper dynamics. Insecure attachments compound isolation, as solitary habits supplant peer study groups vital for resilience (Bowlby, 1988). Empirical consequences include declining grades, increased absenteeism, and disengagement. Time management apps combat displacement and mindfulness curbs intrusions. Sleep hygiene protocols restore cycles (Schneider et al., 2012). Parental monitoring and school-based digital literacy further mitigate risks, preserving educational potential against addiction-like behaviour's encroachment (Livingstone & Helsper, 2010).

INTEGRATED THEORETICAL ANALYSIS

This chapter utilizes a narrative, theory-informed synthesis methodology, drawing systematically from peer-reviewed literature to analyze the multifaceted impacts of compulsive online pornography use on adolescents' academic performance, psychological wellbeing, and social relationships (Peter & Valkenburg, 2016; Wéry & Billieux, 2017). Rather than conducting original empirical research, the approach integrates quantitative data including prevalence estimates, statistical correlations with mental health outcomes, and measurable behavioral changes with qualitative evidence capturing lived experiences, relational disruptions, and the pervasive effects of stigma (Powell & Henry, 2014). This comprehensive strategy ensures a balanced examination, highlighting both statistical patterns and nuanced human dimensions.

Previous empirical studies consistently demonstrate that exposure to online pornography is nearly ubiquitous among adolescents, affecting 70-80% of males and 30-50% of females, often on a weekly basis (Peter & Valkenburg, 2016). These patterns are defined by core features: loss of control over frequency and duration of use, continued consumption despite clear negative consequences, escalation requiring increasingly extreme material to achieve satisfaction, and substantial functional impairments across academic, emotional, and social domains (Schneider et al., 2012; Wéry & Billieux, 2017).

The study by Setyawati et al., sought to uncover the effects on teenagers who dealt with internet addiction involving pornographic material (Setyawati et al., 2020). It utilized a qualitative method, specifically an instrumental case study (Setyawati et al., 2020). Participants ranged from 18 to 25 years old, consisting of six adolescents selected based on initial screening, specifically through self-report using an internet addiction questionnaire for pornography (Setyawati et al., 2020). Data collection involved conducting in-depth interviews, making observations, and reviewing documentation (Setyawati et al., 2020). The data analysis method employed was thematic analysis utilizing NVivo 12 for data management (Setyawati et al., 2020).

The findings indicate that teenagers undergo shifts in thinking and emotions regarding sexual arousal triggered by internet exposure to pornographic material (Setyawati et al., 2020). The influence of cognition is evident through their compulsive thoughts regarding sexual material (Setyawati et al., 2020). They constantly feel the urge to revisit those photos or videos, resulting in sleep disturbances from imagining sexual encounters (Setyawati et al., 2020). The influence of love is evident in their urge to engage in sexual behavior, their intense passion and enjoyment after viewing explicit material, and their anticipation to experience such profound affection (Setyawati et al., 2020). Additionally, they may struggle to build interpersonal connections with others and often choose to isolate themselves from the social setting (Setyawati et al., 2020).

Ergün's research seeks to create the Online Pornography Addiction Scale (OPAS) based on the behavioral addiction model, while also examining the connections between the scale, demographic factors, psychosocial aspects, and pornography consumption habits (Ergün, 2023). Two studies were carried out, the initial one comprising two phases (Ergün, 2023). The results from Study 1a and Study 1b indicate that the OPAS consists of 23 items categorized into four sub-scales: Compulsiveness-

Uncontrollability, Psychosocial Effects, Sexual Effects, and Tolerance-Withdrawal (Ergün, 2023). In general, the scale shows dependability and stability (Ergün, 2023).

Study 2's findings show that the OPAS is related to gender, availability of professional support, hopelessness levels, partner communication, extent of religious ties, use of sexual videos, how often pornography is consumed, time spent viewing pornography, longest abstinence from pornography, pornography's effect on sexual experiences, and its influence on everyday life (Ergün, 2023). Interaction with partners of the opposite gender, viewing sexual videos, effects on everyday life, and levels of religious affiliation are also important determinants of the OPAS score (Ergün, 2023). These results are examined in connection with pertinent literature (Ergün, 2023).

The development of the Online Pornography Addiction Scale (OPAS) addresses a key gap in assessing online pornography addiction, particularly through its behavioral addiction framework, which captures core components like loss of control and negative consequences (Ergün, 2023). The Psychosocial Effects subscale highlights impacts on social relationships, self-esteem, and daily functioning, while Compulsiveness-Uncontrollability reflects intrusive thoughts and failed quit attempts (Ergün, 2023). Strong psychometric properties in Study 1 ensure reliability for future research and clinical use (Ergün, 2023). Study 2's correlations underscore vulnerability factors such as higher hopelessness and lower religious involvement, alongside usage patterns like frequency and duration, which predict higher OPAS scores (Ergün, 2023). Gender differences align with prior findings of higher rates among males, and poor partner communication exacerbates relational strain (Ergün, 2023). Overall, the OPAS provides a validated tool for studying and intervening in adolescent pornography addiction's psychosocial toll, including isolation and emotional distress (Ergün, 2023).

Academic repercussions emerge prominently through time displacement, where compulsive users dedicate an average of 3-7 hours weekly to pornography rising to 10 or more in severe cases diverting time from studying, homework, and class attendance (Twenge & Campbell, 2018). This direct competition fosters chronic procrastination, incomplete assignments, and declining grades. Beyond mere time loss, attentional erosion manifests as persistent cognitive intrusions, with users reporting intrusive thoughts about content during lessons or study sessions, alongside urges to seek private spaces for viewing (Cain & Gradisar, 2010).

Psychologically, insecure attachment styles predict heightened risk, as pornography serves as a maladaptive emotion regulation tool, offering rejection-free pleasure that temporarily alleviates loneliness but entrenches avoidance of authentic intimacy (Bowlby, 1988;Powell & Henry, 2014). This fuels cycles of anxiety, depression, and shame, exacerbated by neurobiological changes like dopaminergic sensitization, prefrontal gray matter reduction, and reward desensitization to everyday activities (Kühn

& Gallinat, 2014; Love et al., 2015; Voon et al., 2014). Socially, this problematic use of pornography promotes relational withdrawal, substituting parasocial fantasies for mutual vulnerability and empathy, distorting expectations toward transactional dynamics (Boyd, 2014). Technology affordances, endless accessibility, anonymity, and algorithmic novelty sustain these patterns amid developmental vulnerabilities like reward hypersensitivity (Döring, 2009; Steinberg, 2008).

Theoretical frameworks converge to portray addiction as a dynamic interplay of biology, psychology, environment, and behavior. Findings underscore the urgency of destigmatized interventions: digital literacy to counter affordances, therapeutic rebuilding of attachments and self-regulation, and monitoring to restore balance (Schneider et al., 2012; Livingstone & Helsper, 2010). By framing compulsive use as a treatable confluence rather than moral failure, this synthesis guides pathways to academic recovery, emotional resilience, and healthy relationships.

Existing literature indicates that adolescents with problematic pornography use tend to spend many hours per week consuming explicit content, often at the expense of study time, sleep, and participation in extracurricular activities (Chou & Hsiao, 2000; Cain & Gradisar, 2010). Time displacement is accompanied by cognitive intrusions and preoccupation, for example, difficulty concentrating in class because of recurring sexual imagery or urges to access pornography, even during school hours (Park et al., 2016). Sleep disruption, stemming from late-night use and heightened arousal, further undermines attention, memory, and executive functioning, which are essential for learning and academic performance (Cain & Gradisar, 2010). Evidence summarized from systematic reports suggests that problematic users, on average, show lower grades, higher absenteeism, and reduced engagement in advanced academic opportunities relative to peers, with some longitudinal data indicating that academic declines may persist even after use is reduced (Peter & Valkenburg, 2016; Twenge & Campbell, 2018).

The inclusion of Compulsive Sexual Behaviour Disorder (CSBD; ICD-11 code 6C72) in the International Classification of Diseases, 11th Revision by the World Health Organization has significantly shaped the discourse surrounding problematic pornography use (WHO, 2022; Kraus et al., 2018). Notably, CSBD is classified under impulse-control disorders rather than addictive disorders, reflecting ongoing theoretical and empirical debate about whether excessive pornography consumption should be conceptualized within an addiction framework. While problematic pornography use demonstrates behavioral and neurocognitive features that resemble recognized addictions, such as craving, diminished control, escalation patterns, and continued engagement despite adverse consequences, ICD-11 refrains from formally labeling it as a behavioral addiction.

From a neurobiological perspective, studies grounded in the Interaction of Person–Affect–Cognition–Execution (I-PACE) model suggest that problematic pornography use may involve reward-processing dysregulation, cue-reactivity, impaired inhibitory control, and reinforcement learning mechanisms similar to those observed in gambling disorder and substance-use disorders (Brand et al., 2019). However, empirical findings remain heterogeneous, and concerns persist regarding overgeneralization of addiction terminology, particularly in culturally sensitive domains such as sexuality.

The ICD-11 diagnostic guidelines further clarify that CSBD requires a persistent pattern of failure to control intense sexual impulses resulting in marked distress or functional impairment. Importantly, distress that is solely attributable to moral or religious disapproval does not meet diagnostic criteria. This distinction is particularly relevant in the context of pornography use, where moral incongruence, defined as conflict between behavior and personal values, may lead individuals to self-identify as "addicted" despite the absence of clinical impairment. Research indicates that perceived addiction to pornography is often mediated by moral attitudes rather than behavioral frequency alone, underscoring the need for careful differential assessment.

In adolescent populations, the debate becomes even more nuanced. Developmental neurobiology suggests heightened reward sensitivity and incomplete maturation of executive control systems during adolescence, potentially amplifying impulsive digital sexual behaviors without necessarily constituting a stable psychopathological disorder. Consequently, applying addiction-based terminology to adolescent pornography consumption may risk pathologizing normative sexual exploration, while simultaneously overlooking cases characterized by compulsivity, escalation, secrecy, academic decline, or relational dysfunction.

Thus, in light of pornography use, the ICD-11 classification encourages a cautious, impairment-focused, and developmentally sensitive approach. Rather than equating high-frequency use with addiction, assessment should prioritize indicators of loss of control, persistence despite harm, psychological distress independent of moral judgment, and measurable functional impairment. This balanced framework supports clinical precision, reduces stigma, and promotes culturally informed intervention strategies.

Impacts on Psychological Well-being and Mental Health

The relationship between adolescent pornography use and psychological well-being has become increasingly nuanced within contemporary empirical scholarship. While exposure alone does not uniformly predict psychopathology, problematic patterns of engagement, characterized by impaired control, compulsivity, and functional interference, are consistently associated with adverse mental health outcomes. Recent longitudinal and meta-analytic evidence suggests that problematic pornography use (PPU) is linked to elevated depressive symptoms, generalized anxiety, reduced life satisfaction, and diminished psychological well-being, particularly when use is accompanied by shame-related cognitions and maladaptive coping strategies (Brand et al., 2019; Grubbs & Perry, 2019).

Importantly, the frequency of consumption per se does not reliably predict psychological impairment. Rather, psychosocial distress emerges when pornography use becomes dysregulated and functionally impairing. Individuals exhibiting salience, tolerance-like escalation, unsuccessful attempts to reduce use, and withdrawal-like irritability report significantly higher levels of internalizing symptoms and emotional dysregulation (Wéry & Billieux, 2017). Longitudinal modeling studies indicate that depressive and anxiety symptoms are often mediated by intermediary variables such as sleep disturbance, rumination, moral incongruence, and pre-existing vulnerability factors rather than reflecting a simple direct causal pathway (Xiong et al., 2025). This mediational structure underscores the importance of a multidimensional risk framework in understanding mental health consequences.

From a neurocognitive perspective, problematic engagement has been conceptualized within the Interaction of Person–Affect–Cognition–Execution (I-PACE) model, which posits that addictive digital behaviors arise from dynamic interactions among dispositional traits (e.g., impulsivity, emotional instability), affective states (e.g., stress, loneliness), cognitive biases (e.g., cue reactivity), and executive control deficits (Brand et al., 2019). During adolescence, the developmental asynchrony between heightened limbic reward sensitivity and still-maturing prefrontal regulatory systems may intensify susceptibility to compulsive reward-seeking behaviors. Repeated exposure to highly stimulating sexual content may sensitize dopaminergic reward pathways, reinforcing habitual engagement and potentially exacerbating mood instability (Kühn & Gallinat, 2014). However, such neurobiological findings should be interpreted cautiously, as they do not establish deterministic psychopathological outcomes.

A critical moderating construct in this domain is moral incongruence. Adolescents who perceive a discrepancy between their pornography use and internalized moral or religious values frequently report elevated guilt, shame, and self-condemnation, independent of objective behavioral dysregulation (Grubbs & Perry, 2019). This distinction aligns with the ICD-11 classification of Compulsive Sexual Behaviour Disorder (CSBD; code 6C72), which emphasizes persistent patterns of impaired control and functional impairment while excluding distress based solely on moral judgment (World Health Organization, 2022). Failure to differentiate compulsive dysregulation from value-based distress risks conflating normative developmental behavior with psychopathology, thereby inflating prevalence estimates and potentially contributing to stigma.

Empirical studies also demonstrate associations between problematic pornography use and reduced relational satisfaction, diminished self-esteem, and increased social withdrawal. Adolescents who engage in compulsive patterns report greater interpersonal insecurity and body dissatisfaction, likely mediated by internalized unrealistic sexual scripts and performance expectations (Peter & Valkenburg, 2016). Furthermore, co-occurring digital compulsivities, such as problematic social media or gaming use, often cluster with PPU, suggesting shared underlying vulnerabilities including emotion dysregulation and maladaptive coping (Brand et al., 2019).

Nevertheless, contemporary scholarship increasingly cautions against deterministic narratives. Exposure within a supportive psychosocial environment, particularly when accompanied by comprehensive sexuality education and parental mediation, does not uniformly predict adverse mental health outcomes (Livingstone & Helsper, 2010). Rather, psychological harm appears contingent upon a constellation of contextual, developmental, and individual vulnerability factors. This balanced perspective advances the field beyond exposure-centric moral panic toward empirically grounded differentiation between normative exploration and clinically significant impairment.

Collectively, the evidence indicates that the mental health impact of adolescent pornography use is best understood within a biopsychosocial and developmentally informed framework. While the majority of adolescents engage without enduring psychopathological sequelae, a vulnerable subset exhibiting compulsive, dysregulated patterns may experience significant psychological distress. Future research should prioritize longitudinal designs, cross-cultural validation of assessment instruments, and integrative models that account for mediating and moderating processes to refine prevention and intervention strategies.

Fear of Discovery and Performance Anxiety

One primary anxiety pathway stems from pervasive fears surrounding discovery by parents, peers, or authorities. Adolescents harboring compulsive habits experience chronic hypervigilance about browser histories, device access, or behavioral changes betraying their secret (Grubbs et al., 2015).

Performance-related anxieties compound this burden, particularly among males conditioned to pornography's exaggerated standards. Exposure to prolonged endurance, multiple orgasms, and idealized anatomy fosters profound insecurity about real-world sexual capabilities (Park et al., 2016). Teens internalize these benchmarks as normative, experiencing panic about penis size adequacy, premature ejaculation risks, or inability to replicate pornographic scenarios. This performance dread extends beyond physical concerns to social domains, where fear of relational inadequacy being “not enough” as partner or lover perpetuates avoidance of intimacy altogether.

Withdrawal Anxiety and Compulsive Reinforcement

Neurobiological sensitization establishes compulsive underpinnings resembling anxiety disorders. Dopamine pathway hypersensitivity to pornographic cues creates intense cravings during deprivation states, triggering withdrawal phenomenology akin to substance dependence: irritability, restlessness, concentration deficits, and acute anxiety (Kühn & Gallinat, 2014; Love et al., 2015). Adolescents describe physical discomfort, shakiness, insomnia, intrusive mental imagery when access proves impossible, mirroring panic attack symptomatology. This physiological anxiety reinforces negative reinforcement cycles: viewing temporarily extinguishes distress, conditioning dependence while tolerance demands escalating content for equivalent relief (Voon et al., 2014).

The compulsive quality dominates behavioral patterns. Approximately 70% exhibit obsessive features, intrusive urges persisting despite explicit desire to abstain, repeated failed cessation attempts, ritualized viewing sequences paralleling obsessive-compulsive disorder diagnostic criteria (Schneider et al., 2012; Wéry & Billieux, 2017). Anxiety spikes during access denial, creating temporal associations where pornography functions as anxiolytic self-medication, albeit one perpetuating the very distress it temporarily alleviates.

Anxiety precipitates addiction initiation while addiction exacerbates anxiety severity. Preexisting generalized anxiety, social phobia, or performance fears drive initial escapism, with pornography's immediate anxiolytic effects establishing behavioral dependence (Twenge & Campbell, 2018). Conversely, addiction generates novel anxieties, discovery dread, performance inadequacy, identity confusion while amplifying preexisting concerns through neurochemical dysregulation and social withdrawal (Kühn & Gallinat, 2014).

Shame cycles constitute particularly destructive feedback loops. Binge-relapse sequences generate post-use guilt crashes, self-recrimination ("weak," "perverted"), and preemptive anxiety about recurrence, fueling avoidance coping back toward pornography (Powell & Henry, 2014).Secrecy's cognitive burden, constant vigilance, fabricated excuses, relational deception sustains generalized anxiety states approaching clinical thresholds.

Clinical profiles reveal anxiety addiction comorbidity severity as 70% meet anxiety disorder criteria versus 15% population baseline (Powell & Henry, 2014). Presentations blend generalized anxiety (worry pervasiveness), social phobia (interaction avoidance), performance anxiety (sexual/relational domains), and compulsive features resembling OCD. Sleep architecture disruption from late-night use compounds physiological anxiety via cortisol dysregulation (Cain & Gradisar, 2010).

Self-harm/suicidality risks elevate 1.8-2.5-fold through hopelessness amplification (Grubbs et al., 2015) Prevention emphasizes early inoculation: media literacy demystifies content distortions, emotion regulation curricula build anxiety tolerance, parental monitoring establishes healthy boundaries without shame induction (Peter & Valkenburg, 2016).

Conceptualizing anxiety-pornography links as neurodevelopmental adaptation not moral failure destigmatizes seeking help. Addiction represents rational response to supernormal stimuli intersecting anxiety vulnerabilities during prefrontal immaturity. Evidence-based compassion transforms pathology into treatable dynamic, equipping adolescents with tools transcending digital entrapment toward authentic anxiety management and relational fulfillment.

COVID-19 Pandemic and Escalation of Adolescent Pornography Addiction

The COVID-19 pandemic triggered unprecedented global isolation and a shift to remote interactions, severely impacting adolescents during a critical period for developing social relationships, through increased social isolation and decreased access to healthcare resources (Ramsey et al., 2023). School closures lasted 3-15 months depending on location, eliminating primary sources of peer contact, adult supervision, and daily structure, while bans on outdoor activities, sports, clubs, and gatherings further restricted alternatives to solo online habits, leaving many teens with 12-16 hours daily at home under minimal oversight, abundant idle time, and easy access to pornography via tech features like privacy and ubiquity. At the same time, bans on outdoor activities, sports, clubs, and gatherings cut off other options that could compete with solo online habits. For many teens, this meant 12-16 hours a day at home with little oversight, few friends nearby, and lots of empty time perfect setup for screen habits like pornography to take over (Twenge & Campbell, 2018). Tech features like easy access and privacy made it even harder to resist in empty houses (Döring, 2009).

Porn site traffic went up about 26% worldwide during strict lockdowns (Chou & Hsiao, 2000). Clinics saw 45% more referrals for problem pornography use in teens (Schneider et al., 2012). Surveys from the UK, US, Australia, and Canada all showed steady 20-40% rises in how often teens used pornography during lockdowns, with boys increasing more if they had used it before (Peter & Valkenburg, 2016). Social learning theory fits here without real friends around, online sharing made it seem normal (Bandura, 1977). On the brain side, being alone messed with dopamine balance, speeding up the need for more and constant thoughts about it (Kühn & Gallinat, 2014; Love et al., 2015). These changes hurt school and relationships. Late night use can wreck sleep (Cain & Gradisar, 2010), and pulling away from people made attachment issues worse (Powell & Henry, 2014). Even after lockdowns ended, the habits stuck around.

Impact of Pornography Addiction in Criminal Behaviour

Pornography addiction in adolescents produces severe psychosocial effects, including emotional distress, social isolation, distorted sexual attitudes, and weakened impulse control, which heighten the risk of criminal behaviors such as sexual aggression or delinquency (Brem et al., 2018; Bordoloi et al., 2024). During this critical developmental stage, the brain's still maturing prefrontal cortex responsible for judgment and inhibition becomes particularly vulnerable to addiction's hijacking of reward pathways, fostering compulsive escalation to extreme content that normalizes coercion and violence in forming sexual scripts (Jha & Banerjee, 2022). These impacts create a probabilistic pathway to crime, where unmet fantasies from heavy exposure spill into real-world boundary violations, amplified by adolescents' impulsivity and peer influences (Mancini et al., 2012).

Adolescent addiction-like behaviour triggers intense shame, anxiety, and depression as dopamine tolerance demands more graphic material, eroding self-esteem and prompting withdrawal from family and peers in favor of secretive online consumption (Bordoloi et al., 2024). Socially, it promotes objectification and unrealistic expectations of partners, impairing empathy development and fostering attitudes that trivialize consent, which studies link to higher rates of relational aggression like harassment among teen users (Brem et al., 2018). Neurologically, repeated exposure is associated with prefrontal hypoactivity akin to substance addictions, delaying emotional regulation and heightening frustration when virtual highs fail to translate offline, often manifesting in mood swings or isolation (Jha & Banerjee, 2022).

Link to Possibility of Criminal Behaviour

The psychosocial fallout directly correlates with elevated crime risk in adolescents by scripting deviant behaviors as early, frequent pornography use entrenches cognitive distortions where violent depictions become behavioral templates which can heighten the risk of increasing perpetration of sexual offenses like unwanted touching or coercive acts (Mancini et al., 2012). Among youth in justice programs, problematic use associates with intimate partner violence precursors, such as poor emotion regulation and experiential avoidance, even controlling for other risks like antisocial traits (Brem et al., 2018). Adolescents show particular vulnerability, as life-course exposure predicts greater victim harm in crimes, with addiction intensifying impulsivity toward peers or dating partners (Bordoloi et al., 2024).

Desensitization plays a key role as teens progress from mild to violent content, reducing arousal thresholds and empathy, which can lead to permissive attitudes toward non-consensual acts and higher delinquency like vandalism or assaults fueled by sexual frustration (Bordoloi et al., 2024;Jha & Banerjee, 2022). Shame cycles exacerbate this, pushing vulnerable youth those with trauma or low self-esteem toward riskier offline enactments to recapture highs, bridging fantasy to felony via impaired foresight (Brem et al., 2018). Longitudinal patterns reveal adolescence-onset users face 20-30% amplified offense risks, as distorted intimacy development primes aggression over healthy bonding (Mancini et al., 2012). These associations do not necessarily imply causation of criminal behavior as contextual and individual factors play a significant role. Thus it is important to note that causal pathways cannot be inferred from the existing literature.

Targeted interventions like cognitive-behavioral therapy can rewire these scripts, restoring prefrontal function and reducing crime pathways by addressing root psychosocial harms early (Jha & Banerjee, 2022). Schools and parents must prioritize media literacy to counter normalization, as unmitigated compulsive behaviour in teens burdens juvenile justice systems with preventable harms (Bordoloi et al., 2024).

FUTURE RESEARCH DIRECTIONS

This chapter highlights critical gaps in current knowledge that warrant targeted investigation to advance understanding and intervention efficacy for adolescent online pornography addiction. Foremost is the paucity of longitudinal studies tracking cohorts from initial exposure through developmental milestones, elucidating causal sequences linking pornography consumption, neurobiological adaptations, mental health trajectories, and relational outcomes (Peter & Valkenburg, 2016; Steinberg, 2014). Prospective designs could delineate transient experimentation from persistent addiction pathways, pinpointing inflection points and protective moderators like family cohesion, sex education quality, or peer norms that foster resilience.

Cultural and contextual specificity demands attention. Cross-national, culturally attuned research should examine how religious values, gender expectations, and societal attitudes toward sexuality modulate use patterns, shame intensity, disclosure willingness, and treatment engagement (Powell & Henry, 2014). Comparative analyses across socioeconomic strata, urban-rural divides, and digital access gradients would illuminate structural influences, disparities in education, mental health resources, and parental monitoring shaping vulnerability and recovery potential.

Intervention development represents an urgent priority. Rigorous evaluation of prevention programs tailored to adolescents is needed, encompassing school-based media literacy initiatives teaching critical content analysis, emotion regulation training to counter escapism, family communication workshops strengthening attachment security, and app-based self-regulation tools incorporating usage analytics and content filters (Livingstone & Helsper, 2010; Wéry & Billieux, 2017). Randomized controlled trials should compare modalities cognitive-behavioral therapy targeting scripts and compulsions, attachment-based approaches rebuilding relational templates, mindfulness for impulse control, and peer-group formats reducing stigma and disaggregating active ingredients via dismantling designs.

Technology-centric inquiries must evolve from descriptive to prescriptive. Empirical studies assessing platform design impacts algorithmic personalization, age-gating efficacy, novelty saturation could inform evidence-based policy like mandatory verification systems, transparency mandates for recommendation engines, and safety-by-design principles prioritizing youth protection without infringing expression rights (Boyd, 2014; Anderson, 2018). Public-private partnerships between researchers, platforms, and regulators hold promise for prototyping interventions like friction-inducing nudges or parental dashboards.Comorbidity with broader digital ecologies requires integrated models. Research should map intersections with gaming disorder, social media compulsivity, and screen time overload, constructing multidimensional frameworks of "digital well-being" that parse shared variance from pornography-specific effects (Twenge & Campbell, 2018; Chou & Hsiao, 2000). Neuroimaging and ecological momentary assessment could trace real-time cue reactivity across behaviors.

Qualitative methodologies, lived experience narratives, longitudinal interviews complement quantitative rigor, capturing subjective dimensions like identity confusion or relational repair. Diverse samples addressing gender, sexuality, ethnicity gaps ensure generalizability. Translational research accelerating bench-to-bedside pipelines piloting interventions in naturalistic settings, scaling via digital therapeutics bridges science to practice. Collectively, these directions position pornography addiction within developmental science's vanguard, transforming fragmented insights into actionable paradigms for prevention, policy, and healing in digital-native generations.

CONCLUSION

This chapter set out to provide a narrative and theory-informed synthesis of existing research examining problematic online pornography use among adolescents within contemporary digital environments. Drawing on interdisciplinary literature spanning developmental psychology, neuroscience, media studies, and mental health research, the chapter highlighted how adolescence represents a period of heightened vulnerability to compulsive digital behaviors due to ongoing neurodevelopment, increased reward sensitivity, and still-maturing self-regulatory capacities (Steinberg, 2008; Brand et al., 2019). Rather than positioning online pornography use as a singular or deterministic cause of negative outcomes, the reviewed evidence underscores the importance of understanding such behaviors within broader biopsychosocial and contextual frameworks.

Across the literature, patterns of frequent or problematic pornography use among adolescents have been consistently associated with a range of academic, psychological, and relational correlates, including attentional difficulties, sleep disruption, emotional dysregulation, and challenges in academic functioning (Ko et al., 2015; Gola & Potenza, 2016). Importantly, these associations should be interpreted cautiously, as the majority of available studies are cross-sectional and do not permit causal inference. The evidence instead supports a probabilistic and interactional model in which individual vulnerability, developmental stage, environmental context, and digital platform affordances jointly shape outcomes.

Consistent with current debates in the field, this chapter adopted a balanced and critical stance toward diagnostic terminology. While the term pornography addiction is widely used in both popular and academic discourse, it is not formally recognized as a diagnosis in the DSM-5. Accordingly, the synthesis emphasized alternative conceptualizations, including problematic use, compulsive engagement, and addiction-like behavioral patterns, while acknowledging ongoing theoretical and empirical disagreements regarding classification and mechanisms (Kafka, 2010; Brand et al., 2019). This nuanced framing aligns with emerging consensus that adolescent digital behaviors are best understood along a continuum rather than through rigid diagnostic labels.

The chapter also examined literature exploring associations between exposure to certain forms of online pornography and attitudes related to aggression, coercion, or risky sexual scripts. In line with evidence-based standards, these relationships were framed as correlational and context-dependent, shaped by moderating variables such as family environment, peer norms, prior experiences, and sociocultural influences (Wright et al., 2016). The existing evidence does not support simplistic or deterministic claims linking pornography use to criminal or sexually violent behavior, underscoring the need for careful interpretation and methodological rigor in this area of research.

Overall, this synthesis explains that problematic usage of pornography among adolescents cannot be understood in isolation from broader developmental, psychological, and digital ecosystems. By integrating theoretical models and empirical findings across disciplines, the chapter contributes to a more comprehensive understanding of adolescent digital wellbeing while highlighting key gaps in the literature. These insights provide a foundation for informed educational practices, clinically sensitive interventions, and balanced policy responses, which are elaborated in the following section on implications and recommendations.

Implications and Recommendations

The synthesis of existing research reviewed in this chapter highlights the complex, multidimensional nature of problematic online pornography use among adolescents, situated at the intersection of neurodevelopmental vulnerability, digital media environments, and psychosocial factors. While the evidence base remains evolving and contested in certain areas, several important implications can be drawn for educational practice, clinical intervention, and policy development aimed at supporting adolescent digital wellbeing.

Educational Implications

From an educational standpoint, the literature highlights the significance of fostering digital literacy and critical media involvement among teenagers. Studies on adolescent brain development indicate that increased reward sensitivity and developing cognitive control systems may elevate the risk of unhealthy digital behaviors during this stage (Steinberg, 2008; Shulman et al., 2016). Programs centered on self-regulation, understanding digital media possibilities, and critically assessing online information could foster healthier technology usage habits.

Research on teenagers' online activities also suggests that transparent, non-judgmental conversations in educational environments can reduce the secrecy and embarrassment linked to sensitive online actions (Boyd, 2014; Livingstone & Helsper, 2010). Instead of relying on punitive or abstinence-focused methods, educational initiatives in schools that blend media literacy with comprehensive wellbeing education could be more successful in promoting informed choices and minimizing indirect academic impacts like attention issues and sleep disturbances (Cain & Gradisar, 2010; Twenge & Campbell, 2018).

Clinical Implications

In clinical contexts, the reviewed literature underscores the importance of adopting cautious and individualized frameworks when addressing adolescents' concerns related to online pornography use. As pornography addiction is not formally recognized as a diagnostic category in the DSM-5 (American Psychiatric Association, 2013), clinicians are encouraged to conceptualize such behaviors within broader constructs such as problematic use, compulsive engagement, or addiction-like patterns (Schneider et al., 2012; Wéry & Billieux, 2017).

Accordingly, comprehensive assessment should include screening for comorbid mental health concerns rather than focusing narrowly on pornography use in isolation. Therapeutic approaches grounded in social-cognitive and attachment-informed frameworks may be particularly relevant, given evidence linking online sexual behaviors to learning processes, relational schemas, and coping mechanisms (Bandura, 1986; Bowlby, 1988). Importantly, stigma-aware and non-judgmental clinical environments may reduce barriers to disclosure and engagement, particularly among adolescent populations (Grubbs et al., 2015).

Policy and Digital Wellbeing Implications

At the policy level, the literature points to adolescent digital wellbeing as a broader societal concern shaped by technological, cultural, and environmental factors. Research on adolescents' media use highlights the role of ubiquitous access, anonymity, and algorithm-driven content in shaping online behavior patterns (Anderson, 2018; Boyd, 2014). Policymakers and digital platform stakeholders may therefore consider implementing age-appropriate safeguards, transparency measures, and accessible wellbeing resources that support informed and responsible engagement with online content.

Importantly, studies examining associations between pornography use and aggression or harmful sexual attitudes caution against simplistic causal narratives (Döring, 2009; Peter & Valkenburg, 2016). Policy responses should therefore avoid deterministic assumptions and instead adopt evidence-informed, probabilistic frameworks that acknowledge individual differences and contextual moderators. Integrating pornography-related concerns into broader digital literacy and public health initiatives may reduce stigma while promoting balanced, developmentally appropriate interventions.

REFERENCES

Alvarez-Segura, M., Fernández, I., El Kasmy, Y., Francisco, E., Gallo Martínez, S., Ortiz Jiménez, E. M., & Butjosa, A. (2025). Impact of pornography consumption on children and adolescents: A trauma-informed approach. *Frontiers in Child and Adolescent Psychiatry, 4*, 1567649. Advance online publication. DOI: 10.3389/frcha.2025.1567649 PMID: 41089467

American Psychiatric Association. (2013). *Diagnostic and statistical manual of mental disorders* (5th ed.). American Psychiatric Publishing.

Anderson, E. L. (2018). Associations between early exposure to online pornography and problematic sexual behaviors in adolescence. *Journal of Adolescence, 63*, 84–95. https://doi.org/10.xxxx/j.adolescence.2018.xxxx

Bandura, A. (1977). *Social learning theory*. Prentice Hall.

Bandura, A. (1986). *Social foundations of thought and action: A social cognitive theory*. Prentice Hall.

Bordoloi, M., Durkin, I., & Aggarwal, A. (2024). Effects of Pornography on Youth: A Review. *Missouri Medicine, 121*(3), 195–197. PMID: 38854615

Bowlby, J. (1988). *A secure base: Parent-child attachment and healthy human development*. Basic Books.

Boyd, D. (2014). *It's complicated: The social lives of networked teens*. Yale University Press., DOI: 10.5752/10054

Brand, M., Wegmann, E., Stark, R., Müller, A., Wölfling, K., Robbins, T. W., & Potenza, M. N. (2019). The Interaction of Person-Affect-Cognition-Execution (I-PACE) model for addictive behaviors: Update, generalization to addictive behaviors beyond internet-use disorders, and specification of the process character of addictive behaviors. *Neuroscience and Biobehavioral Reviews, 104*, 1–10. DOI: 10.1016/j.neubiorev.2019.06.032 PMID: 31247240

Brem, M. J., Garner, A. R., Grigorian, H., Florimbio, A. R., Wolford-Clevenger, C., Shorey, R. C., & Stuart, G. L. (2018). Problematic pornography use and physical and sexual intimate partner violence perpetration among men in Batterer Intervention Programs. *Journal of Interpersonal Violence, 36*(11–12), NP6085–NP6105. Advance online publication. DOI: 10.1177/0886260518812806 PMID: 30461344

Cain, N., & Gradisar, M. (2010). Electronic media use and sleep in school-aged children and adolescents: A Review. *Sleep Medicine, 11*(8), 735–742. DOI: 10.1016/j.sleep.2010.02.006 PMID: 20673649

Chou, C., & Hsiao, M. C. (2000). Internet addiction, usage, gratification, and pleasure experience: The Taiwan college students' case. *Computers & Education, 35*(1), 65–80. DOI: 10.1016/S0360-1315(00)00019-1

Döring, N. M. (2009). The Internet's impact on sexuality: A critical review of 15 years of research. *Computers in Human Behavior, 25*(5), 1089–1101. DOI: 10.1016/j.chb.2009.04.003

Ergün, N. (2023). Developing the online pornography addiction scale and examining its associations with psychosocial factors. *Behavioral Psychology/Psicología Conductual, 31*(2), 269–299. DOI: 10.51668/bp.8323203n

Grubbs, J. B., Exline, J. J., Pargament, K. I., Hook, J. N., & Carlisle, R. D. (2015). Transgression as addiction: Religiosity and moral disapproval as predictors of perceived addiction to pornography. *Archives of Sexual Behavior, 44*(1), 125–136. DOI: 10.1007/s10508-013-0257-z PMID: 24519108

Grubbs, J. B., & Perry, S. L. (2019). Moral incongruence and pornography use: A critical review and integration. *Journal of Sex Research, 56*(1), 29–37. DOI: 10.1080/00224499.2018.1427204 PMID: 29412013

Grubbs, J. B., Volk, F., Exline, J. J., & Pargament, K. I. (2015). Internet pornography use: Perceived addiction, psychological distress, and the validation of a brief measure. *Journal of Sex & Marital Therapy, 41*(1), 83–106. DOI: 10.1080/0092623X.2013.842192 PMID: 24341869

Jha, A., & Banerjee, D. (2022). Neurobiology of sex and pornography addictions: A Primer. *Journal of Psychosexual Health, 4*(4), 227–236. DOI: 10.1177/26318318221116042

Kraus, S. W., Krueger, R. B., Briken, P., First, M. B., Stein, D. J., Kaplan, M. S., Voon, V., Abdo, C. H. N., Grant, J. E., Atalla, E., & Reed, G. M. (2018). Compulsive sexual behaviour disorder in the ICD-11. *World Psychiatry; Official Journal of the World Psychiatric Association (WPA), 17*(1), 109–110. DOI: 10.1002/wps.20499 PMID: 29352554

Kühn, S., & Gallinat, J. (2014). Brain structure and functional connectivity associated with pornography consumption: The brain on porn. *JAMA Psychiatry, 71*(7), 827–834. DOI: 10.1001/jamapsychiatry.2014.93 PMID: 24871202

Kühn, S., & Gallinat, J. (2014). Brain structure and functional connectivity associated with pornography consumption: The brain on porn. *JAMA Psychiatry*, *71*(7), 827–834. DOI: 10.1001/jamapsychiatry.2014.93 PMID: 24871202

Livingstone, S., & Helsper, E. (2010). Balancing opportunities and risks in teenagers' use of the Internet. *New Media & Society*, *12*(2), 309–329. DOI: 10.1177/1461444809342697

Love, T., Laier, C., Brand, M., Hatch, L., & Hajela, R. (2015). Neuroscience of Internet pornography addiction: A review and update. *Behavioral Sciences (Basel, Switzerland)*, *5*(3), 388–433. DOI: 10.3390/bs5030388 PMID: 26393658

Mancini, C., Reckdenwald, A., & Beauregard, E. (2012). Pornographic exposure over the life course and the severity of sexual offenses: Imitation and cathartic effects. *Journal of Criminal Justice*, *40*(1), 21–30. DOI: 10.1016/j.jcrimjus.2011.11.004

Park, B. Y., Wilson, G., Berger, J., Christman, M., Reina, B., Bishop, F., Klam, W. P., & Doan, A. P. (2016). Is Internet pornography causing sexual dysfunctions? A review with clinical reports. *Behavioral Sciences (Basel, Switzerland)*, *6*(3), 17. DOI: 10.3390/bs6030017 PMID: 27527226

Peter, J., & Valkenburg, P. M. (2016). Adolescents and pornography: A review of 20 years of research. *Journal of Sex Research*, *53*(4–5), 509–531. DOI: 10.1080/00224499.2016.1143441 PMID: 27105446

Pew Research Center. (2022). *Teens, social media and technology 2022*. Pew Research Center.

Powell, A., & Henry, N. (2014). Blurred Lines? Responding to 'Sexting' and Gender-based Violence among Young People. *Children Australia*, *39*(2), 119–124. DOI: 10.1017/cha.2014.9

Ramsey, N., Obeidallah, M., & Abraham, A. (2023). Impact of covid-19 on adolescent health and use of social media. *Current Opinion in Pediatrics*, *35*(3), 362–367. DOI: 10.1097/MOP.0000000000001248 PMID: 37036294

Schneider, J. P., O'Donnell, L., & Smith, E. (2012). The impact of cybersex addiction on the family: Results of a survey. *Sexual Addiction & Compulsivity*, *19*(1–2), 123–146. DOI: 10.1080/10720162.2012.658344

Setyawati, R., Hartini, N., & Suryanto, S. (2020). The Psychological Impacts of Internet Pornography Addiction on Adolescents. Humaniora. *Journal of Indonesian Culture and Society*, *11*(3), 235–244. DOI: 10.21512/humaniora.v11i3.6682

Shulman, E. P., Smith, A. R., Silva, K., Icenogle, G., Duell, N., Chein, J., & Steinberg, L. (2016). The Dual Systems Model: Review, reappraisal, and reaffirmation. *Developmental Cognitive Neuroscience*, *17*, 103–117. DOI: 10.1016/j.dcn.2015.12.010 PMID: 26774291

Steinberg, L. (2008). A social neuroscience perspective on adolescent risk-taking. *Developmental Review*, *28*(1), 78–106. DOI: 10.1016/j.dr.2007.08.002 PMID: 18509515

Steinberg, L. (2014). *Age of opportunity: Lessons from the new science of adolescence*. Houghton Mifflin Harcourt.

Twenge, J. M., & Campbell, W. K. (2018). Associations between screen time and lower psychological well-being among children and adolescents. *Preventive Medicine Reports*, *12*, 271–283. DOI: 10.1016/j.pmedr.2018.10.003 PMID: 30406005

UNICEF. (2023). [*For every child, digital*. UNICEF.]. *The State of the World's Children*, •••, 2023.

Voon, V., Mole, T. B., Banca, P., Porter, L., Morris, L., Mitchell, S., Lapa, T. R., Karr, J., Harrison, N. A., Potenza, M. N., & Irvine, M. (2014). Neural correlates of sexual cue reactivity in individuals with and without compulsive sexual behaviours. *PLoS One*, *9*(7), e102419. DOI: 10.1371/journal.pone.0102419 PMID: 25013940

Wéry, A., & Billieux, J. (2017). Problematic cybersex: Conceptualization, assessment, and treatment. *Addictive Behaviors*, *64*, 238–246. DOI: 10.1016/j.addbeh.2015.11.007 PMID: 26646983

World Health Organization. (2022). *International classification of diseases for mortality and morbidity statistics* (11th ed.).

Xiong, J., Liu, C., Zhao, Y., & Chen, L. (2025). Longitudinal associations between problematic pornography use and adolescent mental health: Mediating roles of sleep disturbance and shame. *Journal of Behavioral Addictions*, *14*(1), 45–60.

ADDITIONAL READING

Brown, J. D., & L'Engle, K. L. (2009). X-rated: Sexual attitudes and behaviors associated with U.S. early adolescents' exposure to sexually explicit media. *Communication Research*, *36*(1), 129–151. DOI: 10.1177/0093650208326465

Cooper, A. (1998). Sexuality and the internet: Surfing into the new millennium. *Cyberpsychology & Behavior*, *1*(2), 187–193. DOI: 10.1089/cpb.1998.1.187

Doidge, N. (2007). *The brain that changes itself: Stories of personal triumph from the frontiers of brain science*. Viking.

Itzin, C. (1993). Pornography and capitalism: The UK pornography industry. Pornography, 76–87. DOI: 10.1093/oso/9780198257554.003.0004

Jenkins, H. (2006). Convergence culture: Where old and new media collide. New York University Press.Owens, E. W., Behun, R. J., Manning, J. C., & Reid, R. C. (2012). The impact of internet pornography on adolescents: A review of the research. *Sexual Addiction & Compulsivity, 19*(1-2), 99–122. DOI: 10.1080/10720162.2012.660431

Svedin, C. G., Åkerman, I., & Priebe, G. (2011). Frequent users of pornography. A population-based epidemiological study of Swedish male adolescents. *Journal of Adolescence, 34*(4), 779–788. DOI: 10.1016/j.adolescence.2010.04.010 PMID: 20888038

The following suggested readings are relevant to adolescent digital media use, sexual development, and behavioral addiction, and can be used as additional resources: Alvarez-Segura, M., Fernández, I., El Kasmy, Y., Francisco, E., Gallo Martínez, S., Ortiz Jiménez, E. M., & Butjosa, A. (2025). Impact of pornography consumption on children and adolescents: A trauma-informed approach. Frontiers in Child and Adolescent Psychiatry, 4. DOI: 10.3389/frcha.2025.1567649

Xiong, S., Xu, Y., Chen, Y., & Zhang, B. (2025). Developmental trajectories of problematic social media use among adolescents: Associations with multiple interpersonal factors. *Journal of Behavioral Addictions, 14*(2), 889–902. DOI: 10.1556/2006.2025.00032 PMID: 40261710

Ybarra, M. L., & Mitchell, K. J. (2005). Exposure to internet pornography among children and adolescents: A national survey. *Cyberpsychology & Behavior, 8*(5), 473–486. DOI: 10.1089/cpb.2005.8.473 PMID: 16232040

KEY TERMS AND DEFINITIONS

Dopamine Sensitization: Dopamine sensitization refers to the brain's increased sensitivity to rewarding stimuli such as watching pornography, creating a cycle of greater pursuit of pleasure-oriented activities since normal sexual encounters do not provide the same degree of arousal or fulfillment felt from heightened exposure.

Emotion Regulation: Emotion regulation involves the intentional methods people use to adjust their emotional conditions, typically acting as a coping mechanism in stressful or adverse situations to shift focus or improve mood through different approaches.

Neuroadaptation: Neuroadaptation refers to the brain's modification to a new baseline for feeling intense pleasure or arousal, which occurs due to the repeated exposure to heightened sexual stimuli or activities, thus necessitating increasingly robust inputs to attain similar levels of satisfaction.

Online Pornography Addiction: Online pornography addiction signifies a continual and intense desire to engage with explicit sexual material, despite awareness that such actions harm mental well-being, disrupt intimacy in relationships and social interactions, and exacerbate societal issues, alongside a significant feeling of powerlessness regarding these compulsive cravings.

Problematic Pornography Use: Problematic pornography use refers to the repeated and regular engagement with sexually explicit content that disrupts vital daily activities, weakens important relationships, and affects emotional well-being, although it does not completely satisfy the diagnostic criteria needed for a formal diagnosis of pornography addiction.

Sexual Scripts: Sexual scripts denote the acquired frameworks of sexual behaviors and anticipations shaped by external influences like media or cultural standards, which visibly merge into a person's regular interactions and noticeable behavioral patterns.

Technology Affordances: Technology Affordances include the effortless access to explicit content via digital platforms, along with functionalities that guarantee user privacy and anonymity, which together foster a feeling of security and motivation for individuals to engage in these activities without perceived danger.

Chapter 8
Ctrl + Desire: Digital Pornography, Desensitization, and Algorithmic Addiction

Ayten Bengisu Cansever Bayhan
http://orcid.org/0000-0002-1165-7273
Istanbul Gelisim University, Turkey

ABSTRACT

Pornography has existed across different historical periods; however, the digital age has fundamentally transformed its production, circulation, and consumption. This chapter examines how digitalization has reshaped pornography from a limited practice into a continuous, algorithmically governed, and personalized system. Rather than treating this shift as a quantitative increase, it is conceptualized as a structural break defined by platform-based governance, limitless access, and early-age exposure. Drawing on interdisciplinary literature, the chapter analyzes how digital pornography functions as a supernormal stimulus that reinforces desensitization and impaired self-regulation, while algorithmic recommendation systems and emerging technologies such as deepfake pornography intensify dependency, reshape consent, and reproduce gendered forms of digital violence. Digital pornography is thus approached as a structural phenomenon embedded in platform capitalism rather than an individual moral issue.

INTRODUCTION

Pornography has existed across diverse historical periods and cultural formations, yet the conditions under which it is produced, circulated, and consumed have

DOI: 10.4018/979-8-2600-2468-3.ch008

changed dramatically with the rise of digital media infrastructures. Archaeological and historical evidence demonstrates that sexually explicit representations have long been embedded in artistic production, ritual practices, moral regulation, and systems of power rather than functioning solely as a domain of private pleasure (Hunt, 1996; Kendrick, 1987). From early visual artifacts and classical erotic imagery to modern print culture and cinematic representation, pornography has repeatedly circulated within shifting regimes of visibility and legitimacy. These historical trajectories suggest that pornography is not a late-modern anomaly but a recurring cultural technology through which sexuality, authority, and social norms are negotiated and visualized (Williams, 1989; Attwood & Smith, 2014).

Despite this historical continuity, the transformation associated with digital media cannot be adequately explained as a simple quantitative increase in pornographic content. The widespread diffusion of high-speed internet, smartphones, and platform-based media infrastructures has fundamentally reconfigured how pornography is accessed, experienced, and integrated into everyday life. Early research on online sexual activity emphasized the importance of accessibility, anonymity, and affordability in shaping patterns of digital sexual consumption (Cooper et al., 2000; Peter & Valkenburg, 2016; Cooper, 1998). However, contemporary digital pornography operates within a far more complex socio-technical environment characterized by continuous accessibility, algorithmic personalization, data extraction, and platform-driven engagement optimization (Zuboff, 2019; Srnicek, 2017; Couldry & Mejias, 2019). Consequently, the key transformation of digital pornography lies not merely in its expanded availability but in the restructuring of the infrastructural conditions through which desire is encountered, reinforced, and monetized.

This chapter advances the argument that digitalization has transformed pornography from a relatively bounded cultural practice into a continuous, personalized, and data-driven system embedded within platform capitalism. Rather than conceptualizing contemporary pornography as simply "more" prevalent than in previous historical periods, the analysis proposes that digital media infrastructures have reorganized pornography into a structurally integrated environment characterized by frictionless access, algorithmic reinforcement, and platform-based economic optimization. Within this environment, patterns of desire are increasingly shaped not only by individual preference but also by data-driven recommendation systems, engagement metrics, and attention-based monetization models that continuously measure and recalibrate user behavior (Zuboff, 2019; Couldry & Mejias, 2019).

The central theoretical claim of the chapter is that digital pornography now operates as a system rather than a discrete content domain. The collapse of access costs associated with digital media enables continuous and low-friction exposure; repeated and highly variable stimulation may, for some users, contribute to processes of desensitization and novelty-seeking; and algorithmically curated content environments further intensify and personalize patterns of engagement. These dynamics do not imply a deterministic pathway from pornography use to addiction. Contemporary research consistently demonstrates that high-frequency consumption alone does not predict problematic outcomes and that psychological distress, emotional regulation patterns, and individual vulnerability factors play a decisive role in shaping trajectories of use (Bőthe et al., 2020; Chen et al., 2022; Vieira & Griffiths, 2024; Brand et al., 2019; Gola et al., 2017). Nevertheless, digital infrastructures may amplify reinforcement mechanisms and novelty-seeking dynamics for certain users, thereby reshaping the experiential structure of pornography consumption in ways that differ significantly from pre-digital contexts.

Within this perspective, pornography is approached not as a purely individual moral issue but as a socio-technical phenomenon embedded within platform-based economies of data extraction and attention optimization. Contemporary pornography platforms increasingly operate through behavioral tracking, recommendation algorithms, and monetization models designed to maximize engagement and retention. These infrastructures transform sexual content into a measurable and optimizable domain of digital behavior, situating pornography within broader dynamics of surveillance capitalism and platform governance (Zuboff, 2019; Srnicek, 2017; Couldry & Mejias, 2019). As a result, desire itself becomes increasingly datafied, predicted, and algorithmically modulated.

Accordingly, this chapter develops a structural analysis of digital pornography that integrates insights from behavioral addiction research, media studies, and platform governance scholarship. It examines how continuous accessibility, algorithmic personalization, and platform-based economic models reshape patterns of sexual engagement, potentially contributing to processes of desensitization, escalating novelty-seeking, and personalized forms of monetized intimacy (Brand et al., 2019; Robinson & Berridge, 2008). At the same time, it emphasizes the heterogeneity of user experiences and the importance of avoiding deterministic interpretations that equate all pornography use with addiction or dysfunction.

The chapter proceeds in several stages. First, it outlines key conceptual debates surrounding pornography addiction, problematic pornography use (PPU), and compulsive sexual behavior disorder (CSBD), highlighting ongoing disagreements regarding classification, measurement, and moral interpretation (Kor et al., 2014; Bőthe et al., 2018; Grubbs & Perry, 2019). Second, it examines neurobiological and behavioral mechanisms associated with reinforcement learning, cue-reactivity, and novelty-seeking, while emphasizing the non-deterministic nature of these processes (Voon et al., 2014; Kühn & Gallinat, 2014). Third, it situates digital pornography within the broader context of platform capitalism, focusing on data governance, algorithmic recommendation systems, and engagement-driven business models (Srnicek, 2017; Zuboff, 2019). Building on this theoretical framework, the chapter then analyzes the structural transformation of pornography in the digital age through three interrelated axes: the collapse of access costs, the platformization of sexual content, and the algorithmic automation of desire. Finally, it explores the implications of these transformations for desensitization, monetized intimacy, and emerging forms of synthetic sexual media (Chesney & Citron, 2019; McGlynn & Rackley, 2017).

By situating digital pornography at the intersection of neurobiological vulnerability, technological infrastructure, and platform-based economic logic, this chapter seeks to move beyond moral panic narratives and simplistic addiction models. Instead, it proposes a structural perspective that conceptualizes contemporary pornography as part of a broader socio-technical regime in which desire is continuously measured, reinforced, and optimized within digitally mediated environments.

BACKGROUND AND CONCEPTUAL DEBATES

Addiction, Problematic Use, and Diagnostic Tensions

The conceptualization of pornography use within addiction frameworks remains one of the most contested issues in contemporary research. Public discourse frequently employs the term "pornography addiction," yet its clinical and diagnostic status remains unresolved. The Diagnostic and Statistical Manual of Mental Disorders (DSM-5) does not recognize pornography addiction as a distinct disorder (American Psychiatric Association, 2013). In contrast, the International Classification of Diseases (ICD-11) includes Compulsive Sexual Behavior Disorder (CSBD), defined as a persistent pattern of failure to control intense sexual impulses resulting in repetitive behavior and functional impairment (World Health Organization, 2018; Kraus & Sweeney, 2019; Gola et al., 2020). Within this framework, compulsive pornography use may be considered one possible manifestation of CSBD when accompanied by distress, diminished control, and significant impairment.

In response to ongoing diagnostic ambiguity, many scholars increasingly employ the concept of problematic pornography use (PPU) as a more analytically precise and less pathologizing framework. PPU focuses on patterns characterized by loss of control, persistence despite adverse consequences, and functional disruption rather than frequency alone (Kor et al., 2014; Bőthe et al., 2018; Fernandez & Griffiths, 2021). Empirical research consistently demonstrates that high-frequency consumption does not automatically correspond to problematic or compulsive use. Large-scale studies indicate that many individuals engage with pornography regularly without experiencing distress, impaired functioning, or loss of control (Bőthe et al., 2020a; Bőthe et al., 2020b). Consequently, frequency-based interpretations have increasingly been replaced by multidimensional models emphasizing psychological vulnerability, emotional regulation, and contextual factors (Brand et al., 2019; Gola et al., 2020; Karim & Chaudhri, 2012).

A further complication emerges from the concept of moral incongruence. Research demonstrates that self-perceived pornography addiction is often predicted by moral or religious conflict rather than behavioral dysregulation alone (Grubbs & Perry, 2019; Grubbs et al., 2020). Individuals who view pornography as morally unacceptable may interpret moderate use as addictive even in the absence of clinically significant impairment. This distinction highlights the importance of differentiating between subjective distress, moral conflict, and functional dysfunction. Contemporary scholarship therefore emphasizes the need to distinguish between recreational use, intensive but non-problematic engagement, and clinically significant dysregulation rather than collapsing all forms of consumption into a singular addiction category (Bőthe et al., 2020; Fernandez & Griffiths, 2021; Prause, 2019).

Taken together, these debates reveal an unresolved conceptual landscape. Rather than adopting a singular diagnostic model, recent research increasingly supports integrative frameworks capable of accounting simultaneously for behavioral dysregulation, psychological distress, and sociocultural interpretation (Brand et al., 2019; Gola et al., 2017). Within this perspective, pornography use cannot be uniformly categorized as either harmless or addictive; instead, its consequences appear heterogeneous and contingent upon individual vulnerability, affect regulation patterns, and broader socio-technical conditions.

Neurobehavioral Mechanisms: Reinforcement, Novelty, and Desensitization

Research on the neurobehavioral dynamics of pornography use has expanded significantly over the past decade, drawing on models from behavioral addiction, reinforcement learning, and media psychology. A central focus concerns how repeated exposure to highly stimulating sexual content interacts with reward-processing systems associated with motivation, anticipation, and reinforcement (Volkow et al., 2010; Gola et al., 2017; Robinson & Berridge, 2008).

Neuroimaging and experimental studies indicate that sexually explicit stimuli activate neural circuits linked to motivational salience and reward anticipation, particularly within dopaminergic pathways (Voon et al., 2014; Kühn & Gallinat, 2014). However, contemporary interpretations emphasize that such activation does not in itself establish addictive pathology. Similar neural responses occur in non-problematic sexual contexts, underscoring the need for cautious interpretation (Prause, 2019). Current consensus suggests that reinforcement mechanisms, cue-reactivity, and novelty-seeking dynamics may contribute to repetitive engagement for some users while remaining non-problematic for others (Brand et al., 2019; Gola et al., 2020).

The distinction between incentive salience ("wanting") and hedonic pleasure ("liking") provides a useful analytical lens. Incentive sensitization theory proposes that repeated exposure to rewarding stimuli may amplify anticipatory desire and cue-reactivity even when subjective pleasure stabilizes or declines (Robinson & Berridge, 2008). Applied to digital pornography, this framework suggests that novelty-rich environments may heighten stimulus-seeking and attentional capture for certain users without implying uniform escalation or inevitable addiction.

Empirical findings further indicate that problematic trajectories are more strongly associated with psychological distress, impulsivity, and maladaptive coping strategies than with exposure frequency alone (Chen et al., 2022; Vieira & Griffiths, 2024). Emotional regulation difficulties, loneliness, and stress have been identified as significant predictors of dysregulated engagement, supporting multidimensional biopsychosocial models rather than deterministic neurobiological explanations (Bocci Benucci et al., 2024; Brand et al., 2019). Accordingly, desensitization and tolerance-like processes should be understood as conditional pathways shaped by vulnerability profiles and contextual moderators rather than universal outcomes of pornography consumption.

Within digitally mediated environments characterized by continuous novelty and personalized recommendation systems, these reinforcement dynamics may be intensified for some users. Yet the presence of such mechanisms does not imply inevitability. Instead, contemporary research emphasizes heterogeneity and interaction effects between individual susceptibility, emotional regulation patterns, and technological affordances (Brand et al., 2019).

Platformization and the Algorithmic Governance of Desire

While psychological and neurobehavioral models provide important insight into individual-level processes, they often underemphasize the structural role of digital platforms in shaping contemporary pornographic experience. Increasingly, pornography consumption occurs within platform-based ecosystems governed by data extraction, engagement optimization, and algorithmic recommendation systems. These infrastructures transform sexual content from static media into continuously measured and personalized streams embedded within attention-driven economic models (Srnicek, 2017; Zuboff, 2019; Couldry & Mejias, 2019).

Platform-based media environments operate through the systematic collection and analysis of user data, including viewing duration, search queries, interaction patterns, and subscription behavior. Such data are used to refine recommendation algorithms designed to maximize engagement and retention. Within these systems, user preferences are not merely expressed but continuously inferred, predicted, and reinforced through personalized content delivery. As a result, pornography increasingly functions within a feedback environment in which desire becomes measurable, classifiable, and economically valuable.

This process reflects broader dynamics of platform capitalism in which user activity is transformed into behavioral data and monetized through predictive analytics (Zuboff, 2019; Couldry & Mejias, 2019). In the context of pornography, personalization mechanisms amplify novelty exposure, accelerate content-switching, and encourage extended engagement. Rather than simply responding to pre-existing preferences, algorithmic systems may participate in shaping and intensifying patterns of consumption by structuring the conditions under which sexual content is encountered and repeated.

To conceptualize this transformation, the present chapter introduces the notion of the *automation of desire*. This concept refers to the iterative process through which digital platforms measure, predict, and reinforce patterns of sexual preference through recursive data-feedback loops. Within such environments, desire becomes increasingly datafied and modulated through engagement-driven recommendation architectures. Importantly, this perspective does not assume uniform or inevitable addiction. Instead, it highlights the convergence of neurobehavioral reinforcement processes and platform-based optimization logics that may, under certain conditions, amplify compulsive or dysregulated engagement.

Situating pornography within this platform-mediated framework enables a shift from purely individualistic explanations toward a structural understanding of digitally mediated desire. By foregrounding the role of algorithmic governance, data extraction, and engagement optimization, contemporary pornography can be analyzed not solely as a domain of personal consumption but as part of a broader socio-technical system that organizes visibility, repetition,

METHODOLOGICAL APPROACH: CRITICAL INTEGRATIVE AND CASE-AUGMENTED SYNTHESIS

This chapter adopts a critical integrative synthesis design aimed at developing a theoretically grounded framework for understanding the structural transformation of digital pornography. Rather than presenting original empirical data or conducting a formal meta-analysis, the study synthesizes interdisciplinary scholarship across behavioral addiction research, psychology, media studies, and platform political economy (Brand et al., 2019; Gola et al., 2020; Srnicek, 2017; Zuboff, 2019). The objective is not to quantify prevalence or establish direct causal relationships, but to examine how digital infrastructures reorganize the experiential, psychological, and economic conditions under which pornography is accessed and consumed.

The analytical orientation follows an integrative review model appropriate for conceptually fragmented and rapidly evolving research domains (Torraco, 2016). This approach allows for the identification of structural patterns and emerging dynamics across disciplines while acknowledging ongoing debates and areas of uncertainty. The chapter thus positions itself as a conceptual and theoretically generative contribution rather than a hypothesis-testing empirical investigation.

Literature Selection Strategy

The literature base was constructed through targeted searches of peer-reviewed publications indexed in Scopus, Web of Science, PsycINFO, and Google Scholar. Searches focused primarily on publications between 2010 and 2025, with particular emphasis on post-2018 scholarship reflecting the expansion of platform-based digital ecosystems and AI-mediated media environments (Couldry & Mejias, 2019; Zuboff, 2019).

Core search clusters included:

- "problematic pornography use"
- "pornography addiction debate"
- "compulsive sexual behavior disorder"
- "moral incongruence"
- "cue-reactivity" and "reinforcement learning"
- "platform capitalism" and "algorithmic governance"
- "deepfake pornography" and "image-based sexual abuse"

Priority was given to systematic reviews, meta-analyses, longitudinal and neuroimaging studies, cross-cultural measurement research, and theoretical works addressing datafication and platform governance (Fernandez & Griffiths, 2021; Bőthe et al., 2018; Brand et al., 2019). Empirical claims advanced in this chapter are grounded primarily in peer-reviewed academic literature.

Media reports, policy documents, and journalistic investigations are incorporated selectively and exclusively as illustrative contextual material. They are not treated as primary empirical evidence but as indicators of broader structural developments within digital platform environments (Chesney & Citron, 2019; McGlynn & Rackley, 2017).

Analytical Framework

The chapter employs a structure–mechanism–consequence analytical logic.

Figure 1. structure–mechanism–consequence analytical logic

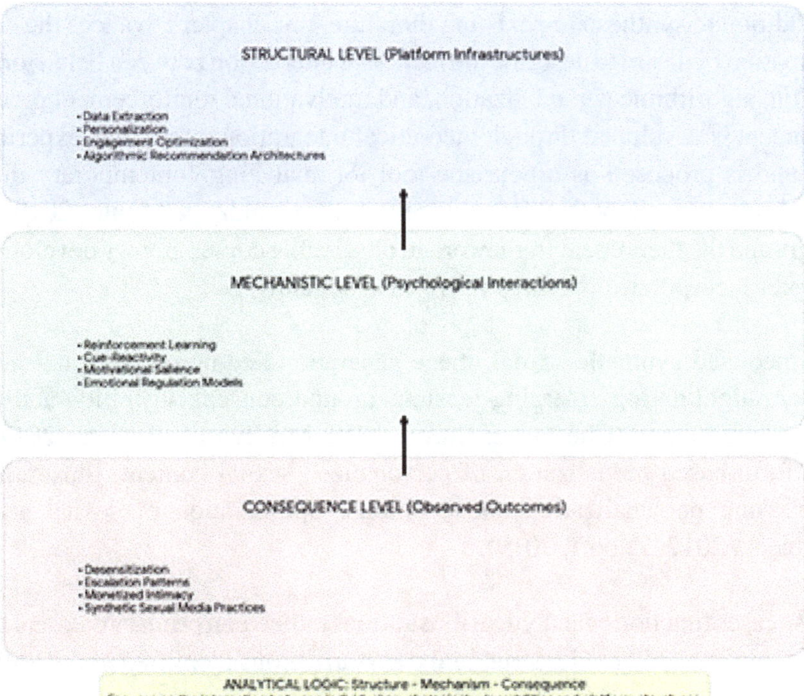

At the structural level, it examines platform infrastructures characterized by data extraction, personalization, engagement optimization, and algorithmic recommendation architectures (Srnicek, 2017; Zuboff, 2019; Couldry & Mejias, 2019).

At the mechanistic level, it integrates findings from reinforcement learning, cue-reactivity research, motivational salience theory, and models of emotional regulation to analyze how digitally mediated environments may interact with psychological vulnerability (Robinson & Berridge, 2008; Brand et al., 2019; Gola et al., 2017).

At the consequence level, it considers how these interacting dynamics may contribute—under specific and non-universal conditions—to desensitization, escalation patterns, monetized intimacy, and the emergence of synthetic sexual media practices (Vieira & Griffiths, 2024; Bocci Benucci et al., 2024).

This layered framework allows the analysis to move beyond binary debates concerning whether pornography is inherently addictive. Instead, it situates problematic engagement within the interaction between individual-level mechanisms and platform-level structural conditions.

Conceptual Contribution and Case-Augmented Analysis

In addition to synthesizing existing literature, this chapter advances the concept of automation of desire to describe the recursive interaction between behavioral data extraction, algorithmic personalization, and motivational reinforcement processes. This concept is developed through theoretical integration rather than experimental testing and is proposed as a heuristic tool for analyzing contemporary digitally mediated sexuality (Zuboff, 2019; Srnicek, 2017; Couldry & Mejias, 2019).

To ground the theoretical framework in observable contemporary developments, the chapter incorporates two illustrative case domains:

1. AI-mediated synthetic sexual image generation and non-consensual manipulation, highlighting emerging tensions around consent, visibility, and digital sexual production (Chesney & Citron, 2019; McGlynn & Rackley, 2017).
2. Platform-based monetization of personalized sexual content, illustrating the increasing personalization and economic optimization of sexual attention (Srnicek, 2017; Zuboff, 2019).

These cases function as analytical illustrations rather than primary datasets and are used to contextualize broader structural transformations identified in the literature.

Scope and Limitations

This chapter does not assume universal harm, inevitability of addiction, or deterministic neurobiological alteration. Desensitization and compulsive engagement are treated as conditional pathways shaped by psychological vulnerability, affect regulation patterns, and socio-technical context.

The analysis complements rather than replaces clinical and psychological research by situating problematic pornography use within broader infrastructural conditions shaped by platform architectures, algorithmic governance, and digital attention economies. As such, the chapter advances a systemic perspective without collapsing complex phenomena into singular moral or diagnostic narratives.

HISTORICAL CONTINUITY, DIGITAL RUPTURE

Pornography is not a recent cultural anomaly but a historically persistent form of representation that has circulated across diverse media systems and cultural formations. Archaeological and art-historical evidence suggests that sexually explicit imagery has long functioned within ritual, symbolic, pedagogical, and regulatory contexts rather than solely as a domain of private pleasure (Hunt, 1996; Kendrick, 1987). From classical Mediterranean frescoes and ceramics to early modern engravings and mass-circulation print culture, representations of sexuality have repeatedly been shaped by available media technologies and regimes of visibility. Pornography has therefore always been mediated—technologically, culturally, and politically—rather than existing as a stable or purely private practice (Williams, 1989; Paasonen, 2011).

Modern visual technologies intensified this mediation. Photography introduced mechanical reproducibility, cinema introduced movement and immersive spectatorship, and twentieth-century print industries embedded erotic imagery within consumer culture. Publications such as Playboy linked sexual display to aspirational lifestyle and consumption, while the brief "porno chic" moment of the 1970s allowed explicit cinema to approach mainstream visibility before renewed regulatory backlash (Williams, 1989). These shifts illustrate that pornography's visibility and legitimacy have historically fluctuated in relation to media infrastructures, regulatory frameworks, and cultural norms rather than following a linear trajectory of expansion.

For this reason, framing the digital era through the question "Is there more pornography today than before?" risks falling into a teleological trap. Historical evidence indicates cycles of normalization, marginalization, and reconfiguration rather than simple quantitative escalation (Hunt, 1996; Kendrick, 1987; Attwood & Smith, 2014). What distinguishes the contemporary moment is not merely volume but the transformation of the conditions under which pornography is accessed, circulated, and experienced.

Prior to the internet, pornography consumption typically involved spatial, economic, and reputational friction. Access required physical mobility, purchase, or exposure to social risk. Digital infrastructures have largely dissolved these barriers. Continuous connectivity, private screens, and anonymous browsing have integrated pornography into everyday digital routines, enabling micro-temporal and on-demand consumption patterns (Cooper et al., 2000; Peter & Valkenburg, 2016). This shift from episodic to continuous accessibility represents a qualitative transformation in the temporal and experiential organization of consumption.

The digital era therefore marks not simply an intensification of existing practices but a structural reorganization. Pornography now operates within platform-mediated environments characterized by persistent availability, data extraction, personalization, and algorithmic recommendation. Rather than functioning as discrete content encountered intermittently, it increasingly forms part of continuous digital environments that measure, predict, and optimize user engagement (Zuboff, 2019; Srnicek, 2017; Couldry & Mejias, 2019). In this sense, the central analytical question is no longer whether pornography has become more prevalent, but how digital infrastructures have reconfigured the architecture of access, repetition, and reinforcement.

Understanding this shift as a structural rupture rather than a quantitative increase enables a more precise analysis of contemporary transformations. Digital pornography does not simply extend earlier media forms; it reorganizes the experiential conditions of desire by embedding sexual content within platform logics of personalization, attention capture, and behavioral prediction (Zuboff, 2019; Gillespie, 2018). The following section examines this transformation as a digital structural break defined by the collapse of access costs, the platformization of sexual content, and the emergence of algorithmically mediated reinforcement environments.

THE DIGITAL STRUCTURAL BREAK: FROM CONTENT TO SYSTEM

The transition from analog to digital media has not merely expanded the availability of pornographic content; it has fundamentally reorganized the infrastructural conditions under which sexual imagery is accessed, circulated, and experienced. Contemporary pornography increasingly operates less as a discrete cultural product and more as a continuously accessible, data-driven, and algorithmically structured system embedded within platform-mediated environments (Paasonen, 2011; Gillespie, 2018; Srnicek, 2017). This transformation can be analytically understood through three interrelated shifts: the collapse of access costs, the platformization of sexual content within data economies, and the emergence of algorithmically reinforced engagement environments.

Rather than representing a linear increase in volume, digitalization has reshaped the temporal, economic, and affective organization of pornography consumption. Pornography is no longer encountered solely as isolated media content but as part of ongoing feedback environments that measure, predict, and modulate user engagement (Zuboff, 2019; Couldry & Mejias, 2019). This shift does not imply uniform or deterministic outcomes. Empirical research consistently demonstrates substantial heterogeneity in motivations, usage patterns, and psychosocial effects (Bőthe et al., 2020; Chen et al., 2022; Fernandez & Griffiths, 2021). Nevertheless, the structural transformation introduced by digital infrastructures reconfigures the conditions under which desire is encountered, repeated, and reinforced.

Collapse of Access Costs: Frictionless Availability and Continuous Exposure

One of the most consequential shifts introduced by digital infrastructures is the dramatic reduction of spatial, economic, and reputational barriers historically associated with pornography consumption. Prior to the diffusion of internet-based media, accessing explicit material often required deliberate effort, including visiting specialized venues, purchasing physical media, or navigating potential social stigma. These forms of friction functioned as structural constraints shaping both the frequency and context of consumption (Williams, 1989).

Digital technologies have largely dissolved these constraints. Smartphones, private screens, and high-speed connectivity allow instantaneous access independent of location or time, enabling pornography to be integrated into micro-temporal intervals of everyday digital life (Cooper et al., 2000; Peter & Valkenburg, 2016; Wright, 2013). This transformation has frequently been summarized through the "Triple-A engine" of online sexual content—accessibility, affordability, and anonymity (Cooper, 1998). Together, these conditions facilitate near-continuous availability and reduce perceived social risk, thereby reshaping the temporal structure of engagement.

Importantly, continuous accessibility does not in itself produce problematic use. Large-scale empirical studies consistently demonstrate that high-frequency consumption alone is not a reliable predictor of loss of control or functional impairment (Bőthe et al., 2020a; Gola et al., 2016; Grubbs et al., 2020). Many individuals engage regularly with pornography without experiencing distress or disruption in personal or relational functioning. However, the removal of structural friction creates an enabling environment in which repetitive engagement can occur with minimal interruption, potentially reinforcing habitual patterns for some users, particularly under conditions of psychological vulnerability.

Continuous availability also alters temporal dynamics. Rather than occurring in discrete sessions, consumption can now unfold across fragmented micro-episodes embedded within everyday digital routines. Rapid transitions between categories and intensities of content become technically effortless, facilitating sustained exposure to novelty. Early exposure has similarly shifted downward in age across many regions due to the ubiquity of internet-enabled devices and largely unsupervised access (Peter & Valkenburg, 2016). While early encounters with explicit material do not uniformly lead to problematic trajectories, developmental timing and contextual factors may influence subsequent patterns of interpretation and engagement.

These dynamics indicate that the most significant transformation lies not in quantitative expansion but in the restructuring of accessibility and temporality. Pornography has shifted from an episodic activity constrained by situational barriers toward a continuously available digital practice embedded within everyday media environments.

Platformization and Data Governance

The second axis of transformation concerns the integration of pornography into platform-based data economies. Contemporary pornography consumption increasingly occurs within digital infrastructures that systematically collect, process, and monetize user behavior. Viewing duration, search queries, interaction patterns, and subscription activity are continuously tracked and translated into engagement metrics. Within surveillance-oriented economic models, such behavioral data become predictive assets used to optimize retention and interaction (Srnicek, 2017; Zuboff, 2019; Couldry & Mejias, 2019).

This platformization situates pornography within broader dynamics of platform capitalism and attention economies (Gillespie, 2018; Srnicek, 2017). Sexual content functions not only as representational material but also as behavioral data. Recommendation systems, personalized feeds, and performance metrics structure how content is encountered and prioritized. Engagement becomes both a behavioral signal and an economic resource, linking individual consumption patterns to platform profitability and algorithmic optimization.

In these environments, user preferences are not merely expressed but continuously inferred and refined through data analytics. Platforms deploy algorithmic sorting and visibility hierarchies that influence which forms of content are encountered, how long users remain engaged, and which categories gain prominence (Bucher, 2018; Gillespie, 2018). Rather than passively responding to pre-existing desires, platform architectures participate in shaping and amplifying patterns of attention through iterative feedback loops. Pornography thus becomes embedded within a datafied economy of attention and affect in which personalization, interaction, and monetization converge.

An additional layer of platformization concerns the transformation of sexual attention into measurable behavioral surplus (Zuboff, 2019). In surveillance-oriented platform economies, user interactions are not merely observed; they are converted into predictive behavioral models. Search queries, dwell time, scrolling speed, interaction frequency, and subscription behaviors become quantifiable indicators of desire. These metrics are subsequently fed back into recommendation systems designed to optimize retention and session duration.

In this configuration, pornography is not only consumed but operationalized. It becomes part of a predictive infrastructure in which desire is modeled probabilistically. Algorithmic systems cluster users into behavioral typologies, anticipate category preferences, and dynamically adjust content hierarchies. This data-driven personalization may increase exposure efficiency by reducing friction between preference and stimulus. While such efficiency can enhance user satisfaction, it may also compress the exploratory distance that historically existed between desire and representation.

The structural novelty lies in the recursive nature of this loop. In earlier media systems, content influenced audiences, but audiences did not immediately restructure the architecture of distribution. In digital platforms, user behavior reorganizes the visibility logic itself (Gillespie, 2018; Bucher, 2018). Thus, pornography becomes co-produced by algorithmic sorting processes that continuously refine what counts as relevant, engaging, or profitable.

This transformation does not imply that algorithms dictate desire. Rather, it situates desire within a cybernetic environment characterized by feedback sensitivity. The boundary between preference formation and preference reinforcement becomes increasingly porous. Such environments may intensify engagement patterns for some users, especially where emotional distress, impulsivity, or novelty-seeking motivations are present (Brand et al., 2019; Vieira & Griffiths, 2024).

Despite these transformations, platformization does not produce uniform behavioral outcomes. Research highlights substantial heterogeneity in motivations and usage trajectories, ranging from recreational engagement to compulsive patterns associated with distress and coping difficulties (Bőthe et al., 2020b; Bőthe et al., 2025; Fernandez & Griffiths, 2021). The significance of platformization therefore lies less in deterministic behavioral effects than in its capacity to reshape the structural conditions under which desire is expressed, measured, and reinforced.

Algorithmic Reinforcement and the Automation of Desire

The third dimension of the digital structural break involves the interaction between algorithmic recommendation systems and neurobehavioral reinforcement processes. Contemporary digital platforms rely on algorithmic curation to personalize content streams based on prior engagement. Viewing histories, search patterns, and interaction metrics feed into recursive feedback loops that continuously refine predictions of user preference. Subsequent exposure is shaped by these predictions, generating personalized content trajectories that may intensify repetition and novelty-seeking (Bucher, 2018; Gillespie, 2018).

Behavioral addiction research emphasizes the role of cue–reward cycles and reinforcement learning in shaping repetitive engagement (Volkow et al., 2010; Brand et al., 2019; Robinson & Berridge, 2008). Within digitally mediated environments characterized by high variability and continuous novelty, algorithmic recommendation systems may amplify these processes by prioritizing stimuli associated with sustained attention. The resulting environment is not inherently pathological but may function as a reinforcement-sensitive ecosystem in which biological reward mechanisms and platform optimization logics interact.

The Interaction of Person–Affect–Cognition–Execution (I-PACE) model conceptualizes problematic digital behaviors as emerging from the interplay between individual vulnerability, affective states, cognitive responses, and executive control processes within reinforcing environments (Brand et al., 2016; Brand et al., 2019). Within such environments, algorithmic personalization can function as an amplifying condition, intensifying exposure to preferred or stimulating content and thereby sustaining engagement loops for some users. Psychological distress, impulsivity, and maladaptive coping strategies appear to operate as moderating variables rather than universal predictors of problematic use (Bocci Benucci et al., 2024; Vieira & Griffiths, 2024).

To conceptualize this emerging configuration, this chapter proposes the notion of automation of desire. Automation of desire refers to the iterative process through which digital infrastructures measure, predict, and reinforce patterns of sexual preference within recursive cycles of data extraction and personalized content delivery (Zuboff, 2019; Couldry & Mejias, 2019). User interactions are translated into behavioral data, processed through algorithmic systems, and reintroduced as curated content streams that shape subsequent engagement. Through these loops, desire becomes increasingly datafied and anticipatory, structured not solely by internal motivations but also by externally mediated recommendation architectures.

This formulation does not assume that algorithmic systems uniformly produce compulsive engagement or addiction. Rather, it highlights a co-amplification environment in which neurobehavioral reinforcement processes and platform optimization logics converge. For some users, this convergence may contribute to escalating novelty-seeking or diminished perceived control, particularly under conditions of psychological vulnerability. For others, engagement remains recreational and contextually bounded.

Taken together, these three dimensions—the collapse of access costs, the platformization of sexual content within data economies, and the emergence of algorithmically mediated reinforcement environments—constitute a structural transformation that distinguishes digital pornography from earlier media forms. Pornography now operates within a continuously functioning socio-technical system that measures, predicts, and optimizes engagement (Srnicek, 2017; Zuboff, 2019). Understanding this transformation provides the analytical foundation for examining how such conditions may contribute, under specific circumstances, to desensitization dynamics, escalation patterns, and emerging forms of personalized and synthetic sexual media.

CORE ANALYSIS: DESENSITIZATION, ESCALATION, AND THE AUTOMATION OF DESIRE

The structural transformations outlined in the previous section do not in themselves determine behavioral outcomes. Continuous accessibility, platform-based personalization, and algorithmic recommendation systems create enabling conditions rather than uniform trajectories. Nevertheless, these infrastructures reshape the experiential and motivational landscape within which pornography is encountered, interpreted, and integrated into everyday digital life (Srnicek, 2017; Zuboff, 2019; Couldry & Mejias, 2019).

Within this environment, three interconnected processes warrant closer examination: desensitization and escalation as conditional dynamics, the co-amplification of biological and algorithmic reinforcement systems, and the economic personalization of intimacy within platform-mediated sexual economies. Together, these processes illustrate how contemporary pornography operates less as a bounded cultural artifact and more as a continuously mediated system embedded within data-driven environments (Attwood & Smith, 2014; Srnicek, 2017).

Desensitization and Escalation as Conditional Processes

Public and scholarly discussions of pornography frequently invoke narratives of tolerance, desensitization, and progressive escalation toward increasingly novel or intense material. While such trajectories are reported by some users, empirical research consistently demonstrates substantial heterogeneity in patterns of engagement and outcome. High-frequency consumption alone does not reliably predict diminished control, distress, or functional impairment (Bőthe et al., 2020; Bőthe et al., 2020b). Instead, problematic trajectories appear more strongly associated with psychological distress, impulsivity, and maladaptive coping patterns than with exposure volume per se (Chen et al., 2022; Vieira & Griffiths, 2024; Bocci Benucci et al., 2024).

Neurobehavioral frameworks provide partial insight into these dynamics. Incentive sensitization theory distinguishes between hedonic pleasure ("liking") and motivational salience ("wanting"), suggesting that repeated exposure to highly stimulating cues may amplify anticipatory desire even when subjective satisfaction stabilizes or declines (Robinson & Berridge, 2008). Neuroimaging studies of compulsive sexual behavior have reported heightened cue-reactivity in reward-related neural circuits among some individuals seeking treatment for problematic use, indicating increased sensitivity to conditioned sexual cues (Voon et al., 2014; Gola et al., 2017; Gola et al., 2020).

However, such findings should be interpreted cautiously. Similar neural activation patterns are observed in non-problematic sexual contexts, and current evidence does not support a uniform neurobiological pathway from exposure to addiction (Prause, 2019). Rather than indicating inevitable progression, desensitization and escalation appear as conditional processes emerging at the intersection of individual vulnerability, emotional regulation dynamics, and environmental reinforcement structures (Brand et al., 2019; Brand et al., 2023).

Digital environments characterized by high variability and continuous novelty may intensify novelty-seeking for some users. The rapid availability of diverse content categories and the ease of switching between them can sustain attentional engagement and exploratory behavior (Cooper, 1998; Cooper et al., 2000). Yet escalation is neither inevitable nor universal. Many users maintain stable consumption patterns without experiencing distress or functional impairment (Bőthe et al., 2020). The analytical focus therefore shifts from deterministic models toward conditional frameworks that examine when and for whom intensified engagement emerges (Fernandez & Griffiths, 2021).

Algorithmic Co-Amplification and the Automation of Desire

The interaction between neurobehavioral reinforcement processes and platform-based recommendation systems introduces a dynamic not present in earlier media environments. Algorithmic systems continuously adjust content streams based on prior engagement, generating feedback loops in which user behavior and platform optimization recursively shape one another (Srnicek, 2017; Zuboff, 2019; Couldry & Mejias, 2019). Within these loops, biological reinforcement mechanisms and algorithmic personalization processes may become mutually amplifying.

Behavioral addiction models emphasize the role of cue–reward cycles and reinforcement learning in shaping repetitive engagement (Volkow et al., 2010; Brand et al., 2019; Robinson & Berridge, 2008). In digitally mediated environments, recommendation systems prioritize content associated with sustained viewing, repeated interaction, and prolonged session duration. Such prioritization may increase exposure to stimuli aligned with prior engagement patterns, thereby reinforcing anticipatory motivation and repetition for susceptible users (Bőthe et al., 2025; Fernandez & Griffiths, 2021).

This interaction can be conceptualized as algorithmic co-amplification: a recursive process in which platform infrastructures and user-level reinforcement processes dynamically interact (Zuboff, 2019; Couldry & Mejias, 2019). The automation of desire emerges within this environment as behavioral data are continuously translated into predictive models of preference and reintroduced as curated content streams. Through these iterative cycles, desire becomes not only expressed but also anticipated and algorithmically modulated.

Importantly, this formulation does not imply technological determinism. Algorithmic systems do not independently generate desire, nor are users passive recipients of technological influence. Rather, the relationship is reciprocal. User behavior informs algorithmic curation, which in turn structures subsequent exposure and engagement opportunities (Srnicek, 2017; Zuboff, 2019). For some individuals, this recursive structure may contribute to intensified engagement, particularly when novelty-rich content intersects with emotional distress or coping-oriented use (Brand et al., 2019; Vieira & Griffiths, 2024). For others, engagement remains recreational and contextually bounded, underscoring the heterogeneity of outcomes within digitally mediated environments (Bőthe et al., 2020a; Bőthe et al., 2020b).

Monetized Intimacy and the Personalization of Sexual Economies

A further dimension of the digital structural transformation concerns the economic personalization of sexual content and the monetization of intimacy. Subscription-based platforms such as OnlyFans, Fansly, and similar creator-centered infrastructures reconfigure pornography from largely anonymous and standardized content into targeted, identity-specific, and financially mediated engagement (Srnicek, 2017; Zuboff, 2019).

Within these environments, users no longer merely access generalized sexual material produced for mass audiences. Instead, they subscribe to individual creators, receive personalized content streams, and often engage in direct interaction through messaging systems and custom requests. Addressing users by name, producing content on demand, and responding to specific fantasies can create a perception of individualized reciprocity. As a result, the pornographic experience may extend beyond visual stimulation into a form of simulated relational proximity.

In the literature, such dynamics are often analyzed through the lens of parasocial relationships and digital intimacy (Kohut et al., 2017; Willoughby et al., 2016). Monetary investment combined with perceived relational interaction may increase sustained engagement and repeated consumption in certain contexts (Campbell & Kohut, 2017; Banet-Weiser, 2018). However, empirical findings remain heterogeneous, and not all forms of personalized engagement translate into dependency or dysfunction. For some users and creators, these platforms provide controlled environments for sexual self-expression, income generation, and negotiated interaction.

Nevertheless, the structural implications are significant. Personalized subscription models integrate pornography into broader platform economies characterized by micro-transactions, attention metrics, and retention strategies (Srnicek, 2017; Zuboff, 2019). Sexual representation becomes embedded within a supply-demand microeconomy structured by algorithmic visibility and financial exchange. Desire in this context is shaped not only through viewing behavior but also through monetary preference and emotional investment.

This convergence of personalization, algorithmic curation, and monetization contributes to what this chapter conceptualizes as the automation of desire. Engagement patterns are continuously measured, translated into data, and used to refine subsequent exposure (Zuboff, 2019; Couldry & Mejias, 2019). In such environments, pornography consumption shifts from episodic viewing toward sustained participation within economically mediated relational ecosystems.

Importantly, this transformation should not be reduced to moral panic or generalized claims of exploitation. Instead, it reflects a broader reorganization of digital intimacy in which attention, identity, and economic exchange intersect (Banet-Weiser, 2018; Srnicek, 2017). The structural question is not whether personalized pornography is inherently harmful, but how monetized intimacy reshapes the feedback conditions through which desire is expressed, sustained, and economically optimized.

Synthetic Sexual Media and the Crisis of Consent

Recent advances in generative artificial intelligence introduce an additional layer of complexity to digitally mediated sexual cultures. AI-powered image and video generation technologies enable the production of highly realistic synthetic sexual content, including deepfake pornography in which individuals' likenesses are manipulated without their knowledge or consent. These developments mark a qualitative shift in the regime of pornographic production.

Unlike traditional pornography, which required filmed participation by performers, synthetic sexual media decouple representation from embodied presence. Photographs, social media posts, or publicly available images can be repurposed as raw material for explicit content generation. Legal scholarship increasingly defines non-consensual deepfake pornography as a form of digital sexual violence, emphasizing its gendered impact and long-term reputational consequences (Chesney & Citron, 2019; McGlynn & Rackley, 2017).

Recent journalistic investigations have illustrated how generative AI systems may be used to sexualize images of ordinary individuals. For example, reporting by Reuters in early 2026 documented instances in which users uploaded publicly available images and requested sexualized modifications through an AI model integrated into a major social media platform (Vicens & Satter, 2026). Such cases demonstrate that synthetic sexual production is no longer confined to public figures or professional performers; everyday online visibility can become subject to algorithmically assisted manipulation.

These developments do not indicate that consent has disappeared from all digital sexual environments. However, they raise profound concerns regarding how consent is negotiated, enforced, and technologically mediated within platform ecosystems. When AI systems can generate explicit imagery without the participation of the depicted individual, the boundaries between fantasy, fabrication, and violation become increasingly blurred.

Testimonial accounts reported in mainstream media describe experiences of shame, reputational harm, and persistent vulnerability among individuals whose likenesses were used in synthetic sexual content (Rolling Stone, 2026). The durability of digital traces and the rapid circulation enabled by platform infrastructures may intensify the psychological and social impact of such violations.

From a structural perspective, synthetic sexual media extend the logic of datafied desire. Fantasy, once confined to imagination, becomes technically producible. Representation no longer requires recording; it can be generated through algorithmic manipulation. This shift potentially expands the range of identities and bodies that can be incorporated into pornographic circulation, not through participation but through extraction and recombination of digital traces (Couldry & Mejias, 2019; Zuboff, 2019).

Understanding these developments within the broader framework of platform governance clarifies that synthetic sexual media are not isolated anomalies but emerging products of data-driven infrastructures (Srnicek, 2017; Zuboff, 2019). They illustrate how the systemization of pornography intersects with questions of consent, gendered harm, and technological accountability. Rather than signaling the end of agency, they highlight the urgency of examining how platform architectures, generative AI systems, and regulatory frameworks shape the conditions under which digital sexual representation is produced and circulated.

From Consumption to Systemic Mediation

Taken together, these dynamics illustrate a broader transformation in the organization of digitally mediated desire. Pornography within contemporary platform environments is no longer confined to discrete acts of consumption. It is embedded within systems that measure engagement, personalize content, monetize interaction, and increasingly generate synthetic representations (Srnicek, 2017; Zuboff, 2019; Couldry & Mejias, 2019).

This transformation does not produce uniform behavioral outcomes, nor does it render addiction inevitable. Rather, it reconfigures the structural conditions under which desire is encountered and sustained. Desensitization and escalation emerge as conditional possibilities rather than universal trajectories (Kühn & Gallinat, 2014; Gola et al., 2017); algorithmic systems participate in shaping exposure and reinforcement patterns without fully determining them (Brand et al., 2019; Robinson

& Berridge, 2008); and personalized sexual economies introduce new intersections between intimacy, attention, and monetization (Banet-Weiser, 2018; Srnicek, 2017).

Understanding pornography as a systemic phenomenon rather than solely as content enables a more nuanced analysis of digitally mediated desire. Such an approach shifts the analytical focus away from singular moral or clinical explanations toward the socio-technical infrastructures that organize visibility, repetition, and engagement in contemporary digital culture (Couldry & Mejias, 2019; Zuboff, 2019).

DISCUSSION: IMPLICATIONS FOR ADDICTION, GOVERNANCE, AND DIGITAL HARM

The analysis developed in this chapter supports a reframing of contemporary pornography: not primarily as a discrete genre of sexual media, but as a socio-technical system embedded within platform infrastructures, data-driven attention economies, and algorithmic governance. This shift from content to system has direct implications for how problematic pornography use (PPU), digital sexual harm, and regulatory responsibility are conceptualized. Instead of treating pornography-related distress either as an individual pathology or as a moral panic, a structural perspective foregrounds the interaction between platform architectures, psychological vulnerability, and evolving digital economies of intimacy.

Rethinking "Addiction" in Platform Environments

One of the central implications concerns the limits of addiction-centered debates when they remain exclusively individualistic. Behavioral addiction frameworks offer useful tools for understanding compulsive patterns—particularly concepts such as reinforcement learning, cue-reactivity, motivational salience, and impaired control (Love et al., 2015; Brand et al., 2016; Kraus et al., 2016; Brand et al., 2019; Gola et al., 2020). However, some neurophysiological studies suggest that responses to sexual stimuli may reflect elevated sexual desire rather than addiction-like mechanisms (Steele et al., 2013). Yet these models can be analytically incomplete if they treat digital environments as neutral backdrops rather than as active infrastructures shaping exposure, repetition, and novelty.

Across contemporary research, the strongest point of convergence is that frequency alone is not an adequate indicator of dysfunction. Clinically relevant cases hinge on loss of control, persistence despite adverse consequences, and functional impairment—rather than sheer exposure volume (Bőthe et al., 2018; Bőthe et al., 2020a; Bőthe et al., 2020b). This is precisely where platform environments matter: pornography is increasingly consumed within recommendation-driven systems designed to maximize engagement, refine predictive accuracy, and sustain attention over time (Srnicek, 2017; Zuboff, 2019). Under these conditions, repetitive use cannot be interpreted solely as a product of individual predisposition, because the environment itself is structured to support continuity, novelty, and frictionless return.

The concept of *desire automation* introduced in this chapter aims to clarify this intersection. It does not claim that platforms "cause" addiction or that users lose agency. Rather, it captures how algorithmic infrastructures may co-amplify existing motivational dynamics by continuously adapting content streams to prior engagement patterns, thereby intensifying exposure to novelty and reinforcing repetition under certain vulnerability conditions (Robinson & Berridge, 2008; Brand et al., 2019). In this sense, the key analytical question shifts away from "Is pornography addictive?" toward: *How do platform-based systems reorganize the conditions under which dysregulated patterns may emerge—and for whom?* This reframing helps explain why diagnostic debates remain unsettled: when repetitive engagement is partly shaped by platform design and feedback loops, purely individual-level classifications risk underestimating structural contributors to compulsive trajectories, while deterministic claims risk overgeneralization (Kraus et al., 2016).

Governance, Accountability, and the Political Economy of Sexual Platforms

A second implication concerns governance. If pornography is increasingly mediated through platforms that extract behavioral data, optimize attention, and algorithmically curate visibility, then regulation cannot be reduced to questions of personal choice or moral discipline. Pornographic content now circulates through infrastructures designed for engagement maximization, positioning sexual media within the broader political economy of platform capitalism and surveillance-oriented datafication (Srnicek, 2017; Zuboff, 2019).

This raises practical and normative governance problems that extend beyond "content moderation." Age verification, recommendation transparency, friction-based design interventions, and AI-generated content policies become central concerns—not because pornography is inherently pathological, but because platform architectures structure the distribution of sexual visibility and the conditions of repeated exposure. Contemporary platform governance also remains uneven and frequently reactive: policies may prioritize takedowns after harm occurs rather than proactive safeguards, especially in relation to non-consensual imagery and synthetic content.

Here, feminist and legal scholarship is especially instructive. Digital sexual harms—such as image-based sexual abuse and deepfake pornography—are not randomly distributed; they are frequently gendered, entangled with misogynistic visibility regimes, and disproportionately borne by women and marginalized groups

(Banet-Weiser, 2018; McGlynn & Rackley, 2017). Accordingly, the governance question is not merely "Is pornography harmful?" but also: *Which infrastructures enable non-consensual circulation, which design choices amplify harassment, and which accountability mechanisms constrain or normalize gendered harms?* Treating pornography as a system reorients responsibility toward platforms as operators of visibility, not merely hosts of content.

At the same time, governance responses must avoid collapsing into moral panic. Regulatory approaches that treat sexual content as inherently corrupting can produce overreach and unintended harms, including punitive surveillance of sexuality and the erosion of sexual autonomy. A structural approach therefore calls for harm-sensitive governance frameworks that focus on consent, safety, and accountability while recognizing heterogeneity in sexual expression and consumption.

Heterogeneity and Differential Vulnerability

A third implication is the centrality of heterogeneity. Even in highly optimized platform environments, outcomes are not uniform. Empirical research repeatedly shows that problematic trajectories are more strongly associated with psychological distress, emotional dysregulation, impulsivity, and coping motives than with exposure frequency alone (Chen et al., 2022; Vieira & Griffiths, 2024). Sociocultural factors—including moral incongruence, religiosity, gender norms, and relational context—also shape how pornography is experienced and interpreted (Grubbs & Perry, 2019; Kohut et al., 2017).

This matters for both scholarship and intervention. If pornography-related distress is sometimes amplified by moral conflict rather than impaired control, then conflating self-perceived addiction with clinical dysfunction risks inflating prevalence and misdirecting clinical attention (Grubbs et al., 2020). Conversely, dismissing all concerns as moral panic risks minimizing experiences of genuine loss of control and impairment among a subset of users. A conditional model—where structural conditions interact with individual vulnerabilities—offers a more accurate account than either "porn harms everyone" or "porn harms no one" (Jeong et al., 2021).

The same logic applies to adolescence and early exposure. Digital environments enable earlier encounters with explicit material, often in unsupervised contexts. Yet early exposure does not automatically imply harm. Rather, it may introduce conditions under which reinforcement, repetition, and identity-related meaning-making occur with fewer protective buffers. This highlights the need for multi-level approaches—digital literacy, consent education, mental health resources, and platform safeguards—rather than blanket prohibition.

From Binary Narratives to Structural Explanation

A structural interpretation also invites a deeper reconsideration of measurement and diagnostic debates within the field. The majority of contemporary instruments assessing problematic pornography use—including the PPCS (Bőthe et al., 2018), PPUS, and related scales—primarily operationalize dysfunction through subjective loss of control, salience, tolerance-like experiences, withdrawal indicators, and functional impairment, reflecting the influence of addiction-based conceptual frameworks within the field (Bőthe et al., 2018; Castro-Calvo et al., 2020). These constructs remain clinically meaningful and have significantly advanced empirical clarity in distinguishing high-frequency use from clinically relevant dysregulation. However, they are largely designed within individual-centered paradigms that conceptualize problematic engagement as emerging from intrapsychic processes rather than socio-technical environments.

Such instruments rarely incorporate platform-level variables, including algorithmic personalization intensity, recommendation feedback density, exposure velocity, or monetized relational engagement. In other words, current measurement models tend to treat the digital environment as a neutral container of behavior rather than as an active shaping force. This omission risks analytically isolating the individual from the infrastructural conditions that structure exposure, repetition, and novelty.

Future empirical research may therefore benefit from incorporating platform exposure metrics into assessment models. Variables such as session fragmentation (micro-episodic engagement patterns), recommendation clustering (content similarity acceleration), exposure acceleration (rapid category-switch capacity), and personalized subscription loops could potentially moderate or mediate problematic trajectories. Integrating such factors would not dilute individual responsibility but rather contextualize it within environments intentionally engineered to optimize engagement and retention. Without such integration, addiction research risks attributing dysregulation solely to internal vulnerability while underestimating environmental amplification mechanisms embedded in platform design.

This shift parallels broader methodological debates in digital media research, where scholars increasingly argue that behavioral outcomes must be understood in relation to design architectures rather than abstracted from them. In attention economies, user behavior is both expressive and responsive. It reflects preference, yet it is simultaneously structured by interface logic, ranking systems, and predictive modeling (Srnicek, 2017; Zuboff, 2019). A purely intrapsychic diagnostic framework may therefore insufficiently capture the recursive feedback loops between user-level reinforcement processes and platform-level optimization strategies.

Moreover, regulatory discussions must contend with the asymmetry between user agency and platform optimization. Users exercise choice, yet those choices unfold within infrastructures intentionally engineered to minimize friction, maximize novelty exposure, and prolong session duration. This asymmetry does not negate agency; rather, it complicates simplistic narratives of individual responsibility. The existence of agency does not eliminate the influence of environmental structuring. Recognizing this layered agency allows for governance models that focus on design accountability—algorithmic transparency, friction-based interventions, and consent-centered safeguards—rather than moral prohibition or blanket censorship.

Importantly, moving toward infrastructural critique does not require pathologizing sexuality or framing pornography as inherently corrupting. A structural approach can simultaneously defend sexual autonomy and interrogate engagement-maximizing architectures. It avoids collapsing the discussion into either moral panic or technological determinism. Instead, it foregrounds how power operates through systems of visibility, prediction, and monetization.

Public discourse often oscillates between two polarized narratives: moral condemnation that frames pornography as socially corrosive, and dismissal that treats concerns as exaggerated panic. The structural perspective advanced here offers a third route. It acknowledges that pornography is historically continuous as a representational practice, while emphasizing that digital infrastructures create a novel regime of access, personalization, monetization, and—via generative AI—synthetic production. The rupture is infrastructural, not merely moral or quantitative.

Within this regime, pornography is increasingly generated, personalized, and economically optimized. The concept of desire automation is proposed as a heuristic for understanding how user preferences are translated into behavioral data, processed through predictive systems, and reintroduced as curated content streams within recursive feedback loops. These loops compress the distance between desire, representation, and reinforcement. This does not imply that desire is externally imposed or that agency disappears. Rather, it highlights how platform architectures participate in structuring exposure patterns, repetition conditions, and attentional rhythms in ways that older media systems could not.

The significance of this systemic frame lies in its capacity to integrate multiple layers of analysis. Neurobehavioral mechanisms such as cue-reactivity and incentive salience interact with platform political economy and algorithmic governance structures. Personalized monetization models intersect with affect regulation dynamics. Synthetic media technologies complicate consent regimes. Instead of reducing these phenomena to a singular cause—addiction, morality, or technology—the systemic perspective situates them within a socio-technical assemblage where psychological processes, economic incentives, and infrastructural design converge.

In sum, the chapter's central contribution is to reposition contemporary pornography within this systemic frame. By foregrounding the interaction between neurobiological reinforcement processes, platform capitalism, and governance conditions, the analysis accommodates ongoing diagnostic uncertainty, preserves recognition of heterogeneity, and sharpens the governance conversation toward consent, accountability, and infrastructural responsibility—without collapsing the field into deterministic or moralized claims. The task moving forward is not to declare pornography universally harmful or harmless, but to analyze how digitally mediated architectures of desire reshape the conditions under which sexuality is encountered, sustained, and economically optimized.

CONCLUSION

Pornography has never been a purely private or purely modern phenomenon; it has historically circulated through the media infrastructures and cultural regimes of each era. What distinguishes the contemporary moment is not simply an increase in explicit material but a transformation in the conditions under which sexual content is encountered, personalized, and sustained. Continuous connectivity, data-driven platforms, and algorithmic recommendation systems have reorganized pornography from a discrete cultural product into a persistent and adaptive digital environment embedded within attention economies.

This chapter has argued that the most consequential transformation introduced by digitalization is structural rather than quantitative. The collapse of access barriers, the platformization of sexual content, and the emergence of algorithmically mediated feedback loops collectively reshape how desire is encountered and repeated. Within such environments, pornography becomes integrated into datafied systems that measure engagement, personalize exposure, and monetize attention. These infrastructures do not uniformly produce harm or compulsive use; rather, they create conditions under which reinforcement dynamics, novelty-seeking, and emotional coping may interact with individual vulnerabilities in heterogeneous ways. Desensitization and escalation therefore appear as conditional trajectories rather than inevitable outcomes, underscoring the need to avoid deterministic or moralizing interpretations.

Reframing pornography as a socio-technical system also repositions ongoing debates about addiction and digital harm. Individual-level diagnostic frameworks remain important but are insufficient on their own when engagement unfolds within environments intentionally designed to optimize retention and personalization. The concept of *desire automation* introduced in this chapter highlights the recursive relationship between behavioral data extraction, algorithmic recommendation, and motivational reinforcement. Within these feedback loops, user preferences are continuously measured, predicted, and reintroduced as curated content streams, shaping exposure patterns without eliminating individual agency. This systemic perspective helps explain why empirical findings remain heterogeneous and why conceptual disagreements within the field persist.

At the same time, the systemization of pornography raises broader governance and ethical questions. Platform infrastructures that host and monetize sexual content also structure visibility, consent, and vulnerability. The rise of personalized creator economies and AI-generated sexual imagery further complicates existing regulatory frameworks, particularly in relation to non-consensual representation and gendered digital harm. Addressing these challenges requires moving beyond binary debates between moral panic and technological determinism toward multi-level approaches that consider platform design, psychological vulnerability, and sociocultural context simultaneously.

Ultimately, the digital transformation of pornography reflects wider shifts in how intimacy, attention, and embodiment are mediated through data-driven technologies. Pornography is no longer only consumed; it is generated, personalized, and economically optimized within platform ecosystems. Recognizing this systemic reorganization does not negate the diversity of user experiences or the persistence of sexual agency. Rather, it provides a conceptual framework for understanding how contemporary architectures of access, repetition, and personalization reshape the conditions under which desire circulates. Future research must therefore continue to examine the intersection of psychological processes, platform governance, and emerging forms of synthetic sexual media in order to better understand the evolving infrastructures of digitally mediated sexuality.

REFERENCES

American Psychiatric Association. (2013). *Diagnostic and statistical manual of mental disorders* (5th ed.). American Psychiatric Publishing.

Attwood, F., & Smith, C. (2014). Porn Studies: An introduction. *Porn Studies, 1*(1-2), 1–6. DOI: 10.1080/23268743.2014.887308

Banet-Weiser, S. (2018). *Empowered: Popular feminism and popular misogyny.* Duke University Press.

Bocci Benucci, S., Di Gesto, C., Ghinassi, S., Casale, S., & Fioravanti, G. (2024). Pornography use, problematic pornography use, impulsivity, and sensation seeking: A meta-analysis. *Journal of Sexual Medicine, 21*(10), 922–939. DOI: 10.1093/jsxmed/qdae101 PMID: 39183145

Bőthe, B., Koós, M., Tóth-Király, I., Orosz, G., & Demetrovics, Z. (2020a). Investigating the associations of pornography use frequency, problematic pornography use, and moral incongruence. *Journal of Sex Research, 57*(4), 442–456. DOI: 10.1080/00224499.2019.1654367

Bőthe, B., Tóth-Király, I., Orosz, G., Potenza, M. N., & Demetrovics, Z. (2020b). High-frequency pornography use may not always be problematic. *Journal of Sexual Medicine, 17*(4), 793–811. DOI: 10.1016/j.jsxm.2020.01.007 PMID: 32033863

Bőthe, B., Tóth-Király, I., Popova, N., Nagy, L., Koós, M., Demetrovics, Z., Potenza, M. N., Kraus, S. W., Ballester-Arnal, R., Batthyány, D., Bergeron, S., Billieux, J., Briken, P., Burkauskas, J., Cárdenas-López, G., Carvalho, J., Castro-Calvo, J., Chen, L., Ciocca, G., & Grubbs, J. B. (2025). Identification and comprehensive characterization of moral disapproval and behavioral dysregulation-based pornography-use profiles across 42 countries. *Journal of Behavioral Addictions, 14*(1), 131–154. DOI: 10.1556/2006.2024.00054 PMID: 39945767

Bőthe, B., Tóth-Király, I., Zsila, Á., Griffiths, M. D., Demetrovics, Z., & Orosz, G. (2018). The Development of the Problematic Pornography Consumption Scale (PPCS). *Journal of Sex Research, 55*(3), 395–406. DOI: 10.1080/00224499.2017.1291798 PMID: 28276929

Brand, M., Wegmann, E., Stark, R., Müller, A., Wölfling, K., Robbins, T. W., & Potenza, M. N. (2019). The interaction of person-affect-cognition-execution (I-PACE) model for addictive behaviors: Update, generalization to addictive behaviors beyond internet-use disorders, and specification of the process character of addictive behaviors. *Neuroscience and Biobehavioral Reviews, 104*, 1–10. DOI: 10.1016/j.neubiorev.2019.06.032 PMID: 31247240

Brand, M., Young, K. S., Laier, C., Wölfling, K., & Potenza, M. N. (2016). Integrating psychological and neurobiological considerations regarding the development and maintenance of specific Internet-use disorders: An Interaction of Person-Affect-Cognition-Execution (I-PACE) model. *Neuroscience and Biobehavioral Reviews, 71*, 252–266. DOI: 10.1016/j.neubiorev.2016.08.033 PMID: 27590829

Bucher, T. (2018). *If...Then: Algorithmic Power and Politics*. Oxford University Press. DOI: 10.1093/oso/9780190493028.001.0001

Campbell, L., & Kohut, T. (2017). The use and effects of pornography in romantic relationships. *Current Opinion in Psychology, 13*, 6–10. DOI: 10.1016/j.copsyc.2016.03.004 PMID: 28813295

Castro-Calvo, J., Gil-Llario, M. D., Giménez-García, C., Gil-Juliá, B., & Ballester-Arnal, R. (2020). Occurrence and clinical characteristics of Compulsive Sexual Behavior Disorder (CSBD): A cluster analysis in two independent community samples. *Journal of Behavioral Addictions, 9*(2), 446–468. DOI: 10.1556/2006.2020.00025 PMID: 32554840

Chen, L., Jiang, X., Wang, Q., Bőthe, B., Potenza, M. N., & Wu, H. (2022). The Association between the Quantity and Severity of Pornography Use: A Meta-analysis. *Journal of Sex Research, 59*(6), 704–719. DOI: 10.1080/00224499.2021.1988500 PMID: 34723731

Chesney, R., & Citron, D. (2019). Deepfakes and the new disinformation war. *Foreign Affairs, 98*(1), 147–155.

Cooper, A. (1998). Sexuality and the Internet: Surfing into the new millennium. *Cyberpsychology & Behavior, 1*(2), 187–193. DOI: 10.1089/cpb.1998.1.187

Cooper, A., Delmonico, D. L., & Burg, R. (2000). Cybersex users, abusers, and compulsives: New findings and implications. *Sexual Addiction & Compulsivity, 7*(1-2), 5–29. DOI: 10.1080/10720160008400205

Couldry, N., & Mejias, U. A. (2019). *The costs of connection: How data is colonizing human life and appropriating it for capitalism*. Stanford University Press., DOI: 10.1515/9781503609754

Fernandez, D. P., & Griffiths, M. D. (2021). Psychometric Instruments for Problematic Pornography Use: A Systematic Review. *Evaluation & the Health Professions, 44*(2), 111–141. DOI: 10.1177/0163278719861688 PMID: 31284745

Gillespie, T. (2018). *Custodians of the Internet: Platforms, Content Moderation, and the Hidden Decisions That Shape Social Media*. Yale University Press.

Gola, M., Lewczuk, K., Potenza, M. N., Kingston, D. A., Grubbs, J. B., Stark, R., & Reid, R. C. (2020). What should be included in the criteria for compulsive sexual behavior disorder? *Journal of Behavioral Addictions, 11*(2), 160–165. DOI: 10.1556/2006.2020.00090 PMID: 34329192

Gola, M., Wordecha, M., Sescousse, G., Lew-Starowicz, M., Kossowski, B., Wypych, M., Makeig, S., Potenza, M. N., & Marchewka, A. (2017). Can Pornography be Addictive? An fMRI Study of Men Seeking Treatment for Problematic Pornography Use. *Neuropsychopharmacology : Official Publication of the American College of Neuropsychopharmacology, 42*(10), 2021–2031. DOI: 10.1038/npp.2017.78 PMID: 28409565

Grubbs, J. B., Kraus, S. W., Perry, S. L., Lewczuk, K., & Gola, M. (2020). Moral incongruence and compulsive sexual behavior: Results from cross-sectional interactions and parallel growth curve analyses. *Journal of Abnormal Psychology, 129*(3), 266–278. DOI: 10.1037/abn0000501 PMID: 32027146

Grubbs, J. B., Perry, S. L., Wilt, J. A., & Reid, R. C. (2019). Pornography Problems Due to Moral Incongruence: An Integrative Model with a Systematic Review and Meta-Analysis. *Archives of Sexual Behavior, 48*(2), 397–415. DOI: 10.1007/s10508-018-1248-x PMID: 30076491

Hunt, L. (1996). *The invention of pornography: Obscenity and the origins of modernity, 1500–1800*. Zone Books.

Jeong, H., Yim, H. W., Lee, S., Lee, H. K., Potenza, M. N., & Park, M. (2021). Joint effects of children's emotional problems and parental depressive symptoms on the occurrence of internet gaming disorder among children and adolescents: A longitudinal study. *Journal of Behavioral Addictions, 10*(2), 244–252. DOI: 10.1556/2006.2021.00030 PMID: 34128830

Karim, R., & Chaudhri, P. (2012). Behavioral addictions: An overview. *Journal of Psychoactive Drugs, 44*(1), 5–17. DOI: 10.1080/02791072.2012.662859 PMID: 22641961

Kendrick, W. (1987). *The secret museum: Pornography in modern culture*. University of California Press.

Kohut, T., Fisher, W. A., & Campbell, L. (2017). Perceived Effects of Pornography on the Couple Relationship: Initial Findings of Open-Ended, Participant-Informed, "Bottom-Up" Research. *Archives of Sexual Behavior, 46*(2), 585–602. DOI: 10.1007/s10508-016-0783-6 PMID: 27393037

Kor, A., Zilcha-Mano, S., Fogel, Y. A., Mikulincer, M., Reid, R. C., & Potenza, M. N. (2014). Psychometric development of the Problematic Pornography Use Scale. *Addictive Behaviors*, *39*(5), 861–868. DOI: 10.1016/j.addbeh.2014.01.027 PMID: 24583276

Kraus, S. W., & Sweeney, P. J. (2019). Hitting the target: Considerations for differential diagnosis when treating individuals for problematic use of pornography. *Archives of Sexual Behavior*, *48*(2), 431–435. DOI: 10.1007/s10508-018-1301-9 PMID: 30229519

Kraus, S. W., Voon, V., & Potenza, M. N. (2016). Should compulsive sexual behavior be considered an addiction? *Addiction (Abingdon, England)*, *111*(12), 2097–2106. DOI: 10.1111/add.13297 PMID: 26893127

Kühn, S., & Gallinat, J. (2014). Brain structure and functional connectivity associated with pornography consumption: The brain on porn. *JAMA Psychiatry*, *71*(7), 827–834. DOI: 10.1001/jamapsychiatry.2014.93 PMID: 24871202

Love, T., Laier, C., Brand, M., Hatch, L., & Hajela, R. (2015). Neuroscience of Internet Pornography Addiction: A Review and Update. *Behavioral Sciences (Basel, Switzerland)*, *5*(3), 388–433. DOI: 10.3390/bs5030388 PMID: 26393658

McGlynn, C., & Rackley, E. (2017). Image-based sexual abuse. *Oxford Journal of Legal Studies*, *37*(3), 534–561. DOI: 10.1093/ojls/gqw033

Paasonen, S. (2011). Revisiting cyberfeminism. *Communications*, *36*(3), 335–352. DOI: 10.1515/comm.2011.017

Peter, J., & Valkenburg, P. M. (2016). Adolescents and Pornography: A Review of 20 Years of Research. *Journal of Sex Research*, *53*(4-5), 509–531. DOI: 10.1080/00224499.2016.1143441 PMID: 27105446

Prause, N. (2019). Porn is for masturbation. *Archives of Sexual Behavior*, *48*(8), 2271–2277. DOI: 10.1007/s10508-019-1397-6 PMID: 30847758

Robinson, T. E., & Berridge, K. C. (2008). Incentive sensitization theory. *Philosophical Transactions of the Royal Society of London. Series B, Biological Sciences*, *363*(1507), 3137–3146. DOI: 10.1098/rstb.2008.0093 PMID: 18640920

Srnicek, N. (2017). *Platform capitalism*. Polity Press.

Steele, V. R., Staley, C., Fong, T., & Prause, N. (2013). Sexual desire, not hypersexuality, is related to neurophysiological responses elicited by sexual images. *Socioaffective Neuroscience & Psychology*, *3*(1), 20770. DOI: 10.3402/snp.v3i0.20770 PMID: 24693355

Stone, R. (2026). *Women targeted by AI-generated sexual imagery describe lasting harm*. Rolling Stone.

Torraco, R. J. (2016). Writing integrative literature reviews: Using the past and present to explore the future. *Human Resource Development Review*, *15*(4), 404–428. DOI: 10.1177/1534484316671606

Vicens, A., & Satter, R. (2026). Investigation reveals misuse of AI image generation for sexualized content. *Reuters*. https://www.reuters.com/world/us/rise-ai-generated-child-sexual-imagery-reports-2026-02-20/

Vieira, C., & Griffiths, M. D. (2024). Problematic pornography use and mental health: A systematic review. *Sexual Health & Compulsivity*, *31*(3), 207–247. DOI: 10.1080/26929953.2024.2348624

Volkow, N. D., Wang, G. J., Fowler, J. S., Tomasi, D., Telang, F., & Baler, R. (2010). Addiction: Decreased reward sensitivity and increased expectation sensitivity conspire to overwhelm the brain's control circuit. *BioEssays : News and Reviews in Molecular, Cellular and Developmental Biology*, *32*(9), 748–755. DOI: 10.1002/bies.201000042 PMID: 20730946

Voon, V., Mole, T. B., Banca, P., Porter, L., Morris, L., Mitchell, S., Lapa, T. R., Karr, J., Harrison, N. A., Potenza, M. N., & Irvine, M. (2014). Neural correlates of sexual cue reactivity in individuals with and without compulsive sexual behaviours. *PLoS One*, *9*(7), e102419. DOI: 10.1371/journal.pone.0102419 PMID: 25013940

Williams, L. (1989). *Hard core: Power, pleasure, and the frenzy of the visible*. University of California Press.

Willoughby, B. J., Carroll, J. S., Busby, D. M., & Brown, C. C. (2016). Differences in Pornography Use Among Couples: Associations with Satisfaction, Stability, and Relationship Processes. *Archives of Sexual Behavior*, *45*(1), 145–158. DOI: 10.1007/s10508-015-0562-9 PMID: 26228990

World Health Organization. (2018). *International classification of diseases (11th revision)*.

Zuboff, S. (2019). *The age of surveillance capitalism*. PublicAffairs.

KEY TERMS AND DEFINITIONS

Algorithmic Addiction: A form of behavioral dependency intensified by algorithmic recommendation systems that predict, reinforce, and escalate user consumption through data-driven content optimization.

Desensitization: A neuropsychological process in which repeated exposure to intense sexual stimuli reduces emotional and physiological responsiveness, leading to diminished arousal and increased demand for extreme content.

Digital Pornography: Pornographic content produced, distributed, and consumed through digital platforms, characterized by unlimited accessibility, algorithmic personalization, and continuous circulation within platform economies.

Neurobiological Tolerance: The gradual reduction of dopaminergic response to repeated sexual stimuli, requiring increased intensity or novelty to achieve the same level of reward activation.

Parasocial Sexual Interaction: A one-sided relational dynamic in which users experience simulated intimacy and emotional connection with pornographic performers, despite the absence of mutual or reciprocal interaction.

Personalized Pornography: A mode of pornographic consumption in which content is tailored to individual users through direct interaction, subscription-based access, and parasocial engagement with specific content creators.

Platform Capitalism: An economic model in which digital platforms extract value from user behavior by transforming attention, desire, and interaction into monetizable data streams.

Pornography Addiction: A pattern of compulsive pornography consumption marked by loss of control, tolerance development, continued use despite negative consequences, and dysregulation of the brain's reward system.

Chapter 9
When Screens Meet Cravings:
Exploring the Intersection of Food and Technology Addiction

Elif Kurtulus Anarat
http://orcid.org/0000-0001-7555-2852
Üsküdar University, Turkey

ABSTRACT

In this era of rapid technological advancement, it is clear that integration with digital devices shapes human behaviour, including consumption habits and eating behaviours. This situation has the potential to pave the way for an increase in addictive tendencies linked to technology use. In this section, the bidirectional link between excessive technology use—specifically online gaming addiction and problematic smartphone use—and emotional eating and food addiction will be examined. In this context, the section will address how digital platforms that are designed to be engaging and encourage connectivity may simultaneously reduce individuals' self-control over eating behaviours and trigger cravings. In examining the relationship between technology use and eating behaviours, the aim is to address common neurobiological foundations and psychological mechanisms such as impulsivity, particularly in the context of addiction. Furthermore, this chapter offers recommendations for future research and practice by exploring the intersections between eating and technology addiction.

DOI: 10.4018/979-8-2600-2468-3.ch009

INTRODUCTION

It has been suggested that problematic internet and smartphone use is associated with disrupted eating behaviour and loneliness, highlighting the complex link between digital engagement and psychological well-being. In particular, it is noted that this relationship manifests itself during adolescence with the increase in smartphone use and the consumption of high-calorie foods (Caninsti & Rahayu, 2024; Liu & Ellis, 2021). On the other hand, it is suggested that another factor potentially playing a mediating role in this situation, which emerges during adolescence—a developmentally critical period—is difficulties in emotion regulation (Domoff et al., 2020). Difficulties with emotional regulation are defined as challenges individuals face in clearly expressing their emotions, employing emotional strategies, controlling their impulses, and engaging in goal-directed behaviour (Gross, 1998). In this context, difficulties with emotion regulation emerge as a significant transdiagnostic factor in the course of substance use disorders and eating disorders. When considered from the perspective of adolescence, a period marked by rapid change and development, it is suggested that individuals in the process of identity formation may be more prone to such behaviours due to their inability to effectively utilise emotional strategies (Domoff et al., 2020; Kim et al., 2020). This supports the view that psychological and environmental factors associated with technology use and problematic eating behaviour may be shared (Attanasi et al., 2021; Kim et al., 2020). Common psychosocial risk and protective factors have been identified for problematic smartphone use, online gaming addiction and eating addiction among adolescents (Mastrobattista et al., 2024).

THE DEFINITION OF EATING ADDICTION IN THE MODERN ERA

Although concepts such as food addiction or eating addiction are not yet classified as substance use disorders in current research, they have emerged as prominent areas of study in recent years (Hebebrand et al., 2014). Although it is not classified as an addiction disorder, it has been suggested that excessive consumption of processed foods may be associated with addiction-like symptoms due to the activation of reward pathways (Mastrobattista et al., 2024). Food addiction, a currently controversial field, is generally considered separately from eating disorders rather than as a substance use disorder ([REMOVED CITATION FIELD]; . It is noted that palatable and ultra-processed foods are associated with the biological and behavioural symptoms of addiction and may lead to obesity by triggering overeating (LaFata & Gearhardt, 2022). The view that neurobiological mechanisms, explained by the influence on dopaminergic reward pathways and executive control functions, are shaped by the interaction of biological sensitivities and environmental factors is supported (Harris & Taillie, 2023; Hebebrand et al., 2014; LaFata & Gearhardt, 2022). The view that fast food can create addiction in a manner similar to psychoactive substances, due to the intersection of obesity and addiction pathways, has gained increasing traction (Lustig, 2020). This perspective, emerging from research, highlights the addictive potential of certain foods in relation to the frequency of use of social media and online food ordering platforms. Consequently, it is argued that the availability of hyper-palatable foods and the use of technology are crucial for understanding contemporary patterns of food addiction (Pretlow et al., 2015). Regarding food addiction, the potential addictive effects of ultra-processed foods are highlighted. As these foods activate reward pathways, individuals may be driven towards compulsive overeating. Rather than nutritional content, the fact that foods are easily accessible, quick and tasty is sufficient to satisfy the reward experience. Research into how technology facilitates the increased accessibility of food—which has become an object of happiness for individuals—suggests that the two fields in question may share common characteristics in their patterns of addiction (Ifland & Brewerton, 2025).

The 'Yale Food Addiction Scale', used to measure food addiction, draws upon symptoms parallel to those of substance use disorders in defining food addiction and measuring addiction-like eating behaviours (LaFata et al., 2024). Although the debate continues as to whether eating addiction is a subtype of an eating disorder or a subtype of substance use disorders, this stems from the lack of universal diagnostic criteria for eating addiction (Meule & Gearhardt, 2014). The absence of established diagnostic criteria also presents challenges in both research and clinical settings (Vasiliu, 2023). Nevertheless, it is argued that the number of studies supporting the validity and clinical significance of food addiction has increased over the years (Gearhardt et al., 2023). In studies using the Yale Food Addiction Scale, significant insights are being gained regarding whether individuals exhibit addiction-like symptoms in response to ultra-processed foods. It is suggested that foods high in fat and sugar activate the brain's reward pathways, thereby acting as addictive substances, and can lead to compulsive overeating behaviour despite their negative consequences. A study by Fletcher and Kenny (2018) found that the consumption of ultra-processed foods, which are high in fat and carbohydrates, increases the hedonic response and activates reward-related regions in the brain. It is noted that this effect observed in the reward system may lead to excessive consumption and subsequently to addiction-like symptoms.

The increase in activation parallels the changes observed in the dopaminergic pathways that encourage the consumption of addictive substances. The neurobiological changes in mesolimbic dopamine pathways, which are associated with tolerance and withdrawal symptoms, strengthen the likelihood that the act of eating could perpetuate an addiction cycle. In addition to shared neurobiological responses, behavioural patterns in food addiction—such as intense cravings, loss of control in the face of excessive consumption, and continued eating despite negative consequences—are also observed to bear similarities to symptoms seen in substance use disorders (Meule & Gearhardt, 2014). Furthermore, previous research has indicated that hyper-palatable foods can induce neurochemical changes in the dopamine and opioid systems, and that this pattern is similar to that seen in substance use and addiction disorders. Given the neurological factors underlying addiction-like symptoms towards specific foods, it is to be expected that the concept of food addiction occupies a controversial position in terms of classification (Morin et al., 2017). On the other hand, a better understanding of neural structures such as the dopamine system and the opioid system is required in order to adopt an appropriate and effective intervention approach for food addiction (Frascella et al., 2010). According to findings from neuroimaging studies, it has been observed that activation in the reward system and the dopaminergic system differs in individuals with food addiction, and that abnormalities are seen in the nucleus accumbens and insula, which are associated with addiction.

NEUROLOGICAL FACTORS ASSOCIATED WITH REWARD AND CRAVINGS

A reduction in the D2 receptor within the dopamine system, in particular, is considered a primary neurological factor in the mimicking of the neuroadaptations observed in substance addiction by hyper-palatable foods. Furthermore, the fact that sugar, as a specific nutrient, can lead to opioid-like withdrawal symptoms highlights the need to consider the addictive potential of different nutrients separately. The fact that impairments in the cognitive inhibition system are associated with an inability to control eating behaviour and excessive consumption also aligns with the sensitivity to external stimuli observed in addiction disorders (Saruco & Pleger, 2021). This neurobiological framework highlights the common neurobiological changes experienced by individuals in both substance-related and non-substance-related addiction disorders (Frascella et al., 2010). In particular, understanding the role of mesolimbic dopamine pathways and the prefrontal cortex in addiction disorders is crucial for comprehending how individuals may develop an addiction to certain foods. For example, research has suggested that in individuals with food addiction, changes in grey matter volume and connectivity in the inferior frontal gyrus may be associated with appetite and inhibition. This structural and functional neuroadaptation explains the extent to which executive functions influence eating behaviour in some individuals. A state of heightened sensitivity to food-related cues, mediated by dopaminergic pathways, is associated with the preference for food as a habit rather than a necessity, and the subsequent loss of control over eating behaviour. Neuroimaging studies support these findings. For example, it has been observed that palatable foods activate brain regions associated with cravings, and that this activity is particularly pronounced in the striatum and prefrontal cortex—areas also implicated in substance use and addiction disorders. This shared mechanism explains the compulsive overconsumption observed in food addiction. Furthermore, it is understood that the absence of inhibitory control in response to food-related cues in obese individuals constitutes a significant risk factor for food intake in terms of addiction. It has been found that altered activation in the dorsomedial prefrontal cortex, ventral striatum and orbitofrontal cortex in response to visual food stimuli is observed in individuals with binge eating behaviour, similar to that seen in substance use and addiction disorders (Frascella et al., 2010; Zhang et al., 2020). On the other hand, it is understood that this neurological overlap manifests itself in areas of impaired decision-making processes and a strong craving for food, and that it follows a similar course to substance use and addiction disorders.

THE EFFECTS OF WIDESPREAD TECHNOLOGY USE ON FOOD CONSUMPTION

It is believed that technology has significantly altered contemporary food consumption habits, particularly in terms of accessibility and the visual appeal of food, and it has been suggested that this may lead individuals to adopt compulsive eating behaviours by stimulating their reward. It is suggested that the increased ease of accessing food, particularly with the rise in technology use, may be linked to compulsive overeating. For example, the ease of ordering food via mobile apps and the prevalence of influencer marketing targeting specific brands and food and beverage establishments on social media, driven by the widespread use of technology, suggest that this risk may be a factor (Davis & Carter, 2014). It is noted that individuals with a sensitivity to rewards may be more vulnerable to this risk due to impulsivity and low levels of self-control (VanderBroek-Stice et al., 2017). It is suggested that, in addition to technology's widespread use shaping behavioural factors related to food and eating, eating behaviour may also exhibit a similar pattern—particularly in social media applications where immediate feedback is available and individuals' reward systems are active—and that the neurological underpinnings of this situation may support both scenarios (Hebebrand et al., 2014). Previous research has also highlighted that difficulties in emotion regulation and weak inhibitory control are significant psychological factors contributing to both the use of technology and the addictive nature of eating behaviour (Cardi et al., 2022). It is known that food addiction, which shares a similar course with addiction disorders but is not officially classified as a type of addiction, is characterised by an inability to resist calorie-rich and hyper-palatable foods (Maqsood et al., 2025; McCausland et al., 2025). In particular, the much easier access to food following the Industrial Revolution has transformed individuals' consumption habits (Moghimi et al., 2021; Moreno-Padilla et al., 2022). Perceptions of food have moved beyond the mere satisfaction of physical needs and have evolved into a behaviour of consuming what is available. Furthermore, the increased production of ultra-processed foods rich in fat, salt and sugar has led individuals to consume food not only to satisfy hunger but also as a source of pleasure. On the other hand, Monosodium Glutamate (MSG), a component of fast food that stands out for its addictive properties, is known to impart umami (the fifth taste) to foods. It is suggested that this may encourage individuals to consume these foods in greater quantities and subsequently exhibit addiction-like symptoms (Rebello & Greenway, 2016) . These foods, which are generally rich in polyunsaturated fatty acids, particularly n-6 linoleic acid, can cause oxidation during processing and storage that disrupts metabolic signalling and increases inflammation; this can impair the brain's ability to control eating behaviour and reinforce reward-driven eating behaviour (Atar, 2026). The high availability of foods and excessive exposure to them via technology can increase individuals' sensitivity to food-related cues beyond their physical needs, leading them to perceive eating as part of a hedonic act (Atalayer, 2017; Atar, 2026). This situation is considered a major lifestyle factor believed to play a significant role in the obesity epidemic. Findings from experimental studies indicate that the hyper-palatability, soft texture and calorie density of foods are decisive factors in consumption habits, the reward system and the pathways of satiety signals in the brain (Juul et al., 2025) . It is argued that high levels of accessibility and the aggressive marketing of ultra-processed foods, particularly via digital platforms, have led to an increase in excessive consumption among individuals (David et al., 2017; Steward & Wierenga, 2022) . Excessive exposure to hyper-palatable foods that trigger a sense of reward leads to the desensitisation of reward pathways and subsequently to increased consumption. This aligns with the cycle of addiction.

DIGITAL PLATFORMS AND FOOD CHOICES: AN OVERVIEW FROM SOCIAL MEDIA TO FOOD DELIVERY APPS

With digitalisation, people are moving away from traditional food and meal habits towards choices that are more practical, accessible and encourage overconsumption (Morin et al., 2017) . With the proliferation of this digital ecosystem, food ordering apps and social media accounts are able to target individuals with advertising and promotions, and this has a decisive influence on dietary habits (Berthoud, 2012) . It is clear that individuals are within the sphere of influence of apps that promote easily accessible and hyper-tasty foods. Furthermore, it is known that these advertisements and promotions targeted at individuals are shaped by advanced algorithms to reflect personal preferences (Cohen, 2008; Lemos et al., 2022) . Consequently, users exposed to such content demonstrate a tendency towards ultra-processed foods that offer quick rewards. Rather than making conscious decisions, individuals' exposure leads them to make automatic choices that allow them to experience the sensation of reward more quickly. This continuous exposure can lead to individuals becoming more sensitive to foods that are accessible, affordable and easy to obtain. These digital cues trigger a cycle of craving and inability to resist, and when combined with neurobiological sensitivity to reward, they increase the tendency to choose high-calorie foods (Sinha, 2017; Yang et al., 2021) . One of the key reasons people enter this cycle so quickly is that the exposure in question is personalised. Personalised content and advertisements targeting specific foods and services can push individuals to a point where they are unable to resist fast-food-type foods (Chew et al., 2023; Jia et al., 2024) . It has been suggested that exposure to personalised content may reach a macro-environmental level and influence the dietary habits of society and the obesogenic system (Yang et al., 2021).

It is noted that food ordering apps via smartphones may be a determining factor in individuals' food choices, and that young adults and adolescents are particularly vulnerable groups regarding this usage habit. When digital access to food is combined with advanced marketing techniques, individuals' tendency to opt for unhealthy foods and beverages increases (Willie et al., 2024) . The selection of these foods—which are high in calories but low in nutritional value—increases the likelihood that individuals will choose larger portions and subsequently experience weight-related issues. In this context, it is understood that this situation may pose a risk as a more general eating behaviour problem that extends beyond food choices; because the increased tendency of individuals to focus on biased attention and rely on facilitative tools may influence their choices, leading to negative outcomes regarding unhealthy eating behaviours and lifestyle habits (Liu & Ellis, 2021). Individuals learn the connection between hyper-palatable foods offering an immediate reward experience and the feedback loop provided by the digital ecosystem (Harris & Taillie, 2024; Molle et al., 2016) . Furthermore, it is noted that marketing strategies targeting children and adolescents, by emphasising the emotional connection to food, may render them unable to resist sugary foods and drinks, fast food, and high-calorie snacks (Fretes et al., 2025; Maksi et al., 2024) . It is noted that this continuous exposure may act as a risk factor, particularly for young individuals who use digital devices most frequently, and that over time, their inability to resist ultra-processed foods may make it increasingly difficult for them to make healthy choices. Based on research on this topic, the link between technology and eating behaviour can be explained by the facilitative functions of technology, changes in food choices, and the resulting cycle of addiction stemming from the pleasure derived from certain food types.

GAMIFICATION OF EATING BEHAVIOUR, REWARDS, PERKS AND ENGAGEMENT

This section examines research findings on how loyalty programmes, virtual rewards and interactive competitions in food ordering apps influence food consumption, and how individuals' consumption habits are shaped through these apps. The aim is to increase user engagement through the rewards offered by social media and mobile apps. This reward system enables users to experience rewards quickly. Furthermore, individuals may place food orders simply to take advantage of the opportunities and benefits offered by the apps, even when they do not physically feel hungry (Choi et al., 2023) . The strategic presentation of points, badges and leaderboards will trigger users' urge to collect rewards, thereby encouraging them to place more food orders and consume more food (Filippone et al., 2022) . It is argued that the gamification strategies employed by food ordering and shopping apps foster loyalty to specific brands, and that this could be a determining factor in dietary habits (Vladimiros, 2025) . This approach, particularly when combined with peer influence among children and adolescents, increases demand for the opportunities offered by gamification techniques and may lead to the consumption of unhealthy food (Harris & Taillie, 2023) .

Through the use of digital marketing techniques enhanced by artificial intelligence and advanced profiling methods, personalised and attractive offers are presented, thereby shaping individuals' preferences, purchasing and consumption behaviours (Driessen et al., 2025; Elliott et al., 2025; Halloran et al., 2021) . It is stated that targeting young consumers, whose decision-making processes are still developing, through personalised marketing techniques brings with it a heightened sensitivity towards digital food marketing (Amson et al., 2024) . It is understood that the combination of digital marketing with peer influence and social media trends is a significant determinant of food choices (Tsochantaridou et al., 2023) . It is known that this dynamic is fuelled by gamification, defined as the incorporation of game design elements into a non-game application or environment (Han et al., 2023; McGloin & Eslami, 2014) . Whilst these techniques could potentially encourage beneficial and healthy choices, when applied specifically to the food sector, gamification increases the tendency towards high-calorie yet nutritionally inadequate foods (Folkvord et al., 2012) .

Gamification is presented to users with features that, by influencing the cognitive processes and psychological sensitivities of adolescents in particular, may lead to compulsive eating behaviour rather than guiding them towards balanced and healthy eating habits. The inclusion of foods that create a sense of reward in this process increases the risk of individuals developing unhealthy and problematic eating behaviours.

A GENERAL OVERVIEW OF TECHNOLOGY ADDICTION: CHARACTERISTICS PARALLEL TO SUBSTANCE USE DISORDERS

In this section, which examines the conceptual and behavioural commonalities between the profile of substance use disorders—derived from previous research and clinical findings on problematic technology use—and problematic technology use, the similar neurobiological pathways and behavioural reinforcers shared by both substance use disorders and problematic technology use are discussed. Through the common characteristics examined, the potential for addiction observed in substance use disorders will be revealed by the way digital stimuli, through intermittent reinforcement, increase individuals' interaction with technology (Albayrak & Özbek, 2025) .

Technology addiction is associated with neurobiological mechanisms, particularly the dopaminergic pathways responsible for the formation of compulsive behaviours (Masri-Zada et al., 2025) . The link between the feedback loop provided by algorithm-generated content and changes in brain physiology may lead to behavioural addiction characteristics similar to those seen in substance use disorders (De et al., 2025) . In essence, research on the subject indicates that technology addiction may lead to symptoms such as mental preoccupation, loss of control, increased usage and withdrawal, which are observed in substance use disorders, and that this is particularly pronounced in the adolescent population, which is neurodevelopmentally vulnerable (Tabish, 2025) . It is suggested that adolescents, whose prefrontal cortex—responsible for executive functions and impulse control—is still immature, are more vulnerable to the rapid sense of gratification offered by digital content (Hutton et al., 2024) . It is noted that this state of vulnerability is exacerbated by the 'algorithmic pleasure structures' offered by digital platforms, which create a cycle of impulsivity that increases the desire for reward; this process is said to operate similarly to the neurobiological processes observed in behavioural addictions (James et al., 2025) .

Findings from neuroimaging studies indicate that excessive use of technology leads to structural and functional changes in brain regions responsible for decision-making, impulse control and emotion regulation, and that these changes are similar in nature to those associated with substance use (Eskandar, 2025; Giansanti, 2025; Lakhan, 2025) . This neural adaptation is associated with changes in regions related to reward experience, cue reactivity and executive control (Wolf et al., 2025) . It is noted that these neural circuits are capable of explaining changes in the brain's reward mechanism, as well as individuals' sensitivity to digital stimuli and the disruption of self-experience mechanisms (Karaköse et al., 2023; Kear & Sasha, 2018) . Consequently, excessive engagement with digital platforms leads to desensitisation of the brain's reward centre and, over time, an increase in the frequency of use required to activate the reward centre (Masri-Zada et al., 2025) . Increased time spent on digital platforms and excessive engagement are characterised by disruptions in the reward mechanism and heightened sensitivity to rewards (Chiu & Chein, 2022) . Hyper-sensitivity to reward, arising from the activation of the ventral-striatal dopamine circuit, is particularly evident in the adolescent population, where cognitive and behavioural control capacities are at a low level (Maza et al., 2023) . Increased reward sensitivity is associated with impairments in the nucleus accumbens and orbitofrontal cortex, which are responsible for reward processing and motivation (Chun et al., 2018) . Furthermore, findings from neuroimaging studies suggest that technology addiction is associated with structural and functional changes in the amygdala, which triggers the dopamine cycle observed in substance use (Patel et al., 2025) .

These changes, proposed by neural adaptation, increase sensitivity to cues that emerge from maladaptive learning processes, as seen in substance addiction (He et al., 2017; Shanmugasundaram & Tamilarasu, 2023) . The role of the mesolimbic reward system is implicated, and the shared neurobiological processes underlying technology use and substance dependence are linked to the activation of similar neural pathways by the consumption of digital content and the associated habits (Tymofiyeva et al., 2020) . This situation impairs behavioural inhibition and increases sensitivity to digital cues (Nesi et al., 2022) .

Based on findings from behavioural and neuroimaging studies, this reinforces the argument that problematic technology use should be addressed from a behavioural addiction perspective. This situation necessitates that intervention programmes developed for problematic technology use address similar neurobiological sensitivities (James et al., 2025; Nesi et al., 2022) . It is anticipated that the shared neural mechanism underlying problematic technology use and behavioural addictions, as well as future studies on diagnostic criteria, will guide future research and contribute to the treatment of problematic technology use and substance addictions, which are becoming increasingly prevalent as public health issues.

BEHAVIOURAL DIAGNOSTIC CRITERIA FOR TECHNOLOGY ADDICTION

Understanding the diagnostic criteria for technology addiction requires an assessment within the framework of behavioural addiction, which manifests as excessive preoccupation with digital content (Chatterjee & Rai, 2023) . This assessment encompasses compulsive use, functional impairment, and withdrawal symptoms associated with the use of digital platforms (Méndez et al., 2024) . The World Health Organisation's International Classification of Diseases, 11th Revision, addresses gaming disorder as a separate category. In the ICD-11, digital gaming disorder is defined by criteria including loss of control over gaming, prioritising gaming over other activities, continuing to game despite negative consequences, and an increase in usage duration (Eskandar, 2025) . Similarly, similar behavioural patterns are observed in other forms of technology addiction, such as problematic social media use. For example, increased preoccupation, craving, and increased stress and functional problems when access is restricted are among the symptoms associated with problematic social media use (Mujica et al., 2022) . These approaches to establishing diagnostic criteria have been structured based on the findings of previous neuroimaging studies, which indicate similarities between internet and substance addiction, and the view has been adopted that technology addiction should be classified among behavioural addictions (Jin et al., 2026).

The fact that changes in the volume of grey and white matter within brain regions associated with the reward experience are of a similar nature is linked to similar changes in functional areas such as reward processing, cognitive control and emotion regulation skills in both technology addiction and substance addiction (Chatterjee & Rai, 2023; Jin et al., 2026) . In this context, it is emphasised that pharmacological and psychotherapeutic interventions developed for technology addiction should take into account neurobiological factors similar to those in substance use disorders (Ekhtiari et al., 2024) . Furthermore, it is thought that the identification of these neurobiological markers could be beneficial in structuring personalised interventions and, consequently, in enhancing treatment efficacy (Liu et al., 2021) . However, despite the findings from existing research, there is no consensus regarding diagnostic criteria that specifically assess technology addiction. There are no established diagnostic criteria for technology addiction, which manifests in various forms such as problematic internet use, smartphone addiction and behavioural addiction (Uma et al., 2014) . This uncertainty is thought to stem from the fact that 'internet gaming disorder' has not yet been formally included as a separate category in the American Psychiatric Association's Diagnostic and Statistical Manual of Mental Disorders, 5th edition (DSM-5), and that assessments continue to be based on the criteria for pathological gambling (Choi et al., 2019) . It is considered that the discussions and uncertainties surrounding this issue necessitate an understanding of at what point the technology widely used in daily life becomes problematic, and that this should be addressed through standardised and evidence-based approaches (Brand et al., 2014) .

It is argued that conceptual uncertainty regarding technology addiction leads to inconsistencies in both research and clinical practice. Therefore, it is necessary to establish the diagnostic validity of this behavioural pathology by presenting neurobiological and psychobiological evidence (Áfra et al., 2023; Courbet et al., 2020; Lin et al., 2016) . It is suggested that, by resolving this uncertainty, it may be possible to develop specific tools such as scales and interventions for technology addiction (Solly et al., 2021; Sun et al., 2025) . Due to the uncertainty surrounding diagnostic criteria, it is emphasised that empirical evidence regarding prevalence rates, long-term effects and risk factors is limited, and that a clearer diagnostic framework needs to be adopted (Tereshchenko, 2023) .

Although pathological gambling is officially defined as a behavioural addiction in the DSM-5, ongoing debates suggest that internet addiction is a condition requiring further research (Bouazza et al., 2022; Brand et al., 2024; Yu & Sussman, 2020) . It is noted that another significant reason behind the uncertainty and debates regarding definition stems from differing views on at what point the use of technology—which is an integral part of daily life—should be classified as addiction beyond its necessary use (Soler et al., 2021) . Furthermore, it is observed that there is no consensus on which aspect of the smartphone can be associated with addiction in this newly studied form of technology addiction, such as smartphone addiction. Whether the smartphone itself is a tool that entirely leads to addiction, or whether one or more of the features it offers (mobile apps, shopping, etc.) are the tools leading to addiction, is a point of disagreement associated with diagnostic uncertainty. For this reason, it is thought that future research, by distinguishing between instrumental attachment to technology and distinct patterns of addiction, could contribute to diagnostic approaches and subsequently to the development of clinical applications.

NEUROCOGNITIVE SIMILARITIES BETWEEN TECHNOLOGY USE AND FOOD CRAVINGS

In order to understand the common neural pathways and cognitive mechanisms underlying technology addiction and food cravings, it is important to examine the background of compulsive behaviours arising from technology use and disordered eating behaviours. Significant activation of the reward system, impaired executive control associated with impulsivity, and alterations in decision-making processes are considered common features (Christensen et al., 2023) . For example, cognitive factors—including increased impulsivity, insufficient top-down executive control, and hypersensitivity to addiction-related stimuli—are observed in both conditions. The neurocognitive limitations described reflect the underlying difficulties in controlling excessive consumption, whether of digital technologies or palatable foods. For instance, in food addiction—where both technology addiction and food cravings are observed—symptoms such as tolerance, withdrawal, and the inability to stop or control use despite negative consequences are evident. It is argued that similarities in neurocognitive factors suggest that theoretical approaches and intervention programmes developed for one area may be applicable to the other, thereby facilitating a more holistic understanding of behavioural addictions.

Conceptual debates regarding the distinction between eating addiction and eating disorders show parallels with discussions in technology addiction concerning whether the issue is behavioural addiction or addiction to devices (Hebebrand et al., 2014) . This notable theoretical parallelism and the presence of shared neurocognitive mechanisms make it possible to compare these disciplines within the research field (Whatnall et al., 2022) . Indeed, the role of dopamine-related reward pathways in food addiction and the neuroadaptations caused by an obesogenic diet are considered to be guiding factors in the study of technology addiction (Whatnall et al., 2022) .

Research indicates that ultra-processed foods, which are rich in fat, sugar and salt, possess addictive properties due to their pharmacokinetic characteristics, and that this aligns with the neurobiological changes observed in substance use disorders and, potentially, in technology addiction (McCausland et al., 2025) . Changes in the mesolimbic dopamine system, similar to those observed with illicit drugs and digital stimuli, have been noted, and it is known that this leads to compulsive consumption (Hough et al., 2026; Pursey et al.,2024) . This neurological overlap has been supported by findings from functional MRI scans based on blood oxygen levels, and it has been suggested that reward sensitivity is similar in obese individuals and those with substance use disorders (Chen et al., 2018) . Similarly, the compulsive consumption of palatable and calorie-rich foods is explained by impairments in dopamine pathways that influence motivation and the reward system (Maqsood et al., 2025; VanderBroek- Stice et al., 2017) . For this reason, the craving observed in technology use and food consumption, along with impaired self-control skills, follow a similar trajectory (Saruco & Pleger, 2021) . Individuals may develop an addiction to hyper-palatable and ultra-processed foods and exhibit impulsive behaviours towards food, or compulsive overconsumption may occur (Atar, 2026) . It has been suggested that understanding these neurological factors in food addiction could make a significant contribution to understanding the potential reinforcing factors in technology addiction (Frascella et al., 2010; Ifland & Brewerton, 2025; Pursey et al., 2024; Wattick et al., 2023) .

It is known that food and technology addiction are characterised by disruptions in the reward system, and that food and digital experiences stimulate similar neural pathways, leading to compulsive behaviour (Lin et al., 2020) . Findings from animal studies have shown that mice exposed to a sugary solution exhibit withdrawal and deprivation symptoms, similar to those seen in substance use (Davis & Carter, 2014) . The initial conceptualisation of these two types of addiction as distinct is important for addressing the frequency of their co-occurrence in subsequent research. As is well known, there is a possibility that these two conditions, which share common neural mechanisms, may co-occur in the same individual; however, prior to identifying this, it is important to understand which condition may constitute a risk factor and to identify the common mechanisms involved (LaFata et al., 2024) . The fact that food and technology can elicit addiction-like biological and behavioural responses, and that they are readily accessible tools capable of enabling individuals to achieve satiety rapidly, strengthens the likelihood of these two behavioural addictions occurring simultaneously. The following section presents research on the extent to which food and technology addiction can influence one another.

THE NEXUS OF FOOD AND TECHNOLOGY ADDICTION: A BIDIRECTIONAL RELATIONSHIP

It is argued that, as technological advancements become an integral part of individuals' lives and individuals integrate these advancements with the demands of daily life, situations may arise where eating behaviours are also affected. Individuals' excessive exposure to food-related content and their engagement with advertisements and influencer marketing on social media can lead to compulsive overeating and food cravings (Mastrobattista et al., 2024) . In particular, the following of social media accounts where visually rich, engaging content—which prioritises the user experience—is shared with users, and exposure to such content, can increase the risk of individuals developing external eating behaviour and subsequently food addiction (Vasiliu, 2023) . In addition to the content shared with users, the prioritisation of user loyalty through gamification, the reinforcement of competition, and the active maintenance of the reward system via bonuses and badges are among other technology-based services that may lead to the continuation of eating behaviour (Whatnall et al., 2022) . The use of these services and exposure to their content increases the likelihood of entering a cycle of engagement and turning to foods that provide instant gratification.

Users exposed to food-related content may develop selective attention towards certain types of food, and this can create a eating cycle where unhealthy foods are preferred simply due to the sight of the food they have been exposed to, even when they do not physically feel hungry (Whatnall et al., 2022) . This exposure can increase sensitivity to food-related cues and lead to compulsive overeating behaviours (Benvegnù et al., 2023) . Furthermore, this persistent digital exposure triggers classical conditioning and conditions an increase in food intake. In such a situation, individuals may choose to eat simply because they have been conditioned to do so, even when they do not feel physically hungry (Humphreys et al., 2020) . This increasingly prevalent digital environment acts as a significant external trigger, and continuous exposure and easy access suggest that food consumption may constitute a potential behavioural addiction (Vasiliu, 2023) .

Findings from studies indicate that food-related content on social media platforms triggers patterns of impulsive eating behaviour and is associated with the act of impulsive eating rather than physical hunger signals (Patwardhan et al., 2024) . It is noted that this situation may also lead to hedonic eating behaviour, where food is used as a means of immediate gratification rather than due to physical hunger. The neural response associated with reward sensitivity aligns with hedonic eating behaviour because individuals do not simply eat to obtain nutrients; they may choose food to derive pleasure and feel rewarded (Ceylan, 2025). Digital food content that activates the brain's dopamine and attention networks can increase hedonic hunger and trigger a bias towards perceiving food as a reward (Cahyani et al., 2023; Uclés-Torrents et al., 2026) . Digital content that triggers an obesogenic environment stimulates appetite and increases addiction-like behaviours to an extent that may override self-control mechanisms (- . This differs from homeostatic hunger, which is felt due to an energy deficit. In the case of homeostatic hunger, individuals prefer to close the energy gap based on physical hunger signals; however, in the case of hedonic hunger, individuals experience an intense craving for specific foods under the influence of environmental cues, even in the absence of physical hunger (Atalayer, 2017; Berthoud, 2012; Boyland et al., 2024) . These environmental cues, which predominantly emerge through digital content, override homeostatic control and activate dopaminergic reward pathways (Teymur & ÖNEY, 2024) . Exposure to food on social media has been linked to body image issues and patterns of unhealthy eating behaviour, and it has been noted that this situation may lead to a cycle of disordered eating and psychological distress (Filippone et al., 2022) . This phenomenon, where the visual presentation of food on social media triggers the desire to eat, is termed 'visual hunger'. When individuals experience visual hunger, they may feel a strong urge to access food without actually feeling physically hungry (Spence et al., 2015) .

Consequently, the co-occurrence of food addiction and technology addiction is becoming increasingly common, as technology serves as a tool through which food can be presented to users as a visual stimulus. In daily life, where access to information is becoming easier by the day thanks to digitalisation, individuals are turning to platforms such as, which are easily accessible and offer instant gratification. As a result of this ease of access and the influence of marketing in social media usage, individuals' preferences are being shaped, and there is an increasing tendency towards objects of pleasure that are easy and quick to obtain. Therefore, it can be argued that problematic use of technology—to the extent that it may exhibit signs of behavioural addiction—is a situation that could lead to individuals being exposed to more digital content, and that it offers algorithms powerful enough to shape the act of eating, which is essential for survival.

THE ROLE OF FOOD IN REINFORCING ENGAGEMENT WITH TECHNOLOGY

As noted in the previous section, the use of technology can serve as a tool that shapes eating behaviours. This is made possible by the content presented to users through sophisticated marketing strategies. When examining the eating behaviour aspect of this two-way relationship, the consumption of particularly hyper-palatable foods can reinforce the reward experience resulting from technology use, thereby demonstrating a reciprocal relationship between eating behaviour and technology use in this direction as well (Vladimiros, 2025) . In this interaction, individuals often turn to fast food and hyper- -tasty foods whilst using technological devices because they are practical and readily available. This situation is widely preferred by users with the proliferation of food ordering apps. Individuals experiencing pleasure from both domains activate dopamine-mediated reward mechanisms in the brain, thereby enhancing the satisfaction derived from both activities (Joseph et al., 2011) . Research indicates that changes in the glycaemic index, which are influenced by eating behaviour, may occur as a result of mental performance during technology use, and that individuals may be inclined towards easily accessible, calorie-rich and tasty foods. Consequently, it is known that this lifestyle habit is prevalent among adolescents, who are the most frequent users of technology.

Individuals establish a learned association where interaction with technology acts as a trigger for eating tasty foods. This situation can trigger a cycle in both behaviours. The problematic nature of eating behaviour and technology use constitutes a symbiotic relationship (Vladimiros, 2025) . Furthermore, the use of screens whilst eating can prevent mindful eating and lead to the adoption of mindless eating behaviour. Screen exposure can create a distraction that prevents individuals from realising how much they are eating. Additionally, due to this distraction, individuals may continue eating rather than following their physical hunger cues. Consequently, this disruption to eating behaviour can impair both physical satiety signals and psychological signals related to fullness (Bai et al., 2025; Liu & Ellis, 2021) . Therefore, it is clear that there is a bidirectional relationship between eating behaviour and technology. In both cases, the first behaviour has the potential to reinforce the other. This situation is shaped by both shared neurobiological mechanisms and the opportunities presented by the environment (Teo et al., 2018). In digital environments, cues related to food and individuals' responses to them demonstrate that technology addiction and eating addiction can be intertwined in some individuals.

FUTURE DIRECTIONS AND RESEARCH GAPS

To gain further insight into the two types of behavioural addiction discussed in this section, it is considered that priority should be given to longitudinal studies. Furthermore, it is believed that examining the long-term neurobiological effects of technology addiction through longitudinal rather than cross-sectional studies is valuable for investigating time-dependent changes (Eskandar, 2025) . Furthermore, it is thought that advanced neuroimaging studies supporting the neurological factors underlying compulsive eating and technology use could make significant contributions, and in particular, could support the literature regarding the changes in brain structure and cortical function caused by excessive screen exposure (Eskandar, 2025) . It is clear that by examining these changes, significant data can be obtained regarding the neurobiological processes underlying technology addiction and eating disorders that are similar to those of substance addiction. In particular, it is thought that changes in the reward system and prefrontal cortex functions can be supported by current studies (He et al., 2017) . These studies may present findings that could play a role in understanding the differences between normal and problematic technology use. Furthermore, it is anticipated that this may help resolve the ongoing debates and uncertainties regarding diagnostic criteria. To address the question of whether technology, in and of itself, can be considered a tool capable of causing addiction, further research is needed to understand the extent to which specific digital content is associated with problematic use (Sun et al., 2025) . One of the reasons for this conceptual ambiguity is that technology is not a tool we can completely cease using in daily life; instead, it is thought that focusing on the platforms and activities provided by technology—and on whether these constitute problematic behaviour depending on the frequency of use—could help resolve this conceptual ambiguity.

Future research should examine the effectiveness of internet-based cognitive behavioural therapy and pharmacotherapeutic approaches targeting disruptions in the reward system, whilst taking into account the individualised nature of digital consumption habits. Furthermore, it is thought that understanding the causal relationship between excessive screen exposure and neurological changes may enable the identification of effective intervention approaches, as existing research generally fails to definitively establish these relationships. In studies examining the links between screen time and neural mechanisms, it is thought that, in addition to self-reported measures, conducting measurements during screen exposure using an experimental design could yield significant findings (Kassa, 2025; Marciano et al., 2021) .

To comprehensively investigate the relationship between digital media habits, eating addiction and neurodevelopment, it is considered necessary to conduct longitudinal neuroimaging studies that integrate multidimensional data, including genetic, behavioural and physiological factors. It is observed that such studies are limited in the literature, and they should be interpretable and generalisable to individuals from different cultures and age groups. Comparative studies across different age groups, from early childhood through adolescence to adulthood, are necessary to understand the developmental trajectory of changes in technology use and eating behaviours, as well as their long-term neurological effects. This comprehensive approach will facilitate the identification of periods of heightened sensitivity and resilience, thereby contributing to the development of age-appropriate interventions and preventive strategies.

Developing Interventions and Prevention Strategies

Future research will focus on designing and evaluating the effectiveness of interventions that address the specific neurocognitive and behavioural mechanisms underlying problematic technology use and eating behaviour. Among intervention programmes, the effectiveness of digital detox programmes and neurofeedback training—aimed at normalising brain activity and enhancing concentration—could be investigated. Furthermore, research into adaptive cognitive training may offer valuable insights into mitigating the harmful effects of eating addiction and excessive screen time on executive functions and attention control. Furthermore, incorporating ecological momentary assessment into intervention studies could provide real-time data on factors influencing eating addiction, technology addiction and patterns of problematic use, thereby facilitating the development of personalised intervention strategies. Furthermore, investigating the effectiveness of campaigns focused on healthy eating behaviour, digital literacy and critical media consumption is crucial for fostering healthier eating habits and digital behaviours from an early age, thereby building resilience against addictions and potential problematic use.

Ethical Considerations in Food and Technology Design

Sensitivity to rewards and issues with executive functions necessitate rigorous research into the ethical dimensions of the design of technologies and food systems, with a view to ensuring responsible innovation and consumer protection. This situation also requires consideration of persuasive design elements and, in particular, their potential to lead to problematic behaviour, especially among vulnerable groups.

Children's executive functions are less developed than those of adults, and they may be more prone to addiction-like behaviours. It is therefore crucial to understand how technology design disrupts underdeveloped executive control functions in young individuals. Future research should examine how persuasive designs influence lifelong addiction-like eating behaviours and how early exposure to such designs via technology persists into adulthood. In particular, the food industry harbours the potential for easily accessible, hyper-palatable, ultra-processed and calorie-dense foods to encourage overeating and increase 'food addiction' in susceptible individuals (Flayelle et al., 2023; James et al., 2025) . Similarly, the technology sector has not focused on the negative consequences of interfaces and interaction designs that could contribute to problematic technology use . It is important to develop ethical guidelines and regulatory frameworks for both the food and technology industries to mitigate risks associated with stimuli and design features that could trigger compulsive behaviours. This implies a re-evaluation of existing industries and a shift towards approaches that prioritise user mental health over interaction metrics and profit maximisation.

The technology and food industries could draw inspiration from the growing body of literature on algorithmic addiction and dark patterns, which explains how design features are deliberately used to trigger addictive user behaviour. Consequently, the ethical framework should be extended to encompass the classification and regulation of highly palatable processed foods, drawing parallels with regulatory efforts regarding substance use, given the potential for addiction. It is known that the design of e-commerce platforms, which utilise personalisation and gamification to increase impulsivity, involves an intense feedback loop, where digital structures create algorithms using behavioural insights and transform user autonomy into mechanisms that drive increased consumption (George & Rupa, 2025) . Developing awareness of this situation is crucial for reducing addiction risks and protecting public health, particularly for adolescents with reduced inhibitory control and heightened sensitivity to rewards. Therefore, an interdisciplinary approach that integrates insights from behavioural economics, neuroethics and public health is essential to develop comprehensive strategies to protect vulnerable groups from technology- and diet-related addictive behaviours (Martin et al., 2019).

Competing Interests: The author(s) declare no competing interest.
Ethics Approval: N/A

REFERENCES

Áfra, E., Janszky, J., Perlaki, G., Orsi, G., Nagy, S., Arató, Á., & Darnai, G. (2023). Altered functional brain networks in problematic Internet use: resting-state fMRI study. *Research Square (Research Square)*. DOI: 10.21203/rs.3.rs-2718429/v1

Albayrak, R., & Özbek, Y. (2025). Determining the relationship of food neophobia, digital addiction, body image perception on social media with dietary inflammatory index among adolescents. *Frontiers in Public Health, 13*, 1683764. Advance online publication. DOI: 10.3389/fpubh.2025.1683764 PMID: 41246100

Amson, A., Bagnato, M., Remedios, L., Pritchard, M., Soulene, S., Gillis, G., & Kent, M. (2024). Beyond the Screen: Exploring the Dynamics of Social Media Influencers, Food Marketing, and Gendered Influences on Adolescent Diets. *Research Square (Research Square)*. DOI: 10.21203/rs.3.rs-3909431/v1

Atalayer, D. (2017). Dürtüsellik ve Aşırı Yeme Arasındaki İlişki: Psikolojik ve Nörobiyolojik Yaklaşımlar. *Psikiyatride Guncel Yaklasimlar -. Psikiyatride Güncel Yaklaşımlar, 10*(2), 1–1. DOI: 10.18863/pgy.358090

Atar, A. (2026). Neurobiological Consequences of High-Fat High-Sugar Diets on the Mesocorticolimbic System: A Narrative Review. *Current Nutrition Reports, 15*(1), 6–6. DOI: 10.1007/s13668-026-00729-5 PMID: 41543783

Attanasi, G., Maffioletti, A., Shalukhina, T., Bel, C., & Chérikh, F. (2021). Gender Differences in the Impact of COVID-19 Lockdown on Potentially Addictive Behaviors: An Emotion-Mediated Analysis. *Frontiers in Psychology, 12*, 703897. Advance online publication. DOI: 10.3389/fpsyg.2021.703897 PMID: 34867588

Bai, J., Zhu, H., Ran, X.-W., Qu, H., He, L., & Zhao, Y. (2025). The time-stamped effects of screen exposure on food intake in adults: A meta-analysis of experimental studies. *Appetite, 206*, 107846–107846. DOI: 10.1016/j.appet.2024.107846 PMID: 39753153

Benvegnù, G., Piva, A., Cadorin, C., Mannari, V., Girondini, M., Federico, A., Tamburin, S., & Chiamulera, C. (2023). The effects of virtual reality environmental enrichments on craving to food in healthy volunteers. *Psychopharmacology, 241*(1), 49–60. DOI: 10.1007/s00213-023-06462-z PMID: 37697163

Berthoud, H.-R. (2012). *The neurobiology of food intake in an obesogenic environment. 71(4), 478-487*. Cambridge University Press., DOI: 10.1017/S0029665112000602

Bouazza, S., Elkinany, S., Abbouyi, S., Rhazi, K., & Zarrouq, B. (2022). Association between problematic use of smartphones and mental health in the Middle East and North Africa (MENA) region: a systematic review. Research Square (United States). DOI: 10.21203/rs.3.rs-1662848/v1

Boyland, E., Spanakis, P., O'Reilly, C., & Christiansen, P. (2024). Associations between everyday exposure to food marketing and hunger and food craving in adults: An ecological momentary assessment study. *Appetite*, *196*, 107241–107241. DOI: 10.1016/j.appet.2024.107241 PMID: 38307297

Brand, M., Antons, S., Bőthe, B., Demetrovics, Z., Fineberg, N., Jiménez-Múrcia, S., King, D. L., Mestre-Bach, G., Moretta, T., Müller, A., Wegmann, E., & Potenza, M. (2024). Current Advances in Behavioral Addictions: From Fundamental Research to Clinical Practice. *The American Journal of Psychiatry*, *182*(2), 155–163. DOI: 10.1176/appi.ajp.20240092 PMID: 39659159

Brand, M., Young, K., & Laier, C. (2014). Prefrontal Control and Internet Addiction: A Theoretical Model and Review of Neuropsychological and Neuroimaging Findings. *Frontiers in Human Neuroscience*, *8*, 375–375. DOI: 10.3389/fnhum.2014.00375 PMID: 24904393

Cahyani, A., Iskandarsyah, A., Cahyadi, S., & Srisayekti, W. (2023). Differences in the Model of Eating in the Absence of Hunger Before and During the COVID-19 Pandemic. *The Open Psychology Journal*, *16*(1), e18743501242291. Advance online publication. DOI: 10.2174/0118743501242291231024071127

Caninsti, R., & Rahayu, S. (2024). The Role of Smartphone Addiction on Bed Procrastination and Mindful Eating Behavior in Adolescents. *Indigenous Jurnal Ilmiah Psikologi*, *9*(1), 1–13. DOI: 10.23917/indigenous.v9i1.2804

Cardi, V., Meregalli, V., Rosa, E., Derrigo, R., Faustini, C., Keeler, J., & Lawrence, N. (2022). A community-based feasibility randomized controlled study to test food-specific inhibitory control training in people with disinhibited eating during COVID-19 in Italy. *Eating and Weight Disorders : EWD*, *27*(7), 2745–2757. DOI: 10.1007/s40519-022-01411-9 PMID: 35666376

Ceylan, J. (2025). The moderating effects of gender and emotional eating on the relationship between social media addiction and hedonic hunger in university students. *Scientific Reports*, *15*(1), 33469–33469. DOI: 10.1038/s41598-025-11668-6 PMID: 41022969

Chatterjee, D., & Rai, R. (2023). Behind the screens: Proposing a mentalization-based theoretical model of problematic Internet use. *Cyberpsychology (Brno)*, *17*(5). Advance online publication. DOI: 10.5817/CP2023-5-6

Chen, R., Peng-Li, D., Turel, O., Sørensen, T., Bechara, A., Li, Y., & He, Q. (2018). Decision Making Deficits in Relation to Food Cues Influence Obesity: A Triadic Neural Model of Problematic Eating. *Frontiers in Psychiatry*, *9*, 264. Advance online publication. DOI: 10.3389/fpsyt.2018.00264 PMID: 29962976

Chew, H., Rajasegaran, N., & Chng, S. (2023). *Effectiveness of interactive technology-assisted interventions on promoting healthy food choices: a scoping review and meta-analysis. 130(7), 1250-1259.* Cambridge University Press., DOI: 10.1017/S0007114523000193

Chiu, M., & Chein, J. (2022). Digital Media and the Developing Brain. *Cambridge University Press eBooks* (s. 104-134). içinde Cambridge University Press. DOI: 10.1017/9781108976237.008

Choi, J.-S., King, D., & Jung, Y.-C. (2019). Editorial: Neurobiological Perspectives in Behavioral Addiction. *Frontiers in Psychiatry*, *10*, 3. Advance online publication. DOI: 10.3389/fpsyt.2019.00003 PMID: 30723426

Choi, R., Park, S., Han, S.-J., & Lee, S.-J. (2023). Impact Ambivalence: How People with Eating Disorders Get Trapped in the Perpetual Cycle of Digital Food Content Engagement. *arXiv (Cornell University)*. doi:/arxiv.2311.05920DOI: 10.48550

Christensen, E., Albertella, L., Chamberlain, S., Brydevall, M., Suo, C., Grant, J., Yücel, M., & Lee, R. (2023). The neurocognitive correlates of non-substance addictive behaviors. *Addictive Behaviors*, *150*, 107904–107904. DOI: 10.1016/j.addbeh.2023.107904 PMID: 37984220

Chun, J.-W., Choi, J., Cho, H., Choi, M.-R., Ahn, K., Choi, J.-S., & Kim, D.-J. (2018). Role of Frontostriatal Connectivity in Adolescents With Excessive Smartphone Use. *Frontiers in Psychiatry*, *9*, 437. Advance online publication. DOI: 10.3389/fpsyt.2018.00437 PMID: 30258373

Cohen, D. (2008). Neurophysiological Pathways to Obesity: Below Awareness and Beyond Individual Control. *57(7)*, 1768-1773. American Diabetes Association. DOI: 10.2337/db08-0163

Courbet, D., Fourquet-Courbet, M.-P., & Amato, S. (2020). "Addictions" and Problematic Behaviors linked to Internet and Social Networks. *HAL (Le Centre pour la Communication Scientifique Directe)*. https://hal-amu.archives-ouvertes.fr/hal-02616325 adresinden alındı

David, I., Krutman, L., Fernández-Santaella, M., Andrade, J., Andrade, E., Oliveira, L., Pereira, M. G., Gomes, F. S., Gleiser, S., Oliveira, J. M., Araújo, R. L., Volchan, E., & Braga, F. (2017). Appetitive drives for ultra-processed food products and the ability of text warnings to counteract consumption predispositions. *Public Health Nutrition*, *21*(3), 543–557. DOI: 10.1017/S1368980017003263 PMID: 29173214

Davis, C., & Carter, J. (2014). If Certain Foods are Addictive, How Might this Change the Treatment of Compulsive Overeating and Obesity? *Current Addiction Reports*, *1*(2), 89–95. DOI: 10.1007/s40429-014-0013-z

De, D., Alsharef, J., Aydemır, E., & Khera, A. (2025). Social Media Algorithms and Teen Addiction: Neurophysiological Impact and Ethical Considerations. *Cureus*, *17*(1). Advance online publication. DOI: 10.7759/cureus.77145 PMID: 39925596

Domoff, S., Sutherland, E., Yokum, S., & Gearhardt, A. (2020). Adolescents' Addictive Phone Use: Associations with Eating Behaviors and Adiposity. *International Journal of Environmental Research and Public Health*, *17*(8), 2861–2861. DOI: 10.3390/ijerph17082861 PMID: 32326344

Driessen, C., Chung, A., Martino, F., Cameron, A., Bhatti, A., Huse, O., & Backholer, K. (2025). Contemporary digital marketing techniques used in unhealthy food campaigns targeting young people. *Appetite*, *211*, 107989–107989. DOI: 10.1016/j.appet.2025.107989 PMID: 40185242

Ekhtiari, H., Sangchooli, A., Carmichael, O., Moeller, F., O'Donnell, P., Oquendo, M., Paulus, M. P., Pizzagalli, D. A., Ramey, T., Schacht, J. P., Zare-Bidoky, M., Childress, A. R., & Brady, K. (2024). Neuroimaging biomarkers of addiction. *Nature Mental Health*, *2*(12), 1498–1517. DOI: 10.1038/s44220-024-00334-x PMID: 39281741

Elliott, C., Truman, E., & Black, J. (2025). Food marketing to teenagers: Examining the digital palate of targeted appeals. *Appetite*, *207*, 107912–107912. DOI: 10.1016/j.appet.2025.107912 PMID: 39956205

Eskandar, K. (2025). The digital trap: Unraveling the neuropsychological impact of technology addiction. *Neuropsychological Trends*, (37), 7–23. DOI: 10.7358/neur-2025-037-eska

Filippone, L., Shankland, R., & Hallez, Q. (2022). The relationships between social media exposure, food craving, cognitive impulsivity and cognitive restraint. *Journal of Eating Disorders*, *10*(1), 184. Advance online publication. DOI: 10.1186/s40337-022-00698-4 PMID: 36434703

Flayelle, M., Brevers, D., King, D., Maurage, P., Perales, J., & Billieux, J. (2023). A taxonomy of technology design features that promote potentially addictive online behaviours. *Nature Reviews Psychology*, *2*(3), 136–150. DOI: 10.1038/s44159-023-00153-4

Folkvord, F., Anschütz, D., Buijzen, M., & Valkenburg, P. (2012). The effect of playing advergames that promote energy-dense snacks or fruit on actual food intake among children. *The American Journal of Clinical Nutrition*, *97*(2), 239–245. DOI: 10.3945/ajcn.112.047126 PMID: 23269821

Frascella, J., Potenza, M., Brown, L., & Childress, A. (2010). Shared brain vulnerabilities open the way for nonsubstance addictions: Carving addiction at a new joint? *1187(1)*, 294-315. Wiley. DOI: 10.1111/j.1749-6632.2009.05420.x

Fretes, G., Véliz, P., Cerezo-Narváez, A., Williams, D., Sibille, R., Arts, M., & Leroy, J. (2025). Digital Marketing of Unhealthy Foods and Non-alcoholic Beverages to Children and Adolescents: A Narrative Review. *Current Developments in Nutrition*, *9*(2), 104545–104545. DOI: 10.1016/j.cdnut.2025.104545 PMID: 40046995

Gearhardt, A., Bueno, N., DiFeliceantonio, A., Roberto, C., Jiménez-Múrcia, S., & Fernández-Aranda, F. (2023). Social, clinical, and policy implications of ultra-processed food addiction. *BMJ (Clinical Research Ed.)*, *383*, e075354. Advance online publication. DOI: 10.1136/bmj-2023-075354 PMID: 37813420

George, A., & Rupa, R. (2025). Swipe, click, regret: An opinion on persuasive e-commerce and consumer autonomy. *Frontiers in Artificial Intelligence*, *8*, 1684841–1684841. DOI: 10.3389/frai.2025.1684841 PMID: 41190037

Giansanti, D. (2025). Smartphone Addiction in Youth: A Narrative Review of Systematic Evidence and Emerging Strategies. *Psychiatry International*, *6*(4), 118–118. DOI: 10.3390/psychiatryint6040118

Gross, J. J. (1998). The emerging field of emotion regulation: An integrative review. *Review of General Psychology*, *2*(3), 271–299. DOI: 10.1037/1089-2680.2.3.271

Halloran, A., Rippin, H., Farrand, C., Wickramasinghe, K., Flore, R., Pires, S., . . . Granheim, S. (2021). *Slide to Order: A Food Systems Approach to Meal Delivery Apps: WHO European Office for the Prevention and Control of Noncommunicable Diseases*. Technical University of Denmark. https://local.forskningsportal.dk/local/dki-cgi/ws/cris-link?src=dtu&id=dtu-c652223c-b60d-4401-9b13-c333c62b730c&ti=Slide%20to%20Order%3A%20A%20Food%20Systems%20Approach%20to%20Meal%20Delivery%20Apps%3A%20WHO%20European%20Office%20for%20the%20Prevention%20and%20Control%20of%20Noncommunicable%20Diseases adresinden alındı

Han, R., Todd, A., Wardak, S., Partridge, S., & Raeside, R. (2023). Feasibility and Acceptability of Chatbots for Nutrition and Physical Activity Health Promotion Among Adolescents: Systematic Scoping Review With Adolescent Consultation. *JMIR Human Factors, 10*, e43227. Advance online publication. DOI: 10.2196/43227 PMID: 37145858

Harris, J., & Taillie, L. (2023). More than a Nuisance: Implications of Food Marketing for Public Health Efforts to Curb Childhood Obesity. *Annual Review of Public Health, 45*(1), 213–233. DOI: 10.1146/annurev-publhealth-090419-102616 PMID: 38109516

Harris, J., & Taillie, L. (2024). More than a Nuisance: Implications of Food Marketing for Public Health Efforts to Curb Childhood Obesity. *Carolina Digital Repository (University of North Carolina at Chapel Hill)*. DOI: 10.17615/whrd-4415

He, Q., Turel, O., Brevers, D., & Bechara, A. (2017). Excess social media use in normal populations is associated with amygdala-striatal but not with prefrontal morphology. *Psychiatry Research. Neuroimaging, 269*, 31–35. DOI: 10.1016/j.pscychresns.2017.09.003 PMID: 28918269

Hebebrand, J., Albayrak, Ö., Adan, R., Antel, J., Diéguez, C., Jong, J., & Dickson, S. (2014). "Eating addiction", rather than "food addiction", better captures addictive-like eating behavior. *Neuroscience and Biobehavioral Reviews, 47*, 295–306. DOI: 10.1016/j.neubiorev.2014.08.016 PMID: 25205078

Hough, K., Friuli, M., Avena, N., & Romano, A. (2026). The addicted brain: How processed foods hijack reward pathways. *Pharmacological Research, 224*, 108097–108097. DOI: 10.1016/j.phrs.2026.108097 PMID: 41525853

Humphreys, G., Evans, R., Makin, H., Cooke, R., & Jones, A. (2020). Identification of Behavior Change Techniques From Successful Web-Based Interventions Targeting Alcohol Consumption, Binge Eating, and Gambling: Systematic Review. *23(2)*. JMIR Publications. DOI: 10.2196/22694

Hutton, J., Piotrowski, J., Bagot, K., Blumberg, F., Canli, T., Chein, J., . . . Potenza, M. (2024). Digital Media and Developing Brains: Concerns and Opportunities. *11(2)*, 287-298. Springer Science+Business Media. DOI: 10.1007/s40429-024-00545-3

Ifland, J., & Brewerton, T. (2025). Binge-type eating disorders and ultra-processed food addiction: Phenomenology, pathophysiology and treatment implications. *Frontiers in Psychiatry, 16*, 1584891–1584891. DOI: 10.3389/fpsyt.2025.1584891 PMID: 40625723

James, S., Karthik, S., & Thomas, B. (2025). Chasing the digital high: Should hedonic consumption be viewed through the lens of behavioral addiction? *Frontiers in Psychiatry*, *16*, 1681307. Advance online publication. DOI: 10.3389/fpsyt.2025.1681307 PMID: 41164096

Jia, S., Todd, A., Vanderlee, L., Farrell, P., Allman-Farinelli, M., Sacks, G., Gibson, A. A., & Partridge, S. (2024). Offline to online: A systematic mapping review of evidence to inform nutrition-related policies applicable to online food delivery platforms. *BMC Medicine*, *22*(1), 542–542. DOI: 10.1186/s12916-024-03747-8 PMID: 39558372

Jin, J., Wei, H., Chai, Y., Wu, L., Chen, M., & Ding, K. (2026). The neurobiology of internet addiction: A scoping review of developmental and gender-specific mechanisms. *Frontiers in Psychology*, *17*, 1729470–1729470. DOI: 10.3389/fpsyg.2026.1729470 PMID: 41768176

Joseph, R., Alonso-Alonso, M., Bond, D., Pascual-Leone, Á., & Blackburn, G. (2011). The neurocognitive connection between physical activity and eating behaviour. *12(10)*, 800-812. Wiley. DOI: 10.1111/j.1467-789X.2011.00893.x

Juul, F., Steele, E., Parekh, N., & Monteiro, C. (2025). The role of ultra-processed food in obesity. *Nature Reviews. Endocrinology*, *21*(11), 672–685. DOI: 10.1038/s41574-025-01143-7 PMID: 40659796

Karaköse, T., Yıldırım, B., Tülübaş, T., & Kardas, A. (2023). *A comprehensive review on emerging trends in the dynamic evolution of digital addiction and depression. 14*. Frontiers Media., DOI: 10.3389/fpsyg.2023.1126815

Kassa, P. (2025). Cognitive benefits and risks of digital technology engagement. *Discover Psychology*, *6*(1), 10. Advance online publication. DOI: 10.1007/s44202-025-00527-0

Kear, A., & Sasha, L. (2018). Digital Technology Disorder: Justification and a Proposed Model of Treatment. *International Journal of Advanced Computer Science and Applications*, *9*(8). Advance online publication. DOI: 10.14569/IJACSA.2018.090882

Kim, K., Lee, I., Kim, J., & Choi, J.-W. (2020). Dietary patterns and smartphone use in adolescents: A large-sample, cross-sectional study. *Research Square (Research Square)*. DOI: 10.21203/rs.3.rs-33267/v1

LaFata, E., Allison, K., Audrain-McGovern, J., & Forman, E. (2024). Ultra-Processed Food Addiction: A Research Update. *13(2)*, 214-223. Springer Science+Business Media. DOI: 10.1007/s13679-024-00569-w

LaFata, E., & Gearhardt, A. (2022). Ultra-Processed Food Addiction: An Epidemic? *Psychotherapy and Psychosomatics*, *91*(6), 363–372. DOI: 10.1159/000527322 PMID: 36349805

Lakhan, S. (2025). Hijacked by the Feed: Social Media Neuroengineering-Induced Digital Anhedonia. *Cureus*, *17*(4). Advance online publication. DOI: 10.7759/cureus.83256 PMID: 40309512

Lemos, T., Coutinho, G., Silva, L., Stariolo, J., Campagnoli, R., Oliveira, L., Pereira, M. G., Mota, B. E. F., Souza, G. G. L., Canella, D. S., Khandpur, N., & David, I. (2022). Ultra-Processed Foods Elicit Higher Approach Motivation Than Unprocessed and Minimally Processed Foods. *Frontiers in Public Health*, *10*, 891546–891546. DOI: 10.3389/fpubh.2022.891546 PMID: 35801235

Lin, C.-Y., Imani, V., Griffiths, M., & Pakpour, A. (2020). Validity of the Yale Food Addiction Scale for Children (YFAS-C): Classical test theory and item response theory of the Persian YFAS-C. *Eating and Weight Disorders : EWD*, *26*(5), 1457–1466. DOI: 10.1007/s40519-020-00956-x PMID: 32676845

Lin, Y.-H., Chiang, C., Lin, P.-H., Chang, L.-R., Ko, C.-H., Lee, Y.-H., & Lin, S.-H. (2016). Proposed Diagnostic Criteria for Smartphone Addiction. *PLoS One*, *11*(11), e0163010. Advance online publication. DOI: 10.1371/journal.pone.0163010 PMID: 27846211

Liu, J., & Ellis, D. (2021). Editorial: Eating in the Age of Smartphones: The Good, the Bad, and the Neutral. *Frontiers in Psychology*, *12*, 796899. Advance online publication. DOI: 10.3389/fpsyg.2021.796899 PMID: 34938246

Liu, Y., Li, L., Wang, Y., Ghahremani, D., Chen, J., Okita, K., Guo, W., & Liao, Y. (2021). Editorial: Neurobiological Biomarkers for Developing Novel Treatments of Substance and Non-substance Addiction. *Frontiers in Psychiatry*, *12*, 811032. Advance online publication. DOI: 10.3389/fpsyt.2021.811032 PMID: 34987436

Lustig, R. (2020). Ultraprocessed Food: Addictive, Toxic, and Ready for Regulation. *Nutrients*, *12*(11), 3401–3401. DOI: 10.3390/nu12113401 PMID: 33167515

Maksi, S., Keller, K., Dardis, F., Vecchi, M., Freeman, J., Evans, R., Boyland, E., & Masterson, T. (2024). The food and beverage cues in digital marketing model: Special considerations of social media, gaming, and livestreaming environments for food marketing and eating behavior research. *Frontiers in Nutrition*, *10*, 1325265. Advance online publication. DOI: 10.3389/fnut.2023.1325265 PMID: 38384857

Maqsood, S., Ahmed, F., Arshad, M., Ikram, A., & Abdullahi, M. (2025). Comparative Analysis of Food Addiction and Obesity. *Critical Reviews in Food Science and Nutrition, 13*(8), e70799. Advance online publication. DOI: 10.1002/fsn3.70799 PMID: 40822524

Marciano, L., Camerini, A.-L., & Morese, R. (2021). *The Developing Brain in the Digital Era: A Scoping Review of Structural and Functional Correlates of Screen Time in Adolescence. 12*. Frontiers Media., DOI: 10.3389/fpsyg.2021.671817

Martin, K., Shilton, K., & Smith, J. (2019). Business and the Ethical Implications of Technology: Introduction to the Symposium. *Journal of Business Ethics, 160*(2), 307–317. DOI: 10.1007/s10551-019-04213-9

Masri-Zada, T., Martirosyan, S., Abdou, A., Barbar, R., Kades, S., Makki, H., . . . Agrawal, D. (2025). The Impact of Social Media & Technology on Child and Adolescent Mental Health. *PubMed, 9*(2), 111-130. https://pubmed.ncbi.nlm.nih.gov/40520349 adresinden alındı

Mastrobattista, L., Pérez, L., Gallimberti, L., Genetti, B., Andreotti, A., Fassinato, D., & Mortali, C. (2024). Psychosocial risk and protective factors for youth problem behavior are associated with food addiction in the Generation Z. *Frontiers in Public Health, 12*, 1414110. Advance online publication. DOI: 10.3389/fpubh.2024.1414110 PMID: 38859893

Maza, M., Fox, K., Kwon, S.-J., Flannery, J., Lindquist, K., Prinstein, M., & Telzer, E. (2023). Association of Habitual Checking Behaviors on Social Media With Longitudinal Functional Brain Development. *JAMA Pediatrics, 177*(2), 160–160. DOI: 10.1001/jamapediatrics.2022.4924 PMID: 36595277

McCausland, H., Gearhardt, A., Peralta, J., & LaFata, E. (2025). A Critical Evaluation of the Terms Used To Describe Foods Implicated in Addictive-Like Eating. *Current Addiction Reports, 12*(1), 71. Advance online publication. DOI: 10.1007/s40429-025-00689-w

McGloin, A., & Eslami, S. (2014). *Digital and social media opportunities for dietary behaviour change. 74(2), 139-148*. Cambridge University Press., DOI: 10.1017/S0029665114001505

Méndez, M., Padrón, I., Fumero, A., & Marrero, R. (2024). Effects of internet and smartphone addiction on cognitive control in adolescents and young adults: A systematic review of fMRI studies. *Neuroscience and Biobehavioral Reviews, 159*, 105572–105572. DOI: 10.1016/j.neubiorev.2024.105572 PMID: 38320657

Meule, A., & Gearhardt, A. (2014). Food Addiction in the Light of DSM-5. *Nutrients, 6*(9), 3653–3671. DOI: 10.3390/nu6093653 PMID: 25230209

Moghimi, E., Davis, C., Bonder, R., Knyahnytska, Y., & Quilty, L. (2021). Exploring women's experiences of treatment for binge eating disorder: Methylphenidate vs. cognitive behavioural therapy. *Progress in Neuro-Psychopharmacology & Biological Psychiatry, 114*, 110492–110492. DOI: 10.1016/j.pnpbp.2021.110492 PMID: 34863926

Molle, R., Fatemi, H., Dagher, A., Levitan, R., Silveira, P., & Dubé, L. (2016). *Gene and environment interaction: Is the differential susceptibility hypothesis relevant for obesity? 73, 326-339*. Elsevier BV., DOI: 10.1016/j.neubiorev.2016.12.028

Moreno-Padilla, M., Alacreu-Crespo, A., Guillaume, S., & Paso, G. (2022). The outcome-representation learning model: Impairments in decision-making in adolescents with excess weight. *Current Psychology, 42*(26), 22404–22414. DOI: 10.1007/s12144-022-03299-1

Morin, J.-P., Rodríguez-Durán, L., Guzmán-Ramos, K., Perez-Cruz, C., Ferreira, G., Díaz-Cintra, S., & Pacheco-López, G. (2017). *Palatable Hyper-Caloric Foods Impact on Neuronal Plasticity. 11*. Frontiers Media., DOI: 10.3389/fnbeh.2017.00019

Mujica, A., Crowell, C., Villano, M., & Uddin, K. (2022). ADDICTION BY DESIGN: Some Dimensions and Challenges of Excessive Social Media Use. *Medical Research Archives, 10*(2). Advance online publication. DOI: 10.18103/mra.v10i2.2677

Nesi, J., Subrahmanyam, K., Valkenburg, P., Morita, H., Ehrenreich, S., Chiu, M., & Weinstein, E. (2022). *Handbook of Adolescent Digital Media Use and Mental Health*. Cambridge University Press., DOI: 10.1017/9781108976237

Patel, D., Kshatri, A., Kommuru, S., & Javvaji, C. (2025). A Narrative Review of Digital Addiction and Health: A New Challenge for Modern Medicine. *Cureus, 17*(12). Advance online publication. DOI: 10.7759/cureus.100491 PMID: 41625856

Patwardhan, V., Mallya, J., Kaliappan, S., & Kumar, D. (2024). Influence of social media on young adults' food consumption behavior: Scale development. *Cogent Social Sciences, 10*(1), 2391016. Advance online publication. DOI: 10.1080/23311886.2024.2391016

Pretlow, R., Stock, C., Allison, S., & Roeger, L. (2015). Treatment of Child/Adolescent Obesity Using the Addiction Model: A Smartphone App Pilot Study. *Childhood Obesity, 11*(3), 248–259. DOI: 10.1089/chi.2014.0124 PMID: 25760813

Pursey, K., Babicola, L., Ventura, R., & Segni, M. (2024). Editorial: Dysfunctional motivation in eating behaviors: a complex gene x environment interplay. *Frontiers in Behavioral Neuroscience, 18,* 1367256. Advance online publication. DOI: 10.3389/fnbeh.2024.1367256 PMID: 38405038

Pursey, K., Yokum, S., Brain, K., & Burrows, T. (2024). Neural Responses in Addictive Eating: a Systematic Review. *11(2),* 173-190. Springer Science+Business Media. DOI: 10.1007/s40429-023-00538-8

Rebello, C., & Greenway, F. (2016). Reward-Induced Eating: Therapeutic Approaches to Addressing Food Cravings. *33(11),* 1853-1866. Adis, Springer Healthcare. DOI: 10.1007/s12325-016-0414-6

Saruco, E., & Pleger, B. (2021). A Systematic Review of Obesity and Binge Eating Associated Impairment of the Cognitive Inhibition System. *Frontiers in Nutrition, 8,* 609012–609012. DOI: 10.3389/fnut.2021.609012 PMID: 33996871

Shanmugasundaram, M., & Tamilarasu, A. (2023). *The impact of digital technology, social media, and artificial intelligence on cognitive functions: a review. 2.* Frontiers Media., DOI: 10.3389/fcogn.2023.1203077

Sinha, R. (2017). *Role of addiction and stress neurobiology on food intake and obesity. 131, 5-13.* Elsevier BV., DOI: 10.1016/j.biopsycho.2017.05.001

Soler, I., Sánchez, C., & Quiles-Soler, M. (2021). Nomophobia in teenagers: Digital lifestyle, social networking and smartphone abuse. *Communicatio Socialis, 34*(4), 17–32. DOI: 10.15581/003.34.4.17-32

Solly, J., Hook, R., Grant, J., Cortese, S., & Chamberlain, S. (2021). Structural gray matter differences in Problematic Usage of the Internet: a systematic review and meta-analysis. *27(2),* 1000-1009. Springer Nature. DOI: 10.1038/s41380-021-01315-7

Spence, C., Okajima, K., Cheok, A., Petit, O., & Michel, C. (2015). Eating with our eyes: From visual hunger to digital satiation. *Brain and Cognition, 110,* 53–63. DOI: 10.1016/j.bandc.2015.08.006 PMID: 26432045

Steward, T., & Wierenga, C. (2022). Foreword to the special issue on the neuroscience of obesity and related disorders. *23(4),* 679-681. Springer Science+Business Media. DOI: 10.1007/s11154-022-09739-4

Sun, H., Wu, D., Liu, W., Yu, G., & Yao, M. (2025). Emotionally Vulnerable Subtype of Internet Gaming Disorder: Measuring and Exploring the Pathology of Problematic Generative AI Use. *arXiv (Cornell University).* doi:/arxiv.2510.06908DOI: 10.48550

Tabish, S. (2025). From Evolution to Obsession: Understanding Digital Addiction Among Youth in the Modern Age. *American Journal of Health Research, 13*(4), 248–258. DOI: 10.11648/j.ajhr.20251304.17

Teo, E., Goh, D., Vijayakumar, K., & Liu, J. (2018). To Message or Browse? Exploring the Impact of Phone Use Patterns on Male Adolescents' Consumption of Palatable Snacks. *Frontiers in Psychology, 8*, 2298. Advance online publication. DOI: 10.3389/fpsyg.2017.02298 PMID: 29358925

Tereshchenko, S. (2023). Neurobiological risk factors for problematic social media use as a specific form of Internet addiction: A narrative review. *World Journal of Psychiatry, 13*(5), 160–173. DOI: 10.5498/wjp.v13.i5.160 PMID: 37303928

Teymur, Z., & ÖNEY, B. (2024). HEDONİK AÇLIK VE OBEZİTE. *DergiPark (Istanbul University).* https://dergipark.org.tr/tr/pub/arsagbil/issue/86259/1460606 adresinden alındı

Tsochantaridou, A., Sergentanis, T., Grammatikopoulou, M., Merakou, K., Vassilakou, T., & Kornarou, E. (2023). Food Advertisement and Dietary Choices in Adolescents: An Overview of Recent Studies. *Children (Basel, Switzerland), 10*(3), 442–442. DOI: 10.3390/children10030442 PMID: 36980000

Tymofiyeva, O., Yuan, J., Kidambi, R., Huang, C.-Y., Henje, E., Rubinstein, M., Jariwala, N., Max, J. E., Yang, T. T., & Xu, D. (2020). Neural Correlates of Smartphone Dependence in Adolescents. *Frontiers in Human Neuroscience, 14*, 564629. Advance online publication. DOI: 10.3389/fnhum.2020.564629 PMID: 33132878

Uclés-Torrents, M., Ruiz-Gamarra, G., & Aparicio-Martinez, P. (2026). Social Media Use, Affect, and Dietary Choices Across Age Groups—Insights from the Special Issue "The Impact of Social Media on Eating Behavior". *Nutrients, 18*(2), 335–335. DOI: 10.3390/nu18020335 PMID: 41599948

Uma, P., Buzana, T., & Iluzija, B. (2014). PSIHOLOGIJA, https://citeseerx.ist.psu.edu/viewdoc/summary?doi=10.1.1.461.8490 adresinden alındı

VanderBroek-Stice, L., Stojek, M., Beach, S., vanDellen, M., & MacKillop, J. (2017). Multidimensional assessment of impulsivity in relation to obesity and food addiction. *Appetite, 112*, 59–68. DOI: 10.1016/j.appet.2017.01.009 PMID: 28087369

Vasiliu, O. (2023). An integrative model as a step toward increasing the awareness of eating disorders in the general population. *Frontiers in Psychiatry, 14*, 1184932. Advance online publication. DOI: 10.3389/fpsyt.2023.1184932 PMID: 37205977

Vladimiros, P. (2025). The Edible Interface: How Mass-Market Foods Became Sophisticated Delivery Systems for Biological Influence. Zenodo *(CERN European Organization for Nuclear Research).* DOI: 10.5281/zenodo.17815936

Wattick, R., Olfert, M., Claydon, E., Hagedorn, R., Barr, M., & Brode, C. (2023). Early life influences on the development of food addiction in college attending young adults. *Eating and Weight Disorders : EWD, 28*(1), 14. Advance online publication. DOI: 10.1007/s40519-023-01546-3 PMID: 36807705

Whatnall, M., Skinner, J., Leary, M., & Burrows, T. (2022). Food Addiction: A Deep Dive into 'Loss of Control' and 'Craving'. *Current Addiction Reports, 9*(4), 318–325. DOI: 10.1007/s40429-022-00431-w

Willie, M., Maqbool, M., & Qadir, A. (2024). From click to calories: Navigating the impact of food delivery apps on obesity. *Open Health, 5*(1), 20230022. Advance online publication. DOI: 10.1515/ohe-2023-0022

Wolf, N., Henemann, G., Schmitgen, M., Koenig, J., Bach, P., & Wolf, R. (2025). Screens and brains: Multimodal neuroimaging insights into mechanisms of problematic smartphone use. *Progress in Neuro-Psychopharmacology & Biological Psychiatry, 142*, 111531–111531. DOI: 10.1016/j.pnpbp.2025.111531 PMID: 41120086

Yang, Y., Wu, Q., & Morys, F. (2021). Brain Responses to High-Calorie Visual Food Cues in Individuals with Normal-Weight or Obesity: An Activation Likelihood Estimation Meta-Analysis. *Brain Sciences, 11*(12), 1587–1587. DOI: 10.3390/brainsci11121587 PMID: 34942889

Yu, S., & Sussman, S. (2020). Does Smartphone Addiction Fall on a Continuum of Addictive Behaviors? *International Journal of Environmental Research and Public Health, 17*(2), 422–422. DOI: 10.3390/ijerph17020422 PMID: 31936316

Zhang, H.-B., Zheng, H., Zhang, Y., & Zhao, D. (2020). *Commentary: Compulsive drug use is associated with imbalance of orbitofrontal- and prelimbic-striatal circuits in punishment-resistant individuals. 14, 49-49.* Frontiers Media., DOI: 10.3389/fncir.2020.00049

KEY TERMS AND DEFINITIONS

Food Addiction: A pattern of eating behaviour characterised by compulsive consumption of palatable foods, loss of control over intake, and continued eating despite negative consequences. The construct draws on the diagnostic criteria for substance use disorders — tolerance, withdrawal, and failed attempts to reduce consumption — and is typically assessed using the Yale Food Addiction Scale. Its classification remains contested: some researchers treat it as a subtype of eating disorder, others as a form of substance-related pathology, and a substantial body of literature argues it should be distinguished from both.

Yale Food Addiction Scale (YFAS): A standardised psychometric instrument designed to operationalise food addiction by mapping DSM criteria for substance use disorders onto eating behaviour. Items assess phenomena such as tolerance, withdrawal symptoms, inability to cut down, and continued use despite harm.

Online Gaming Disorder: Classified by the World Health Organization in ICD-11 as a formal diagnostic category, online gaming disorder is defined by impaired control over gaming, the persistent prioritisation of gaming over other activities, and continuation of gaming behaviour despite clear negative consequences. The DSM-5 lists "internet gaming disorder" as a condition warranting further research, stopping short of full diagnostic recognition.

Mesolimbic Dopamine System: A subcortical circuit connecting the ventral tegmental area to the nucleus accumbens, prefrontal cortex, amygdala, and hippocampus. It is the primary substrate of reward learning and motivational salience.

Hyper-palatable Foods: Foods engineered to produce maximal hedonic response through combinations of fat, sugar, salt, and flavour-enhancing additives, a profile that exceeds the palatability of naturally occurring foods.

Gamification: The incorporation of game design elements including points, badges, leaderboards, progress bars, and reward streaks — into non-game environments, including food ordering and delivery applications. In the food context, gamification exploits the reward system by creating structures of intermittent reinforcement that encourage repeat engagement and purchasing.

Inhibitory Control: The capacity to suppress automatic, habitual, or prepotent responses in favour of deliberate, context-appropriate behaviour. In eating behaviour research, impaired inhibitory control is associated with increased consumption of palatable foods, difficulty resisting food cues, and binge eating. In technology addiction research, equivalent deficits predict compulsive checking, prolonged screen time, and inability to disengage from digital content despite intention to stop.

Algorithmic Pleasure Structures: A conceptual term referring to the computational systems embedded in digital platforms that selectively surface content predicted to maximise user engagement. By delivering emotionally resonant or rewarding content at variable intervals, these structures replicate the conditions of intermittent reinforcement and exploit dopaminergic reward circuitry in ways functionally analogous to the mechanisms underlying behavioural addiction.

Obesogenic Environment: An environment, physical, social, economic, or digital — that promotes energy intake and discourages energy expenditure, thereby increasing population-level obesity risk. The digital dimension of obesogenic environments has grown substantially with the proliferation of food delivery applications, food-adjacent social media content, and targeted digital marketing of energy-dense products.

Craving: An intense, subjectively experienced urge to consume a specific substance or engage in a specific behaviour, typically triggered by exposure to conditioned cues. In both food addiction and technology addiction research, craving is understood as the motivational expression of sensitised reward circuitry — the result of repeated pairings between environmental stimuli and rewarding outcomes. It is one of the most reliably reported subjective features of addictive disorders.

Chapter 10
Nocturnal Screen Exposure and Sleep Disturbance

M. Balamurugan
http://orcid.org/0000-0001-9737-2035
Dayananda Sagar College of Engineering, India

Karimov Abror
Karshi State Technical University, Uzbekistan

Meyliqulova Manzura
Termez University of Economics and Service, Uzbekistan

Safarova Svetlana
Mamun University, Uzbekistan

Mastona Gozieva
Alfraganus University, Uzbekistan

Sadikov Iskandar
Tashkent State University of Economics, Uzbekistan

Oteuliyev Zhaksylyk
Karakalpak State University, Uzbekistan

N. Raghu
http://orcid.org/0000-0002-2091-8922
Jain University, India

ABSTRACT

In the digital era, social media has become an integral part of everyday life, particularly among adolescents, young adults, and working professionals. While these platforms provide numerous benefits, including social connectivity, entertainment, and access to information, they also pose significant challenges to users' sleep health. This chapter explores the detrimental impact of late-night social media usage on sleep quality and overall well-being. As screen time during nighttime hours becomes increasingly common, users are exposed to blue light emissions, algorithm-driven content, and cognitive stimulation that delay sleep onset and reduce sleep duration. Biologically, the disruption of circadian rhythms and suppression of melatonin

DOI: 10.4018/979-8-2600-2468-3.ch010

caused by prolonged exposure to screens lead to poor sleep architecture and neural fatigue. Psychologically, users report heightened anxiety, mood swings, and depressive symptoms linked to both insufficient sleep and online social comparison.

INTRODUCTION

In the 21st century, social media has evolved from a niche networking tool to a global cultural and behavioral phenomenon. Platforms such as Instagram, TikTok, X (formerly Twitter), Facebook, YouTube, and Snapchat have amassed billions of users worldwide. According to recent data from Statista (2024), the average global user spends over 2.5 hours daily on social media, with higher usage rates reported among adolescents and young adults. The ubiquity of smartphones and affordable data access have transformed social media into a round-the-clock activity, accessible from virtually anywhere, at any time. As platforms for social interaction have now expanded into ecosystems for entertainment, business, activism, and education. The boundaries between offline and online life are increasingly blurred, and social media has emerged as a dominant force in shaping identity, relationships, values, and worldviews. However, as digital engagement deepens, concerns about its impact on mental, emotional, and physical health have grown, especially regarding how it affects sleep.

Figure 1. Year wise social media usage with respect to time

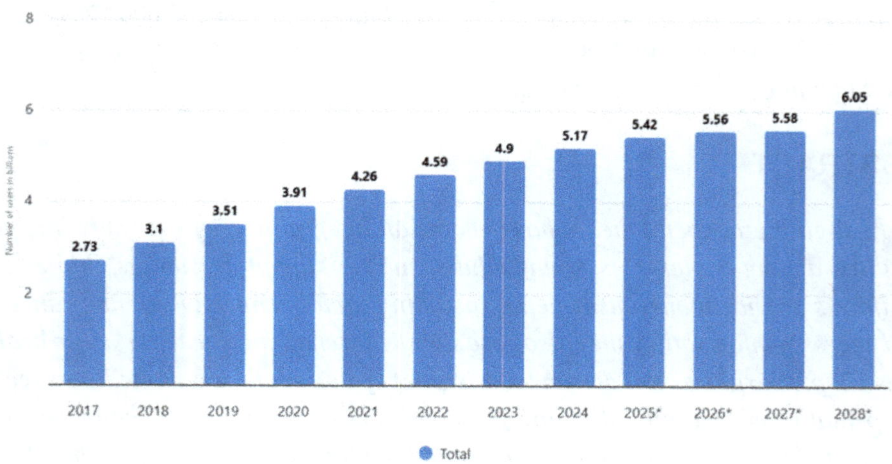

(Whatley, 2026).

As of 2024, the average daily social media usage of internet users worldwide amounted to 143 minutes per day, down from 151 minutes in the previous year. Currently, the country with the most time spent on social media per day is Brazil, with online users spending an average of three hours and 49 minutes on social media each day. In comparison, the daily time spent with social media in the U.S. was just two hours and 16 minutes as shown in fig [1]. Currently, the global social network penetration rate is 62.3 percent. Northern Europe had an 81.7 percent social media penetration rate, topping the ranking of global social media usage by region. Eastern and Middle Africa closed the ranking with 10.1 and 9.6 percent usage reach, respectively. People access social media for a variety of reasons. Users like to find funny or entertaining content and enjoy sharing photos and videos with friends, but mainly use social media to stay in touch with current events friends.

Social media has a wide-reaching and significant impact on not only online activities but also offline behaviour and life in general. During a global online user survey in February 2019, a significant share of respondents stated that social media had increased their access to information, ease of communication, and freedom of expression. On the flip side, respondents also felt that social media had worsened their personal privacy, increased a polarization in politics and heightened everyday distractions.

Rise of Late-Night Screen Time Behaviour

One of the most alarming behavioural patterns associated with modern social media use is the significant increase in screen time during late-night hours. Studies have shown that users often engage with their phones just before bed, leading to a delay in sleep onset and a decrease in overall sleep duration (Lin et al., 2024). The concept of "revenge bedtime procrastination" where individuals deliberately delay sleep to reclaim personal time lost to daily obligations, has gained traction particularly among students and working professionals who feel deprived of leisure during the day.

Figure 2. Social Media usage and its effects on sleep.

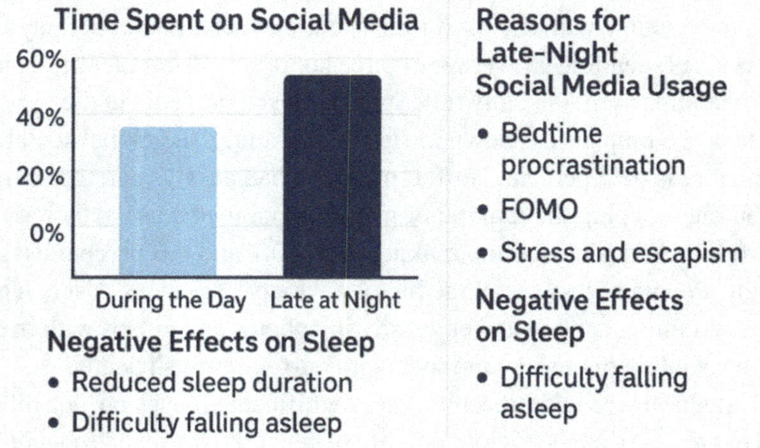

Late-night social media use is fueled by various psychological triggers: the desire for social validation, fear of missing out (FOMO), escapism from real-world stress, and the irresistible pull of endless scrolling and algorithmic content. Notifications, trending content, and late-night live streams entice users to stay awake longer than intended. Many people do not realize how the dopamine-driven design of social media platforms subtly reinforces prolonged engagement, even at the cost of rest (Y. Lee, 2024). Furthermore, bedtime usage is often considered "me time" providing emotional comfort or entertainment after a stressful day. Unfortunately, this practice becomes self-defeating when the immediate gratification of scrolling interferes with the longer-term need for restorative sleep as shown in fig [2].

Importance of Sleep for Mental and Physical Health

Sleep is not a passive state it is a fundamental biological process that is crucial for cognitive functioning, emotional stability, physical health, and overall well-being. The human body follows a circadian rhythm a roughly 24-hour internal clock regulated by light and hormonal cues. Quality sleep facilitates memory consolidation, muscle repair, immune system function, emotional regulation, and decision-making capabilities (Van Den Eijnden et al., 2021). Chronic sleep deprivation, defined as consistently getting less than the recommended 7–9 hours of sleep per night, can result in a range of health issues, including weakened immunity, obesity, diabetes, cardiovascular diseases, anxiety, depression, and impaired brain function. For adolescents and young adults, who are already navigating significant developmental, academic and emotional changes, insufficient sleep can have lasting repercussions on both their personal growth and social adaptation. Numerous global health organizations, including the World Health Organization (WHO) and the Centers for Disease Control and Prevention (CDC), have flagged sleep deprivation as a public health epidemic. In this context, the rise in digital distractions particularly late-night social media usage emerges as a key contributor to the sleep crisis (Ren et al., 2026).

Figure 3. Different social media platform usage

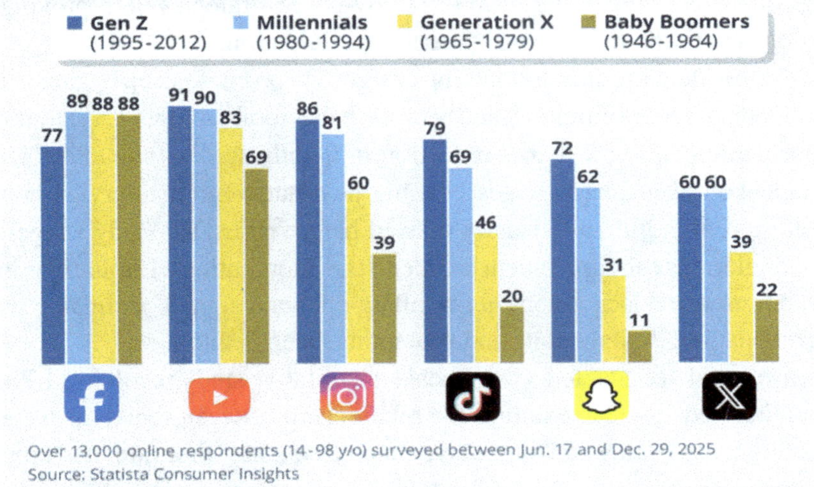

(Link: https://www.statista.com/topics/1164/social-networks/ Date: 16/05/2026 Time: 08:03PM)

Social media advertising worldwide continues to grow rapidly, with Facebook and Instagram remaining the key players driving this expansion. Their global reach, paired with powerful targeting and data capabilities, makes them essential platforms for advertisers aiming to engage audiences across regions and demographics. Instagram, in particular, has seen rising prominence as a hub for influencer marketing, visual storytelling, and social commerce making it especially appealing for lifestyle, fashion, and consumer brands. Facebook, while more established, still commands massive engagement globally and offers extensive tools for advertisers to reach users in both mature and emerging markets (Levenson et al., 2017). As businesses increasingly shift their marketing strategies toward digital-first approaches, Facebook and Instagram are positioned at the center of global social media advertising spend, consistently delivering strong performance and return on investment for brands worldwide. Here is a graph illustrating the average daily time spent on major social media platforms in 2023.Facebook and Instagram lead in usage, with users spending close to 3 hours daily, highlighting their significant role in contributing to late-night screen time behavior and potential sleep disruption as shown in fig [3].

LITERATURE SURVEY

Van Den Eijnden et al. surveyed 2,200 adolescents, examining the impact of nighttime social media usage and parental digital rules. Teens with enforced evening screen curfews slept on average 40 minutes more per night and reported fewer mood disturbances. The study highlighted that parental modelling parents adhering to their own digital limits amplified the positive effects (Bourke et al., 2026). Although reliant on self-reported behaviors, the large, diverse sample strengthens its validity. Findings underscore the importance of family-based strategies in improving sleep through behavioral boundaries and parental participation.

Fino et al. evaluated a smartphone app designed to promote sleep hygiene through timed reminders, screen dimming, and bedtime behavioral prompts. Over four weeks, 150 adult participants saw a 20% reduction in nightly screen time and a 15-point improvement on sleep quality scales. Notably, post-intervention interviews revealed users felt more mindful and visually relaxed before bed. This study suggests that app-based solutions can supplement broader sleep interventions. Limitations include its short duration and lack of long-term follow-up, but it signals promising scalable tools for managing digital habits and promoting sleep health.

Levenson et al., conducted a large-scale quantitative study involving 1,788 U.S. young adults aged 19–32 to examine the relationship between social media use and sleep disturbances. Using self-reported data on frequency, duration, and emotional engagement with various social media platforms, the study revealed that participants in the highest quartile of usage were nearly twice as likely to experience disrupted sleep patterns. Notably, both the frequency of social media engagement and the emotional investment in content were significant predictors of sleep quality. The findings emphasized the importance of understanding how not only the quantity but the nature of social media interaction affects sleep. While the study offers strong statistical significance due to its large sample size and thorough demographic representation, its cross-sectional design and reliance on self-reporting limit its ability to establish causality. Nevertheless, it provides compelling evidence for including digital media use as a factor in behavioral sleep health assessments.

Carter et al. presented a systematic review studies exploring the relationship between portable screen use (e.g., smartphones, tablets) and sleep outcomes in children and adolescents. The review consistently found that screen-based media use before or during bedtime significantly affected sleep onset, duration, and quality. Interestingly, even the presence of media devices in the bedroom regardless of active use was associated with sleep disruption, likely due to psychological cues or interrupted routines. The analysis highlighted screen time as a modifiable risk factor, reinforcing the need for behavioral interventions such as screen curfews or restricted bedroom device access. Though comprehensive, the review's limitations include variation in the definitions of screen use, reliance on subjective measures across studies, and its restriction to English-language publications.

Twenge et al. analyzed longitudinal survey data from over 360,000 U.S. adolescents spanning the years 2009 to 2017, aiming to uncover trends linking digital media use with declining sleep duration. The researchers found that as smartphone usage surged, especially among teenagers, average nightly sleep duration dropped significantly, with more adolescents reporting less than seven hours of sleep. The correlation was particularly strong for those using screens for more than two hours daily. This large-scale study highlighted a generational shift toward digital engagement at the expense of sleep, which may have lasting implications on adolescent development. The research's key strength lies in its expansive dataset and temporal scope, allowing for trend analysis over nearly a decade. While causality remains unproven, the temporal alignment between rising smartphone uses and sleep deprivation strengthens the inference. The authors advocate for policy-level interventions to reduce screen exposure in adolescents, particularly during nighttime hours.

Alfonsi et al. conducted an experimental study involving Italian adolescents to assess the impact of pre-sleep social media use on sleep patterns. Using a combination of sleep diaries and behavioral surveys, the researchers found that adolescents who engaged in social media activities within one hour before bedtime experienced delayed sleep onset and disrupted sleep continuity. The role of cognitive arousal, suggesting that even passive browsing could keep the brain mentally engaged and delay the body's transition into rest. The combination of subjective reports and semi-controlled conditions adds strength to the findings. However, the study's limitations include its relatively small, homogeneous sample and short observation window, which may affect generalizability. Despite this, it contributes to the literature by highlighting the importance of timing and mental state in understanding how digital behavior affects sleep, particularly in adolescent populations prone to bedtime procrastination.

Woods et al. explored the impact of nighttime social media use on sleep quality and emotional well-being in a sample of 467 UK adolescents. Their findings revealed a strong association between high bedtime engagement on platforms and poor sleep quality, as well as increased levels of anxiety and depression. A key variable in this study was Fear of Missing Out (FOMO), which was found to significantly mediate the relationship between late-night social media use and emotional distress. Adolescents who frequently checked their phones after going to bed exhibited not only poorer sleep but also heightened psychological distress. The study provides valuable insight into how psychosocial factors interact with digital behaviors to influence sleep. Although limited by its moderate sample size and reliance on self-reporting, it underscores the emotional underpinnings of social media addiction and supports the development of interventions that address both technological habits and emotional needs.

Exelmans et al. investigated the relationship between media consumption and sleep efficiency in adults, using data from 844 participants aged 18 to 94. The study found that individuals who used smartphones and social media extensively before bed experienced longer sleep latency, lower sleep efficiency, and overall poorer rest quality. Notably, it differentiated between types of media, finding that interactive devices (smartphones) disrupted sleep more than passive devices (TV). This finding suggests that cognitive engagement plays a larger role than screen exposure alone. Using validated sleep quality scales, the study adds credibility to its claims. However, it relies heavily on self-reporting and doesn't factor in physiological data, such as melatonin levels or heart rate. Still, it provides a broader perspective by focusing on an adult demographic, supporting the notion that sleep disturbances due to social media are not limited to adolescents.

Kuss and Griffiths conducted a literature review focused on the addictive nature of social networking and its psychological consequences, particularly sleep deprivation. Their analysis drew from studies linking excessive use of platforms like Facebook and Instagram with increased anxiety, stress, and poor sleep outcomes. The authors introduced the term "social media fatigue", describing a state of mental exhaustion resulting from constant connectivity. They highlighted how addictive design features such as infinite scrolling, push notifications, and algorithmic content delivery perpetuate compulsive usage, especially before bedtime. The review also emphasized the bidirectional relationship between mental health and screen use, where poor sleep worsens anxiety, and anxiety encourages more screen time. While the paper does not present new empirical data, its synthesis of existing literature offers a theoretical framework for understanding how social media disrupts sleep. It calls for interdisciplinary approaches that incorporate digital wellness into mental health and sleep treatment plans.

R. Alonzo et al., examined how social media use affects sleep quality and mental health problems through research from multiple clinical and behavioral studies. The authors studied how screen time before bedtime and social media use during the night and notification frequency and body clock disturbances and psychological effects interact with each other. The study found that continuous blue light exposure from devices leads to reduced melatonin production which results in longer time needed to fall asleep and less efficient REM sleep. People who spend too much time on social media sites tend to experience heightened cognitive function and emotional attachment and stress reactions which lead to anxiety and depression symptoms. The connection between sleep loss and social media addiction through two research methods which included longitudinal studies and cross-sectional studies. The studies which used machine learning enabled researchers to forecast sleep disturbances and mental stress based on data from users' online activities.

BIOLOGICAL IMPACT OF SLEEP DEPRIVATION

The human body is biologically programmed to follow certain rhythms that govern fundamental functions, one of the most important being the sleep-wake cycle. This cycle, tightly linked to external cues such as light and darkness, is crucial for maintaining mental clarity, emotional stability, immune defense and overall physical health. However, with the rise of digital screens and the increasing tendency to use social media late into the night, our natural biological processes particularly those related to sleep are facing unprecedented disruption (Reichenberger et al., 2026). In this section, we explore three major biological consequences of sleep deprivation caused by late-night screen use: circadian rhythm disruption due to blue light exposure, melatonin suppression, and sleep cycle disturbances leading to neural fatigue.

Circadian Rhythm and Blue Light Exposure

At the core of the sleep-wake regulation system lies the circadian rhythm, a 24-hour internal clock that governs various physiological and behavioral processes such as body temperature, hormone secretion, digestion, and most importantly sleep. This rhythm is controlled by a tiny region in the brain called the suprachiasmatic nucleus (SCN), located in the hypothalamus. The SCN responds to light signals received through the eyes and helps synchronize the body's activities with the day-night cycle. One of the most significant environmental cues for the SCN is light, especially natural sunlight. During the day, exposure to sunlight tells the SCN that it's time to stay awake and alert. As the day ends and natural light fades, the SCN signals the pineal gland to begin producing melatonin, a hormone that facilitates sleep.

However, this finely tuned system is disrupted by exposure to artificial blue light, which is abundantly emitted by the screens of smartphones, tablets, and computers. Blue light has a short wavelength and high energy, mimicking the intensity and quality of daylight. When users engage with their devices during nighttime particularly for extended periods on social media platforms the brain is tricked into believing it's still daytime (Langdon et al., 2026). This confuses the SCN and delays the onset of the sleep signal cascade. Scientific studies have shown that blue light exposure, even for just two hours before bedtime, can significantly shift circadian rhythms by up to 90 minutes. This circadian misalignment doesn't just lead to difficulty falling asleep it can also affect the quality and depth of sleep achieved once a person does fall asleep. Over time, repeated disruption of this biological clock can contribute to chronic sleep disorders, metabolic imbalances, and increased vulnerability to diseases such as diabetes and hypertension.

Melatonin Suppression and Its Consequences

Melatonin is often referred to as the "sleep hormone." Secreted by the pineal gland, melatonin production typically begins in the evening as light levels drop, peaking in the middle of the night and tapering off toward morning. This hormone plays a critical role in signaling to the body that it's time to wind down and prepare for rest. Importantly, melatonin doesn't induce sleep directly but facilitates the transition from wakefulness to sleep by lowering body temperature, slowing metabolic processes, and reducing alertness. Exposure to artificial light especially blue light from screens suppresses melatonin production (Carter et al., 2017). The brighter and more prolonged the light exposure, the more significant the suppression. Research has shown that screen use can suppress melatonin production by up to 50%, depending on the brightness and proximity of the screen to the eyes. This suppression not only delays sleep onset but also reduces the duration and quality of REM (Rapid Eye Movement) sleep, the phase most closely associated with dreaming, emotional processing, and memory consolidation.

A deficiency in REM sleep can lead to emotional volatility, poor concentration, and reduced ability to retain new information effects that are particularly detrimental for students and working professionals. Over time, disrupted melatonin cycles can also impact immune function, increase the risk of infections and even contribute to long-term health issues such as depression, anxiety disorders, and cancer. Furthermore, melatonin levels naturally decline with age (Shochat et al., 2010). For adolescents and young adults groups who are among the most avid late-night users of social media external suppression of melatonin during a time when their sleep patterns are already shifting due to biological changes can create a perfect storm of delayed sleep phase syndrome and daytime dysfunction. Here is a visual representation of the biological impacts of sleep deprivation caused by late-night social media use. The graph highlights the severity of each consequence, with melatonin suppression and sleep cycle disruption ranking among the most significant as shown in fig [4].

Figure 4. Biological impacts of late-night screen usage.

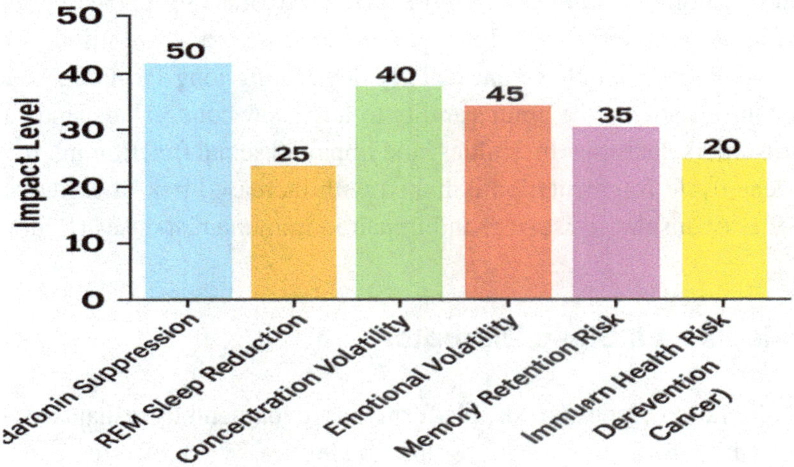

Sleep Cycle Disruption and Neural Fatigue

A normal sleep cycle consists of multiple stages: NREM (Non-Rapid Eye Movement) stages 1 through 3, followed by REM sleep. Each complete cycle lasts about 90 minutes and repeats multiple times throughout the night. During these stages, the brain and body engage in essential maintenance processes. For instance, stage 3 (deep sleep) is crucial for physical restoration, while REM sleep is essential for emotional balance, learning, and creativity. Late-night social media use interferes with both the duration and quality of these cycles. First, delayed sleep onset leads to a shortened total sleep duration, especially if individuals still need to wake early for school or work. Second, screen-induced arousal both cognitive and emotional prevents the user from descending quickly into the deeper stages of sleep (Twenge et al., 2017). Instead, sleep becomes lighter and more fragmented, with frequent awakenings and reduced time spent in restorative stages. This leads to a condition known as neural fatigue, in which the brain does not have adequate time to recharge, reorganize neural connections, or clear out metabolic waste products (such as beta-amyloid, associated with Alzheimer's disease). Neural fatigue manifests as difficulty concentrating, slower reaction times, impaired decision-making, and poor emotional regulation. It also reduces executive functioning, the brain's ability to plan, prioritize, and resist impulses functions that are vital in academic and professional environments.

Moreover, sleep deprivation negatively affects the prefrontal cortex, the brain region responsible for higher-order thinking and impulse control. This creates a paradoxical loop: sleep-deprived individuals often find it harder to resist the urge to continue scrolling, making it even more difficult to break the cycle of poor sleep hygiene (Fino & Mazzetti, 2019). In adolescents, whose brains are still developing, sleep cycle disruption can have particularly devastating long-term consequences. It affects neuroplasticity, the brain's ability to form new connections, and can lead to mood disorders, learning difficulties, and impaired social functioning. In adults, chronic sleep cycle fragmentation is linked with increased risk of cardiovascular disease, obesity, insulin resistance, and impaired immune responses (Reiter et al., 2014).

Social Media as a Sleep Disruptor

The proliferation of social media platforms has fundamentally reshaped how people engage with information, relationships, and leisure. While offering a multitude of benefits, social media has also introduced significant challenges to sleep health, particularly through late-night usage. Unlike traditional forms of media consumption, such as reading a book or watching a television program with a defined endpoint, social media platforms are designed for infinite consumption. They employ behavioral design techniques that tap into psychological vulnerabilities, encouraging users to remain engaged well past the point of intended use (Orben & Przybylski, 2019). This section explores how specific features of social media—namely endless scrolling, algorithmic content personalization, notifications, and cognitive stimulation act as powerful sleep disruptors.

The Role of Endless Scrolling and Algorithm Design

Social media platforms are deliberately engineered to keep users engaged for as long as possible. One of the most powerful design elements contributing to this is endless scrolling a feature that removes stopping cues by allowing content to load continuously without the need for user action. Unlike flipping a book's last page or watching the end of a television episode, infinite scroll provides no natural conclusion, making it far easier for users to lose track of time. These behavioral psychologists call the "Zeigarnik effect", where people tend to remember and focus on unfinished tasks. In the case of social media, the "unfinished task" is the next video, photo, or post constantly dangled in front of the user by a system designed to optimize for attention. The user interface delivers intermittent rewards through a mix of emotionally resonant content, humor, social validation (likes, comments, shares), and breaking news. The result is a feedback loop similar to that seen in slot machine gambling, with dopamine-driven engagement keeping users hooked.

Behind this experience is an intricate algorithmic engine that tracks user behavior, preferences, and interaction history to curate a hyper-personalized feed. The more a user engages, the better the algorithm becomes at predicting what will keep them engaged next. This personalization increases the emotional relevance of content, making it more difficult to disengage even when users are aware that they should be sleeping. Popular platforms like TikTok, Instagram Reels, facebook and YouTube Shorts exemplify this pattern, offering short, snackable content optimized for virality and compulsive consumption. This work poses a particular challenge late at night, when users seek to "unwind" by mindlessly scrolling. Ironically, this relaxation strategy backfires as users get caught in the loop of one more post, one more video until minutes turn into hours (Alfonsi et al., 2020). The result is delayed sleep onset, shortened sleep duration, and compromised next-day functioning.

Notifications and the Fear of Missing Out

The users put their phones down, social media continues to exert influence through push notifications pings, buzzes, banners, and badges that signal new messages, reactions, or updates. These notifications trigger a psychological and physiological response, elevating alertness and increasing the likelihood that users will check their devices again. This is especially disruptive at night, when the body and mind should be preparing for rest. The constant presence of notifications cultivates a "fear of missing out" (FOMO). The anxiety that others are having rewarding experiences or accessing information from which one is excluded. FOMO is a powerful emotional motivator that drives users to re-engage with social media even when they intend to sleep. It generates mental restlessness, making it difficult to achieve the sense of closure necessary for relaxation (Scott et al., 2019). FOMO is not a vague cultural concept but a well-documented psychological phenomenon. Studies have shown that individuals with high levels of FOMO are significantly more likely to engage in bedtime procrastination and experience sleep disturbances, including insomnia and fragmented sleep. Social media's real-time nature reinforces this behavior by creating the illusion that important interactions are always happening and could be missed if one logs off.

The anticipation of notifications is often enough to disturb sleep. Users may leave their phones next to their pillows, frequently glancing at the screen or waking up during the night to check for updates. This hypervigilance undermines the deep, uninterrupted rest needed for the brain to consolidate memories and regulate emotions (Exelmans & Van den Bulck, 2016). Even when notifications are turned off, the habit of checking becomes so deeply ingrained that users may unconsciously reach for their phones, disrupting their sleep cycles further. Here's a circular analysis graph showing the key contributors to sleep disruption caused by social media usage. "Endless Scrolling & Algorithm Design" accounts for the largest share, followed by "Notifications & FOMO" and "Cognitive Arousal & Overstimulation" as shown in fig [5].

Figure 5. Key Disruptors of sleep from social media usage.

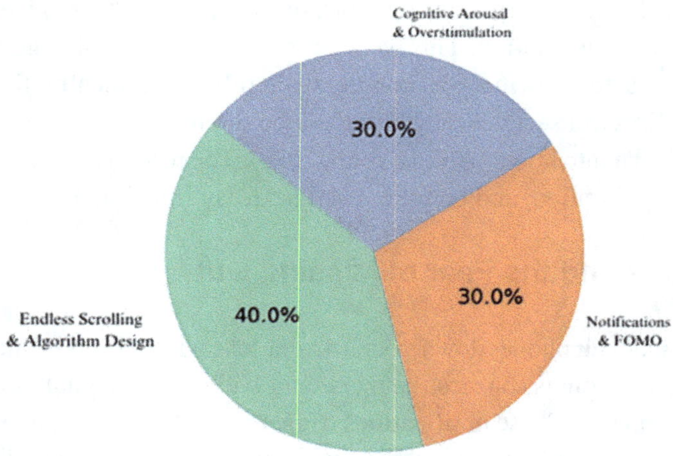

PSYCHOLOGICAL AND BEHAVIORAL CONSEQUENCES

The biological disruptions caused by late-night social media use are deeply concerning, the psychological and behavioral consequences are equally profound. Sleep is intricately linked to mental well-being, emotional regulation, and functional capacity in everyday life. When digital engagement especially social media use interferes with sleep, it sets off a cascade of psychological effects that impair mood, cognition, and behavior.

Anxiety, Depression and Mood Swings

Sleep is essential for maintaining emotional stability and mental clarity. Disrupted sleep patterns caused by late-night social media use can exacerbate psychological conditions such as anxiety and depression and lead to frequent mood swings. These conditions are not merely side effects of sleep deprivation; they are often worsened by the emotional content and dynamics of social media itself. Users are frequently exposed to negative news cycles, online arguments, cyberbullying, and social comparison all of which elevate stress and contribute to emotional exhaustion (Kuss & Griffiths, 2015). Platforms like Instagram, TikTok, and Facebook promote idealized portrayals of people's lives highlight reels filled with curated success, beauty, wealth, and popularity. For vulnerable users, especially adolescents and young adults, these portrayals can induce feelings of inadequacy, loneliness, and self-doubt. When combined with insufficient sleep, the ability to manage and recover from these negative emotions is significantly impaired (Yu et al., 2024).

Furthermore, lack of sleep affects the amygdala, the brain region responsible for processing emotions, and weakens the connection with the prefrontal cortex, which helps regulate emotional responses. This neurological imbalance results in heightened emotional reactivity, making users more susceptible to irritability, sadness, and even panic attacks. Over time, poor emotional regulation due to sleep deprivation can lead to chronic mood disorders (Zhang et al., 2023). Numerous studies have drawn a direct link between late-night screen use, especially involving social media, and increased symptoms of depression and anxiety. For instance, a study published in the Journal of Youth and Adolescence found that adolescents who used social media for more than three hours per night were significantly more likely to report symptoms of major depressive disorder. Another study from the Sleep Research Society revealed that sleep-deprived individuals showed increased threat perception and social rejection sensitivity, which worsened their anxiety and social withdrawal.

Decline in Academic and Workplace Productivity

The consequences of late-night social media use extend beyond personal well-being and into academic and professional performance. Sleep is essential for concentration, memory consolidation, learning, creativity, and problem-solving all of which are critical for success in school and the workplace. When these cognitive functions are impaired by inadequate or poor-quality sleep, performance inevitably suffers (Khan et al., 2024). For students, especially those in high school or college, staying up late on social media reduces both the quantity and quality of sleep, leaving them fatigued and mentally foggy the next day. This affects their ability to retain information, participate meaningfully in class discussions, and perform well in exams or assignments. Sleep deprivation is particularly harmful during periods of intense academic demand, such as exam seasons, when students ironically increase their screen time as a coping mechanism, compounding the problem. In the workplace, professionals who engage in late-night scrolling often report reduced motivation, slower decision-making, and lower task efficiency. The cognitive burden caused by sleep loss makes it harder to meet deadlines, manage stress, or innovate traits that are highly valued in modern work environments (F. Lafontaine-Poissant, 2024). Furthermore, individuals may experience microsleeps, brief and involuntary episodes of sleep that can last a few seconds but significantly impact attention and safety, particularly in high-stakes professions like healthcare, transportation, or engineering.

In both academic and professional contexts, the inability to function at full mental capacity also affects self-esteem and confidence, further reinforcing feelings of anxiety, frustration, and helplessness (Nicholson et al., 2023). It becomes a self-perpetuating cycle: the more one's performance declines, the more they turn to social media for distraction or escape, which further compromises sleep and deepens the problem. Here is a circular analysis graph depicting the psychological and behavioral consequences of late-night social media use. The impact is distributed across anxiety and mood-related issues, reduced productivity, and the development of addictive behaviors, all of which contribute to a cycle of digital overuse and poor sleep.

ADDICTIVE BEHAVIORS AND DIGITAL DEPENDENCY

Perhaps the most insidious consequence of late-night social media use is the development of addictive behaviours and digital dependency. Social media platforms are engineered to be habit-forming, employing mechanisms such as intermittent rewards, variable reinforcement schedules, and personalized content loops (Kuss & Griffiths, 2011). These features tap into the brain's dopaminergic reward system, making users crave the next like, comment, or update. Over time, this leads to compulsive checking, even when it disrupts essential activities such as sleep. Late-night use, in particular, becomes a ritualistic behaviour. Users often engage with social media as part of a winding-down routine, falsely believing it will help them relax. However, this pattern quickly morphs into digital dependency, where the individual feels discomfort or anxiety when not connected. This results in bedtime procrastination, where users actively delay sleep to continue engaging with their devices, despite being aware of the negative consequences (Giumetti & Kowalski, 2022).

This compulsive behaviour reduces self-regulation, a key executive function that allows individuals to make choices aligned with long-term goals rather than immediate gratification. Over time, the ability to resist late-night scrolling diminishes, even when users experience chronic fatigue or declining mental health. The feedback loop is self-reinforcing: users stay up late using social media, wake up tired and stressed, seek relief through more screen time, and repeat the cycle. Digital dependency can also lead to nomophobia (the fear of being without a mobile phone), phantom vibration syndrome, and withdrawal symptoms similar to substance addiction, including irritability, restlessness, and difficulty concentrating when deprived of device access.

These symptoms become more pronounced at night, when the world quiets down, and individuals are alone with their thoughts making the allure of digital escape all the more tempting. For many users, especially adolescents, nighttime may be the only unstructured time available to them free from school, family, or work obligations. Unfortunately, without boundaries or interventions, this time becomes a breeding ground for unhealthy digital consumption patterns, resulting in long-term behavioural dependency that is difficult to reverse (Sampasa-Kanyinga et al., 2022).

Coping Mechanisms and Healthy Habits

The profound impact of late-night social media use on sleep health, it is critical to identify and implement practical solutions. While awareness of the problem is the first step, long-term improvement hinges on adopting healthy habits and digital boundaries that promote restful sleep. Coping strategies must be holistic, addressing behavioral, environmental, and technological factors. In this section, we explore evidence-based coping mechanisms including digital detox strategies, structured bedtime routines, and technology-assisted sleep enhancement to help individuals reclaim their nights and restore their sleep quality.

Digital Detox Strategies and Sleep Hygiene

A digital detox is not about rejecting technology altogether but about mindfully managing screen time, especially in the hours leading up to bedtime (Alonzo et al., 2020). The goal is to reduce cognitive stimulation, minimize blue light exposure, and create a psychological association between nighttime and rest. Here are several effective strategies that support this process:

- Set Screen Curfews: Establish a fixed "digital sunset" a time after which all screen-based activities stop, typically 1–2 hours before bedtime. This curfew helps the brain unwind and re-establishes natural melatonin production. For many, an effective cutoff time is 9:00 PM or one hour before their intended sleep time.
- Remove Devices from the Bedroom: Keeping phones, tablets, and laptops out of the bedroom reduces temptation and interruptions. Instead, use traditional alarm clocks to eliminate the "need" for a phone nearby. This simple boundary can significantly reduce midnight checking behavior and anxiety around notifications.
- Enable Night Mode or Blue Light Filters: Most modern smartphones, tablets, and computers now offer "night shift," "night light," or "dark mode" settings. These features reduce blue light emission by warming the screen tone. While

not a replacement for reduced screen time, they can mitigate melatonin suppression when screen use is unavoidable.

- Create a No-Screen Zone: Designate areas in your home especially the bedroom as screen-free zones. This helps reinforce psychological boundaries between work/leisure and rest. Couples and families can agree on shared screen-free time to promote relationship-building and sleep hygiene.
- Digital-Free Wind-Down Rituals: Replace social media scrolling with offline nighttime activities such as reading physical books, light stretching, or listening to calming music. A structured pre-sleep routine sends signals to the brain that it is time to relax.

Setting Screen Time Limits and Bedtime Routines

Creating a healthy bedtime routine involves transitioning the brain from stimulation to relaxation. This shift requires intentional actions and the removal of distracting digital content. Built-In Screen Time Tools: Both iOS and Android offer Screen Time and Digital Wellbeing features that allow users to monitor and limit their app usage. Users can set daily usage caps for specific apps (such as Instagram or YouTube) and schedule "downtime" when only essential apps are accessible. These features provide automated nudges that support self-regulation.

- Schedule App Locks or Content Restrictions: Third-party apps like Freedom, Forest, and Stay Focused offer additional control, allowing users to block social media apps during specific times of day. For users prone to compulsive checking, these apps can help break habitual loops and enforce screen-free time.
- Replace Scrolling with Offline Routines: Substitute nighttime screen use with analog activities known to promote relaxation. These include:
- Reading a printed book (preferably fiction or non-stimulating content)
- Mindfulness meditation or breathing exercises, which activate the parasympathetic nervous system
- Go to Bed at the Same Time Every Night: Consistency reinforces the circadian rhythm. Even on weekends, maintaining a regular bedtime can improve overall sleep efficiency and reduce sleep debt accumulation.

Use of Technology for Sleep Enhancement (Apps, Wearables)

Paradoxically, while technology can disrupt sleep, it can also be a valuable ally in improving sleep hygiene when used intentionally. Many tools are available that track, support, and enhance sleep behaviors using biofeedback, guided relaxation, and habit-forming frameworks.

a) Sleep Apps
   - Calm: Offers guided meditations, sleep stories, breathing exercises, and music designed to induce relaxation. Its bedtime stories are particularly effective for users transitioning from mental overactivity to sleep readiness.
   - Headspace: A well-known mindfulness app with a dedicated sleep section. Headspace features guided wind-downs, "sleepcasts," and audio experiences that help users mentally disconnect from daily stressors.
   - Pzizz: Uses psychoacoustic principles to deliver dynamic soundscapes that adapt over time, helping users fall asleep faster and stay asleep longer.
   - Insight Timer: Free meditation app with sleep-specific playlists, ambient music, and guided sessions led by sleep therapists and psychologists.

b) Wearable Devices
   - Fitbit: Provides detailed sleep analytics including time spent in light, deep, and REM stages. Fitbit's sleep score and smart alarm features help users understand their sleep cycles and wake up during lighter stages for optimal energy.
   - Oura Ring: A sleek ring that offers high-fidelity data on heart rate variability (HRV), body temperature, and sleep stages. It also includes daily readiness scores to guide activity and rest balance.
   - Apple Watch and Samsung Galaxy Watch: These offer sleep tracking, reminders to wind down, and silent alarms. When paired with built-in apps like Apple's "Wind Down" feature, they provide a structured transition into bedtime.
   - Whoop Strap: Popular among athletes and high-performers, this device offers advanced insights into recovery and strain, helping users optimize their sleep schedules for peak performance.

These technologies do more than monitor, to promote accountability and offer real-time feedback, helping users recognize poor patterns and build better habits. However, it's important to note that these tools work best when paired with behavioural changes rather than used in isolation.

POLICY RECOMMENDATIONS AND PARENTAL GUIDANCE

The individual actions and self-regulation are critical in mitigating the adverse effects of late-night social media use on sleep, systemic support through policy, education, and corporate responsibility is equally essential. The growing crisis of sleep deprivation particularly among adolescents, students, and professionals calls for a collaborative, multi-stakeholder approach. Educational institutions, families, and tech companies all have a role to play in fostering a healthier digital environment. This section outlines practical and scalable recommendations across three pillars: school and college-level interventions, parental guidance and control, and responsible design by social media corporations.

School and College-Level Interventions

Educational institutions are uniquely positioned to influence young people during their formative years. Schools and colleges can play a central role in promoting digital literacy and sleep health awareness by incorporating them into the curriculum and campus culture. Here are several impactful strategies:

- Integrate Digital Wellness into the Curriculum: Schools should introduce age-appropriate modules on digital hygiene, emphasizing not only cyber safety but also the impact of screen time on mental health and sleep. This can be included in life skills education, health science, or as part of technology courses.
- Conduct Awareness Campaigns on Sleep and social media: Regular workshops, posters, assemblies, and guest lectures can create a culture of mindfulness around digital use. Campaigns could focus on themes such as "Power Down for Better Sleep," "No Scroll Zones," or "Screens Off, Minds On".
- Screen-Free Hours on Campus: Institutions can establish screen-free study periods or zones, especially in dormitories or libraries, to encourage students to disconnect and engage in non-digital relaxation activities.
- Flexible Morning Schedules: Where possible, particularly for high schools and colleges, institutions should explore delaying start times. Research shows that adolescents have delayed circadian rhythms and benefit from later school start times, which can compensate for sleep lost to late-night screen use.
- Digital Usage Assessments: Incorporating digital health check-ins during counselling sessions allows educators and support staff to identify at-risk students who might be suffering from excessive nighttime digital use and provide timely guidance.

School-based interventions can normalize healthy tech use and provide students with tools and knowledge to self-regulate, forming lifelong habits that promote both academic success and personal well-being.

Parental Control and Modelling Behaviour

Parents and guardians have a profound influence on their children's digital behaviour both through explicit rules and implicit modelling. The home environment must reflect the digital habits that families wish to instil. Here's how parents can be empowered to create sleep-positive digital routines:

- Set Household Tech Boundaries: Parents should enforce screen curfews, such as turning off devices at least one hour before bedtime, and make bedrooms device-free zones. These consistent household rules help reduce temptation and reinforce sleep-friendly behaviour.
- Use Parental Control Tools: Mobile platforms like iOS and Android offer built-in settings to restrict access to certain apps during specific times, monitor screen time, and control the types of content children can view. Third-party parental control apps like Bark, Qustodio, or Norton Family offer even more customizable options.
- Model Responsible Digital Behaviour: Children often imitate the behaviour of their caregivers. When parents set aside devices during dinner, avoid scrolling in bed, and prioritize relaxation over digital engagement, they set a powerful example. A family-wide commitment to screen-free evenings can be both bonding and beneficial to everyone's health.
- Discuss the Risks Openly: Open conversations about the impact of technology on sleep, stress, and health can help children understand why certain restrictions are necessary. Framing rules as acts of care, rather than punishment, encourages cooperation and long-term internalization of healthy habits.
- Provide Alternatives to Digital Entertainment: Encourage hobbies such as reading, drawing, journaling, or board games that serve as offline substitutes for screen-based entertainment. Especially for younger children, bedtime stories or calming music can be effective sleep cues.

Corporate Responsibility of Social Media Platforms

Tech companies that design and maintain social media platforms also bear ethical responsibility for the behavioural impact of their products. Given the persuasive technologies embedded in social media such as infinite scroll, algorithmic content delivery, and push notifications, it is imperative that platforms include design features that prioritize user well-being, especially related to sleep. Several corporate interventions can make a meaningful difference:

- Auto-Disable Features After Set Hours: Platforms could allow users (or parents) to schedule periods during which the app becomes temporarily inaccessible, especially during late-night hours. TikTok, for instance, has trialed bedtime reminders and brief pauses, but these should be made default for younger users and customizable for adults.
- Built-In Sleep Reminders: Apps should include behavioural nudges that alert users when they've exceeded healthy usage thresholds late at night. These reminders could be tied to usage analytics and even offer a "sleep now" mode that hides non-essential notifications and stops video autoplay.
- Limit Algorithmic Stimulation at Night: Social media feeds could be designed to reduce emotionally arousing or addictive content after a certain time. For instance, platforms might shift the algorithm to prioritize calming, positive, or less engaging content during late hours.
- Daily and Weekly Usage Reports: Similar to Apple's Screen Time and Google's Digital Wellbeing dashboards, platforms could offer in-app insights into time spent on the app, especially during night hours, and suggest break intervals or digital detox plans.
- Youth-Focused Protective Defaults: For users under 18, platforms should implement automatic screen limits, nighttime restrictions, and enhanced privacy settings. These could be opt-out rather than opt-in, encouraging safer default behavior.
- Transparency and Research Funding: Social media companies can also support independent research into the mental and sleep health effects of their platforms, and share anonymized usage data with public health researchers for the development of best practices.

Longitudinal Studies on Social Media and Sleep Health

Most current research on the relationship between social media and sleep is cross-sectional it captures data at a single point in time. While such studies are helpful in identifying correlations, they fall short in establishing causal relationships or tracking long-term health outcomes. This limitation poses a significant research gap, especially given that the effects of sleep deprivation often accumulate over months or years. There is a pressing need for longitudinal studies that track individuals over extended periods, observing how patterns of social media use influence sleep quality, emotional well-being, cognitive function, and even physical health outcomes such as obesity, hypertension, and immune suppression. For example, multi-year studies could monitor adolescents from high school through college to assess how their evolving digital habits shape their sleep and mental health trajectories. Such studies could also shed light on critical developmental windows, identifying the age ranges or life transitions (e.g., adolescence, college entry, first jobs) when individuals are most vulnerable to sleep disturbances due to digital overuse. Longitudinal research would enable more predictive modeling, helping clinicians and policymakers develop targeted interventions based on usage patterns and risk factors.

Additionally, including diverse populations across geography, culture, socio-economic status, and neurodiversity would help generalize findings and avoid a one-size-fits-all approach. For instance, how might screen-induced sleep disruption differ between urban youth with high digital access versus rural youth with limited connectivity. Funding and institutional support for such studies are essential, as longitudinal research requires sustained resources, consistent participation, and robust data collection over time.

Role of AI and Personalization in User Addiction

Artificial Intelligence (AI) and machine learning now form the backbone of most social media platforms. These technologies enable personalized content delivery, adaptive advertising, and dynamic user interfaces. While personalization enhances user experience, it also poses significant ethical and psychological challenges, particularly in relation to sleep health.

AI algorithms are designed to maximize user engagement, often by delivering emotionally provocative, novel, or high-reward content. This design leads to the creation of "scroll traps," where users continue interacting with the platform far beyond their intended duration especially during vulnerable periods such as nighttime. Algorithms learn from user behavior what we click, pause on, or engage with to serve increasingly irresistible content, creating a feedback loop that deepens dependency. The addictive design driven by AI is particularly problematic before bedtime, when users seek a moment of distraction or relaxation but instead find themselves cognitively stimulated and emotionally aroused. This contributes to delayed sleep onset, reduced sleep duration, and disrupted circadian alignment. Future research must critically examine how algorithmic design influences nighttime behavior, and whether certain personalization models are more likely to promote compulsive use. Moreover, AI could also be reprogrammed for wellness, offering possibilities for positive disruption.

- Wellness-focused algorithms could prioritize calming, positive, or low-engagement content during late-night hours.

- AI could be trained to detect signs of digital fatigue or bedtime procrastination and respond with gentle nudges or auto-disable functions.
- Personalized sleep hygiene recommendations, based on user patterns, could be integrated into apps to guide healthier nighttime routines.

Emerging Tech (e.g., VR) and Its Future Impact on Sleep

As we move beyond smartphones and into more immersive technologies like Virtual Reality (VR), Augmented Reality (AR), and Mixed Reality (MR), the relationship between digital environments and sleep may become even more complex. These technologies offer novel forms of interaction that are visually stimulating, spatially engaging, and emotionally intense all factors that could significantly affect sleep cycles. VR holds potential for disrupting sleep health:

- High levels of sensory immersion can lead to overstimulation and difficulty transitioning into a relaxed state.
- Evening or nighttime VR gaming could delay melatonin release even more intensely than standard screens.
- Users may experience lingering cognitive arousal after exposure to action-oriented or emotionally charged virtual experiences.
- On the other hand, VR also presents opportunities for enhancing sleep quality, if used intentionally:
- VR meditation and mindfulness apps (e.g., Tripp, Guided Meditation VR) offer immersive calming environments that promote relaxation.
- VR could help train the brain to follow sleep rituals or engage in cognitive behavioral therapy for insomnia (CBT-I) through gamified formats.
- Simulated natural environments (e.g., forests, oceans, night skies) may provide soothing alternatives to urban noise or mental clutter before bed.

The wearable technology integrated with AR/VR (like smart headbands or haptic devices) may provide real-time feedback on stress, heart rate, or sleep latency, helping users recognize when it's time to disengage from digital activities.

- As these technologies become more mainstream, future research should investigate:
- Their short-term and long-term effects on sleep architecture and circadian rhythms.
- How content type, duration, and time of use impact sleep latency and quality.
- Guidelines for responsible usage windows, especially among younger or more vulnerable populations.

The regulations and ethical standards must evolve alongside these technologies to ensure their development aligns with user well-being, not just entertainment or engagement metrics. The key findings of literature review with respect to the methodology and limitations are shown in table 1.

Table 1. Comparative Analysis of different studies of social media usage.

Study	Methodology	Population Studied	Key Findings	Limitations
Levenson et al.	Quantitative survey (cross-sectional)	1,788 U.S. young adults (ages 19–32)	Higher frequency and emotional engagement with social media significantly associated with sleep disturbance	Self-reported data; no causal inference due to cross-sectional design
Carter et al.	Systematic review of 20 studies	Children and adolescents	Bedtime screen use linked to delayed sleep onset, shorter sleep duration, and poor quality; even access to devices impacts sleep	Variation in screen time definitions; limited to English publications
Twenge et al.	Quantitative (national survey data)	360,000 U.S. adolescents (2009–2017)	Teen sleep duration declined as screen time increased; <7 hrs sleep now common	Correlation-based; can't isolate individual behaviors
Orben & Przybylski	Quantitative with statistical modeling	120,000+ UK teens	Found modest, nonlinear effects of digital tech on sleep and well-being	Minimal effect sizes; doesn't address late-night use specifically
Alfonsi et al.	Experimental + sleep diaries	Italian adolescents	Social media use in the hour before bed linked to poor sleep continuity and later sleep onset	Small national sample; lacks long-term outcomes

CONCLUSION

To effectively tackle the rising concern of sleep deprivation linked to social media use, a collective cultural reset is necessary, one that places greater value on digital boundaries and sleep hygiene. Late-night scrolling must no longer be dismissed as harmless downtime. Instead, it should be recognized as a behavior that carries real costs to cognitive performance, emotional regulation, and physical health. By integrating these insights into public awareness campaigns, educational programs, and policy initiatives, we can begin shifting habits on a broader scale. True progress, however, will depend on the intentional collaboration of all stakeholders from tech companies designing more humane interfaces to educators teaching responsible usage, and from parents modeling healthy digital habits to individuals making conscious choices about when and how to engage online. At the core of this change is the idea of mindful technology using digital tools to enrich, not exhaust. Prioritizing rest and mental clarity over algorithm driven content is not just an individual act of self-care, it's a step toward a healthier, more balanced digital society.

Future Research Directions

As technology continues to evolve, the intersection between social media use and sleep health will remain a vital area of interdisciplinary research. Future studies should prioritize longitudinal and experimental designs to establish causal relationships between late-night screen exposure and long-term health outcomes. With the rise of AI-driven personalization, understanding how algorithms contribute to digital addiction and how they can be reprogrammed to promote healthier behaviors offers a critical avenue for innovation. There is also a need to expand the demographic reach of research to include middle-aged professionals, neurodiverse populations, and non-Western cultures, ensuring more inclusive and globally relevant findings. Emerging technologies like virtual reality (VR), augmented reality (AR), and wearable biofeedback tools present both risks and opportunities; their impact on circadian rhythms and mental rest must be closely examined. On the policy front, future efforts should explore the development of ethical design standards for social media platforms that prioritize user wellness, particularly during nighttime hours. Education systems and healthcare providers can collaborate to incorporate digital wellness and sleep literacy into mainstream curricula and counseling. By addressing these areas, we can build a more balanced relationship with technology that supports, rather than disrupts, the fundamental human need for sleep.

ADDITIONAL READINGS

Aljomaa, S. S., Qudah, M. F. A., Albursan, I. S., Bakhiet, S. F., & Abduljabbar, A. S. (2016). Smartphone addiction among university students in the light of some variables. *Computers in Human Behavior, 61*, 155–164. https://www.sciencedirect.com/science/article/pii/S0747563216302126. DOI: 10.1016/j.chb.2016.03.041

Bert, F., Giacometti, M., Gualano, M. R., & Siliquini, R. (2014). Smartphones and health promotion: A review of the evidence. *Journal of Medical Systems, 38*(1), 9995. DOI: 10.1007/s10916-013-9995-7 PMID: 24346929

Parasuraman, S., Sam, A. T., Yee, S. W. K., Chuon, B. L. C., & Ren, L. Y. (2017). Smartphone usage and increased risk of mobile phone addiction: A concurrent study. *International Journal of Pharmaceutical Investigation, 7*(3), 125. https://pmc.ncbi.nlm.nih.gov/articles/PMC5680647/. DOI: 10.4103/jphi.JPHI_56_17 PMID: 29184824

Paul, M., Maglaras, L., Ferrag, M. A., & Almomani, I. (2023). Digitization of healthcare sector: A study on privacy and security concerns. *ICT Express, 9*(4), 571–588. DOI: 10.1016/j.icte.2023.02.007

REFERENCES

Alfonsi, V., Scarpelli, S., D'Atri, A., Stella, G., & De Gennaro, L. (2020). Later school start time: The impact of sleep on academic performance and health in the adolescent population. *International Journal of Environmental Research and Public Health, 17*(7), 2574. DOI: 10.3390/ijerph17072574 PMID: 32283688

Alonzo, R., Hussain, J., Stranges, S., & Anderson, K. K. (2020). Interplay between social media use, sleep quality, and mental health in youth: A systematic review. *Sleep Medicine Reviews, 56*, 101414. DOI: 10.1016/j.smrv.2020.101414 PMID: 33385767

Bourke, M., Maddren, C. I., Sippel, F., & Thomas, G. (2026). Within-person association between daily screen use and sleep in youth: A systematic review and meta-analysis. *JAMA Pediatrics, 180*(5), 500. Advance online publication. DOI: 10.1001/jamapediatrics.2025.6490 PMID: 41770550

Carter, G., Milner, A., McGill, K., Pirkis, J., Kapur, N., & Spittal, M. J. (2017). Predicting suicidal behaviours using clinical instruments: Systematic review and meta-analysis of positive predictive values for risk scales. *The British Journal of Psychiatry : The Journal of Mental Science*, *210*(6), 387–395. DOI: 10.1192/bjp.bp.116.182717 PMID: 28302700

Exelmans, L., & Van den Bulck, J. (2016). Bedtime mobile phone use and sleep in adults. *Social Science & Medicine*, *148*, 93–101. DOI: 10.1016/j.socscimed.2015.11.037 PMID: 26688552

Fino, E., & Mazzetti, M. (2019). Monitoring healthy and disturbed sleep through smartphone applications: A review of experimental evidence. *Sleep & Breathing = Schlaf & Atmung*, *23*(1), 13–24. DOI: 10.1007/s11325-018-1661-3 PMID: 29687190

Giumetti, S., & Kowalski, R. (2022). Cyberbullying via social media and well-being. *Current Opinion in Psychology*, *45*, 101314. DOI: 10.1016/j.copsyc.2022.101314 PMID: 35313180

Khan, G., Thomas, S., Karatela, S., Morawska, A., & Werner-Seidler, A. (2024). Intense and problematic social media use and sleep difficulties of adolescents in 40 countries. *Journal of Adolescence*, *96*(5), 1116–1125. DOI: 10.1002/jad.12321 PMID: 38570320

Kuss, D. J., & Griffiths, M. D. (2011). Online social networking and addiction—A review of the psychological literature. *International Journal of Environmental Research and Public Health*, *8*(9), 3528–3552. DOI: 10.3390/ijerph8093528 PMID: 22016701

Kuss, D. J., & Griffiths, M. D. (2015). Social networking sites and addiction: Ten lessons learned. *International Journal of Environmental Research and Public Health*, *12*(3), 1286–1306. DOI: 10.3390/ijerph14030311 PMID: 28304359

Lafontaine-Poissant, F., Lang, J. J., McKinnon, B., Simard, I., Roberts, K. C., Wong, S. L., Chaput, J.-P., Janssen, I., Boniel-Nissim, M., & Gariépy, G. (2024). Social media use and sleep health among adolescents in Canada. *Health Promotion and Chronic Disease Prevention in Canada : Research, Policy and Practice*, *44*(7–8), 338–346. DOI: 10.24095/hpcdp.44.7/8.05 PMID: 39141617

Langdon, R., Gioia, G., & Law, E. (2026). Digital media use in adolescents with migraine: A topical review. *Current Pain and Headache Reports*, *30*(1), 2. DOI: 10.1007/s11916-025-01444-6 PMID: 41396410

Levenson, J. C., Shensa, A., Sidani, J. E., Colditz, J. B., & Primack, B. A. (2017). Social media use before bed and sleep disturbance among young adults in the United States: A nationally representative study. *Sleep (Basel)*, *40*(9), zsx113. Advance online publication. DOI: 10.1093/sleep/zsx113 PMID: 28934521

Lin, S., Longobardi, C., Gastaldi, F. G. M., & Fabris, M. A. (2024). Social media addiction and aggressive behaviors in early adolescents: The mediating role of nighttime social media use and sleep quality. *The Journal of Early Adolescence*, *44*(1), 41–58. DOI: 10.1177/02724316231160142

Nicholson, D., Bohnert, A., & Crowley, S. (2023). A developmental perspective on sleep consistency. *Behavioral Sleep Medicine*, *21*(1), 97–116. DOI: 10.1080/15402002.2021.2024192 PMID: 35014925

Orben, A., & Przybylski, A. K. (2019). Screens, teens, and psychological well-being: Evidence from three time-use-diary studies. *Psychological Science*, *30*(5), 682–696. DOI: 10.1177/0956797619830329 PMID: 30939250

Reichenberger, D. A., Snyder, C. K., & Chang, A. M. (2026). Screen use, sleep, and circadian disruption. In *Sleep and Health* (pp. 207–215). Academic Press.. DOI: 10.1016/B978-0-443-13954-3.00018-8

Reiter, R. J., Tan, D. X., & Galano, A. (2014). Melatonin: Exceeding expectations. *Physiology (Bethesda, MD)*, *29*(5), 325–333. DOI: 10.1152/physiol.00011.2014 PMID: 25180262

Ren, Z., Lu, H., Ma, X., Min, G., Liu, L., Wu, L., Xu, R., & Yu, K. (2026). Longitudinal association between problematic social media use and sleep problems among adolescents: A random intercept cross-lagged panel model and sex differences. *Journal of Youth and Adolescence*, *55*(1), 119–134. DOI: 10.1007/s10964-025-02310-9 PMID: 41452419

Sampasa-Kanyinga, H., Lien, A., Hamilton, H. A., & Chaput, J. P. (2022). Cyberbullying involvement and short sleep duration among adolescents. *Sleep Health*, *8*(2), 183–190. DOI: 10.1016/j.sleh.2021.11.009 PMID: 35120851

Scott, H., Biello, S. M., & Woods, H. C. (2019). Social media use and adolescent sleep patterns: Cross-sectional findings from the UK millennium cohort study. *BMJ Open*, *9*(9), e031161. DOI: 10.1136/bmjopen-2019-031161 PMID: 31641035

Shochat, T., Cohen-Zion, M., & Tzischinsky, O. (2010). Functional consequences of inadequate sleep in adolescents: A systematic review. *Sleep Medicine Reviews*, *14*(5), 303–312. DOI: 10.1016/j.smrv.2013.03.005 PMID: 23806891

Twenge, J. M., Krizan, Z., & Hisler, G. (2017). Decreases in self-reported sleep duration among U.S. adolescents 2009–2015 and association with new media screen time. *Sleep Medicine*, *39*, 47–53. DOI: 10.1016/j.sleep.2017.08.013 PMID: 29157587

Van Den Eijnden, R. J., Geurts, S. M., Ter Bogt, T. F., van Der Rijst, V. G., & Koning, I. M. (2021). Social media use and adolescents' sleep: A longitudinal study on the protective role of parental rules regarding internet use before sleep. *International Journal of Environmental Research and Public Health*, *18*(3), 1346. DOI: 10.3390/ijerph18031346 PMID: 33540882

Whatley, S. (2026). Predictive modeling in social media deepfake identification. *Scholars Crossing (Liberty University)*. https://doi.org/DOI: 10.13140/rg.2.2.20551.97449

Yu, D. J., Wing, Y. K., Li, T. M., & Chan, N. Y. (2024). The impact of social media use on sleep and mental health in youth: A scoping review. *Current Psychiatry Reports*, *26*(3), 104–119. DOI: 10.1007/s11920-024-01481-9 PMID: 38329569

Zhang, P., Li, Y., & Zhao, Y.. (2023). Effect of social media addiction on executive functioning: Mediating roles of sleep quality. *Psychology Research and Behavior Management*, *16*, 1911–1920. DOI: 10.2147/PRBM.S414625 PMID: 37255996

KEY TERMS AND DEFINITIONS

Social Media Analytics: The process of gathering and studying how people interact on social networks, to figure out behavior patterns, communication trends and psychological effects.

Sleeping Quality: A way to rate how well someone sleeps, including sleep duration, time to fall asleep REM cycles continuity and how rested they feel.

Circadian Rhythm: The internal body clock that sets the sleep wake cycle and other bodily rhythms over about a 24-hour span.

Melatonin Suppression: Less melatonin production caused by blue light from phones and screens, leading to later sleep onset and broken sleep patterns.

Insomnia: A sleep problem where you can't fall asleep, stay asleep or get deep, restorative sleep often linked to too much screen time and stress.

Digital mental Health: A mixed field that uses digital tech, data analysis and watching online behaviour to evaluate, predict and try to improve mental health problems.

Digital Dependency: Heavy reliance on digital gadgets, internet services, or tech stuff for everyday tasks, which can make independent thinking fade out and also cut down on real life social contact.

Chapter 11
Digital Addictions and Public Health From Theoretical Models to Community-Based Interventions: Exploring the Nexus Between Technology Use and Mental Well-Being

Kadriye Olğaç Ak
http://orcid.org/0009-0006-8957-2524
Mardin Artuklu University, Turkey

ABSTRACT

This chapter presents a comprehensive public health perspective on digital addictions, focusing on problematic behaviors associated with smartphones, social media, online gaming, and other digital platforms. It explores a range of adverse physical, psychological, and social outcomes linked to these behaviors, including sleep disturbances, mental health challenges, and impaired functioning. The chapter reviews key theoretical frameworks such as behavioral addiction models, cognitive-behavioral approaches, and socio-ecological perspectives to clarify mechanisms and risk factors. It also addresses the influence of social determinants, digital environments, and vulnerable populations. Building on these foundations, the chapter outlines evidence-based, community-level prevention and intervention strategies,

DOI: 10.4018/979-8-2600-2468-3.ch011

emphasizing family, school, and healthcare settings. Interdisciplinary collaboration, health literacy, and policy development are underscored as essential to promoting sustainable and equitable public health responses to digital addictions.

1. INTRODUCTION

Digital technologies offer significant opportunities in many areas such as education, communication, access to healthcare services and social participation, while also revealing patterns of 'problematic use' characterised by loss of control, impaired functionality and psychosocial harm. Digital products such as smartphones, social media platforms, and online games are optimised to increase user engagement through design features such as instant reward loops, personalised feeds, notifications, and infinite scrolling. Within this ecosystem, usage in some individuals may exhibit behavioural addiction characteristics such as inability to manage time, shifting priorities in favour of digital activities, and persistence despite negative consequences. The World Health Organisation (WHO) has defined 'gaming disorder' within the ICD-11 framework, emphasising the clinical significance of a subset where gaming behaviour is accompanied by significant functional impairment. It specifies that the impairment must typically last at least 12 months and result in marked impairment in personal, family, social, educational, or occupational domains (WHO, 2020; Darvesh et al., 2020).

Conceptual clarity in the field of digital addictions is still developing. Under the umbrella of 'digital addiction(s)' in the literature, sub-phenomena such as internet gaming disorder, problematic social media use, problematic smartphone use, and, more broadly, problematic internet use are discussed. Particularly with regard to smartphone use, recent review studies indicate that problematic use is associated with outcomes such as anxiety, depressive symptoms, and sleep problems; the mechanisms may be shaped through difficulties in emotion regulation, impulsivity, reward sensitivity, and digital escape behaviour as a coping mechanism for stress (Ndayambaje & Okereke, 2025). In terms of gaming behaviour specifically, differences in diagnostic criteria (DSM and ICD approaches) may affect prevalence estimates; meta-analytic findings suggest that IGD rates vary depending on the sample and criteria, but indicate a significant public health burden (Zhou et al., 2024; Gisbert-Pérez et al., 2025).

These findings demonstrate that addressing digital addictions solely through the lens of individual 'willpower' or 'self-discipline' is insufficient; rather, they represent a multi-layered public health risk shaped by social determinants, the digital environment, and lifestyle factors. Social media use among young people has reached near-universal levels; the potential harms of this intense exposure have drawn the attention of public authorities and professional organisations. The US Surgeon General's Advisory highlights both the potential benefits and risks of social media for children and adolescents, emphasising that current evidence is insufficient to declare social media sufficiently safe and underscoring the urgent need for action to create safer digital environmentsb (Office of the Surgeon General (OSG), 2023; U.S. Department of Health and Human Services & Office of the Surgeon General, 2023). Similarly, the American Psychological Association (APA) recommends routine screening for signs of 'problematic social media use' in adolescents and strengthening protective approaches at the family, school, and community levels (American Psychological Association, 2023).

Another dimension that increases the public health importance of digital addictions is their indirect effects on sedentary behaviour and sleep patterns. The WHO's physical activity and sedentary behaviour guidelines position reducing sedentary time and increasing regular physical activity throughout the life cycle as a fundamental protective strategy (Bull et al., 2020). In particular, the disruption of sleep hygiene by screen-based activities, their substitution for physical activity, and their conflict with daily roles (school/work, family responsibilities, social relationships) may create a context that strengthens the link between digital addictions and chronic stress, emotional problems, and reduced quality of life. Therefore, digital addictions are not merely a matter of 'individual psychopathology'; they are a public health issue that must be addressed within the framework of behavioural risks, environmental exposure, and inequalities.

In recent years, interventions aimed at reducing digital use have also increased. Systematic reviews and meta-analyses of 'digital detox' programmes indicate the possibility of improvement in some mental health outcomes, although intervention types, durations, and measures are heterogeneous (Ramadhan et al., 2024). However, as a significant portion of the evidence is based on short-term, self-reported studies with limited sample diversity, multi-level (individual–family–school–community–policy) and context-sensitive programmes are needed for effective and sustainable results. Furthermore, the burden of digital addictions can exacerbate inequalities by interacting with factors such as socio-economic conditions, family functioning, school climate, neighbourhood safety, digital literacy, and access to mental health services. Therefore, it is critical that interventions do not merely tell individuals to "reduce usage", but rather generate healthy alternatives (safe social spaces, sports/games/peer activities), ensure that digital platform designs are aligned with harm reduction principles, and strengthen primary/community-based services.

This book chapter aims to address digital addictions along a continuum from theoretical models (behavioural addiction frameworks, cognitive-behavioural explanations, self-regulation and reward mechanisms, socio-ecological approaches) to community-based interventions. First, discussions on the definition and measurement of digital addictions, risk and protective factors, and possible mechanisms will be summarised. Subsequently, school-based programmes, family-focused approaches, peer support models, digital literacy and health literacy initiatives, primary care screening and referral strategies, and harm reduction practices at the policy level will be evaluated. Thus, the chapter aims to contribute to the design of evidence-based, equity-focused, and sustainable public health actions in the fight agonist digital addictions.

2. THEORETICAL AND CONCEPTUAL FRAMEWORKS

2.1. Behavioral Addiction Models

Behavioral addiction models conceptualize certain excessive digital behaviors (e.g., gaming, social media engagement, smartphone checking) as sharing core features with substance-related addictions: impaired control, salience/priority, continued use despite harm, and, in some cases, tolerance-like escalation and withdrawal-like distress. Within this perspective, digital platforms can operate as powerful reinforcers through variable-ratio reward schedules (e.g., unpredictable likes, wins, notifications), promoting habit formation and repetitive checking. Contemporary behavioral addiction frameworks emphasize that "addiction-like" patterns are not defined by high use alone, but by functional impairment and the persistence of behavior despite negative consequences.

A clinically anchored example is the WHO's ICD-11 description of gaming disorder, which specifies impaired control, increased priority given to gaming over other activities, and continuation or escalation despite negative consequences, with a requirement for significant impairment in functioning and typically a 12-month pattern (WHO, 2020). This approach supports a public health framing: the goal is not to pathologize normative digital engagement, but to identify the subgroup experiencing measurable harm and requiring prevention and care pathways.

In summary, behavioral addiction models help explain how certain digital behaviors can become compulsive, particularly when reinforced by platform design, and why not all high usage indicates addiction.

2.2. Cognitive-Behavioral Model of Digital Addictions

Cognitive-behavioral approaches propose that problematic digital use is sustained by a reciprocal loop between maladaptive cognitions (e.g., "I am only valued online," "I can't cope offline," "I must check now"), negative affect (stress, loneliness, anxiety), and reinforcing online experiences. A foundational contribution is Davis's cognitive-behavioral model of pathological Internet use, which distinguishes generalized versus specific problematic use and highlights the central role of maladaptive cognitions as proximal drivers of dysregulated behaviors (Schimmenti, 2023).

More recent process-oriented models extend this logic across different digital applications. The I-PACE model (Interaction of Person–Affect–Cognition–Execution) describes how individual predispositions (e.g., impulsivity, psychopathology symptoms), affective and cognitive responses (e.g., craving, attentional bias, coping expectancies), and executive functions interact over time, producing escalating loss of control in specific internet-use behaviors (gaming, social media, pornography, shopping, etc.) (Brand et al., 2016). Complementary theories, such as Compensatory Internet Use, argue that some individuals engage online to compensate for offline stressors or unmet psychological needs; problematic use can thus represent a coping strategy that becomes self-reinforcing when it temporarily reduces distress (Kardefelt-Winther, 2014).

2.3. Neurobiological Mechanisms

Neurobiological accounts do not reduce digital addictions to "brain causes," but they help explain why certain digital activities can become compelling and difficult to regulate. Addiction neuroscience highlights interacting systems related to reward/incentive salience, stress/negative affect, and executive control. Reviews of addiction neurocircuitry emphasize that dysregulation across these systems can promote compulsive seeking and diminished inhibitory control—mechanisms that are plausibly relevant to some forms of compulsive digital engagement (especially when paired with vulnerability factors such as stress, depression, or sleep deprivation) (Koob & Volkow, 2016).

Key syntheses in the brain disease model literature describe how repeated exposure to highly reinforcing stimuli can alter motivational learning and executive control processes, increasing cue reactivity and making "stopping" harder even when the individual intends to reduce use (Volkow et al., 2016). In the context of digital addictions, these mechanisms are often discussed as transdiagnostic: cue-driven attention capture (notifications), habit learning (automatic checking), and stress-related escalation (using digital media to downregulate distress). Importantly, neurobiological explanations should be integrated with social and environmental drivers rather than treated as stand-alone causes.

In summary, neurobiological explanations provide valuable insights into the compulsive nature of certain digital behaviors, especially when combined with psychological vulnerabilities. However, these should be considered alongside social and environmental factors to avoid reductionist interpretations.

2.4. Social-Ecological and Public Health Perspectives

A public health framing situates digital addictions within layered determinants that extend beyond the individual. Social-ecological models emphasize that health behaviors are shaped by interactions across individual, interpersonal, organizational, community, and policy levels (Golden et al., 2015). Applied to digital addictions, this means that family routines, peer norms, school climate, workplace expectations, neighborhood safety (which may limit offline activities), and platform design/policy all influence risk and protection.

From this perspective, prevention and intervention should not rely solely on individual self-control strategies. Instead, it prioritizes multi-level action: digital literacy and coping skills (individual), parent/caregiver mediation and family media plans (interpersonal), school-based prevention and supportive climates (organizational), accessible youth/community activities as healthy alternatives (community), and regulation/industry standards that reduce exploitative engagement design and strengthen protections for minors (policy). This aligns with the broader shift in public health toward structural and systems-level approaches when behaviors are shaped by commercial, technological, and social environments.

This framework illustrates how digital addictions are not only individual choices, but behaviors shaped by broader social and environmental structures, requiring multi-level interventions.

2.5. WHO and APA Conceptualizations of Problematic Digital Use

The WHO's approach is most explicit in relation to gaming: gaming disorder is classified in ICD-11 under "disorders due to addictive behaviours," with diagnostic emphasis on functional impairment and persistence over time (typically ≥12 months). This conceptualization supports health system responses (recognition, standardized assessment, treatment development) while underscoring that only a small proportion of gamers are likely to meet disorder thresholds (WHO, 2020).

The APA, in contrast, has focused recent guidance on adolescent social media exposure and has explicitly highlighted "problematic social media use" as a pattern that can impair functioning. The APA's health advisory recommends that adolescents be routinely screened for signs of problematic social media use that interfere with daily roles and routines and may increase risk for more serious harms over time (APA, 2023). Together, these frameworks converge on two key principles for population health: (1) differentiate high use from harmful, impairing use, and (2) pair individual-level guidance with systemic supports and safer digital environments.

3. DETERMINANTS AND RISK FACTORS

3.1. Individual-Level Factors

Individual characteristics play a fundamental role in the emergence of digital addictions. In terms of personality traits, impulsivity, sensation seeking, low self-control, and neuroticism are the traits most frequently associated with problematic digital use. These traits increase sensitivity to digital applications that offer instant gratification and heighten the risk of loss of control.

Factors related to mental health are also decisive. Depression, anxiety, loneliness, stress, and low subjective well-being can pave the way for the use of digital platforms as a means of escape, emotion regulation, and temporary relief. The literature shows that this relationship is often bidirectional; problematic digital use can increase mental health symptoms, while existing mental health problems can also increase the risk of digital addiction.

From a developmental perspective, adolescence and young adulthood are particularly risky periods. During these periods, while areas of brain development related to executive functions and impulse control are not yet fully mature, the reward system is more sensitive, increasing vulnerability to digital environments (Dumontheil, 2016). Therefore, age should be considered not only as a demographic but also as a biopsychosocial determinant of digital addictions.

3.2. Social and Interpersonal Determinants

The social context in which an individual finds themselves strongly shapes digital usage patterns. At the family level, weak parental supervision, inconsistent media rules, parents' own problematic digital usage patterns, and low family functionality are identified as risk factors, particularly for children and adolescents. In contrast, open communication, shared family activities, and structured digital media plans play a protective role.

Peer influence is particularly evident in the context of social media and online gaming. Peer norms, online visibility, the search for social approval, and fear of exclusion can cause young people to spend more time on digital platforms. In the school environment, academic pressure, school climate, and teacher-student relationships; and in the workplace, the expectation of constant availability, performance pressure, and remote working arrangements can increase the risk of problematic digital use.

In this context, digital addictions should be considered not only as individual preferences but also as behavioural patterns shaped by social roles and expectations (Odgers & Jensen, 2020).

3.3. Environmental and Structural Drivers

Environmental and structural factors play a critical role in the increasing risk of digital addiction. The prevalence of smartphones, high-speed internet access, and the constant availability of digital platforms are key factors that increase usage frequency and duration.

In addition, the design features of digital platforms (e.g. infinite scrolling, autoplay, notifications, personalised algorithms) aim to maximise user engagement and reinforce behavioural addiction mechanisms (Montag et al., 2019). These structures, developed in line with commercial interests, pose a significant public health problem, particularly for vulnerable groups such as children and adolescents.

Digital marketing strategies, micro-targeting, and gamification techniques can also reinforce problematic use. Therefore, digital addictions are increasingly being highlighted as an area that should be addressed within the framework of "commercial determinants of health".

3.4. Sociocultural and Economic Influences

Socio-cultural norms and economic conditions directly and indirectly influence the risk of digital dependency. In societies where digital technologies are equated with productivity, success, and social status, excessive use can be more easily normalised. Furthermore, the perception of an 'online presence obligation' can create pressure, particularly on young people and the working population.

From an economic perspective, low socio-economic status is associated with risk due to limited access to safe physical activity areas, limited cultural and sporting opportunities, and digital tools becoming the most accessible form of entertainment. However, intense academic and professional expectations in high-income groups can also increase the risk of excessive digital use. This situation demonstrates that digital addictions are not a one-sided poverty issue, but rather a context-sensitive, multidimensional phenomenon (van Deursen & Helsper, 2015; Robinson et al., 2015).

3.5. Vulnerable and High-Risk Groups

Evidence suggests that certain groups are at higher risk of digital addiction. Children and adolescents are the most highlighted groups due to their developmental vulnerabilities. In addition, individuals with a history of mental illness, those with neurodevelopmental differences (e.g. ADHD), those experiencing social isolation, and groups under chronic stress are at higher risk (Panagiotidi & Overton, 2018).

In the post-pandemic period, remote education and remote working arrangements have increased digital exposure, particularly for young adults and white-collar workers, and have made problematic usage patterns visible. For migrants, refugees, and disadvantaged communities, digital tools can both provide opportunities for social connection and pose a risk of excessive use.

Therefore, a public health approach should prioritise vulnerable group-sensitive, equity-focused, and context-specific strategies over 'one-size-fits-all' interventions (Boer et al., 2021).

4. EPIDEMIOLOGY OF DIGITAL ADDICTIONS

4.1. Global Prevalence and Cross-National Comparisons

Epidemiological findings on digital addictions present a variable picture due to criteria, scales, sample characteristics, and cultural context, rather than providing a "single global prevalence." One of the best-studied areas is internet gaming disorder/ internet gaming addiction. A recent meta-analysis, evaluating DSM-5-based IGD and ICD-11-based GD studies together, reported a pooled prevalence of 6.7%; it also showed that prevalence rates can differ significantly according to DSM-5 and ICD-11 criteria (Zhou et al., 2024). This finding highlights that "definition/criterion" inconsistencies in cross-country comparisons directly impact epidemiological interpretations.

One of the strongest comparative data sources for problematic social media use (PSMU) is the HBSC (Health Behaviour in School-aged Children) study. The latest WHO/HBSC report states that in a sample covering Europe, Central Asia, and Canada, problematic social media use rose from 7% in 2018 to 11% in 2022; by gender, it was 13% among girls and 9% among boys (Boniel-Nissim et al., 2024). Such standardized international monitoring systems are critical for understanding temporal trends as well as differences between countries.

4.2. Trends in Children, Adolescents, and Young Adults

The epidemiological literature shows that the risk is particularly concentrated during adolescence and young adulthood. WHO/HBSC data reveal that problematic social media use among adolescents increased during the 2018–2022 period and was higher in certain subgroups (especially among adolescent girls) (Boniel-Nissim et al., 2024).

Furthermore, a large-sample study examining concurrent risk patterns at the country/context level (41 countries/regions; n≈171,000) showed that PSMU among adolescents clustered into heterogeneous classes, with the "high problematic use" group representing a small but clinically and public health-relevant subgroup (Lu,

2025). Such findings point to the importance of identifying and targeting high-risk subgroups rather than focusing on "average prevalence."

Adult data on smartphone use is also increasing. For example, a study conducted on a household sample in Singapore reported that the risk of problematic smartphone use was higher in the 21–30 age group and that PSU was associated with anxiety, depressive symptoms, and poor sleep quality (Ong et al., 2024). This suggests that digital addictions are not limited to adolescents; however, they may become more pronounced during developmental transition periods (adolescence, transition to college, early adulthood).

4.3. Gender, SES, and Cultural Variations

Gender differences may exhibit a pattern that varies according to the type of digital addiction. In HBSC reporting, the fact that problematic social media use is higher among girls is evaluated in conjunction with mechanisms such as social approval/peer interaction and online visibility pressure (Boniel-Nissim et al., 2024). On the other hand, while some samples in the gaming disorder literature report higher risk among boys (especially in game-focused measurements), diagnostic criteria and sample type can significantly influence the magnitude of this difference (Zhou et al., 2024).

In terms of socioeconomic status (SES) and cultural context, multi-country analyses show that economic deprivation can increase risk at the individual level; at the national level, structural indicators such as educational inequality and gender inequality can be associated with higher risk profiles (Lu, 2025). This finding demonstrates that epidemiology provides answers not only to the question "Who has more?" but also to the question "Which social conditions increase the risk?"

4.4. Measurement Tools and Challenges in Assessment

The greatest challenge in the epidemiology of digital addictions is the heterogeneity of measurement tools and cutoff points. The use of different scales for the same behavioral domain, different time windows (past 12 months / past 3 months / past week), self-report-based biases, and the lack of validation through clinical interviews directly affect prevalence estimates.

Examples of commonly used scales in this field:

- **Gaming**: IGDS9-SF (Internet Gaming Disorder Scale–Short Form) is a widely used psychometric measure (Monacis et al., 2016; Evren et al., 2018).

· **Social media**: The Social Media Disorder Scale (SMD-9) and Bergen Social Media Addiction Scale (BSMAS) are common in international Studies (van den Eijnden et al., 2016; Lin et al., 2017; Zarate et al., 2022).
· **Smartphone**: The Smartphone Application-Based Addiction Scale (SABAS) stands out for its short length and suitability for screening purposes (Csibi et al., 2018; Peng et al., 2023).

However, the distinction between "high use" and "problematic/disruptive use" must be epidemiologically clear: While monitoring systems such as WHO/HBSC attempt to standardize PSMU based on "addictive-like symptoms" (World Health Organization & International HBSC Network, 2023), the different conceptualizations of DSM-5 and ICD-11 in the gaming field can directly lead to prevalence differences (Zhou et al., 2024). Therefore, when reporting epidemiological results, the definition/scale used, cutoff point, time window, and sample characteristics must be clearly specified.

5. PUBLIC HEALTH IMPACTS OF DIGITAL ADDICTIONS

5.1. Mental Health Outcomes

One of the most visible public health burdens of problematic digital use is mental health outcomes. Systematic reviews and meta-analyses examining problematic social media use (PSMU) among adolescents and young adults show that PSMU is associated with higher levels of depression and anxiety symptoms and higher stress levels (Shannon et al., 2022). Similarly, meta-analytic evidence focusing on problematic smartphone use (PSU) reports that PSU is significantly associated with depression and anxiety risk (Yang et al., 2020).

In terms of policy and practice, the U.S. Surgeon General's Advisory and the APA's health advisory on social media use in adolescents emphasize that adolescence is a developmentally vulnerable period, that the distinction between "high use" and "problematic/disruptive use" is important, and that screening for risky patterns is necessary (American Psychological Association, 2023; Office of the Surgeon General (OSG), 2023).

Beyond adolescents, problematic digital use increasingly affects the adult workforce. Expectations of constant online availability, digital multitasking, and blurred work–life boundaries may contribute to reduced productivity, burnout, and occupational stress. From a public health perspective, these patterns represent indirect economic costs through decreased work efficiency, increased absenteeism, and rising demand for mental health services.

5.2. Physical Health Consequences

The most consistent relationships in terms of physical health are seen through sleep and sedentary behavior. Systematic reviews and meta-analyses on the relationship between PSU and sleep problems show that PSU is associated with poor sleep quality and risk of sleep disorders (Akbari et al., 2023). These patterns are further reinforced by behaviors such as increased nighttime use, sleep interruptions due to notifications, and bedtime delay (An & Zhang, 2024).

A sedentary lifestyle and reduced physical activity are considered indirect but critical consequences of digital addiction. The WHO positions reducing sedentary time and increasing regular physical activity as a fundamental public health priority for protecting health; this framework also guides efforts to reduce risks associated with screen-based lifestyles (Bull et al., 2020).

5.3. Cognitive and Developmental Implications

Problematic digital use during childhood and adolescence is associated with negative effects in developmental areas such as attention processes, impulse control, emotion regulation, and social cognition. Clinically, the issue is not the high amount of "screen time" alone, but rather that usage interferes with developmental tasks (sleep, learning, face-to-face relationships, physical activity) to a disruptive degree and is accompanied by loss of control. At this point, APA and Surgeon General documents draw attention to developmental sensitivity, safety/protection measures, and early recognition of problematic patterns (American Psychological Association, 2023; Office of the Surgeon General (OSG), 2023).

5.4. Academic, Occupational, and Social Functioning

Educational and functional outcomes represent the "invisible" but costly part of the public health burden. Recent systematic reviews and meta-analyses examining the relationship between problematic smartphone use and academic achievement report a statistically significant (usually small to moderate) negative association between PSU and lower academic achievement (Sunday et al., 2021; Paterna et al., 2024).

Evidence is similar regarding gaming behavior: a systematic review examining the relationship between "problematic gaming/IGD" and students' academic performance generally points to a trend of negative academic outcomes (Alzahrani & Griffiths, 2025).

In the workplace, problematic digital use can trigger processes such as distraction, loss of productivity, work-home conflict, and burnout. These effects become more pronounced when combined with the norms of "always being available" and the pressure of digital communication (organizational expectations, remote work, after-hours messaging, etc.).

5.5. Family and Community-Level Effects

The effects of digital addiction are not limited to the individual; they also have consequences on family interactions, home routines, caregiver-child relationships, and social participation. At the family level, conflict, reduced shared time, and unclear household rules can fuel risk cycles; at the community level, school climate, peer norms, and the availability of safe/accessible activity spaces in the neighborhood (sports, culture, safe social spaces) can either prevent or accelerate digital use becoming the "only option." Therefore, the Surgeon General and APA frameworks emphasize the importance of multi-layered protective actions at the family-school-community and policy levels, not just individual Recommendations (American Psychological Association, 2023; Office of the Surgeon General (OSG), 2023).

6. PREVENTION AND EARLY INTERVENTION STRATEGIES

6.1. Health Promotion Approaches

Preventing digital addictions, when addressed through a health promotion approach in public health, aims not only to reduce risky behaviors but also to strengthen psychosocial well-being, self-regulation skills, and healthy lifestyles. The health promotion principles emphasized in the World Health Organization's Ottawa Charter provide guidance for preventing digital addictions in terms of developing individual skills, creating supportive environments, and implementing healthy public policies (WHO, 1986).

In this context, effective approaches include programs focused on coping with stress, regulating emotions, managing time, and strengthening social bonds. Encouraging physical activity, supporting sleep hygiene, and increasing offline social activities stand out as key protective strategies that can indirectly reduce excessive digital use (Bull et al., 2020). The health promotion perspective makes it possible to address digital addictions as a preventable and modifiable behavioral risk rather than an "individual weakness."

It is critical to distinguish between clinically diagnosed Gaming Disorder, as defined in ICD-11, and broader patterns of problematic digital use such as social media or smartphone overuse. While Gaming Disorder requires structured clinical assessment and, in many cases, specialized treatment pathways, interventions targeting problematic social media use should primarily focus on digital hygiene, health promotion, and preventive strategies. Maintaining this distinction is essential to avoid over-pathologizing normative digital behaviors.

6.2. School-Based Prevention Programs

Schools are one of the most critical settings for preventing digital addiction among children and adolescents. School-based programs can be structured at universal (for all students), selective (for at-risk groups), and indicator-based (for students showing early signs) levels. Evidence shows that social-emotional learning (SEL)-based programs reduce the risk of problematic digital use by developing self-regulation, problem-solving, and healthy relationship skills (Durlak et al., 2011). For instance, the "Media Heroes" program implemented in several European schools integrates social-emotional learning with digital literacy to reduce problematic media use among adolescents. Evaluations have shown improvements in self-regulation and peer relationships (Agbakoba et al., 2016).

School-based interventions targeting problematic social media use and gaming behavior include components such as digital awareness, coping with peer pressure, online risks, and encouraging offline activities. WHO and UNICEF recommend supporting digital well-being in the school environment, integrating it with mental health services, and empowering teachers to recognize early warning signs (UNICEF, 2021; WHO, 2022). The success of school-based programs is closely related to family involvement and school climate.

6.3. Family-Oriented Interventions

The family plays a central role in shaping digital usage patterns, especially for children and adolescents. Family-focused interventions focus on parental guidance, media parenting (parental mediation), and strengthening family communication. Research shows that consistent rules, age-appropriate limits, and open communication reduce the risk of problematic digital use (Nikken & Schols, 2015).

Effective family-based strategies include shared "family media plans," increasing screen-free time together, and parents modeling healthy digital behaviors. The APA recommends that families evaluate the dimensions of content, context, and functionality together, rather than focusing solely on time limits (APA, 2023). This approach emphasizes the goal of balance and responsible use rather than completely banning digital technologies.

6.4. Digital Literacy and Responsible Use Education

Digital literacy is increasingly recognized as an important public health tool in preventing digital addictions. Digital literacy education encompasses not only technical skills, but also dimensions such as critical thinking, algorithmic awareness, privacy and security, digital footprint, and ethical use. UNESCO and the OECD position digital literacy among the essential life skills of the 21st century (OECD, 2021; UNESCO, 2018).

Responsible digital use education supports individuals in monitoring their own usage patterns, recognizing risky behaviors, and setting healthy boundaries in the digital environment. Such education contributes to understanding the difference between "high usage" and "problematic usage," particularly among young people, and prevents stigmatizing approaches.

6.5. Screening and Early Detection in Community Settings

Early diagnosis and intervention are critical in reducing the public health burden of digital addictions. Primary care services, school health services, university health centers, and community mental health units are appropriate points of contact for screening and early intervention. The use of brief and valid screening tools (e.g., BSMAS, IGDS9-SF, SABAS) enables the early identification of at-risk individuals (Monacis et al., 2016; van den Eijnden et al., 2016).

In community settings, peer-led workshops that combine digital hygiene education with sports and social activities have been piloted in urban youth centers in Canada and Australia, showing promising reductions in screen time and improvements in sleep routines.

APA and Surgeon General guidelines recommend integrating indicators of problematic digital use, particularly in adolescents, into routine mental health assessments (APA, 2023; Office of the Surgeon General, 2023). Using screening results for risk identification and referral rather than clinical diagnosis aligns with a preventive public health approach that reduces stigma. Early interventions should include brief counseling, psychoeducation, and referral to specialized services when necessary.

7. CLINICAL AND PSYCHOSOCIAL TREATMENT APPROACHES

7.1. Cognitive Behavioral Therapy (CBT) for Digital Addictions

CBT is the most frequently used and most evidence-based approach in the clinical management of digital addictions. The focus of the intervention is on recognizing triggering situations, restructuring dysfunctional thoughts, managing urges/cravings, behavioral activation, time management, and relapse prevention. Meta-analytic evidence indicates that CBT can reduce symptom severity and associated anxiety/depression, particularly in the field of internet gaming disorder (IGD/GD) (Stevens et al., 2019; Núñez-Rodríguez et al., 2025).

However, differences in sample size, definition/criterion heterogeneity, and follow-up duration across studies necessitate context-sensitive interpretation of the "effect size." (Reangsing et al., 2025). In clinical practice, it is recommended that CBT be adapted in a modular manner according to comorbidities (depression, anxiety, ADHD, sleep disorders) and level of functional impairment.

Clinical interventions described in this section are primarily applicable to individuals meeting diagnostic thresholds or experiencing significant functional impairment. In contrast, individuals exhibiting subclinical or self-reported problematic digital use may benefit more from low-intensity, preventive, and community-based interventions.

It is important to distinguish between preventive interventions aimed at individuals with subclinical or early-risk patterns and clinical treatments designed for those who meet diagnostic criteria for disorders such as Gaming Disorder. While CBT and integrated care models are typically reserved for clinically significant cases, mindfulness and motivational interviewing may be adapted for early intervention or preventive contexts depending on severity and functional impairment.

7.2. Mindfulness and Emotion Regulation Interventions

Mindfulness-based approaches and emotion regulation interventions target the avoidance/emotion regulation-driven use cycle, a key mechanism underlying digital addictions. Mindfulness practices can provide protective/remedial benefits by fostering awareness of automatic, uncontrolled use, developing the ability to "pause" when urges arise, and regulating stress responses. A recent meta-analysis examining the relationship between mindfulness and problematic smartphone use indicates that mindfulness-focused approaches can lead to meaningful improvement in problematic use (Ru et al., 2025).

Furthermore, an RCT meta-analysis showing that mindfulness/self-compassion/acceptance-based content can be taught via smartphone apps suggests that digital health tools may be a scalable option (Linardon, 2020).

7.3. Motivational Interviewing and Behavioral Contracting

Motivational Interviewing (MI) is an appropriate approach for working with the ambivalence (wanting to quit but also wanting to continue) commonly seen in digital addictions. MI aims to increase readiness for change, clarify goals, and strengthen self-efficacy (participation–focus–evocation–planning steps) (Miller & Rollnick, 2013).

Regarding digital addictions, MI-based intervention protocols conducted online/remotely and school-based group MI applications show promising findings that they may improve change motivation and some behavioral outcomes; however, more high-quality RCTs and long-term follow-ups are needed (Dieris-Hirche et al., 2021; Tse et al., 2024).

Behavioral contracting and "staged goals" (e.g., reducing weeknight use, limiting notifications, screen-free alternative routines) are particularly applicable in adolescents with family/school collaboration; monitoring the contract and planning positive reinforcements can increase the sustainability of the intervention.

7.4. Technology-Assisted Interventions

Technology-based interventions for digital addictions (apps, online counseling/telemedicine, digital monitoring, and feedback) are rapidly increasing. A systematic review examining technology-based interventions for internet-related addictive behaviors highlights the advantages of this approach in terms of accessibility and scalability, while noting heterogeneity in study quality and outcome measures (Peñafiel Mora et al., 2025).

However, adherence is a fundamental challenge in digital interventions: meta-analytic evidence on smartphone-based mental health interventions shows high dropout rates and low participation are common (Linardon & Fuller-Tyszkiewicz, 2020). Therefore, in app-based programs, "micro-habits," personalization, balanced use of reminders, and user-friendly design are crucial.

While AI-based tools (e.g., psychoeducation via chatbots, self-monitoring, and referral) have been explored in substance use, security, privacy, clinical boundaries, and crisis referral protocols must be clarified when adapting them for digital addictions (Lee et al., 2024).

7.5. Integrated Public Health and Clinical Pathways

Because the burden of digital addictions is widespread at the societal level, an effective response requires integrated care pathways that combine clinical and public health components. The WHO's inclusion of gaming disorder in ICD-11 provides a framework that supports identification, assessment, and service development processes in health systems (WHO, 2020). Field studies examining the clinical applicability of the ICD-11 diagnostic guidelines provide evidence of the guidelines' clinical reliability (Ma et al., 2021).

In practice, an integrated roadmap can be designed in the following steps:

- Community/school/primary care screening (short scales + functional impairment inquiry),
- Brief intervention (psychoeducation, sleep hygiene, behavioral goals, MI-based interview),
- Referral (CBT/emotion regulation-based psychotherapy; comorbidity management),
- Follow-up and relapse prevention (family/school support, digital environment adjustments, technology-assisted follow-up if necessary).

This integration helps to manage clinical service needs more rationally by promoting low-intensity interventions in the early stages while maintaining the distinction between "high use" and "dysfunctional/problematic use."

8. COMMUNITY-BASED INTERVENTIONS

8.1. Community Needs Assessment and Risk Mapping

The first step for community-based interventions to be effective is the systematic identification of local needs and mapping of risks. Community needs assessment (CNA) processes aim to reveal digital usage patterns, at-risk groups, existing resources, and service gaps. In this process, it is recommended to use quantitative data (surveys, school/health records, screening scales) together with qualitative data (focus group interviews, stakeholder meetings) (Minkler & Wallerstein, 2008).

Risk mapping in the context of digital addictions may include variables such as age groups, school districts, socioeconomic indicators, access to digital infrastructure, and the availability of alternative social/recreational spaces. This approach enables the development of context-sensitive, targeted community-based strategies rather than a "one-size-fits-all" intervention, thereby strengthening the principle of equity in public health (WHO, 2014).

8.2. Community Empowerment and Peer Support Programs

Community-based interventions focus on empowerment. The empowerment approach aims to enable individuals and communities to gain control over factors that affect their health. Peer support programs in preventing digital addiction enable young people to develop awareness and model healthy digital behaviors based on their own experiences.

Peer-based interventions are particularly effective in reshaping social norms among adolescents and young adults. There is strong public health evidence that school- and community-based peer leadership programs are effective in reducing risky behaviors and improving psychosocial well-being (Campbell & Cornish, 2010). In the field of digital addiction, these programs can target healthy digital habits, the promotion of offline social activities, and the strengthening of supportive social networks.

8.3. School–Family–Community Collaboration Models

Digital addictions are a multidimensional problem that cannot be solved by the intervention of a single institution. Therefore, school-family-community cooperation models are of critical importance. Based on a socioecological approach, these models involve the coordination of school policies, family media guidance, and community resources (youth centers, sports clubs, libraries) (McLeroy et al., 1988).

Effective collaboration models include regular communication channels, shared goals, and role sharing. UNICEF and WHO recommend integrating school-based programs with family and community support to protect the mental health of children and adolescents (UNICEF, 2021; WHO, 2022). In terms of digital addictions, this integration ensures that risks identified early in school are referred to family and community services in a timely manner.

8.4. Local Government and NGO-Led Initiatives

Local governments and civil society organizations (CSOs) have the capacity to produce structural and sustainable solutions to prevent digital addiction. Youth centers, sports and cultural programs, and safe public spaces run by municipalities offer alternative channels for social participation to digital environments. At the same time, local governments can develop policies that support digital well-being (school environment regulations, youth services, social awareness campaigns).

CSOs are important actors in terms of advocacy, education, and access to vulnerable groups. The WHO's commercial determinants of health framework emphasizes the importance of public-NGO partnerships to balance the impact of digital platforms' commercial interests on public health (WHO, 2023). In this context, initiatives at the local level contribute to addressing digital addiction not only as an individual but also as a social problem.

8.5. Community-Based Monitoring and Evaluation

The sustainability of community-based interventions depends on the effectiveness of monitoring and evaluation (M&E) systems. M&E processes aim to monitor the reach, implementation quality, and short- and long-term outcomes of interventions. Monitoring indicators in the field of digital addictions may include problematic use frequency, intermediate outputs such as sleep and physical activity, academic/ functional indicators, and subjective well-being measurements.

Participatory monitoring approaches encourage active participation of community members in evaluation processes and increase program ownership (Minkler & Wallerstein, 2008). WHO's community mental health and health promotion guidelines emphasize that M&E systems based on local data and incorporating feedback loops strengthen the effectiveness and scalability of interventions (WHO, 2014). This approach enables the continuous improvement of community-based programs developed for digital addictions.

9. POLICY, REGULATION, AND ETHICAL CONSIDERATIONS

9.1. National Policies Targeting Digital Well-Being

National policies for digital well-being are generally shaped around three axes:

1. Online protection of children,
2. Early recognition of problematic use/addiction-like patterns and access to services,
3. Risk reduction through design and data governance.

The inclusion of gaming disorder in ICD-11 provides a framework that could strengthen countries' clinical service planning and epidemiological surveillance capacity; the WHO emphasizes that for diagnosis, the behavioral pattern must cause significant functional impairment and typically last at least 12 months. This approach supports a policy focus on dysfunctional/problematic use rather than "high use." (WHO, 2020).

Effective policy design at the national level requires a cross-sectoral perspective that acknowledges that digital harms cannot be explained by individual choice alone; education, social welfare, the media ecosystem, and platform design must be addressed together. At this point, the WHO's "Health in All Policies (HiAP)" framework provides a roadmap that recommends the systematic integration of health into other sector policies (Health in All Policies (HiAP) framework for country action, 2014).

To translate conceptual insights into practice, public health authorities should focus on multi-level implementation: from brief intervention models in primary care, to cross-sectoral coordination with education, mental health, and technology governance bodies.

9.2. Regulation of Social Media Platforms and Gaming

The EU's Digital Services Act (DSA) framework is one of the most recent examples of regulating the platform and gaming ecosystem. The DSA imposes obligations on online intermediaries and platforms regarding risk management, transparency, accountability, and the protection of minors (European Commission, 2025). In the implementation of the DSA, topics such as "addictive design," "dark patterns," advertising transparency, and researchers' access to data are particularly prominent on the regulatory agenda (European Parliament, 2024).

In the United Kingdom, the Online Safety Act 2023 defines new obligations aimed at protecting children and adults in the online environment; it imposes risk reduction and system/process-based security responsibilities on platforms. These regulations show that "harmful design and interaction architecture" has become as much a policy issue as "harmful content" in digital addictions (GOV.UK., 2024).

9.3. Data Privacy, Surveillance Risks, and Ethical Challenges

One of the most sensitive areas of digital well-being policies is balancing data privacy and surveillance risks with public health objectives. The EU General Data Protection Regulation (GDPR) centers on principles such as lawfulness, fairness/transparency, purpose limitation, data minimization, security, and accountability in the processing of personal data (European Union, 2016). These principles are particularly relevant in terms of protecting children's data, targeted advertising, behavioral tracking, and "addictive" personalization practices.

Furthermore, the ethical principles developed by the WHO for digital health solutions emphasize the need to uphold values such as human rights, do no harm, fairness, transparency, and accountability in the design and implementation of digital systems (WHO, 2024). WHO guidelines on the use of generative AI/LMMs in health and public health also highlight ethical challenges such as privacy and security risks, as well as mis/malicious outputs, explainability, and responsibility (WHO, 2025).

9.4. Intersectoral Policy Frameworks

The policy response to digital addictions often remains fragmented when limited to a single ministry/agency. Therefore, effective frameworks include: health (screening–early intervention–clinical referral), education (school-based programs and digital literacy), telecom/BTK-like regulators (access, advertising, data governance), and justice/child protection (abuse, bullying, illegal content, age verification). The HiAP approach offers a practical "country action framework" to institutionalize this coordination (WHO, 2014).

A rights-based approach to the digital environment for children suggests that regulations should not only aim to "restrict" but also to support participation, protection, and development. The Council of Europe's guidelines on children's rights in the digital environment elaborate on this rights-based balance (Council of Europe, 2018).

9.5. Global Guidelines and WHO Recommendations

Three main reference points stand out for global policy:

WHO: By defining gaming disorder within the scope of ICD-11, it provides a common language for monitoring, comparability, and service planning; it also supports efforts to develop diagnostic/classification and screening tools (WHO, 2020).

OECD: Proposes "risk-proportionate" policy principles to balance children's safety and benefits in the digital environment and emphasizes multi-stakeholder governance (Organisation for Economic Co-operation and Development, 2025).

UNICEF: Provides policy guidance on platform regulation for child safety and analysis of current global regulatory trends; highlights design, accountability, and implementation/monitoring components centered on children's rights (UNICEF, 2025).

In summary, an effective regulatory response to digital addictions requires coherence across multiple domains—platform design standards, data governance, children's rights protections, and ethical AI deployment. While sector-specific policies are essential, their integration under a unified public health and digital wellbeing framework remains critical for sustainable impact.

10. FUTURE DIRECTIONS AND INNOVATIONS

10.1. Artificial Intelligence and Predictive Analytics in Prevention

In the prevention field, artificial intelligence (AI) and predictive analytics hold the potential to capture the early signs of problematic digital use and personalize interventions. This approach can generate risk scores by combining;

1. Self-report surveys (scales),
2. Passive digital traces (screen time, nighttime usage patterns, notification intensity), and
3. Contextual data (school term stress, exam weeks, shifts/work hours).

For example, studies aimed at predicting addiction risk in VR users show that predictive models can be developed using variables such as usage time and type of use (He et al., 2025).

However, ethical governance is critical for the use of such systems in public health: data minimization, explainability, reduction of bias risks, protection of children, and clarification of clinical liability boundaries must be ensured. The WHO's "AI ethics and governance" guide for large multi-modal models (LMM) provides comprehensive recommendations for governments, technology companies, and healthcare providers, laying the foundation for the safe scaling of this field (WHO, 2025).

10.2. Human–Technology Interaction and Design for Digital Well-Being

The focus of the future innovation agenda will shift from the goal of "keeping users engaged longer" to interaction design that supports digital well-being. HCI (human–computer interaction) literature highlights "behavioral science-based" design interventions to enhance digital well-being:

- Transparent feedback (time tracking dashboards),
- Deliberate friction (e.g., "suggesting a break before continuing"),
- Redesigning notification architecture (mindful notifications),
- Default settings optimized for well-being (e.g., silencing notifications in night mode) (Al-Mansoori et al., 2023).

In parallel, work at the intersection of "addictive design" and "dark patterns" argues that hyper-interactive designs can erode user autonomy and should therefore be subject to regulatory/ethical scrutiny. The innovation track is therefore not only focused on creating new "digital well-being applications," but also on aligning the core design of platforms with harm reduction principles (Esposito et al., 2024; Ye, 2025).

10.3. Emerging Addictions

While concerns regarding addiction-like dynamics are emerging, AI companions and immersive technologies have also shown potential therapeutic benefits, particularly in reducing loneliness and providing psychosocial support, when appropriately designed, regulated, and ethically governed.

The metaverse, VR/AR, and AI companion systems possess three characteristics that could increase the risk of digital addiction: high immersion, intense social rewards, and personalized recommendation systems. The literature on the Metaverse's addiction potential emphasizes that interaction and immersiveness can reinforce "classic" social media/gaming addiction mechanisms; however, epidemiological evidence specific to the Metaverse is still limited (Jia & Nkoulou Mvondo, 2025).

In contrast, systematic/qualitative review studies published in 2025 show that metaverse use has been reported to be associated with negative experiences such as loneliness, depressive mood, and social anxiety for some users; they also indicate that the concept of "metaverse addiction" has begun to be discussed (Aboul-Yazeed et al., 2025). On the VR side, both analytical studies predicting addiction risk (He et al., 2025) and publications addressing the therapeutic benefits and risks of VR/AR together necessitate a "double-edged sword" (benefit + harm) approach (Buragohain et al., 2025).

Specifically for AI companions (chat bots/emotional support bots), addiction dynamics can develop through attachment, coping with loneliness, and reward/reinforcement cycles. As this field is growing rapidly, safety, privacy, age appropriateness, and crisis referral standards will be key innovation topics in clinical and public health approaches (especially for children).

10.4. Equity-Centered Public Health Approaches

In the future, the most critical aspect of combating digital dependencies will be the institutionalization of equality-centered approaches rather than solutions designed for the "average user." Digital inequalities manifest not only in terms of access (internet/devices) but also in terms of digital literacy, quality of use, capacity to benefit, and exposure to risks. Therefore, digital well-being interventions require a design that strengthens infrastructure and literacy in low-resource areas, adapts to the needs of vulnerable groups, and monitors the risk of discrimination. A recent scoping review summarizing digital health equity frameworks shows that principles ensuring equity throughout "intervention design + implementation + evaluation" are becoming increasingly clear in this field (Hatef et al., 2024; Kim & Backonja, 2025).

Furthermore, at the policy level, the "equity-by-design" approach is also emerging in digital mental health and digital well-being regulations (e.g., equity-centered regulatory tools). regulatoryrapporteur.org This orientation reaffirms that digital addictions are not merely individual clinical problems; they are public health issues that interact with structural conditions and commercial drivers.

11. FUTURE RESEARCH DIRECTIONS

Despite rapid growth in the literature, several critical gaps remain in digital addiction research. One of the most pressing needs is for longitudinal and life-course studies that clarify causal pathways between digital use patterns and mental, physical, and social health outcomes. Much of the existing evidence relies on cross-sectional, self-reported data, limiting the ability to distinguish antecedents from consequences. Long-term cohort studies would enable a more precise understanding of risk trajectories, resilience factors, and critical developmental windows.

Future research should also prioritize the refinement and harmonization of measurement tools. Variability in definitions, diagnostic thresholds, and screening instruments continues to hinder comparability across studies and countries. Developing consensus-driven, functionally oriented assessment frameworks that clearly differentiate high engagement from harmful or impairing use is essential for both epidemiological surveillance and clinical practice.

Another important direction involves evaluating the effectiveness and sustainability of multi-level interventions. While short-term improvements have been reported for school-based programs, digital detox interventions, and psychosocial treatments, evidence on long-term outcomes, scalability, and equity impacts remains limited. Implementation research that examines contextual factors, community participation, and policy integration will be critical for translating evidence into sustainable public health practice.

Emerging technologies also warrant careful investigation. Artificial intelligence, immersive virtual environments, and AI-based social agents may introduce new forms of digital engagement with both therapeutic potential and addiction risk. Future studies should adopt a balanced, ethics-informed approach that examines benefits and harms simultaneously, with particular attention to vulnerable populations such as children, adolescents, and socially disadvantaged groups.

Finally, equity-centered research agendas are needed to address digital addictions as a social and structural phenomenon. Future studies should examine how digital inequalities, commercial determinants, and policy environments interact to shape risk and protection, ensuring that prevention and intervention strategies do not inadvertently widen existing health disparities.

12. CONCLUSION

Digital addictions have emerged as a complex and evolving public health challenge shaped by rapid technological innovation, individual vulnerabilities, social contexts, and structural determinants. As this chapter has demonstrated, problematic digital use cannot be reduced to excessive screen time alone; rather, it reflects patterns of impaired control, functional impairment, and continued use despite harm, with consequences that extend from individual mental and physical health to families, communities, and broader social systems.

Drawing on theoretical models, epidemiological evidence, and public health frameworks, this chapter highlights that digital addictions are multidimensional phenomena. Behavioral and cognitive-behavioral models, neurobiological mechanisms, and socio-ecological perspectives collectively underscore the need for integrated explanations that move beyond individual blame. Epidemiological data reveal substantial cross-national and developmental variation, while persistent challenges in measurement remind us that policy and practice must be grounded in transparent, context-sensitive assessment approaches.

The public health impacts of digital addictions are far-reaching. Associations with anxiety, depression, sleep disturbance, sedentary lifestyles, cognitive and developmental concerns, and impairments in academic, occupational, and social functioning underscore the importance of early, preventive action. Importantly, these harms are not evenly distributed: children, adolescents, young adults, and socially disadvantaged groups bear a disproportionate burden, reinforcing the necessity of equity-centered strategies.

Prevention and response efforts are most effective when they are multi-level and coordinated. Health promotion initiatives, school-based and family-oriented programs, digital literacy education, and early screening in community settings provide complementary entry points for action. At the clinical level, evidence-based psychosocial interventions—particularly cognitive behavioral therapy, mindfulness-based approaches, and motivational interviewing—offer meaningful benefits when embedded within integrated care pathways that link community services with specialized treatment.

At the policy level, national regulations, platform governance, and global guidance—especially those led by the World Health Organization—play a critical role in shaping safer digital environments. Regulatory attention to platform design, data privacy, ethical use of artificial intelligence, and intersectoral collaboration across health, education, telecommunications, and justice sectors is essential for sustainable impact. Looking ahead, innovations in artificial intelligence, predictive analytics, and human-centered design offer new opportunities for prevention, provided they are implemented with robust ethical oversight and a commitment to reducing digital health inequities.

Public health systems can operationalize these insights by integrating digital addiction screening into primary care protocols, supporting school- and community-based prevention programs, and collaborating across sectors to address commercial drivers through regulation and policy design.

In conclusion, addressing digital addictions requires a shift from fragmented, individual-level responses toward coherent public health strategies that integrate theory, evidence, community action, clinical care, and policy. By aligning prevention and intervention efforts with principles of equity, participation, and ethical governance, public health systems can better mitigate the harms of digital addictions while preserving the undeniable benefits of digital technologies. This integrated approach is critical for promoting digital well-being and safeguarding population health in an increasingly connected world.

REFERENCES

Aboul-Yazeed, R. S., Darwish, A., & Hassanien, A. E. (2025). Flourish the mood: A systematic review on the impacts of metaverse on psychological and mental health. *Frontiers in Virtual Reality*, *6*, 1429038. DOI: 10.3389/frvir.2025.1429038

Agbakoba, R., McGee-Lennon, M., Bouamrane, M.-M., Watson, N., & Mair, F. S. (2016). Implementation factors affecting the large-scale deployment of digital health and well-being technologies: A qualitative study of the initial phases of the 'Living-It-Up' programme. *Health Informatics Journal*, *22*(4), 867–877. DOI: 10.1177/1460458215594651 PMID: 26276795

Akbari, M., Seydavi, M., Sheikhi, S., & Spada, M. M. (2023). Problematic smartphone use and sleep disturbance: The roles of metacognitions, desire thinking, and emotion regulation. *Frontiers in Psychiatry*, *14*, 1137533. DOI: 10.3389/fpsyt.2023.1137533 PMID: 37593452

Al-Mansoori, R. S., Al-Thani, D., Ali, R., & Yan, Z. (2023). Designing for digital wellbeing: From theory to practice — a scoping review. *Human Behavior and Emerging Technologies*, *9924029*, 1–24. Advance online publication. DOI: 10.1155/2023/9924029

Alzahrani, A. K. D., & Griffiths, M. D. (2025). Problematic gaming and students' academic performance: A systematic review. *International Journal of Mental Health and Addiction*, *23*(5), 4062–4095. DOI: 10.1007/s11469-024-01338-5

American Psychological Association. (2023, May 9). *Health advisory on social media use in adolescence*. American Psychological Association. https://www.apa.org/topics/social-media-internet/health-advisory-adolescent-social-media-use

An, Y., & Zhang, M. X. (2024). Relationship between problematic smartphone use and sleep problems: The roles of sleep-related compensatory health beliefs and bedtime procrastination. *Digital Health*, *10*, 20552076241283338. DOI: 10.1177/20552076241283338 PMID: 39291154

Boer, M., Stevens, G. W. J. M., Finkenauer, C., de Looze, M. E., & van den Eijnden, R. J. J. M. (2021). Social media use intensity, social media use problems, and mental health among adolescents. *Computers in Human Behavior*, *116*, 106645. DOI: 10.1016/j.chb.2020.106645

Boniel-Nissim, M., Marino, C., Galeotti, T., Blinka, L., Ozoliņa, K., Craig, W., Lahti, H., Wong, S. L., Brown, J., Wilson, M., Inchley, J., & van den Eijnde, R. (Eds.). (2024). *A focus on adolescent social media use and gaming in Europe, Central Asia and Canada: Health Behaviour in School-aged Children international report from the 2021/2022 survey* (Vol. 6). World Health Organization Regional Office for Europe.

Brand, M., Young, K. S., Laier, C., Wölfling, K., & Potenza, M. N. (2016). Integrating psychological and neurobiological considerations regarding the development and maintenance of specific Internet-use disorders: An Interaction of Person-Affect-Cognition-Execution (I-PACE) model. *Neuroscience and Biobehavioral Reviews, 71*, 252–266. DOI: 10.1016/j.neubiorev.2016.08.033 PMID: 27590829

Bull, F. C., Al-Ansari, S. S., Biddle, S., Borodulin, K., Buman, M. P., Cardon, G., Carty, C., Chaput, J. P., Chastin, S., Chou, R., Dempsey, P. C., DiPietro, L., Ekelund, U., Firth, J., Friedenreich, C. M., Garcia, L., Gichu, M., Jago, R., Katzmarzyk, P. T., & Willumsen, J. F. (2020). World Health Organization 2020 guidelines on physical activity and sedentary behaviour. *British Journal of Sports Medicine, 54*(24), 1451–1462. DOI: 10.1136/bjsports-2020-102955 PMID: 33239350

Buragohain, D., Khichar, S., Deng, C., Meng, Y., & Chaudhary, S. (2025). Analyzing metaverse-based digital therapies, their effectiveness, and potential risks in mental healthcare. *Scientific Reports, 15*(1), 17066. DOI: 10.1038/s41598-025-00916-4 PMID: 40379748

Campbell, C., & Cornish, F. (2010). Towards a "fourth generation" of approaches to HIV/AIDS management: Creating contexts for effective community mobilisation. *AIDS Care, 22*(sup2, S2), 1569–1579. DOI: 10.1080/09540121.2010.525812 PMID: 21161761

Council of Europe. (2018). *Guidelines to respect, protect and fulfil the rights of the child in relation to the digital environment*. Council of Europe. https://rm.coe.int/guidelines-to-respect-protect-and-fulfil-the-rights-of-the-child-in-th/16808d881a

Csibi, S., Griffiths, M. D., Cook, B., Demetrovics, Z., & Szabo, A. (2018). The Psychometric Properties of the Smartphone Application-Based Addiction Scale (SABAS). *International Journal of Mental Health and Addiction, 16*(2), 393–403. DOI: 10.1007/s11469-017-9787-2 PMID: 29670500

Darvesh, N., Radhakrishnan, A., Lachance, C. C., Nincic, V., Sharpe, J. P., Ghassemi, M., Straus, S. E., & Tricco, A. C. (2020). Exploring the prevalence of gaming disorder and Internet gaming disorder: A rapid scoping review. *Systematic Reviews, 9*(1), 68. DOI: 10.1186/s13643-020-01329-2 PMID: 32241295

Dieris-Hirche, J., Bottel, L., Pape, M., Te Wildt, B. T., Wölfling, K., Henningsen, P., Timmesfeld, N., Neumann, A., Neusser, S., Beckers, R., & Herpertz, S.OMPRIS study group. (2021). Effects of an online-based motivational intervention to reduce problematic internet use and promote treatment motivation in internet gaming disorder and internet use disorder (OMPRIS): Study protocol for a randomised controlled trial. *BMJ Open*, *11*(8), e045840. DOI: 10.1136/bmjopen-2020-045840 PMID: 34344675

Dumontheil, I. (2016). Adolescent brain development. *Current Opinion in Behavioral Sciences*, *10*, 39–44. DOI: 10.1016/j.cobeha.2016.04.012

Durlak, J. A., Weissberg, R. P., Dymnicki, A. B., Taylor, R. D., & Schellinger, K. B. (2011). The impact of enhancing students' social and emotional learning: A meta-analysis. *Child Development*, *82*(1), 405–432. DOI: 10.1111/j.1467-8624.2010.01564.x PMID: 21291449

Esposito, F., & Maciel Cathoud Ferreira, T. (2024). Addictive design as an unfair commercial practice: The case of hyper-engaging dark patterns. *European Journal of Risk Regulation*, *15*(4), 999–1016. DOI: 10.1017/err.2024.8

European Commission. (2025). Digital Services Act. European Commission. https://digital-strategy.ec.europa.eu/en/policies/digital-services-act

European Parliament. (2024). *Digital markets and digital services: The Digital Services Act and the Digital Markets Act — Implementation and enforcement* (EPRS_ATA(2024)766256). European Parliamentary Research Service. https://www.europarl.europa.eu/thinktank/en/document/EPRS_ATA(2024)766256

European Union. (2016). Article 5: Principles relating to processing of personal data. In *Regulation (EU) 2016/679 (General Data Protection Regulation)*. European Union. https://gdpr-info.eu/art-5-gdpr/

Evren, C., Dalbudak, E., Topcu, M., Kutlu, N., Evren, B., & Pontes, H. M. (2018). Psychometric validation of the Turkish nine-item Internet Gaming Disorder Scale-Short Form (IGDS9-SF). *Psychiatry Research*, *265*, 349–354. DOI: 10.1016/j.psychres.2018.05.002 PMID: 29793049

Gisbert-Pérez, J., Longobardi, C., Martí-Vilar, M., Mastrokoukou, S., & Badenes-Ribera, L. (2025). Prevalence of Internet gaming disorder in young adults: A systematic review and meta-analysis. *Addictive Behaviors*, *174*, 108576. DOI: 10.1016/j.addbeh.2025.108576 PMID: 41317410

Golden, S. D., McLeroy, K. R., Green, L. W., Earp, J. A., & Lieberman, L. D. (2015). Upending the social ecological model to guide health promotion efforts toward policy and environmental change. *Health Education & Behavior : The Official Publication of the Society for Public Health Education, 42*(1, Suppl), 8S–14S. DOI: 10.1177/1090198115575098 PMID: 25829123

GOV.UK. (2024). *Online Safety Act: explainer.* https://www.gov.uk/government/publications/online-safety-act-explainer/online-safety-act-explainer#:~:text=The%20Act%20requires%20social%20media,are%20shielded%20from%20harmful%20content

Hatef, E., Hudson Scholle, S., Buckley, B., Weiner, J. P., & Austin, J. M. (2024). Development of an evidence- and consensus-based digital healthcare equity framework. *JAMIA Open, 7*(4), ooae136. Advance online publication. DOI: 10.1093/jamiaopen/ooae136 PMID: 39553827

He, J., Yu, S., & Zhang, J. (2025). Analysis and prediction of addiction among virtual reality users. *PLoS One, 20*(3), e0318117. DOI: 10.1371/journal.pone.0318117 PMID: 40072966

Health in All Policies (HiAP) framework for country action. (2014). *Health promotion international, 29 Suppl 1*, i19–i28. https://doi.org/DOI: 10.1093/heapro/dau035

Jia, Y., & Nkoulou Mvondo, G. F. (2025). Exploring the adverse effects of the metaverse on users' psychological well-being and self-esteem: A mixed-methods study. *Journal of Retailing and Consumer Services, 86*, 104321. DOI: 10.1016/j.jretconser.2025.104321

Kardefelt-Winther, D. (2014). A conceptual and methodological critique of internet addiction research: Towards a model of compensatory internet use. *Computers in Human Behavior, 31*(1), 351–354. DOI: 10.1016/j.chb.2013.10.059

Kim, K. K., & Backonja, U. (2025). Digital health equity frameworks and key concepts: A scoping review. *Journal of the American Medical Informatics Association : JAMIA, 32*(5), 932–944. DOI: 10.1093/jamia/ocaf017 PMID: 39936843

Koob, G. F., & Volkow, N. D. (2016). Neurobiology of addiction: A neurocircuitry analysis. *The Lancet. Psychiatry, 3*(8), 760–773. DOI: 10.1016/S2215-0366(16)00104-8 PMID: 27475769

Lee, S., Yoon, J., Cho, Y., & Chun, J. (2024). A systematic review of chatbot-assisted interventions for substance use. *Frontiers in Psychiatry, 15*, 1456689. DOI: 10.3389/fpsyt.2024.1456689 PMID: 39319358

Lin, C. Y., Broström, A., Nilsen, P., Griffiths, M. D., & Pakpour, A. H. (2017). Psychometric validation of the Persian Bergen Social Media Addiction Scale using classic test theory and Rasch models. *Journal of Behavioral Addictions*, *6*(4), 620–629. DOI: 10.1556/2006.6.2017.071 PMID: 29130330

Linardon, J. (2020). Can Acceptance, Mindfulness, and Self-Compassion Be Learned by Smartphone Apps? A Systematic and Meta-Analytic Review of Randomized Controlled Trials. *Behavior Therapy*, *51*(4), 646–658. DOI: 10.1016/j.beth.2019.10.002 PMID: 32586436

Linardon, J., & Fuller-Tyszkiewicz, M. (2020). Attrition and adherence in smartphone-delivered interventions for mental health problems: A systematic and meta-analytic review. *Journal of Consulting and Clinical Psychology*, *88*(1), 1–13. DOI: 10.1037/ccp0000459 PMID: 31697093

Lu, Z. (2025). Mapping adolescent problematic social media use patterns across 41 countries/regions: A multilevel latent class analysis with social determinants. *Addictive Behaviors*, *172*, 108523. DOI: 10.1016/j.addbeh.2025.108523 PMID: 41110245

Ma, C., Wang, Z., Li, C., Lu, J., Long, J., Li, R., Wu, Q., Jiang, H., Du, J., Li, R., Wang, P., Ma, L., Li, H., Hui, S., Zhao, W., Zhong, N., & Zhao, M. (2021). The clinical consistency and utility of ICD-11 diagnostic guidelines for gaming disorder: A field study among the Chinese population. *Frontiers in Psychiatry*, *12*, 781992. DOI: 10.3389/fpsyt.2021.781992 PMID: 35002801

McLeroy, K. R., Bibeau, D., Steckler, A., & Glanz, K. (1988). An ecological perspective on health promotion programs. *Health Education Quarterly*, *15*(4), 351–377. DOI: 10.1177/109019818801500401 PMID: 3068205

Miller, W. R., & Rollnick, S. (2013). *Motivational interviewing: Helping people change* (4th ed.). Guilford Press.

Minkler, M., & Wallerstein, N. (2008). *Community-based participatory research for health: From process to outcomes* (2nd ed.). Jossey-Bass.

Monacis, L., Palo, V., Griffiths, M. D., & Sinatra, M. (2016). Validation of the Internet Gaming Disorder Scale - Short-Form (IGDS9-SF) in an Italian-speaking sample. *Journal of Behavioral Addictions*, *5*(4), 683–690. DOI: 10.1556/2006.5.2016.083 PMID: 27876422

Montag, C., Lachmann, B., Herrlich, M., & Zweig, K. (2019). Addictive features of social media/messenger platforms and freemium games against the background of psychological and economic theories. *International Journal of Environmental Research and Public Health, 16*(14), 2612. DOI: 10.3390/ijerph16142612 PMID: 31340426

Ndayambaje, E., & Okereke, P. U. (2025). The Psychopathology of Problematic Smartphone Use (PSU): A Narrative Review of Burden, Mediating Factors, and Prevention. *Health Science Reports, 8*(5), e70843. DOI: 10.1002/hsr2.70843 PMID: 40415982

Nikken, P., & Schols, M. (2015). How and why parents guide the media use of young children. *Journal of Child and Family Studies, 24*(11), 3423–3435. DOI: 10.1007/s10826-015-0144-4 PMID: 26472932

Núñez-Rodríguez, S., Burgos-González, D., Mínguez-Mínguez, L. A., Menéndez-Vega, F., Antoñanzas-Laborda, J. L., González-Bernal, J. J., & González-Santos, J. (2025). Effectiveness of therapeutic interventions in the treatment of internet gaming disorder: A systematic review. *European Journal of Investigation in Health, Psychology and Education, 15*(4), 49. DOI: 10.3390/ejihpe15040049 PMID: 40277866

Odgers, C. L., & Jensen, M. R. (2020). Annual research review: Adolescent mental health in the digital age. *Journal of Child Psychology and Psychiatry, and Allied Disciplines, 61*(3), 336–348. DOI: 10.1111/jcpp.13190 PMID: 31951670

OECD. (2021). *21st-century readers: Developing literacy skills in a digital world.* OECD Publishing. https://www.oecd.org/content/dam/oecd/en/publications/reports/2021/05/21st-century-readers_26f2b462/a83d84cb-en.pdf

Office of the Surgeon General (OSG). (2023). *Social Media and Youth Mental Health: The U.S. Surgeon General's Advisory.* US Department of Health and Human Services. https://www.hhs.gov/sites/default/files/sg-youth-mental-health-social-media-advisory.pdf

Ong, R. H. S., Sim, H. S., Bergman, M. M., How, C. H., Png, C. A. L., Lim, C. S., Peh, L. H., & Oh, H. C. (2024). Prevalence and associations of problematic smartphone use with smartphone activities, psychological well-being, and sleep quality in a household survey of Singapore adults. *PLoS One, 19*(12), e0315364. DOI: 10.1371/journal.pone.0315364 PMID: 39693321

Organisation for Economic Co-operation and Development. (2025). Children in the digital environment. OECD. https://www.oecd.org/en/topics/children-in-the-digital-environment.html

Panagiotidi, M., & Overton, P. G. (2018). The relationship between internet addiction, attention deficit hyperactivity disorder symptoms and online activities. *Comprehensive Psychiatry*, *87*, 7–11. DOI: 10.1016/j.comppsych.2018.08.004 PMID: 30176388

Paterna, A., Alcaraz-Ibáñez, M., Aguilar-Parra, J. M., Salavera, C., Demetrovics, Z., & Griffiths, M. D. (2024). Problematic smartphone use and academic achievement: A systematic review and meta-analysis. *Journal of Behavioral Addictions*, *13*(2), 313–326. DOI: 10.1556/2006.2024.00014 PMID: 38669081

Peñafiel Mora, V. F., Granda, M. F., & Parra, O. (2025). Technology-based interventions to address internet addictive behaviors: Systematic review. *Discover Mental Health*, *5*(1), 167. DOI: 10.1007/s44192-025-00187-5 PMID: 41171525

Peng, P., Chen, Z., Ren, S., Liu, Y., He, R., Liang, Y., Tan, Y., Tang, J., Chen, X., & Liao, Y. (2023). Determination of the cutoff point for Smartphone Application-Based Addiction Scale for adolescents: A latent profile analysis. *BMC Psychiatry*, *23*(1), 675. DOI: 10.1186/s12888-023-05170-4 PMID: 37716941

Ramadhan, R. N., Rampengan, D. D., Yumnanisha, D. A., Setiono, S. B., Tjandra, K. C., Ariyanto, M. V., Idrisov, B., & Empitu, M. A. (2024). Impacts of digital social media detox for mental health: A systematic review and meta-analysis. *Narra J*, *4*(2), e786. DOI: 10.52225/narra.v4i2.786 PMID: 39280291

Reangsing, C., Wongchan, W., Trakooltorwong, P., Thaibandit, J., & Oerther, S. (2025). Effects of cognitive behavioral therapy (CBT) on addictive symptoms in individuals with internet gaming disorders: A systematic review and meta-analysis. *Psychiatry Research*, *348*, 116425. DOI: 10.1016/j.psychres.2025.116425 PMID: 40054044

Robinson, L., Cotten, S. R., Ono, H., Quan-Haase, A., Mesch, G., Chen, W., Schulz, J., Hale, T. M., & Stern, M. J. (2015). Digital inequalities and why they matter. *Information Communication and Society*, *18*(5), 569–582. DOI: 10.1080/1369118X.2015.1012532

Ru, Y., Norlizah, H. C., Burhanuddin, N. A. N., Liu, H., & Dong, J. (2025). The correlation between mindfulness and problematic smartphone use: A meta-analysis. *Addictive Behaviors*, *164*, 108272. DOI: 10.1016/j.addbeh.2025.108272 PMID: 39923383

Schimmenti, A. (2023). Beyond Addiction: Rethinking Problematic Internet use from a Motivational Framework. *Clinical Neuropsychiatry*, *20*(6), 471–478. DOI: 10.36131/cnfioritieditore20230601 PMID: 38344462

Shannon, H., Bush, K., Villeneuve, P. J., Hellemans, K. G., & Guimond, S. (2022). Problematic Social Media Use in Adolescents and Young Adults: Systematic Review and Meta-analysis. *JMIR Mental Health, 9*(4), e33450. DOI: 10.2196/33450 PMID: 35436240

Stevens, M. W. R., King, D. L., Dorstyn, D., & Delfabbro, P. H. (2019). Cognitive-behavioral therapy for Internet gaming disorder: A systematic review and meta-analysis. *Clinical Psychology & Psychotherapy, 26*(2), 191–203. DOI: 10.1002/cpp.2341 PMID: 30341981

Sunday, O. J., Adesope, O. O., & Maarhuis, P. L. (2021). The effects of smartphone addiction on learning: A meta-analysis. *Computers in Human Behavior Reports, 4*, 100114. DOI: 10.1016/j.chbr.2021.100114

Tse, N., Siu, A., & Tsang, S.. (2024). Group motivational interviewing for adolescents at risk of internet gaming disorder: A mixed-methods preliminary evaluation. *Clinical Social Work Journal.* Advance online publication. DOI: 10.1007/s10615-024-00968-5

UNESCO. (2018). *Global framework of reference on digital literacy skills.* UNESCO. https://unesdoc.unesco.org/ark:/48223/pf0000265403

UNICEF. (2021). *The state of the world's children 2021: On my mind.* UNICEF. https://www.unicef.org/reports/state-worlds-children-2021

UNICEF. (2025). *Keeping children safe online: trends in online platform regulation and emerging lessons.* UNICEF. https://www.unicef.org/media/177636/file/FINAL_Policy%20brief_online%20platform%20regulation.pdf.pdf

U.S. Department of Health and Human Services & Office of the Surgeon General. (2023). *Surgeon General's advisory on youth mental health and social media.* U.S. Department of Health and Human Services. https://www.hhs.gov/sites/default/files/sg-youth-mental-health-social-media-advisory.pdf

van den Eijnden, R. J. J. M., Lemmens, J. S., & Valkenburg, P. M. (2016). The Social Media Disorder Scale: Validity and psychometric properties. *Computers in Human Behavior, 61*, 478–487. DOI: 10.1016/j.chb.2016.03.038

van Deursen, A. J. A. M., & Helsper, E. J. (2015). The third-level digital divide: Who benefits most from being online? *Communication and Information Technologies Annual, 10*, 29–52. DOI: 10.1108/S2050-206020150000010002

Volkow, N. D., Koob, G. F., & McLellan, A. T. (2016). Neurobiologic Advances from the Brain Disease Model of Addiction. *The New England Journal of Medicine, 374*(4), 363–371. DOI: 10.1056/NEJMra1511480 PMID: 26816013

World Health Organization. (1986). *Ottawa Charter for Health Promotion.* World Health Organization. https://www.who.int/teams/health-promotion/enhanced-wellbeing/first-global-conference

World Health Organization. (2014). *Preventing suicide: A global imperative* (community-based approaches section). World Health Organization. https://www.who.int/publications/i/item/9789241564779

World Health Organization. (2020). *Addictive behaviours: Gaming disorder.* https://www.who.int/news-room/questions-and-answers/item/addictive-behaviours-gaming-disorder

World Health Organization. (2022). *Guidelines on mental health at work.* World Health Organization. https://www.who.int/publications/i/item/9789240053052

World Health Organization. (2023). *Commercial determinants of health.* World Health Organization. https://www.who.int/news-room/fact-sheets/detail/commercial-determinants-of-health

World Health Organization. (2024). *Global brief for World Mental Health Day 2024: Mental health is a universal human right.* World Health Organization. https://www.who.int/publications/i/item/9789240029200

World Health Organization. (2025). *Ethics and governance of artificial intelligence for health: Guidance on large multi-modal models.* World Health Organization. https://iris.who.int/server/api/core/bitstreams/e9e62c65-6045-481e-bd04-20e206bc5039/content

World Health Organization & International HBSC Network. (2023). *Problematic social media use. HBSC Data Browser.* World Health Organization. https://data-browser.hbsc.org/measure/problematic-social-media-use/

Yang, J., Fu, X., Liao, X., & Li, Y. (2020). Association of problematic smartphone use with poor sleep quality, depression, and anxiety: A systematic review and meta-analysis. *Psychiatry Research, 284*, 112686. DOI: 10.1016/j.psychres.2019.112686 PMID: 31757638

Ye, X. (2025). Dark patterns and addictive designs. *Weizenbaum Journal of the Digital Society, 5*(3), Article 2.

Zarate, D., Hobson, B. A., March, E., Griffiths, M. D., & Stavropoulos, V. (2022). Psychometric properties of the Bergen Social Media Addiction Scale: An analysis using item response theory. *Addictive Behaviors Reports, 17*, 100473. DOI: 10.1016/j.abrep.2022.100473 PMID: 36536822

Zhou, R., Morita, N., Ogai, Y., Saito, T., Zhang, X., Yang, W., & Yang, F. (2024). Meta-Analysis of Internet Gaming Disorder Prevalence: Assessing the Impacts of DSM-5 and ICD-11 Diagnostic Criteria. *International Journal of Environmental Research and Public Health, 21*(6), 700. DOI: 10.3390/ijerph21060700 PMID: 38928946

KEY TERMS AND DEFINITIONS

Behavioral Addiction: A category of addictions involving compulsive engagement in rewarding non-substance-related behaviors (e.g., gambling, gaming), sharing core features such as impaired control, salience, and persistence despite harm.

Commercial Determinants of Health: The systems, practices, and strategies through which commercial actors influence health, including product design, marketing, and regulatory environments that may contribute to health risks such as digital addiction.

Digital Addiction: An umbrella term used to describe patterns of excessive or dysregulated engagement with digital technologies (e.g., social media, gaming, smartphones) characterized by impaired control, functional impairment, and continued use despite negative consequences. The term is primarily used in public health and research contexts rather than as a formal diagnostic category.

Digital Well-Being: A multidimensional concept referring to the balanced, healthy, and intentional use of digital technologies in ways that support mental, physical, and social well-being, rather than undermine it.

Gaming Disorder: A diagnosable condition recognized in the ICD-11, defined by impaired control over gaming, increasing priority given to gaming over other activities, and continuation or escalation of gaming despite negative consequences, typically present for at least 12 months and associated with significant functional impairment.

Problematic Digital Use: A pattern of digital technology use that interferes with daily functioning, well-being, or social roles but does not necessarily meet clinical diagnostic criteria. This concept emphasizes functional impact rather than time spent online.

Problematic Social Media Use (PSMU): A form of problematic digital use characterized by addiction-like symptoms (e.g., preoccupation, loss of control, withdrawal-like experiences) related specifically to social media platforms, often assessed using standardized self-report scales in epidemiological research.

Social-Ecological Model: A public health framework that conceptualizes health behaviors as shaped by interactions across multiple levels, including individual, interpersonal, organizational, community, and policy contexts.

Chapter 12 Technology Addictions and Digital Diseases: Economic Consequences and Policy Perspectives

Constantinos Challoumis
http://orcid.org/0000-0002-7436-0506
National and Kapodistrian University of Athens, Greece

ABSTRACT

The rapid diffusion of digital technologies has generated new forms of compulsive use, commonly described as technology addictions or "digital diseases," including smartphone addiction, social media addiction, online gaming addiction, digital hyperstimulation, and compulsive online consumption. While these phenomena are usually examined within medical and psychological frameworks, their broader economic implications remain insufficiently systematized. This chapter develops a purely theoretical and conceptual analysis of the economic consequences of digital diseases, emphasizing their systemic effects at both microeconomic and macroeconomic levels. Drawing on behavioral economics, public economics, health economics, and labor and growth theory, it identifies key economic transmission channels—productivity loss, healthcare costs, human capital erosion, household financial stress, and macro-level distortions. These relationships are organized in a conceptual matrix and visualized through a heatmap used as an interpretive, non-empirical tool.

DOI: 10.4018/979-8-2600-2468-3.ch012

1. INTRODUCTION

Digital technology is a ubiquitous element of everyday life, leading to psychological dependence and even addiction in some cases. Many people use their cell phones every 10 minutes. Insistent cell phone ringing that interrupts major events is dangerous. A cell phone has been identified as a “dangerous killer”. Not listening to cell phone calls or text messages increases anxiety. Even in the work environment where concentration is most important, the influence of cell phone use is huge. It is said that 30% of people have been addicted to games. Game addiction can hinder mental and physical development and normal social life. The Internet has brought great changes to human life. However, the negative effect, Internet addiction, has attracted the attention of the whole of society and the media. The use and dependence on computers is similar to computers. Psychologically, dependence and addiction are two extreme conditions of behavior. Behavior is mixed and psychologically negative, and it is considered dependence, while more extreme negativity is recognized as addiction. Internet and computer addiction are rapidly spreading and the causes are several. Ache noted that person characteristics, social psychology environment, family background, and temporary stresses could lead to acquisition of addiction. Emotional neglect by family, attempts in upbringing control during child care, uncontrollable environment, social neurological pressure, abusive parent behavior, and other cyber accompaniment could lead someone being addicted. The digital revolution reshapes the world economy along with the rise of associated risks for compulsive use of technologies and related “digital diseases” – smartphone addiction, social media addiction, online gaming addiction, digital hyperstimulation, etc. These new disease-describing terms capture risks that transcend personal medicine and health psychology paradigms and direct attention at their underlying economic effects that are systemic. Digital economy pathologies cause the following effects at the microeconomic level: digital addictions reduce productive potential due to cyberloafing, multitasking fatigue, and attention bric-a-brac; households face excessive spending on digital consumption and high out-of-pocket expenditures on the treatment of digital consuming diseases that reduce savings and investments. With the long-term digital overstimulation leads to the human capital adverse effect due to academic underperformance and the decline of workplace skills, particularly capital destruction within youth cohorts. At the macroeconomic level, these microeconomic phenomena result in the lower total factor productivity growth, high healthcare spending, depreciation of labor force quantity and quality, distortions of welfare estimation due to excessive contribution of “attention economy” digital industries to the classical GDP (Challoumis, 2025d, 2025c). Growth of digital addiction correlates with relevant long-term trends of economic development – low productivity growth, demographic crisis, labor market deterioration, low fertility, stagnation of physical and human capital, etc. From the public and health economics perspective, the increasing burden of digital diseases treatment on universal health insurance systems, pension funds, and state budgets raises a clear question about the prioritization of methods and tools for diseases prevention and treatment. From the industrial and public economics viewpoint, the creation of digital industries and platforms generates positive effects for the national economy, and the systemic spreading of their negative externalities threatens the "invisible hand" of the market to reallocate costs onto society. Therefore, questions arise regarding the preventive policies of regulation of addictions-explicit features of design, fiscal policy of direct taxation of digital goods and services, labor relations policy oriented on workplace- and family-friendly working hours, information campaigns on digital hygiene, policy of digital detoxification, and digital rights interrogation. Comparison of selected examples of international digital economy pathologies regulation such as various restrictions on digital gaming in Asian countries, digital rights concepts in the European Union, and others illustrates the variety of strategies employed to address digital economy pathologies across different jurisdictions. In this chapter, tools of behavioral and public economics will be used alongside some cross-country datasets analysis and international case studies of states' strategies dealing with "digital diseases". The hypothesis will be tested that digital diseases create systemic economic impact, and the pathology nature of risk for compulsive use of technologies is an individual, medical, psychological, etc. Consequently, measures against digital economy pathologies are proposed to preserve economic growth, human capital formation, and welfare in the digital economy (Challoumis, 2023, 2024b). Recommended policy measures include the development of industrial policies aimed at encouraging the production of digital goods, the reduction of fiscal pressures in favoritism of electronic commerce, digital detox campaigns, and the integration of social and labor market policies.

Digital addictions are usually framed as individual mental-health issues, but their most policy-relevant impacts operate as economic externalities that affect productivity, human capital formation, household financial resilience, and public budgets. The analytical problem is that these economy-wide effects are not consistently integrated into standard digital-economy and public-economics frameworks, leaving regulation fragmented and welfare assessment incomplete.

Research objectives of the current research:

- Conceptually map major forms of technology addiction ("digital diseases") to key economic transmission channels.
- Reframe digital addiction as a market- and institutional-design problem involving externalities, time-inconsistency, and welfare loss.

- Provide a heuristic economic intensity framework (ordinal scoring + heat-map) to organize policy priorities transparently.
- Derive policy instruments (taxation, design constraints, consumer protection, education/labor coordination) consistent with welfare economics.

In addition, the chapter explicitly addresses three core analytical questions that are central to contemporary debates in the digital economy and public economics. First, it examines the channels through which digital addictions translate from individual-level behavioral patterns into macro-level economic distortions, including productivity losses, human capital erosion, labor market inefficiencies, and increased pressure on public welfare systems. Second, it evaluates which policy instruments are most defensible under Pigouvian and welfare-economic logic, while also acknowledging their distributional consequences and equity limits, particularly for vulnerable populations. Third, it identifies the institutional failures that explain the persistence of digital addictions, focusing on platform incentive structures within the attention economy, information asymmetries between users and digital service providers, and systematic self-control problems that undermine individual welfare. By moving beyond clinical and psychological framings, the chapter advances a systemic economic interpretation of digital addiction, offering a unified conceptual framework that links micro-level behavioral mechanisms to macro-level outcomes. Finally, it introduces a transparent visualization and ordinal-intensity framework designed to support policy reasoning and comparative assessment, without making empirical or causal claims.

Existing research on digital addiction is extensive in terms of psychological and clinical measurement, yet it remains comparatively weak in its integration of economy-wide effects and macroeconomic implications. While individual-level outcomes such as cognitive overload, anxiety, or compulsive behavior are well documented, fewer studies systematically connect these behavioral patterns to broader economic outcomes, including productivity dynamics, human capital accumulation, labor market efficiency, and long-run growth trajectories. This micro–macro linkage gap limits the ability of current scholarship to inform comprehensive economic and public policy responses. A second gap concerns the limited application of welfare-economic frameworks to digital addiction. Although behavioral anomalies are frequently acknowledged, key distinctions between experienced utility and decision utility, the role of internalities, and the normative conditions under which paternalistic interventions may be justified are often underdeveloped. As a result, policy discussions tend to oscillate between laissez-faire and restrictive approaches without a consistent welfare-theoretic foundation. Furthermore, institutional and regulatory dimensions remain insufficiently integrated into the analysis. Platform incentive structures and market design features associated with the attention economy—such as engagement-maximizing algorithms, notification architectures, and data-driven personalization—are not consistently treated as economic governance problems. This institutional gap obscures the extent to which digital addictions are shaped by endogenous market incentives rather than solely by individual behavioral predispositions. Distributional considerations are frequently secondary in the literature. Vulnerable populations, including children, adolescents, low-income users, and individuals with limited digital literacy, are disproportionately exposed to the adverse effects of compulsive digital use, yet access asymmetries and equity implications are rarely placed at the center of economic analysis. This omission weakens the connection between digital addiction research and broader human capital and social policy debates. In response to these gaps, the present chapter contributes a coherent economic framing of digital addiction and introduces a structured heuristic approach—based on conceptual intensity scoring and heatmap visualization—to systematically organize behavioral mechanisms, economic transmission channels, and policy responses. This framework is designed to enhance analytical clarity and policy reasoning while remaining explicitly non-empirical in nature.

2. THEORETICAL FRAMEWORK

2.1 Literature Review: Technology Addictions And Digital Deseases

The adapted term 'digital diseases' originates in Mental Health in the Digital Age and refers to altered patterns of thinking and behavior in relation to technology. 'Diseases' can also refer to excessive technology exposure and use that has a deleterious impact on the well-being of individuals and society. The classic medical definition refers to disease as "a condition of the living animal or plant body or one of its parts that impairs normal functioning and is typically manifested by distinguishing signs and symptoms" and "a harmful deviation from the normal structural or functional state of an organism, or any of its parts". The term 'added technology' describes behaviors not traditionally regarded as involving an addictive substance—like gambling, sex, Internet browsing, technology, and work . Such behaviors are recognized as meeting addiction criteria, including mood modification, salience, conflict, and relapse.

Technology addiction is often linked to such digital diseases as Internet Gaming and social networking addictions. These several science-based formulations of technology addiction—the most commonly researched types—together with Internet Addiction and Problematic Mobile Phone Use are sufficient for the classification of technology-related disease and disorder concepts. The largest body of research on the neurophysiology of technology addiction and digital disease comes from neuroscience where brain scannings show neural networks of people during gaming visual stimulation are similar to those of substance-addicted individuals. Other studies suggest that affective or impulse disorders may prompt a search for pleasurable experiences in a gaming world and that any increase in gaming is a negative development for adults and children. Several studies confirm positive associations between components of technology addiction and negative bulimia effects including attention deficit, academic failure, and lower life satisfaction (Challoumis & Eriotis, 2025). Liss and Erchull show that women who focus on the appearance of others while using Facebook report lower body-image and life satisfaction and higher social-movement concerns, while Udris and Kantera find that susceptibility to video-game addiction depends on motivation rather than the addictive nature of games themselves. Mobile-data traffic is projected to increase at a higher rate than predicted by models of previous years, which together with high-frequency keywords such as smartphone, self-service, and mobile indicate a glittering future for mobile and online services worldwide.

From an economic standpoint, technology addictions can be interpreted through (i) rational addiction dynamics (Becker–Murphy), where past consumption raises current marginal utility; (ii) time-inconsistency and self-control problems (hyperbolic discounting), where individuals overconsume relative to long-run welfare; and (iii) bounded rationality and information asymmetries, where platforms exploit predictable behavioral biases. These mechanisms motivate a shift from "individual pathology" toward internalities and externalities, implying that private choices may deviate from socially efficient outcomes even without classic market power. Across disciplines, there is convergence that compulsive digital use is associated with attention fragmentation, sleep disruption, anxiety/depression comorbidity, and reduced educational outcomes; economically, these map to productivity loss and human capital erosion. However, empirical findings diverge on net productivity and innovation effects: digital tools can raise output and access to services while simultaneously increasing distraction and cyberloafing. This contradiction suggests the need for frameworks that distinguish productive digital adoption from addictive engagement driven by platform revenue models. A regulatory-economics interpretation treats these harms as partly endogenous to incentive design (notifications, endless scroll, variable rewards), implying that policy should target market design features rather than digital technology per se. The evidence base is comparatively OECD-centric. In low- and middle-income settings, digital addiction may interact differently with labor informality, weaker mental-health service capacity, lower digital literacy, and different household budget constraints. This matters for policy transfer: interventions that rely on costly clinical pathways may be infeasible, increasing the relevance of prevention, consumer protection, and low-cost educational instruments.

This chapter is subject to several limitations that should be acknowledged. First, the analysis is purely conceptual and theoretical, and therefore does not provide empirical estimation or causal inference regarding the magnitude of economic costs associated with digital addictions. Second, the ordinal intensity scoring and heatmap visualization are heuristic devices intended to structure complex relationships rather than measurement tools, and they inevitably involve a degree of author judgement, which may affect replicability. Third, while the framework integrates insights from welfare economics, behavioral economics, and public policy, it does not formally model dynamic interactions or general equilibrium effects, limiting its capacity to capture feedback loops and long-term adaptation. Fourth, the discussion relies primarily on evidence and regulatory contexts from advanced economies, which may constrain the generalizability of policy implications to low- and middle-income settings. Finally, although the chapter adopts the term "digital diseases" for analytical clarity, this terminology may raise normative and ethical concerns regarding medicalization, which are acknowledged but not fully explored within the present scope. The term "digital diseases" is used as an analytical umbrella to describe persistent compulsive-use patterns with measurable welfare and economic consequences. It is not intended to medicalize normal digital use or impose stigma; rather, it serves as a policy-relevant shorthand for conditions where self-control problems and platform incentives jointly generate harms that justify public intervention. Despite the breadth of existing research on technology addiction, important analytical gaps remain. Much of the literature focuses on individual psychological or clinical outcomes, while offering limited integration of these findings into economy-wide frameworks that link attention capture and compulsive use to productivity dynamics, human capital formation, and long-run growth. Moreover, welfare-economic perspectives—particularly distinctions between experienced and decision utility, the role of internalities, and the normative conditions for paternalistic intervention—are unevenly applied. Institutional dimensions of the digital economy, including platform incentives and market design within the attention economy, are also insufficiently treated as regulatory-economics problems. Finally, distributional considerations, such as differential exposure among vulnerable populations and access asymmetries, are often secondary. This chapter addresses these gaps by advancing a systemic economic interpretation of digital addiction and introducing a structured heuristic framework that links micro-level behavioural mechanisms to macro-level economic outcomes and policy responses.

2.2 Methodology

This study adopts a purely theoretical and conceptual research design, grounded in economic theory, behavioral economics, and public economics. No original empirical dataset, econometric estimation, causal inference, or statistical testing is employed. The objective of the methodology is not measurement or hypothesis testing, but analytical synthesis and structured interpretation of existing theoretical insights and well-established empirical findings from the interdisciplinary literature on technology addiction, digital diseases, and their economic consequences. The methodological approach proceeds in three stages. First, the study conducts a systematic conceptual mapping of technology addictions—such as smartphone addiction, social media addiction, online gaming addiction, digital hyperstimulation, and compulsive online consumption—to their principal economic transmission channels. These channels are derived from the literature and include productivity loss, direct healthcare costs, human capital erosion, household financial stress, and macro-level economic distortions. The selection of these dimensions reflects recurrent themes in public finance, labor economics, health economics, and growth theory, as discussed throughout the chapter. Second, based on this mapping, the study applies a theoretical intensity scoring framework. Each combination of addiction type and economic channel is assigned a relative intensity value on an ordinal scale (0–5), where higher values indicate stronger conceptual economic pressure (Challoumis, 2019, 2025a). These scores do not represent observed data, probabilities, or marginal effects. Instead, they reflect comparative theoretical severity, informed by the consistency, breadth, and strength of arguments in the existing literature, as well as by economic reasoning regarding externalities, human capital formation, and productivity dynamics. Third, the resulting conceptual matrix is visualized using a heatmap representation. The heatmap serves as an analytical visualization device, designed to condense multidimensional theoretical relationships into a single, interpretable graphical form. Its purpose is heuristic and explanatory: it allows the reader to identify dominant impact patterns, asymmetries across addiction types, and clusters of economic vulnerability. Importantly, the heatmap does not claim causal ranking, quantitative magnitude, or empirical validation. It functions as an authorial synthesis tool, analogous to a conceptual diagram or schematic framework.

The use of heatmaps in this context follows a growing methodological practice in theoretical and policy-oriented economic research, where visualization is employed to clarify complex systemic interactions rather than to present estimated results. By translating abstract theoretical arguments into a structured visual format, the methodology enhances transparency, internal coherence, and policy interpretability, while remaining fully consistent with the non-empirical nature of the analysis. This methodological design ensures that the chapter's conclusions are theory-driven, logically consistent, and policy-relevant, while clearly avoiding claims of statistical causality or empirical generalization. The heatmap visualization complements the textual analysis by illustrating the systemic nature of digital diseases and reinforcing the argument that their economic consequences operate through multiple, interacting channels that cannot be adequately addressed by healthcare policy alone.

Figure 1. Technology Addictions and Digital Diseases

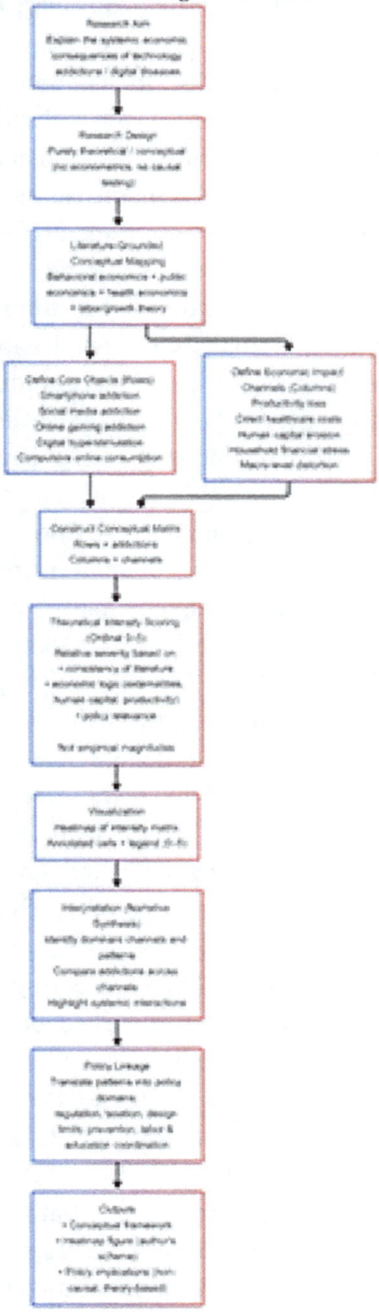

(author's scheme).

This figure summarizes the logical sequence of the chapter's methodology, showing how the analysis moves from abstract research objectives to concrete conceptual outputs in a transparent and non-empirical way. The process begins with the research aim, which is to explain the systemic economic consequences of technology addictions and "digital diseases." This starting point clarifies that the focus is not on individual pathology alone, but on economy-wide effects such as productivity loss, human capital degradation, and welfare distortions. From the outset, the aim frames technology addiction as an economic phenomenon with structural implications. The next step defines the research design as purely theoretical and conceptual. This box is crucial because it explicitly excludes econometric modeling, causal testing, or original data analysis. By doing so, the flowchart signals methodological boundaries and prevents misinterpretation of the results as empirical measurement. The chapter instead relies on economic theory and synthesis of existing knowledge. The methodology then proceeds to literature-grounded conceptual mapping. Here, insights from behavioral economics, public economics, health economics, and labor and growth theory are integrated. This step establishes the analytical lenses used throughout the chapter and explains why particular economic mechanisms—such as externalities, attention allocation, productivity dynamics, and human capital formation—are emphasized. Following this theoretical grounding, the flowchart splits into two parallel steps. One branch defines the core objects of analysis, namely the main forms of technology addiction examined in the chapter (smartphone addiction, social media addiction, online gaming addiction, digital hyperstimulation, and compulsive online consumption). The other branch defines the economic impact channels, that is, the pathways through which these addictions affect the economy (productivity loss, healthcare costs, human capital erosion, household financial stress, and macro-level distortion). This parallel structure highlights that the analysis is explicitly multidimensional. These two branches converge in the construction of a conceptual matrix, where addiction types form the rows and economic channels form the columns. This matrix represents the analytical backbone of the chapter, as it systematically organizes complex interactions that would otherwise remain fragmented across the text. The next step introduces theoretical intensity scoring. Each cell of the matrix is assigned an ordinal score (0–5) reflecting relative economic severity. The flowchart emphasizes that these scores are not empirical magnitudes but are based on three criteria: consistency in the literature, economic logic (externalities, productivity, human capital), and policy relevance. This step translates qualitative theory into a structured comparative framework. The scored matrix is then transformed into a heatmap visualization. The heatmap provides a visual synthesis of the theoretical framework, allowing dominant patterns and asymmetries to be identified at a glance. Importantly, the flowchart makes clear that visualization serves interpretive clarity rather than statistical inference.

The methodology then moves to interpretation through narrative synthesis. In this stage, the heatmap is analytically read: dominant channels are identified, addiction types are compared across dimensions, and systemic interactions are highlighted. This step reconnects the visual output with economic reasoning and theoretical discussion. The flowchart culminates in policy linkage and outputs. The identified patterns are translated into policy-relevant domains such as regulation, taxation, platform design constraints, prevention strategies, and labor and education coordination. The outputs consist of a coherent conceptual framework, an author-designed heatmap, and theory-based policy implications. The flowchart thus demonstrates how the chapter progresses logically from theory to visualization to policy insight, while remaining explicitly non-causal and conceptually grounded.

2.3 Economic Burden: Direct And Indirect Costs

Where specific studies or prevalence estimates are mentioned below, they are used illustratively to motivate channels, not to produce new aggregate cost estimates. Excessive use or addiction to technology creates several economic burdens, the most important being direct and indirect costs. The term direct medical costs means the cost of treating the clinical manifestations of addiction (mental health problems; injuries caused by distracted driving; burns and fallout due to social media hoaxes; etc.) and the costs of restorative services associated with use by individuals: the personnel of 119, police or other protective services and doctors. Costs that cannot be traced back to treatment or restoration of victims are classified as indirect costs. These include general service disruptions (blackouts, traffic jams, etc.), indirect costs of the treatment of the addicted, the lost output of the addicted, their underproductivity and the distress of those around them. Many studies have duplicated such costs in relation to gambling addiction and smoking behaviors. No solid conclusions have yet been formulated regarding the economic consequences of other technology addictions or the use of technology for criminal activity: child pornography, fraud, hacking or phishing, etc. Some kind of conceptualization or direction can be indicated using the analytical structure of direct and indirect costs. Recent research, for instance, has found that individuals with gambling disorders have higher annualized medical spending than the average person, and that the excess spending is attributed to both Medicare and private payers. An increase in the unemployment rate during the preceding working-age life might place individuals at a higher risk of gambling disorders in later life, and that a poor Gold Scale assessment is linked to a greater tendency to remain gambling quite later in life. The economic consequences of digital addiction are not evenly distributed across populations. Individuals from lower-income households, younger users, and groups with limited digital literacy are often more exposed to engagement-intensive platforms while having fewer resources to mitigate adverse effects. These asymmetries translate into unequal impacts on educational attainment, labour market participation, and financial resilience, thereby reinforcing existing socio-economic inequalities. From a policy perspective, digital addiction therefore represents not only an efficiency problem but also a distributional challenge, with implications for equity-oriented interventions in education, consumer protection, and social policy.

2.3.1 Healthcare Expenditures And Productivity Loss

Technology addictions and digital diseases increase healthcare expenditures and decrease productivity, which in turn reduce national economic growth and overall welfare. Affected individuals tend to habitually consume substances for instance cigarettes and alcohol that may lead to shortening their life expectancy. Similarly, they also devote significant time to screen-based entertainment such as video games and social platforms, which may lead to either a stagnant or lower level of mental maturity. These actions are expected to have feedbacks on purchasing demands for both types of products. The loss due to earlier death will generate the economic consequence. More obviously, the time devoted to work-related and production activities is decreased, harming productivity. Technology addictions and digital diseases thus have negative impacts on both the supply-side and demand-side of economics. The estimation of economic damages caused by deaths from technology addictions and digital diseases are consummated within a partial equilibrium setting. Based on the earlier assumption of market equilibrium, the equilibrium price for screen-based entertainment is further defined by relating the supply-side function with the demand-side function (Challoumis, 2024c, 2024d). The evaluation of loss in national productivity due to healthcare disorders linked to digital disease and technology addiction is decomposed into three categories: screened media disorders, other health diseases, and indirect loss arising from the treatment of oneself. The former case directly counts the loss in labor productivity and the consequent loss in the long-term economic growth caused by the earlier retirement of those who play screen-based games from a very young age.

2.3.2. Labor Market Implications And Output Gaps

The labor market is one of the key pillars of the economy and it is through labor that the economy grows. Therefore, the shortage of labor in the economy affects the output of the economy negatively. Even though a few studies on the implications of technology addiction (TA) for health have identified transcriptional biomarkers, the effect of TA on the labor market has not been examined. Unemployment resulting from TA decreases the effective working-age population and thus has a contractionary effect on potential output. The income effect, failure to satisfy co-workers, and a reduced number of available working hours cause a fall in actual output in the short run, leading to a negative short-term output gap. A shortage of physical fatigue capital widow workers, in combination with a negative physical capital gap, causes a negative long-term output gap as well.

TA also leads to a lower level of well-being in youth, increases street crimes, decreases workforce participation, and increases early school dropouts. Although additional elements like social harmony and crime are put aside in the analysis, they nevertheless exist and are serious issues in the economy. Thus, tau can be regarded as an unseen factor. Long-term investments are normally made after observing the short-term result, while businesses work on the basis of expected long-term net advantage. Hence, both capital accumulation and the public sector play key roles in future situations.

2.4. Sectoral Impacts: Education Finance And Public Services

Sectoral examples are included as documented cases from the literature and do not constitute new empirical testing within this chapter. The education sector is often afflicted by technology addictions, especially among students and young people. Among students in Taiwan, the prevalence of behavioral addiction is alarmingly high, at 27.3 percent. It has been argued that when the Chinese-language vocabulary of a language learner is small, the impact of smartphone applications on language learning might be used to reaffirm the psychological loss of leisure in cyberspace. Also, teachers believe that learning is less interesting among students with problematic cellphone use, with gender differences existing in teachers' survey assessments. The drivers of smartphone addiction among students and adolescents include internal, external, and sociodemographic variables. Education has been identified as the most powerful protective factor against cellphone addiction. Moderate cellphone use is positively associated with academic performance, while Internet gaming disorder is negatively associated with academic performance. When expanded to transactional distance theory, high perceptions of community in online learning and low perceptions of external regulation diminish the risk of smartphone addiction. School engagement has a mediating effect between smartphone addiction and school life adjustment. The online financial sector has long been considered a vulnerable sector for fraud, but behavioral addiction also appears to be a driver of financial losses. A study using the Taiwan Financial Data Center shows that an increase in the number of online gambling transactions, as well as Internet pathologic use and pathologic social online, imposes a negative impact on financial performance. In Taiwan and in many other economies, gambling sites using the domain have seen their information technology bear the negative impact of online gambling. Fraudsters use various means to trick the public into online gambling risk.

2.5. Policy Instruments And Public Interventions

Several policies are proposed to mitigate technology addictions and associated digital diseases: a tax on the technology industry to finance educational programs to raise awareness of the problems and effects caused by technology addictions; restrictions on advertising for addictive technologies and products to minors; a ban on contracts with celebrities for advertising addictive technologies and products; and a ban on attention-seeking behavioral practices (personalization of content, notifications, reward systems) and gamification in the design of websites and applications targeted at minors (Challoumis, 2022, 2024a). The goal of these interventions is to mitigate the negative externalities associated with technology addictions by reducing the consumption of attention-seeking products and promoting healthier and more elevated products.

2.5.1. Prevention And Early Intervention Programs

University-wide prevention and early intervention programs that target technology addictions (technology use that is harmful for well-being), such as the Responsible Use of Technology Initiative and the Personal Development and Well-Being Initiative of the University of Bern, are important to foster student resilience, well-being, and healthy use of technology. For example, the preventive offer of the Personal Development and Well-Being Initiative comprises workshops on general well-being, on developing resilience and self-efficacy, and on the development of social and emotional skills to prevent and to protect students against anxiety disorders, depression, and other affective disorders, all of which are associated with technology use. Other strategies integrate the 2-hour "Digital Detox" workshop into the first-year seminars of all university programs. Based on a conceptual framework, the workshop provides students with basic knowledge about the potential costs and benefits of technology use and highlights risk factors for technology addiction. Together with helpful suggestions for a healthy and responsible technology use, such as a technology-free dinner with the family, a conscious use of screens, and a technology diet, the workshop intends to raise awareness of healthy/responsible technology use (Allcott, 2020; Bhargava & Velasquez, 2020; Cho et al., 2018; Y. Gao et al., 2025; Gül, 2025; Kuss & Billieux, 2017; Kuss & Gainsbury, 2021; Olaya-Cotera et al., 2025).

There is preliminary evidence suggesting that this approach may have a positive effect on students' well-being: First students with higher risk factors for technology addiction, such as low self-regulation, high loneliness, and a high demand for social interaction, report a lower impact of bad technological habits on their well-being. Second, technology addiction symptoms in students who have visited the workshop are ranked as less severe than in students who have not attended this workshop. Third, students confirm the practical and useful content of the workshop. University-specific interventions also exist that are focused on creating a general awareness of technology-related issues among students, staff, and the general public.

2.5.2. Regulation, Digital Sanitasion, And Platform Design

Given the economic, social, and health hazards of technology addiction and related digital diseases, specific regulatory interventions are warranted. Development of the digital environment should evolve past the "free-for-all" ecosystem pioneered by the American Internet era. Some light regulation encompasses Internet addiction treatment facilities in China and recent claims by the U.S. Surgeon General regarding serious risks arising from excessive screen time among children and teenagers. Increasing attention should focus on the structural, Digital Sanitation, and Design approaches. The first seeks to eliminate addictive, malicious, and other harmful applications from the digital ecosystem. Effective Digital Sanitation would establish sanctions for individuals and organizations that create harmful applications.

Efforts should also concentrate on changing teenagers' screen time and usage pattern preferences, perhaps encouraging them to write novels, poems, and other forms of creative expression. Development of engaging health-oriented applications that build health habits, foster exercise, deepen knowledge, develop marketing capability, and create savings and investment awareness is also essential. The Design approach advocates that social media, smartphone apps, and online games adopt design protocols to limit excessive use. Mindful of the addiction and public health risks posed by excess screen time, Google, Apple, and other technology giants are pioneering the establishment of such protocols in their products (Andrade & Viñán-Ludeña, 2025; Błachnio et al., 2019; Duradoni, Colombini, Barucci, et al., 2025; Karakose et al., 2023; Kaye et al., 2025; Lam & Harcourt, 2024; Rumpf et al., 2022; Small et al., 2020).

2.5.3. Labor Education Policy Coordination

Technology addictons and digital diseases: Economic consequences and policy perspectives. Technology addictions and digital diseases result in various negative economic effects, creating a substantial need for policies to remedy these addictions. Potential labor policy considerations and educational policy adaptations include coordination of both policies (Abbas et al., 2023; Aftabi & Bahramjerdi, 2023; Cain et al., 2024; Clare et al., 2019; Dechezleprêtre & Sato, 2017; J. Gao et al., 2020; Hidalgo-Sánchez et al., 2022; Mazzucato, 2023; Ouyang et al., 2020; Petrolia et al., 2020; Yoo & Lee, 2010). Policymakers deserve to consider the labor market challenges posed by teenage technology addictions that could have implications for the future productivity of the economy. The natural cure of outgrowing the addiction may be the best option, given the educational and labor issues. Attempting to suppress the addiction seems a much poorer second choice, with a possibly high social cost. But such consideration presumes that the inherent tendency is to outgrow these addictions-remain healthy. Certainly, not all workers who exhibit these addictions will suffer a decline in productivity. Technology addictions and digital diseases represent an unusually clear-cut case in which short-term and long-term economic efficiencies are irreconcilable. The near-term economic ineficiencies could point to the long-term benets of a stable-funding preventive policy.

2.6. Economic Efficiency Equity Considerations

With respect to economic efficiency, analysts must grapple with the following questions: To what extent should society devote resources to combating technology addictions? Is it possible to determine an efficient level of such addictions? If so, how? As previously discussed, technology addictions exert negative spillovers on unengaged third parties similar to pollution effects. The classic Pigovian model (wherein taxes are levied on activities generating negative spillovers) can shed light on optimal public policy responses. In this instance, the optimal tax is equal to the change in the aggregate non-engaged utility due to unit changes in the consumption of technology-addictive goods and services. If an additional unit of consumption reduces these utility levels by $500, for example, a tax equal to $500 is warranted (Agasalim, 2024; Bateman & Kling, 2020; Csereklyei, 2020; Duffield, 1997; Guo et al., 2022; Huseynli, 2024; Rogers et al., 2015; Susilo et al., 2024; Teeli et al., 2024; Theodora, 2020). The previous section also highlighted equity considerations that complicate efficiency analysis. In particular, the cumulative disadvantages faced during childhood can lead to outcomes in which individuals supportive of Pigovian taxes would not invest optimally in the human-capital formation that enables coping with technology addictions. Consequently, the compensatory transfers required to restore (Challoumis, 2023, 2024b) Pigovian taxation's efficiency plausibly exceed the negative externalities induced by such addictions. Those transfers could take one of two forms: offering in-kind subsidies (for public schooling, parental training, and parental schooling) that reduce the consumption of technology addictions, or (unions-managed) reducing labor-hours (thereby rewarding union workers who devote less time to technology).

2.6.1. Cost Benefit Frameworks And Welfare Implications

Cost-benefit frameworks typically used in Health Economics for the analysis of Public Health Policies can be applied here to study technology addictions and digital diseases. The confronting sets of behavioural problems and medical disorders arise in society when the new addictive technologies are available and widely diffused. Therefore, they should be considered as disutilities that must be contrasted with the returns usually known from the adoption of technologies, mainly in terms of a more productive life. In such equilibrium, the policy-maker, besides the duty to support research which increases the knowledge about these sets of effects, has to account for a second-order, constitutive, determinant. Such determinant bridges the research agenda on addictions and disorders in studies of economic welfare of technology beckons offering only psychological rewards. Therefore, in case of irrational addictions, non-experienced-purchaser behaviours become typical, while the existence of irrational disorders makes any corrective action indispensable (Chauhan & Raj, 2025; Gkargkavouzi & Halkos, 2024; Jiang et al., 2023; Kontoleon, 2003; Li et al., 2025; Magio et al., 2021; Nadić, 2021; Saputra, 2024).

Technology addictions cannot derive exclusively from the hyperbolic utility function. They were already considered in the Ascmann's (demand-side) model of the ADDictive Electronic Game–DEAG (credit-side) Market based on the Becker-Murphy investing function for normal addictions. The model also coped with empirical tests aimed at determining how many people had suffered in the past from this addiction (Dong et al., 2025; Dresp & Hutt, 2022; Duradoni, Colombini, Battistoni, et al., 2025; Moqbel & Kock, 2018; Turel et al., 2021; Wang & Wang, 2023; Zhang et al., 2022). These tests had become possible thanks to Aschmann's own experience in this regard, confirmed by family strengthens on the whole suffering symptoms but without any ratification or rejection of these findings by other empirical tests. Actually, these addictions are not yet inelastic or highly elastic demand nor supply functions. Their existence would simply speed up the onset of Ricardian normal technology demand (mainly or only for young consumers with low bargaining power, which were flexibly replaced in young-associates laboratories after some years).

2.6.2. Equity Dimensions: Vulnerable Populations And Acess To Care

Access to quality and timely mental health and substance abuse services is critical in addressing these problems. More than 25% of the population in OECD countries experiences such problems at some point in their lives, but only a small fraction obtains appropriate care, and rates of serious mental health issues from addiction are rising. Failure of policy to invest adequately in mental health and addiction treatment will incur long-term economic consequences for productivity and fiscal sustainability, and neglected symptoms of problems must not be treated merely within the criminal justice system. In particular, the stigmas associated with these issues increases sensitivity of vulnerable subpopulations to access barriers (Berthon et al., 2019; Eskandar, 2025; Hanna, 2020; Manyazewal et al., 2023; Minari, 2025; Scott et al., 2017; Sémanne, 2025; Shetty et al., 2022). Latest estimates suggest that between 10% and 15% of Internet users suffer considerable psychosocial impairments due to their online activities, and that these levels are higher among adolescents and young adults. The lack of resources or ability to pay increases access barriers for these groups. While much of the empirical literature examines both issues among adolescents and young adults, drug-related disorders are often considered in older adults alone owing to the fact that drug-related problems affect a limited proportion of youth compared to their elder counterparts. Furthermore, urban cities often provide better access to treatment facilities than rural areas.

3. FINDINGS

3.1 Case-Studies And Comparative Perspectives

Health economists often make a distinction between diseases that cause structural damage to the body and those, such as obesity, smoking and alcohol, that lead to conditions encompassing overweight or related clinical risks, such as adiposity. The emergence of these conditions may be brought together under the umbrella concept of behavioural or addictive consumption. Psychological and economic motives often push individuals to reduce immediate costs, and they cannot resist temptation to consume despite clear negative consequences. Government policies have thus mainly encouraged health-promotion activities that explicitly target the prevention or reduction of negative externalities. These problems are highlighted by the youth market, typically responsible for the diffusion of some regulations. Risky behaviours pose both individual and social consequences: the smoker damages her own health, the non-smoker nearby is indirectly harmed, and, although natural for an external observer, the non-smoker herself tends to underestimate risks when deciding to initiate. Given the distinction between a disease (e.g. stupidity, shortsightedness) and a disability (i.e. the inability to bear costs), the prudence of a smoker should take into account the compensation by others (Andreassen et al., 2016; Anghel, 2025; Xiong et al., 2023). These examples show that both a narrower and a broader concepts of digital disease can be delineated from a case study perspective. Smoking, when initiated in youth, belongs to both categories: the smoking addict typically pays for the damage caused to her lungs, eyes and for the contributions to the health-related costs of others linked to passive smoke. Still, her environment would prefer that she stops smoking not only for her own health and life expectancy, but also for others' health. Precise information on the risk of initiation and risk-reduction strategies of smoking is important for designing a common good investment in activities promoting H.

3.2. National Strategies And Program Evaluations

A strategic assessment of knowledge focused on national-level efforts—namely those of the European Commission, the United Kingdom, Canada, and Australia—also reveals growing concern about the effects of technology addiction on vulnerable populations, particularly children and adolescents. Canada was the first country to directly recognize these concerns, announcing in 2019 that it would develop a national strategy to combat excessive screen time among children. As part of this strategy, the Canadian government commissioned an Expert Advisory Council Report offering a comprehensive analysis of the influence of screen time on the health and well-being of Canadian children, the impact of the COVID-19 pandemic, and a series of recommendations for policy action to help prevent various forms of technology addiction. The Canadian Minister of Health stated that, "With this Strategy, Canada joins the United Kingdom and Australia in recognizing the threats to the health of children and youth from technology addiction, and the need to create the conditions that enable and encourage healthier screen use."

The influence of technology on youngsters is, therefore, a growing concern among national governments, and national strategies focusing on approval for "healthy" technology use are in development. The Canadian report also supports the establishment and evaluation of pilot programs to promote healthy technology use among youth. Hence, the evaluation of existing national and community pilot programs on technology addiction should provide meaningful insights for new international endeavors (Atkinson et al., 2018; Berthon et al., 2019; Chen et al., 2025; Foster & Azmeh, 2019; Kuss & Gainsbury, 2021; Lam & Harcourt, 2024). The search for such evaluations is more complicated, as there is no widely accepted definition of technology addiction or technology disease. However, comparing existing national programs with the proposed framework of technology diseases can shape a better understanding of international perspectives.

3.3. International Cooperation And Knowledge Sharing

Enhancing international cooperation and knowledge sharing remains central to effective policy responses to technology addictions and digital diseases. As with digital-business risks and harms, many such global challenges—child sexual exploitation, hate speech, and non-consensual intimate images—cross borders and require actions that are effective and not just location-based. Participants in at-risk groups share a common vulnerability but may be distinguished by risk exposure and incident prevalence in different jurisdictions. Priorities therefore differ: some jurisdictions wish to manage the cross-border impact of others' content policies—fearing excessive regulation and/or content restrictions and loss of business attractiveness—whereas others wish to end exploitation of specially prioritized groups, such as children. Recent years also saw an upsurge of focus on misinformation and disinformation, further complicating an already-heavy policy agenda for technology intermediaries (Challoumis, 2025b; De Jesus Correa et al., 2025; Foster & Azmeh, 2019; "Impact of Social Media Addiction on Employees' Wellbeing and Work Productivity," 2020; Matanana et al., 2024; Pang et al., 2022; Yılmaz et al., 2025). On the supply-side, online platforms pledge to avert, detect, and swiftly remove illegal content, often while taking more substantive proactive steps on legal but potentially harmful content. On the demand-side, a broad range of steps aim to bolster both resilience against and preparedness for exposure to potentially damaging experiences on the internet. Both supply and demand responses require underlying regulatory, educational, and judicial frameworks, a span of processes that calls for effective international cooperation, both operational and conceptual.

4. FUTURE RESEARCH DIRECTIONS

Policy Mismatch. In countering new addictions and diseases, government responses increasingly do not pursue the innovation-driving principle of Schumpetarian economics. The focus has switched from promoting free market creative destruction to from identifying and stemming negative externalities. From a public finance perspective, the resulting costs may actually prove higher than any benefits. Indeed, many new technologies are not even benign: virtual and augmented worlds with their encapsulating muck become addictive for many sensitive individuals, remaining in these worlds potentially affecting their physical and mental health. Although information about such risks now presents even in popular newspapers, research into such negative externalities remains virtually absent. Only relatively wealthy societies, willing and able to extent their policies even beyond their own geographical borders, are facing and dealing with these problems. Other countries allocacating only a fraction of their oftentimes insufficient R&D budgets, or even neglecting R&D funding shift their priorities toward creating a comparatively attractive climate for spurting, sustaining and exploiting their creative destruction processes. Priority-setting depends to great extent on complementing considerations of investments and investments on satisfying information needs. Even private enterprises are loath to undertake and bear been assignments (Allcott, 2020; Cho et al., 2018; Y. Gao et al., 2025; Gül, 2025; Kuss & Billieux, 2017; Olaya-Cotera et al., 2025).

Figure 2. Economic Consequences of Technology Addictions.

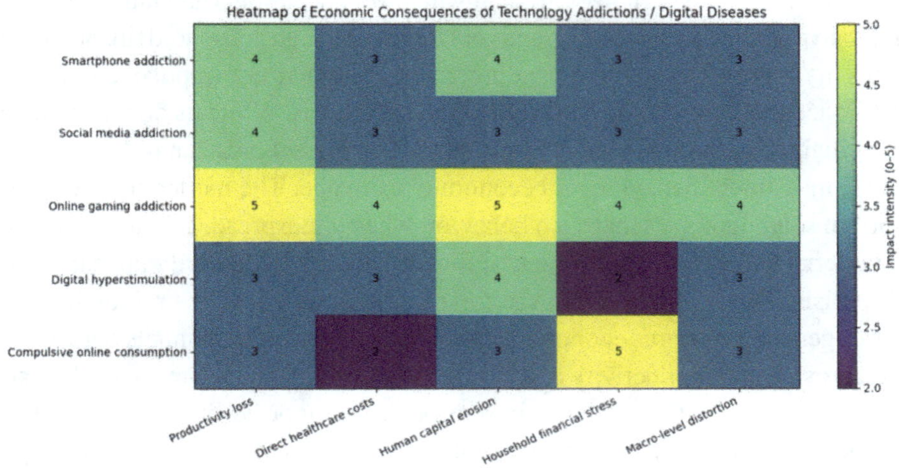

(author's scheme, see Appendix I).

This figure provides a synthetic overview of the relative economic intensity associated with different forms of technology addiction across five key economic transmission channels. Its purpose is not to establish causality, but to visually consolidate the conceptual arguments of the current research, highlighting where digital diseases exert stronger or weaker pressures within the economic system. First, online gaming addiction clearly emerges as the most economically burdensome phenomenon across almost all dimensions. It exhibits the highest intensity in productivity loss and human capital erosion, reflecting prolonged disengagement from education, skill formation, and labor market participation. Elevated healthcare costs are also visible, consistent with the need for psychological treatment and the management of comorbid mental health conditions. The strong macro-level distortion score indicates that, when aggregated, these effects can contribute to lower potential output and structural inefficiencies in the economy. Second, smartphone addiction and social media addiction show pronounced productivity losses, confirming the role of attention fragmentation, multitasking fatigue, and cyberloafing in reducing workplace efficiency. However, their healthcare and household financial impacts remain moderate compared to gaming addiction. This pattern supports the interpretation that these forms of addiction generate diffuse but widespread productivity externalities, which are individually mild yet collectively significant at the macroeconomic level. Third, digital hyperstimulation is characterized by moderate productivity and healthcare effects but relatively strong human capital erosion. This reflects long-term cognitive impacts—such as reduced concentration capacity and learning efficiency—rather than immediate financial or medical costs. The comparatively low household financial stress score suggests that its primary damage occurs through latent capability degradation, which materializes gradually in lower educational and labor outcomes. Compulsive online consumption stands out for its very high household financial stress score. This captures excessive spending, micro-transactions, impulsive purchases, and debt accumulation associated with digital platforms. While its direct healthcare costs remain low, the financial pressure placed on households can indirectly affect savings, investment behavior, and economic resilience. The moderate macro-level distortion score indicates that such behavior, when widespread, can alter consumption patterns and distort welfare measurement without necessarily appearing as a health crisis. The heatmap reinforces the central argument of the research: digital diseases generate systemic economic effects through multiple channels, with human capital erosion and productivity loss acting as the dominant long-term mechanisms. The visualization clarifies why policy responses cannot be limited to healthcare alone but must integrate labor policy, education, consumer protection, and digital market regulation to address the full economic footprint of technology addiction. The conceptual framework and heatmap presented in this chapter highlight how individual-level behavioral distortions can aggregate into macroeconomic trends of broader concern. Productivity slowdowns, erosion of human capital, and rising fiscal pressures emerge not as isolated outcomes but as interconnected effects of sustained attention misallocation and compulsive digital engagement. By explicitly mapping these transmission channels, the framework clarifies how digital addiction can contribute to long-term growth challenges and public finance stress, thereby reinforcing its relevance for macroeconomic and policy analysis. The analysis is conceptual and does not provide empirical estimation of economic costs or causal relationships. The ordinal scoring and heatmap visualisation are heuristic tools that involve informed judgement and may affect replicability. Additionally, the framework does not model dynamic feedback effects or general equilibrium interactions. These limitations point to avenues for future research, including empirical validation, cross-country comparative studies, and integration with formal economic modelling.

5. CONCLUSION

The dramatic growth of Internet-based technological development has generated a significant impact on the social behaviour of technology users. The digital revolution is changing not only the way people communicate, work, learn, play, and socialise but also how they feel and think. A rising number of adolescents are communicating through chats or Facebook rather than via face-to-face interactions, exerting addictive behaviour and losing the ability to interact with real people. The Internet is not only the largest source of information but also the largest source of boredom. Many users are spending an extraordinary amount of time accessing digital-based games or virtual worlds rather than engaging in real-life activities. A new condition named Internet addiction syndrome was found to exist for some Internet users. The situation is becoming serious enough for psychologists to attribute the growing incidence of Attention Deficit Hyperactivity Disorder (ADHD) among adolescents to digital-based distractions that are undermining their ability to concentrate on single tasks. A growing number of studies show the negative impact of video games on children, the association of addiction problems with changes in brain structures in teenagers and young adults, and the role of the digital revolution as a causal factor of psychiatric disorders. A rising number of teenagers are seeking treatment for behaviours and disorders originating from Internet-related activities; more requests for treatment as a consequence of addiction problems are observed in psychotherapeutic centres. Evidence is emerging on the influence of technology addiction on adolescents' health, relationships, study performance, and ability to control impulses and desires. The digital revolution reshapes the world economy along with the rise of associated risks for compulsive use of technologies and related "digital diseases" – smartphone addiction, social media addiction, online gaming addiction, digital hyperstimulation, etc. These new disease-describing terms capture risks that transcend personal medicine and health psychology paradigms and direct attention at their underlying economic effects that are systemic. Digital economy pathologies cause the following effects at the microeconomic level: digital addictions reduce productive potential due to cyberloafing, multitasking fatigue, and attention bric-a-brac; households face excessive spending on digital consumption and high out-of-pocket expenditures on the treatment of digital consuming diseases that reduce savings and investments. With the long-term digital overstimulation leads to the human capital adverse effect due to academic underperformance and the decline of workplace skills, particularly capital destruction within youth cohorts. At the macroeconomic level, these microeconomic phenomena result in the lower total factor productivity growth, high healthcare spending, depreciation of labor force quantity and quality, distortions of welfare estimation due to excessive contribution of "attention economy" digital industries to the classical GDP. Growth of digital addiction correlates with relevant long-term trends of economic development – low productivity growth, demographic crisis, labor market deterioration, low fertility, stagnation of physical and human capital, etc. From the public and health economics perspective, the increasing burden of digital diseases treatment on universal health insurance systems, pension funds, and state budgets raises a clear question about the prioritization of methods and tools for diseases prevention and treatment. From the industrial and public economics viewpoint, the creation of digital industries and platforms generates positive effects for the national economy, and the systemic spreading of their negative externalities threatens the "invisible hand" of the market to reallocate costs onto society. Therefore, questions arise regarding the preventive policies of regulation of addictions-explicit features of design, fiscal policy of direct taxation of digital goods and services, labor relations policy oriented on workplace- and family-friendly working hours, information campaigns on digital hygiene, policy of digital detoxification, and digital rights interrogation. Comparison of selected examples of international digital economy pathologies regulation such as various restrictions on digital gaming in Asian countries, digital rights concepts in the European Union, and others illustrates the variety of strategies employed to address digital economy pathologies across different jurisdictions. In this chapter, tools of behavioral and public economics will be used alongside some cross-country datasets analysis and international case studies of states' strategies dealing with "digital diseases". The hypothesis will be tested that digital diseases create systemic economic impact, and the pathology nature of risk for compulsive use of technologies is an individual, medical, psychological, etc. Consequently, measures against digital economy pathologies are proposed to preserve economic growth, human capital formation, and welfare in the digital economy. Recommended policy measures include the development of industrial policies aimed at encouraging the production of digital goods, the reduction of fiscal pressures in favoritism of electronic commerce, digital detox campaigns, and the integration of social and labor market policies.

Duffield, J. (1997). NONMARKET VALUATION AND THE COURTS: THE CASE OF THE EXXON VALDEZ. *Contemporary Economic Policy*, *15*, 98–110. https://doi.org/10.1111/j.1465-7287.1997.tb00493.x

REFERENCES

Abbas, Z., Javied, U., & Pratt, S. (2023). Exploring the energy intensity – per capita income nexus: Evidence from middle-income and high-Income countries. *Journal of Environmental Economics and Policy*, *13*(1), 70–82. DOI: 10.1080/21606544.2023.2212367

Aftabi, P., & Bahramjerdi, S. F. N. (2023). Developing a decision-making framework within the management of historical cities: Towards integrated conservation and development of the Roudaki neighbourhood. *Land Use Policy*, *129*, 106653. Advance online publication. DOI: 10.1016/j.landusepol.2023.106653

Agasalim, A. A. (2024). Empirical Findings on the Relationship of Energy Consumption, Gross Domestic Product Per Capita and Carbon Dioxide (CO2) Emissions. *International Journal of Energy Economics and Policy*. DOI: 10.32479/ijeep.14062

Allcott, H. (2020). *Digital Addiction*. AEA Randomized Controlled Trials., DOI: 10.1257/rct.5796-1.2000000000000002

Andrade, L., & Viñán-Ludeña, M. (2025). Mapping research on ICT addiction: A comprehensive review of Internet, smartphone, social media, and gaming addictions. *Frontiers in Psychology*, *16*, 1578457. Advance online publication. DOI: 10.3389/fpsyg.2025.1578457 PMID: 40443730

Andreassen, C. S., Billieux, J., Griffiths, M., Kuss, D., Demetrovics, Z., Mazzoni, E., & Pallesen, S. (2016). The relationship between addictive use of social media and video games and symptoms of psychiatric disorders: A large-scale cross-sectional study. *Psychology of Addictive Behaviors : Journal of the Society of Psychologists in Addictive Behaviors*, *30*(2), 252–262. DOI: 10.1037/adb0000160 PMID: 26999354

Anghel, O. (2025). INTERNET ADICTION AND ITS EFFECTS (FROM ARTS). *Review of Artistic Education*. DOI: 10.35218/rae-2025-0050

Atkinson, G., Groom, B., Hanley, N., & Mourato, S. (2018). Environmental Valuation and Benefit-Cost Analysis in U.K. Policy. *Journal of Benefit-Cost Analysis*, *9*(1), 97–119. DOI: 10.1017/bca.2018.6

Bateman, I., & Kling, C. (2020). Revealed Preference Methods for Nonmarket Valuation: An Introduction to Best Practices. *Review of Environmental Economics and Policy, 14*(2), 240–259. DOI: 10.1093/reep/reaa009

Berthon, P., Pitt, L., & Campbell, C. (2019). Addictive De-Vices: A Public Policy Analysis of Sources and Solutions to Digital Addiction. *Journal of Public Policy & Marketing, 38*(4), 451–468. DOI: 10.1177/0743915619859852

Bhargava, V., & Velasquez, M. (2020). Ethics of the Attention Economy: The Problem of Social Media Addiction. *Business Ethics Quarterly, 31*(3), 321–359. DOI: 10.1017/beq.2020.32

Błachnio, A., Przepiorka, A., Gorbaniuk, O., Benvenuti, M., Ciobanu, A., Senol-Durak, E., Durak, M., Giannakos, M., Mazzoni, E., Pappas, I., Popa, C., Seidman, G., Wu, A., Yu, S., & Ben-Ezra, M. (2019). Cultural Correlates of Internet Addiction. *Cyberpsychology, Behavior and Social Networking, 22*(4), 258–263. DOI: 10.1089/cyber.2018.0667 PMID: 30958038

Cain, L., Hernández-Cortés, D., Timmins, C., & Weber, P. (2024). Recent Findings and Methodologies in Economics Research in Environmental Justice. *Review of Environmental Economics and Policy, 18*(1), 116–142. DOI: 10.1086/728100

Challoumis, C. (2019). The R.B.Q. (Rational, Behavioral and Quantified) Model. *Ekonomika (Niš), 98*(1), 6–18. DOI: 10.15388/Ekon.2019.1.1

Challoumis, C. (2022). Conditions of the CM (Cycle of Money). In *Social and Economic Studies within the Framework of Emerging Global Developments, Volume -1, V. Kaya* (pp. 13–24). DOI: 10.3726/b19907

Challoumis, C. (2023). FROM SAVINGS TO ESCAPE AND ENFORCEMENT SAVINGS. *Cógito (Salvador), XV*(4), 206–216.

Challoumis, C. (2024a). Approach on Arm's Length Principle and Fix Length Principle Mathematical Representations. In *Innovations and Contemporary Trends in Business & Economics* (pp. 25–44). Peter Lang., https://www.peterlang.com/search?searchstring=Approach+on+Arm's+Length+Principle+and+Fix+Length+Principle+Mathematical+Representations

Challoumis, C. (2024b). From Economics to Economic Engineering (The Cycle of Money): The case of Romania. *Cógito (Salvador), XVII*(2), 161–170.

Challoumis, C. (2024c). Integrating Money Cycle Dynamics and Economocracy for Optimal Resource Allocation and Economic Stability. *Journal of Risk and Financial Management, 17*(9), 1–25. DOI: 10.3390/jrfm17090422

Challoumis, C. (2024d). The Index of the Cycle of Money: The Case of Switzerland. *Journal of Risk and Financial Management, 17*(4), 1–24. https://doi.org/https://doi.org/10.3390/jrfm17040135. DOI: 10.3390/jrfm17040135

Challoumis, C. (2025a). QUANTIFICATION OF EVERYTHING METHOD IN ECONOMICS. *INDeCS, 23*(4), 323–339. https://www.indecs.eu/2025/indecs2025-pp323-339.pdf

Challoumis, C. (2025b). The Economic Dimensions of Technology and Media in Digital Social Innovation. In *Examining the Intersection of Technology, Media, and Social Innovation.* IGI Global., https://www.igi-global.com/book/examining-intersection-technology-media-social/381810#table-of-contents DOI: 10.4018/979-8-3373-5307-4.ch013

Challoumis, C. (2025c). The impact factor of Tangibles and Intangibles of controlled transactions on economic performance. *Economic Alternatives, 31*(1), 64–76. https://www.unwe.bg/doi/eajournal/2025.1/EA.2025.1.04.pdf

Challoumis, C. (2025d). THE INFLATION ACCORDING TO THE CYCLE OF MONEY (C.M.). *Economic Alternatives, 2025*(2), 324–353. https://doi.org/https://doi.org/10.37075/EA.2025.2.03

Challoumis, C., & Eriotis, N. (2025). The Impact of Artificial Intelligence on the Greek Economy. *Journal of Open Innovation, 11*(3), 1–13. https://doi.org/https://doi.org/10.1016/j.joitmc.2025.100578. DOI: 10.1016/j.joitmc.2025.100578

Chauhan, P., & Raj, T. (2025). *Optimizing Indian Tourism and Cultural Heritage: Bridging Policy Gaps through Integrated Governance, Agrotourism, and Regenerative Development.* International Journal For Multidisciplinary Research., DOI: 10.36948/ijfmr.2025.v07i04.54654

Chen, Y., Wang, Z., Zhao, J., Zhao, X., Zuo, S., & Liu, W. (2025). Paths to Policy Sustainability for Protecting Cultural Heritage: A Quantitative Analysis of Conservation Policies for the Great Wall Within the "Instrument–Objective–Stakeholder" Framework. *Sustainability (Basel), 17*(10), 4378. Advance online publication. DOI: 10.3390/su17104378

Cho, D.-J., Kim, H., Lee, J., & Park, S. (2018). Economic cost–benefit analysis of the addictive digital game industry. *Applied Economics Letters, 25*(9), 638–642. DOI: 10.1080/13504851.2017.1355528

Clare, B., Walter, E., & Harold, E. (2019). Free market for the environment. *Economic Policy, 14*(1), 116–125. Advance online publication. DOI: 10.18288/1994-5124-2019-1-116-125

Csereklyei, Z. (2020). Price and income elasticities of residential and industrial electricity demand in the European Union. *Energy Policy*, *137*, 111079. DOI: 10.1016/j.enpol.2019.111079

De Jesus Correa, J., Souza, J., & Da Silva, P. R. (2025). PSIQUIATRIA DA ADIÇÃO DIGITAL: IMPACTOS DO USO EXCESSIVO DE TECNOLOGIA NO SISTEMA DE RECOMPENSA. *Revista Ft.* DOI: 10.69849/revistaft/dt10202506041027

Dechezleprêtre, A., & Sato, M. (2017). The Impacts of Environmental Regulations on Competitiveness. *Review of Environmental Economics and Policy*, *11*(2), 183–206. DOI: 10.1093/reep/rex013

Dong, R., Yuan, D., Wei, X., Cai, J., Ai, Z., & Zhou, S. (2025). Exploring the relationship between social media dependence and internet addiction among college students from a bibliometric perspective. *Frontiers in Psychology*, *16*, 1463671. Advance online publication. DOI: 10.3389/fpsyg.2025.1463671 PMID: 40144033

Dresp, B., & Hutt, A. (2022). Digital Addiction and Sleep. *International Journal of Environmental Research and Public Health*, *19*(11), 6910. Advance online publication. DOI: 10.3390/ijerph19116910 PMID: 35682491

Duradoni, M., Colombini, G., Battistoni, V., Zagaglia, V., & Guazzini, A. (2025). Exploring the Role of Online Social Capital in Differentiating Technology Addiction Effect on Well-Being. *Human Behavior and Emerging Technologies*, *2025*(1), 6211572. Advance online publication. DOI: 10.1155/hbe2/6211572

Eskandar, K. (2025). *The digital trap: unraveling the neuropsychological impact of technology addiction.* Neuropsychological Trends., DOI: 10.7358/neur-2025-037-eska

Foster, C., & Azmeh, S. (2019). Latecomer Economies and National Digital Policy: An Industrial Policy Perspective. *The Journal of Development Studies*, *56*(7), 1247–1262. DOI: 10.1080/00220388.2019.1677886

Gao, J., Peng, B., & Smyth, R. (2020). On Income and Price Elasticities for Energy Demand: A Panel Data Study. *EnergyRN: Other Energy Policy & Economics (Topic).* DOI: 10.2139/ssrn.3674641

Gao, Y., Yang, Y., Lu, J., Chen, C., & Liang, X. (2025). Does digital economy development enhance Chinese residents' health? Impact and mechanism. *BMC Public Health*, *25*(1), 1154. Advance online publication. DOI: 10.1186/s12889-025-22325-y PMID: 40140993

Gkargkavouzi, A., & Halkos, G. (2024). The Psychology of Non-Market Environmental Valuation: An integrative review of research evidence, theoretical insights, and policy considerations. *Journal of Environmental Psychology*. Advance online publication. DOI: 10.1016/j.jenvp.2024.102510

Gül, G. (2025). The effects of digital engagement in the workplace on employee performance. *Business & Management Studies: An International Journal.* DOI: 10.15295/bmij.v13i1.2514

Guo, M., Wang, H., & Kuai, Y. (2022). Environmental Policy and Green Innovation: Evidence from Heavily Polluting Firms in China. *Finance Research Letters*. Advance online publication. DOI: 10.1016/j.frl.2022.103624

Hanna, N. (2020). Assessing the digital economy: Aims, frameworks, pilots, results, and lessons. *Journal of Innovation and Entrepreneurship*, *9*(1), 16. Advance online publication. DOI: 10.1186/s13731-020-00129-1 PMID: 32923308

Hidalgo-Sánchez, F., Carrascal-Pérez, M., Pérez, J. R., Plaza, C., & Mascort-Albea, E. (2022). Cultural Heritage, Sustainability, Conservation, and Social Welfare. A Management Plan for the Historic Municipal Buildings of Seville (Andalusia, Spain). *The Historic Environment*, *13*(4), 426–458. DOI: 10.1080/17567505.2022.2146332

Huseynli, B. (2024). Analyzing the Relationship between Renewable Energy Sources, Economic Growth and Energy Consumption in Greece. *International Journal of Energy Economics and Policy*. DOI: 10.32479/ijeep.15356

Impact of Social Media Addiction on Employees' Wellbeing and Work Productivity. (2020). *The Qualitative Report.*, DOI: 10.46743/2160-3715/2020.4099

Jiang, J., Zhang, Q.-H., & Hui, Y. (2023). The Impact of Market and Non-Market-Based Environmental Policy Instruments on Firms' Sustainable Technological Innovation: Evidence from Chinese Firms. *Sustainability (Basel)*, *15*(5), 4425. Advance online publication. DOI: 10.3390/su15054425

Karakose, T., Yildirim, B., Tülübaş, T., & Kardaş, A. (2023). A comprehensive review on emerging trends in the dynamic evolution of digital addiction and depression. *Frontiers in Psychology*, *14*, 1126815. Advance online publication. DOI: 10.3389/fpsyg.2023.1126815 PMID: 36844332

Kaye, A., Islam, R., Tong, V., Sorrel, M., Allen, K., Nguyen, I., Miller, B., Sharpe, M., Ahmadzadeh, S., Griffin, P., Shekoohi, S., & Varrassi, G. (2025). A Narrative Inquiry Into Problematic Internet Use Among Young Adults: A Narrative Review. *Cureus*, *17*. Advance online publication. DOI: 10.7759/cureus.85705 PMID: 40642670

Kontoleon, A. (2003). *Essays on non-market valuation of environmental resources: policy and technical explorations.* https://consensus.app/papers/essays-on-nonmarket-valuation-of-environmental-resources-kontoleon/c0ffb545a0a355c6879de7545cb39883/

Kuss, D., & Billieux, J. (2017). Technological addictions: Conceptualisation, measurement, etiology and treatment. *Addictive Behaviors*, *64*, 231–233. DOI: 10.1016/j.addbeh.2016.04.005 PMID: 27136694

Kuss, D., & Gainsbury, S. M. (2021). Debate: Behavioural addictions and technology use - risk and policy recommendations for problematic online gambling and gaming. *Child and Adolescent Mental Health*, *26*(1), 76–77. Advance online publication. DOI: 10.1111/camh.12449 PMID: 33426713

Lam, H., & Harcourt, M. (2024). Digital Addiction in Organizations: Challenges and Policy Implications. *Employee Responsibilities and Rights Journal*, *36*(4), 1–15. DOI: 10.1007/s10672-024-09493-6

Li, J., Wu, X., & Du, Y. (2025). Reframing Cultural Heritage Policy Through Place-Based Perspectives: The Evolution of China's ICH Governance Amid Historical Continuity and Global Convergence. *Land (Basel)*, *14*(7), 1425. Advance online publication. DOI: 10.3390/land14071425

Magio, K., Aranda, L. L., González, L., & Alpuche, C. (2021). *Analysis and Identification of Sustainable Public Policy for Management of Cultural and Natural Heritage in the Maya Region in Line with the Sustainable Development Goals.* Heritage., DOI: 10.3390/heritage4040229

Manyazewal, T., Ali, M., Kebede, T., Magee, M., Getinet, T., Patel, S., Hailemariam, D., Escoffery, C., Woldeamanuel, Y., Makonnen, N., Solomon, S., Amogne, W., Marconi, V., & Fekadu, A. (2023). Mapping digital health ecosystems in Africa in the context of endemic infectious and non-communicable diseases. *NPJ Digital Medicine*, *6*(1), 97. Advance online publication. DOI: 10.1038/s41746-023-00839-2 PMID: 37237022

Matanana, N., Denhere, P., Chibhoyi, D., Mutumwa, A., Morgen, S., & Mutongoreni, N. (2024). *An Assessment on the Impact of Technological Addiction on Workplace Productivity: Case of the Public Sector in Zimbabwe.* World Journal of Engineering and Technology., DOI: 10.4236/wjet.2024.123040

Mazzucato, M. (2023). Governing the economics of the common good: From correcting market failures to shaping collective goals. *Journal of Economic Policy Reform*, *27*(1), 1–24. DOI: 10.1080/17487870.2023.2280969

Minari, T. (2025). Intersectoral Strategies for Type 2 Diabetes Prevention and Management in Emerging Countries: A Narrative Review of Food Sovereignty, Digital Health, and Syndemic Dynamics. *International Journal of Environmental Research and Public Health*, *22*(10), 1572. Advance online publication. DOI: 10.3390/ijerph22101572 PMID: 41154976

Moqbel, M., & Kock, N. (2018). Unveiling the dark side of social networking sites: Personal and work-related consequences of social networking site addiction. *Information & Management*, *55*(1), 109–119. DOI: 10.1016/j.im.2017.05.001

Nadić, D. (2021). Understanding the public and common good in the contemporary environmental policy. *Socioloski Pregled*, *55*(4), 1590–1609. Advance online publication. DOI: 10.5937/socpreg55-35441

Olaya-Cotera, S., Iparraguirre-Villanueva, O., & Flores-Castañeda, R. O. (2025). Technological Addiction Exploring the Risks of Excessive Use of Mobile Devices and Social Networks in Adolescents: A Systematic Review. *Academic Journal of Interdisciplinary Studies*. DOI: 10.36941/ajis-2025-0014

Ouyang, X., Li, Q., & Du, K. (2020). How does environmental regulation promote technological innovations in the industrial sector? Evidence from Chinese provincial panel data. *Energy Policy*, *139*, 111310. Advance online publication. DOI: 10.1016/j.enpol.2020.111310

Pang, J., Jiao, F., & Zhang, Y. (2022). An Analysis of the Impact of the Digital Economy on High-Quality Economic Development in China—A Study Based on the Effects of Supply and Demand. *Sustainability (Basel)*, *14*(24), 16991. Advance online publication. DOI: 10.3390/su142416991

Petrolia, D., Guignet, D., Whitehead, J., Kent, C., Caulder, C., & Amon, K. (2020). Nonmarket Valuation in the Environmental Protection Agency's Regulatory Process. *Applied Economic Perspectives and Policy*. Advance online publication. DOI: 10.1002/aepp.13106

Rogers, A., Kragt, M., Gibson, F., Burton, M., Petersen, E., & Pannell, D. (2015). Non-Market Valuation: Usage and Impacts in Environmental Policy and Management in Australia. *Agricultural & Natural Resource Economics EJournal*. DOI: 10.1111/1467-8489.12031

Rumpf, H., Effertz, T., & Montag, C. (2022). The cost burden of problematic internet usage. *Current Opinion in Behavioral Sciences*, *44*, 101107. Advance online publication. DOI: 10.1016/j.cobeha.2022.101107

Saputra, R. (2024). Governance Frameworks and Cultural Preservation in Indonesia: Balancing Policy and Heritage. *Journal of Ethnic and Cultural Studies*, *11*(3), 25–50. Advance online publication. DOI: 10.29333/ejecs/2145

Scott, D., Valley, B., & Simecka, B. (2017). Mental Health Concerns in the Digital Age. *International Journal of Mental Health and Addiction*, *15*(3), 604–613. DOI: 10.1007/s11469-016-9684-0

Sémanne, A. (2025). State Primary Socialization Indoctrination: A Libertarian Critique of Youth Digital Regulation. *The Journal of Libertarian Studies*, *29*(2). Advance online publication. DOI: 10.35297/001c.142734

Shetty, K., Tewathia, N., Bamney, U., & Rawat, V. (2022). Micro- and macro-level economic implications of digital addictions: A case study. *MGM Journal of Medical Sciences*, *9*(4), 588–590. DOI: 10.4103/mgmj.mgmj_199_22

Small, G., Lee, J., Kaufman, A., Jalil, J., Siddarth, P., Gaddipati, H., Moody, T., & Bookheimer, S. (2020). Brain health consequences of digital technology use. *Dialogues in Clinical Neuroscience*, *22*(2), 179–187. DOI: 10.31887/DCNS.2020.22.2/gsmall PMID: 32699518

Susilo, Y., Kartawinata, M., & Herawan, J. (2024). The Effect of Energy Consumption Towards Economic Growth: The Case of 11 Asian Countries. *International Journal of Energy Economics and Policy*. DOI: 10.32479/ijeep.15676

Teeli, A. A., Bhat, M. A., & Subhan, M. (2024). Empirical insights into India's energy demand: Unveiling elasticity dynamics for strategic policy initiatives. *Environmental Science and Pollution Research International*, *31*(55), 63895–63909. DOI: 10.1007/s11356-024-35423-y PMID: 39514078

Theodora, Y. (2020). *Cultural Heritage as a Means for Local Development in Mediterranean Historic Cities—The Need for an Urban Policy*. Heritage., DOI: 10.3390/heritage3020010

Turel, O., Qahri-Saremi, H., & Vaghefi, I. (2021). Special Issue: Dark Sides of Digitalization. *International Journal of Electronic Commerce*, *25*(2), 127–135. DOI: 10.1080/10864415.2021.1887694

Wang, F., & Wang, Z. (2023). The impact of the digital economy on occupational health: A quasi-experiment based on "Broadband China" pilot. *Frontiers in Public Health*, *10*, 1007528. Advance online publication. DOI: 10.3389/fpubh.2022.1007528 PMID: 36761332

Xiong, S., Lu, H., Peoples, N., Duman, E., Najarro, A., Ni, Z., Gong, E., Yin, R., Østbye, T., Palileo-Villanueva, L., Doma, R., Kafle, S., Tian, M., & Yan, L. (2023). Digital health interventions for non-communicable disease management in primary health care in low-and middle-income countries. *NPJ Digital Medicine*, *6*(1), 12. Advance online publication. DOI: 10.1038/s41746-023-00764-4 PMID: 36725977

Yılmaz, R. C., Karaoba, D. D., & Candiri, B. (2025). *Digital Addiction and Sedentary Life Pandemic*. TOGÜ Sağlık Bilimleri Dergisi., DOI: 10.52369/togusagbilderg.1511985

Yoo, S., & Lee, J. (2010). Electricity consumption and economic growth: A cross-country analysis. *Energy Policy*, *38*(1), 622–625. DOI: 10.1016/j.enpol.2009.05.076

Zhang, J., Zhao, W., Cheng, B., Li, A., Wang, Y., Yang, N., & Tian, Y. (2022). The Impact of Digital Economy on the Economic Growth and the Development Strategies in the post-COVID-19 Era: Evidence From Countries Along the "Belt and Road.". *Frontiers in Public Health*, *10*, 856142. Advance online publication. DOI: 10.3389/fpubh.2022.856142 PMID: 35669751

ADDITIONAL READINGS

Arenas-Escaso, J., Folgado-Fernández, J., & Palos-Sanchez, P. (2024). Internet interventions and therapies for addressing the negative impact of digital overuse: A focus on digital free tourism and economic sustainability. *BMC Public Health*, *24*(1), 176. Advance online publication. DOI: 10.1186/s12889-023-17584-6 PMID: 38218759

Challoumis, C. (2023a). Utility of Cycle of Money without the Escaping Savings (Protection of the Economy). In *Social and Economic Studies within the Framework of Emerging Global Developments* (Vol. 2, pp. 53–64). V. Kaya., DOI: 10.2139/ssrn.4403915

Challoumis, C. (2023b). Impact Factor of Liability of Tax System According to the Theory of Cycle of Money. In *Social and Economic Studies within the Framework of Emerging Global Developments* (Vol. 3, pp. 31–42). V. Kaya., DOI: 10.2139/ssrn.4616728

Challoumis, C. 2023c. A comparison of the velocities of minimum escaped savings and financial liquidity, in: Social and Economic Studies within the Framework of Emerging Global Developments, Volume - 4, V. Kaya. pp. 41–56. DOI: 10.3726/b21202

Gega, L., Janković, D., Saramago, P., Marshall, D., Dawson, S., Brabyn, S., Nikolaidis, G., Melton, H., Churchill, R., & Bojke, L. (2022). Digital interventions in mental health: Evidence syntheses and economic modelling. *Health Technology Assessment*, *26*(1), 1–182. DOI: 10.3310/RCTI6942 PMID: 35048909

Kuş, Ö. A. (2016). *Bir pazarlama aracı olarak mobil pazarlama: İstanbul ili kapsamında y kuşağının mobil pazarlamaya bakış açısı*. Yayınlanmamış Yüksek Lisans Tezi, Okan Üniversitesi Sos. Bilim. Enstitüsü.

Kuş, Ö. A. (2023a). *Oyun, dijital oyun, bağımlılık ve motivasyon kavramları arasındaki ilişkiler*. Urzeni Yayınevi.

Kuş, Ö. A. (2023b). *İnteraktif bir iletişim alanı olarak dijital oyunlar; oyun oynama motivasyonlarının dijital oyun bağımlılığına etkileri üzerine bir araştırma Doktora Tezi*. İstanbul Üniversitesi Sos. Bilim. Enstitüsü.

Petruželka, B., Vacek, J., Gavurová, B., Kubák, M., Gabrhelík, R., Rogalewicz, V., & Barták, M. (2020). Interaction of Socioeconomic Status with Risky Internet Use, Gambling and Substance Use in Adolescents from a Structurally Disadvantaged Region in Central Europe. *International Journal of Environmental Research and Public Health*, *17*(13), 4803. Advance online publication. DOI: 10.3390/ijerph17134803 PMID: 32635320

Singh, C. B., Sharma, N., & Pandey, S. (2025). *How Digital Addiction Fuels Youth Consumerism in India?* Involv. Int. J. Bus., DOI: 10.62569/iijb.v2i2.72

KEY TERMS AND DEFINITIONS

Digital Addiction: Digital addiction refers to a persistent pattern of compulsive engagement with digital technologies or platforms that reduces an individual's ability to allocate attention optimally, resulting in measurable economic, social, or welfare losses beyond voluntary or productive use.

Digital Diseases: Digital diseases denote a conceptual category of technology-induced behavioural conditions that generate systematic economic distortions—such as productivity loss, human capital degradation, and fiscal pressure—rather than being limited to clinical or psychological pathology.

Attention Economy: The attention economy describes a market structure in which digital platforms compete to capture and monetise user attention, often through design mechanisms that prioritise engagement maximisation over user welfare or long-term efficiency.

Internalities: Internalities are welfare losses borne by individuals themselves due to systematic self-control problems, time inconsistency, or bounded rationality, where private decision-making deviates from long-run personal welfare even in the absence of external harm.

Behavioural Externalities: Behavioural externalities arise when individual behavioural distortions—such as compulsive digital use—aggregate to impose costs on others or on the economy as a whole, including reduced productivity, increased healthcare expenditure, and public fiscal burdens.

Human Capital Erosion: Human capital erosion refers to the gradual reduction in cognitive capacity, skills accumulation, or educational outcomes caused by sustained attention fragmentation and reduced deep learning associated with excessive digital engagement.

Productivity Distortion: Productivity distortion denotes the divergence between potential and realised output that occurs when digital technologies shift from efficiency-enhancing tools to sources of distraction, task fragmentation, and labour misallocation.

Ordinal Intensity Scoring: Ordinal intensity scoring is a non-empirical heuristic method used to rank the relative strength of relationships between behavioural phenomena and economic outcomes without assigning quantitative magnitudes or causal estimates.

Policy Heuristic Framework: A policy heuristic framework is a structured analytical tool designed to organise complex interactions between behaviour, economic outcomes, and policy instruments in order to support reasoning and prioritisation rather than prediction or measurement.

Welfare Misalignment: Welfare misalignment refers to the systematic divergence between individually perceived benefits of digital engagement and its actual long-term economic and social costs, arising from behavioural biases, information asymmetries, and platform-driven incentive structures that distort optimal choice.

APPENDIX I

```
# Constantinos Challoumis ©® 2025 All Rights Reserved
import numpy as np
import pandas as pd
import matplotlib.pyplot as plt
# -----------------------------
# 1) Conceptual intensity matrix (0–5)
# -----------------------------
rows = [
“Smartphone addiction”,
“Social media addiction”,
“Online gaming addiction”,
“Digital hyperstimulation”,
“Compulsive online consumption”
]
cols = [
“Productivity loss”,
“Direct healthcare costs”,
“Human capital erosion”,
“Household financial stress”,
“Macro-level distortion”
]
# Intensity scores (0–5): illustrative synthesis consistent with the chapter logic
M = np.array([
[4, 3, 4, 3, 3], # Smartphone addiction
[4, 3, 3, 3, 3], # Social media addiction
[5, 4, 5, 4, 4], # Online gaming addiction
[3, 3, 4, 2, 3], # Digital hyperstimulation
[3, 2, 3, 5, 3], # Compulsive online consumption
], dtype=float)
df = pd.DataFrame(M, index=rows, columns=cols)
# -----------------------------
# 2) Plot
# -----------------------------
plt.figure(figsize=(12, 6))
im = plt.imshow(df.values, aspect=”auto”) # default colormap; do not hardcode colors
# Axis labels / ticks
plt.xticks(range(len(cols)), cols, rotation=25, ha=”right”)
plt.yticks(range(len(rows)), rows)
# Cell annotations
for i in range(df.shape[0]):
for j in range(df.shape[1]):
plt.text(j, i, f”{df.iloc[i, j]:.0f}”, ha=”center”, va=”center”)
# Colorbar + title
plt.colorbar(im, label=”Impact intensity (0–5)”)
```

```
plt.title("Heatmap of Economic Consequences of Technology Addictions / Digital Diseases")
plt.tight_layout()
# Optional: save high-resolution figure for a book chapter
# plt.savefig("heatmap_digital_diseases.png", dpi=300, bbox_inches="tight")
plt.show()
```

Chapter 13

Innovations and Strategies for Treating Digital Addictions

Pawan Pant
http://orcid.org/0000-0003-1774-5650
Chandigarh University, Mohali, India

ABSTRACT

Digital addictions, encompassing compulsive behaviors involving smartphones, gaming, social media, and digital platforms, have emerged as a significant public health challenge in the digital age. The impacts of digital addictions on mental health, social relationships, and productivity will challenge individuals and communities in every corner of the world. In this chapter, we investigate treatment options from traditional paradigms, such as cognitive-behavioural therapy (CBT) and digital detox programs, to forward-looking, technology-based alternatives like AI-powered mental health apps, wearables, and virtual reality therapies. The chapter will highlight community-based interventions, engagement in policy development, and illustrative case studies of global examples of digital addictions, including South Korea's national digital detox programs and gaming restrictions in China. This chapter offers a broad view of how different types of interventions - clinical psychological, technological, and policy approaches have been integrated to manage and prevent digital addictions.

1. INTRODUCTION

In the past twenty years, rapid advances in digital technology and the widespread migration to the digital world have transformed communication, entertainment,

DOI: 10.4018/979-8-2600-2468-3.ch013

education, and work. However, rapid digitalisation was not without noting the existence of a new suite of behavioural health problems, called digital addictions. Digital addictions involve compulsive and excessive use of one specific digital platform or device, characterised by impaired behavioural control, preoccupation, withdrawal, and a tendency to engage even with negative consequences (American Psychiatric Association, 2013; World Health Organisation [WHO], 2019). The new class of mental illness and addiction habitually includes smartphones, social media, gaming disorder, and internet addiction. It thus exhibits identifiable, distinct behavioural patterns associated with different psychological traits (Kuss & Lopez-Fernandez, 2016).

The recognition of the clinical relevance of digital addictions has developed over a period of time. A significant point in that development was the inclusion of Internet Gaming Disorder (IGD) as a condition for further study in the Diagnostic and Statistical Manual of Mental Disorders, Fifth Edition (DSM-5). The DSM-5 outlines nine criteria for IGD and include: preoccupation with gaming; withdrawal symptoms; tolerance; unsuccessful efforts to reduce the amount of use; loss of interest in a prior activity unrelated to gaming; use continues despite damage or harm occurring related to that use; lies to conceal amount of gaming; using gaming to escape negative feelings or moods; and jeopardizing or loosing a social function (American Psychiatric Association, 2013). In 2019, building on the DSM-5 foundation, the WHO officially recognised Gaming Disorder (GD) in the International Classification of Diseases, Eleventh Revision (ICD-11), thereby bringing global recognition of the disorder. The ICD-11 has defined GD as a pattern of persistent and recurrent gaming behaviours, characterised by impaired control of gaming behaviour, prominence of gaming behaviour, and continued gaming behaviour despite adverse consequences (WHO, 2019). This inclusion has legitimised a global move towards research and treatment (King & Delfabbro, 2019).

Newer research performed finds that digital addictions (for instance, phone addiction, social media addiction, gaming addiction, and Internet addiction) have become a widespread public health issue globally. Through a meta-analysis of more than 500 addiction studies, in 64 different countries and nearly 2.1 million subjects, researchers found a global prevalence of 27% smartphone addiction, 17.4% social media addiction, and 14.2% general internet addiction (Meng et al., 2022). Gaming addiction is estimated to affect about 3-6% of people around the world, but the numbers are much higher for children, adolescents, and young adults (Fam, 2018). In India, the rise in smartphone usage has resulted in some concerning rates of potential addiction. A study that thoroughly reviewed the evidence on internet addiction among Indian university students found that the prevalence rates, depending on different diagnostic criteria, ranged from 19.9% to 40.7% (Gupta et al., 2021). Depression, insomnia, quality of sleep, lower grades, and even sleep have connections with smartphone overuse, especially in adolescents aged between 6 and 18 (Solankure et al., 2025). There are also similar international findings; many studies found a correlation of digital addictions to mental distress such as anxiety, depression, feelings of isolation, and inadequate health-related quality of life (Elhai et al., 2017; Rajpurohit & Yadav, 2024). Although digital addictions are gaining recognition, treatment of these conditions is still a complicated task. First, diagnostic uncertainty exists, as except for Gaming Disorder, most digital addictions do not have universally accepted diagnostic definitions (Starcevic et al., 2021). For instance, definitions vary widely of "problematic social media use" and/or "smartphone addiction," which causes difficulty in standardising treatments (Billieux et al., 2015).

Second, the rapid and ever-changing nature of technology means new forms of addiction, like compulsive scrolling on short-form video platforms or virtual reality addiction, are constantly evolving, frequently outpacing clinical research and treatment development (Montag et al., 2021).

Third, there is a lack of qualified clinicians and/or treatment facilities, especially in low- and middle-income countries. Apart from simply favouring abandonment of a problematic use, even where resources and clinicians are available, stigma and a general lack of awareness may prevent people from seeking help (Griffiths et al., 2016).

Lastly, culture influences how digital additions develop and how treatment should be informed by culture. Interventions designed in one culture may not be broadly applicable, demonstrating the need for culturally appropriate and amenable treatment strategies (Kuss et al., 2019).

Therefore, there will be a need for innovative, multi-modal treatment strategies that incorporate psychological, technological, educational, and policy approaches. The previously mentioned traditional forms of treatment (e.g., cognitive-behavioural therapy (CBT) and motivational interviewing (MI)) are important, as are innovative approaches, including AI-assisted therapeutic tools, wearables, virtual reality (VR) exposure therapy, and digital detox programs (King et al., 2019).

There is also a role for governments and community interventions. For example, South Korea has national digital detox camps and counselling centres, whereas authorities in China have instituted limits on youth gaming and hobby hours (Xanidis & Brignell, 2016). Both examples represent systemic approaches in addition to individual therapy approaches.

This chapter has considered the history of interventional strategies to address digital addictions and reviewed both traditional and innovative treatments in practice. This chapter will include case studies, study analyses, and an analysis of implementation effectiveness for future research and practice. In this chapter, the phenomenon of digital addiction is not just a consequence of excessive tech use (i.e., a behavioural problem) but rather encompasses multiple social, psychological, technological, and policy challenges arising from platform design, behavioural reinforcement systems, and changing technological environments. There will be an analysis through international examples and a critical view of therapy, AI products, government and institutional support, and ethics to explore alternative or new ways of treating digital addiction.

2. BACKGROUND

Digital addiction is becoming a significant concern in behavioural health as people engage with technology more for social, educational, and recreational purposes. While digital technologies have vastly improved global connectivity and ease, misuse of digital technologies has created maladaptive behaviours that resemble substance-related addictions (Kuss & Griffiths, 2017). These behaviours often stem from compulsively engaged and uncontrollable behaviour that typically results in adverse psychosocial outcomes, including social isolation, diminished academic or occupational functioning, and poorer mental health (Andreassen et al., 2016).

The emerging recognition of digital addictions has raised calls for new theoretical frameworks that can help to explain the emergence and persistence of, and to treat, Internet Gaming Disorder (IGD) (American Psychiatric Association, 2013) and problematic social media use. In this section, we highlight the main theoretical frameworks underpinning digital addiction research and development, which stem from classical addiction development theories, behavioural and cognitive models, and cultural models, and relate these frameworks to ideas for future treatment innovations. The idea of addictive behaviour in the context of the internet and technology first surfaced in the late 1990s when Young (1998) developed the term "Internet Addiction Disorder (IAD)" and suggested criteria for IAD that were similar to pathological gambling. Young was motivated to do so by the growing body of anecdotal reports from people describing compulsive online behaviours (e.g., online gaming and chatting) that were negatively affecting their day-to-day functioning (see Young, 1998).

At first, there was some contention about whether or not excessive digital engagement was a real psychiatric disorder. However, after further research, evidence began to show that behavioural addictions were similar to substance use disorders in terms of their neurobiological mechanisms and similar psychological features (i.e., craving and withdrawal; Brand et al., 2019; Griffiths, 2016). With this evidence, Internet Gaming Disorder was eventually included in the DSM-5 as a condition for further study (American Psychiatric Association [APA], 2013), and Gaming Disorder (GD) was included as an official diagnosis in the ICD-11 (World Health Organisation [WHO], 2019). These developments have helped advance the public perception of digital addictions as legitimate public health issues that require systematic prevention and treatment (King & Delfabbro, 2019a).

Table 1. Types of Digital Addiction

Type	Characteristics	Common Platforms
Social Media Addiction	Compulsive social engagement	Instagram, TikTok
Gaming Disorder	Excessive gaming behavior	MMORPGs
Smartphone Addiction	Constant device dependency	Mobile applications
Streaming Addiction	Continuous content consumption	Netflix, YouTube
Online Gambling Addiction	Risk-oriented digital behavior	Betting platforms

3. TRADITIONAL TREATMENT APPROACHES

Digital addictions, which include problematic internet use, gaming disorder, social media addiction, and smartphone addiction, are now seen as legitimate public health concerns internationally (Kuss & Griffiths, 2017; WHO, 2019). Prior to advances in technology and technology-based interventions, these issues were treated using traditional psychological and behavioural therapies that have been adapted from models for other substance use or behavioural addictions. In their traditional forms, the primary base of these treatments is psychological counselling, behavioural modification, and/or structured clinical interventions, with aims of decreasing compulsive digital behaviours, promoting self-regulation, and/or addressing co-occurring mental health illnesses (King et al., 2019).

Traditional treatment approaches serve as a foundational option, utilising established, evidence-based interventions that underlie modern, technology-based interventions. Examples of traditional treatments include Cognitive-Behavioural Therapy (CBT), Motivational Interviewing (MI), Family-Based Therapy (FBT), Psychoeducation, and Digital Detox Programs.

Figure 1. Traditional Treatment Approaches for Digital Addictions

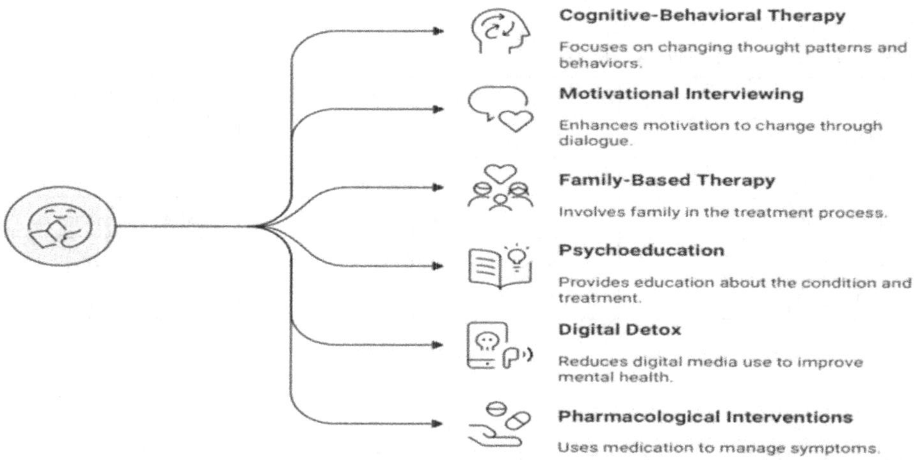

A. Cognitive-Behavioural Therapy (CBT)

Cognitive-Behavioural Therapy (CBT) is the most thoroughly researched and utilised traditional intervention strategy for digital addiction disorders, and was derived from cognitive-behavioural models of addiction (Davis, 2001). CBT takes the view that problematic technology use is a by-product of maladaptive thinking patterns and the behavioural cycles that reinforce them. This perspective suggests people may engage in excessive digital or online activities to cope with stress, boredom, social engagement, loneliness, or negative affect (King & Delfabbro, 2019b).

CBT can include different approaches, and for the treatment of digital addictions, CBT may include the following core concepts:

- Cognitive restructuring – identifying irrational beliefs about the need to be online or game excessively.
- Behaviour change – putting in place pragmatic solutions using concrete situations and ideas around technology use, such as using a time management strategy to manage limits around technology use, or offline (non-digital) alternatives to replace online time (Young, 2011).
- Resilience skills training - training individuals to develop coping (resilience) skills to manage their triggers and stresses that cause excessive and compulsive use of technology.

- Relapse prevention involves recognising possible early signs of relapse and developing personalised skills to enhance positive behaviour change and recovery.

There is a substantial body of literature showing efficacy for CBT in managing internet and gaming disorders. For example, King et al. (2017) showed a significant decrease in hours of gaming and improvement in psychosocial functioning in individuals who completed a structured CBT program. Furthermore, a randomised controlled trial that was completed in China reported evidence from a group-based CBT approach found considerable improvements in adolescent overall scores related to internet addiction (Li et al., 2016).

Recent clinical studies indicate that CBT-based interventions significantly reduce problematic internet usage and improve emotional regulation among adolescents and university students.

B. Motivational Interviewing (MI)

Motivational Interviewing (MI) is a client-centred approach to therapy aimed at increasing a person's internal motivation to change their behaviour (Miller & Rollnick, 2013). Many individuals with a digital addiction may not recognise the full extent of their problems or may feel conflicted about decreasing their use of technology. MI assists with that process by helping clients examine personal values and work through ambivalence. Important aspects of MI, when implementing an approach for digital addiction treatment, include:

- Expressing Empathy: Create a supportive, non-judgmental therapeutic atmosphere.
- Developing Discrepancy: Help clients identify the discrepancy between their behaviours, their digital use, and their life goals.
- Rolling with Resistance: Provide the gravity of debate without pressure and confrontation, empowering self-efficacy.
- Supporting Autonomy: Connect clients to their solutions and action plans.

MI is often utilised with CBT in the field of addiction to promote retention and decrease discharge rates (King et al., 2019). Moreover, evidence indicates that MI strategies led to greater engagement with treatment and improved outcomes in a research setting for gaming disorder (Stevens et al., 2021a).

C. Family-Based Therapy (FBT)

Family dynamics are instrumental for the formation and perpetuation of digital addictions, specifically for children and adolescents (Young, 2009). Family-Based Therapy (FBT) addresses family dynamics by involving parents, caregivers, and siblings throughout the treatment process.

Primary Goals of FBT:

- Improving family communication by highlighting arguments that may have led to a resolution for excessive use of digital devices.
- Parental involvement involves teaching parents how to establish healthy limits and monitor digital use effectively.
- Systemic change, reducing internal and external environmental triggers that contribute to compulsion.
- Supportive relationships help create emotional bonds and provide healthy social interaction.

Research supports the efficacy of FBT in reducing gaming disorder symptomology and enhancing family functioning. Specifically, studies have shown that FBT is more effective when implemented well, with multiple participants demonstrating significantly greater improvements after treatment than with individual therapy alone (Han & Renshaw, 2012).

D. Psychoeducation and Awareness Programs

Psychoeducation educates individuals, families, and communities about the nature of digital addictions, the dangers of digital addictions, and ways to cope. Psychoeducation is most helpful in early intervention, education, and prevention. Psychoeducation includes:

- inform individuals about the psychological mechanisms of digital addiction,
- inform individuals about the negative impact of excessive screen time on mental and physical health,
- provide suggestions on how to self-monitor and self-regulate their digital usage, and
- Provide individuals with a safe space to discuss their feelings about their digital use, helping to reduce stigma when seeking treatment (Griffiths et al., 2016).

School-based evaluation programs and widespread public awareness campaigns have been shown to help reduce excessive digital use or increase awareness among adolescents. For example, national education initiatives in South Korea have been credited with increasing the "awareness and early identification" of cases of digital addiction (Kim, 2017).

E. Digital Detox Programs

Digital detox programs involve temporarily stopping or limiting the use of digital devices to disrupt the habit of compulsively engaging with them. These detox programs, which are generally offered as retreats/camps, provide participants with an itinerary that prioritises offline activities, mindfulness, or socialising with other participants (Xanidis & Brignell, 2016).

Countries such as South Korea and China have developed government-sponsored digital detox camps where adolescents, for example, with severe gaming addictions receive intensive counselling and outdoor programs (Park et al., 2018). While digital detox on its own is not a cure-all, it can offer a reset before proceeding to more structured therapies with individuals to reshape their relationship with technology.

F. Pharmacological Interventions

While psychological therapies remain the primary modality for treating digital addiction, some exploration has been done on pharmacological approaches in the treatment of overlapping psychiatric conditions, namely ICD-10: F43.21 (depression); ICD-10: F41.0 (anxiety); ADHD (disorder) that contribute to compulsive technology use (Müller et al., 2015).

- SSRIs (Selective Serotonin Reuptake Inhibitors) are currently believed to be a possible treatment option for an individual with comorbid anxiety/depression.
- Stimulant medications are also showing to be a promising treatment option and may also be appropriate for individuals displaying symptoms of ADHD as well as Gaming disorder.

It should be noted that pharmacological treatment of digital addiction is considered best practice as a component of having psychological treatment under the careful eye of an expert (Petry et al., 2018).

Table 2. Traditional Treatment Approaches

Treatment Approach	Primary Goal	Key Techniques	Evidence of Effectiveness
Cognitive-Behavioural Therapy (CBT)	Restructure maladaptive thoughts and behaviours	Cognitive restructuring, relapse prevention	Strong evidence from multiple RCTs (King et al., 2019)
Motivational Interviewing (MI)	Increase readiness to change	Empathy, discrepancy, self-efficacy	Effective when combined with CBT (Stevens et al., 2021b)
Family-Based Therapy (FBT)	Improve family dynamics and support	Parent training, conflict resolution	High success rates with adolescents (Han & Renshaw, 2012)
Psychoeducation	Increase awareness and self-regulation	Workshops, public campaigns	Useful for prevention and early intervention (Kim, 2017)
Digital Detox Programs	Break the cycle of compulsive use	Abstinence, mindfulness, and offline activities	Effective as an initial intervention (Park et al., 2018)
Pharmacological Interventions	Manage comorbid conditions	SSRIs, ADHD medications	Limited, adjunctive role (Müller et al., 2015)

Although the principal and varied therapeutic methods of digital health treatment will continue to include CBT, mindfulness-based therapies, and behavioural counselling, they will also be implemented in different ways depending on which country or organisation is utilising them; these will be explained in more detail in Section 7. Traditional therapies are mainly focused on the person's or individual´s recovery from addiction through their behaviour and psychological support. Technological advancements have allowed for earlier detection of pain associated with Digital Addictions, creating new tools for monitoring and providing support to those with a digital addiction.

4. INNOVATIONS IN TREATMENT STRATEGIES

The rapid growth of technological development has greatly impacted the formation of digital addictions and how they are treated. The treatment modalities CBT, MI, and psychoeducation provide a strong initial base for addressing problematic digital use (King et al., 2019). However, these approaches can be practical at times but often barely address scalability, personalisation, and engagement (Stevens et al., 2021b). As digital addictions, including Internet Gaming Disorder (IGD), social media addiction, and smartphone addiction, continue to proliferate throughout the globe, the need for creative, technology-enabled, and multidisciplinary treatment methods also grows (Kuss & Griffiths, 2017; WHO, 2019).

Emerging technologies have already started to transform treatment, providing a range of treatment modalities including digital health tools, artificial intelligence (AI), virtual reality (VR), wearable technologies, and gamification, in addition to policies, initiatives, or community-based interventions that can now be integrated indirectly into treatment. These types of solutions improve accessibility, cost-effectiveness, and treatment adherence while addressing the complex nature of digital dependencies in modern society (Montag et al., 2021).

Figure 2. Innovative Treatment Strategy for Digital Addiction

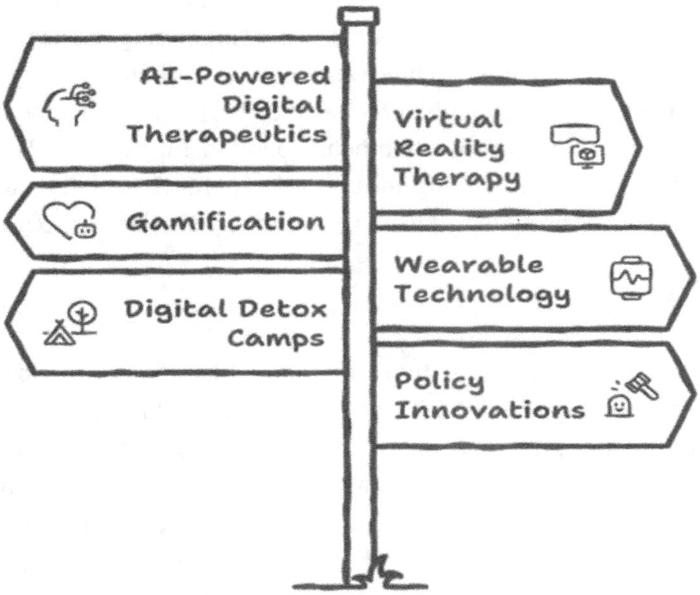

A. AI-Powered Digital Therapeutics

Artificial Intelligence (AI) is transforming the treatment of digital addictions through tools such as mobile applications, chatbots, and machine learning algorithms that provide real-time monitoring and individualised feedback (Torous et al., 2020). At scale, AI enables individualised monitoring of screen time (Montag et al., 2021), provides 24/7 access to therapeutic chats with chatbots (Fulmer et al., 2018), and offers clinicians more information through data-driven insights. Woebot, an app that uses AI and employs evidence-based strategies derived from Cognitive Behavioural Therapy (CBT), aims to alleviate the anxiety and depression related to digital withdrawal (Fitzpatrick et al., 2017). In summary, the inclusion of AI in the treatment of digital addiction increases access to care for all, especially for individuals in a broadly unexpected hierarchical situation to engaging with mental health support, while simultaneously introducing ethical considerations related to privacy, ownership of data, and algorithm implementation (Torous et al., 2020).

B. Virtual Reality (VR) Therapy

Virtual Reality (VR) offers a secure, controlled environment to help confront the triggers of digital addiction (e.g., gaming and social media) and develop self-regulation (Peris et al., 2020). VR is used in exposure therapy and creates simulated environments, such as virtual gaming rooms, to develop coping and decision-making skills (Park et al., 2022). VR-based interventions can facilitate recovery by alleviating cravings and supporting healthier habits, thus becoming a therapeutic adjunct, especially in connection with cognitive-behavioural therapy (CBT). The VR-based intervention process is a compelling and effective approach to developing healthier gaming habits and fostering long-term digital literacy (Park et al., 2022).

C. Gamification

GAmplification is the application of a game-like framework in therapeutic contexts to enhance motivation and engagement, particularly among video game players (Johnson et al., 2016). Examples of video game mechanics can help the client understand and assess their progress, motivate engagement in the process, and support accountability by using point systems, progress challenges, and competitive elements. Researchers report that gamification improves self-awareness and engagement while decreasing dropout rates in treatment programs (Lister et al., 2014). Applications like Forest and Habitica utilise these enhancements to foster beneficial daily habits. They are also designed to be non-digital activities, which can benefit patients with digital addictions by providing context-aware therapeutic recovery experiences.

D. Wearable technology

Wearable devices, such as smartwatches and biometric wearables, are important for tracking biological and behavioural indicators of digital addiction, including heart rate, sleep, and stress (Montag et al., 2021). Wearable devices allow individuals to identify early signs of relapse, coordinate with their clinician regarding their data, and enhance self-awareness through self-monitoring of their progress. For example, a user could wear a device that alerts them when their screen time reaches an unhealthy level, thereby promoting timely self-management and ultimately fostering healthier digital habits (Gao et al., 2020). Therefore, wearable devices represent a valuable advancement in prevention and intervention strategies for digital addiction.

E. Digital Detox Camps and Community-Based Initiatives

Additionally, new community-based initiatives (both virtual and in-person), such as digital detox camps, group therapy, and awareness campaigns, are receiving increased support from government and non-profits to help individuals reflect on and improve their digital habits. For example, national detox centres are operated by South Korea for youth who suffer from severe gaming addiction (Kim, 2017), while China has implemented national measures to limit minors' gaming time (Li et al, 2022). In Europe and North America, companies are pushing back against worker screen fatigue by promoting digital wellness programs. These treatment models supplement individualised treatment outcomes, as they tackle broader social and contextual components of digital addiction (Griffiths et al, 2016).

F. Policy and Regulatory Innovations

Policymaking is key to establishing safer conditions for the prevention and treatment of digital addiction. Governments are attempting to protect vulnerable groups (i.e., children and teens) through legislation, including establishing gaming age and time limits (Li et al., 2022); requiring apps or devices to include warnings or parental-control options; and funding public health campaigns on gaming addiction. The inclusion of Gaming Disorder in the ICD-11 by the WHO is an important milestone for standardised diagnosis, tracking, and treatment support (WHO, 2019). Policies can raise awareness about digital addiction while holding users accountable and addressing access to care.

Table 3. Innovative Treatment Strategies

Innovative Strategy	Core Focus	Key Benefits	Example/Case Study
AI-Powered Digital Therapeutics	Personalised, adaptive interventions	Scalable, real-time support	Woebot AI-CBT app
Virtual Reality Therapy (VR)	Simulated exposure to triggers	Safe, controlled environment	VR-based gaming disorder treatment (Park et al., 2022)
Gamification	Increasing motivation and engagement	Reduces dropout rates and is user-friendly	Forest, Habitica apps

continued on following page

Table 3. Continued

Innovative Strategy	Core Focus	Key Benefits	Example/Case Study
Wearable Technology	Physiological and behavioural tracking	Early relapse detection	Smartwatch-based alerts
Digital Detox Camps	Offline reset and recovery	Holistic, group-based interventions	South Korea detox centres
Policy Innovations	Regulation and public health advocacy	Prevention and societal support	China's gaming time limits

Table 4. AI-Based Intervention Tools and Ethical Risks

Technology	Benefit	Ethical Concern
Wearables	Continuous monitoring	Privacy invasion
AI Chatbots	Accessibility	Data misuse
Predictive Analytics	Early intervention	Algorithmic bias

4.1 Ethical Challenges in AI-Driven Digital Therapeutics

Although AI-assisted interventions are increasingly effective and scalable, several substantial ethical concerns regarding privacy, surveillance, informed consent, and data ownership remain. Numerous wearable monitoring systems and behavioural tracking applications frequently collect highly sensitive psychological and behavioural data, creating a high risk of misuse, commercial exploitation, and insufficient consent. Predictive behaviour systems also potentially diminish users' autonomy by encouraging the continual monitoring and algorithm-based intervention in users' average daily behaviour. The rapid expansion of AI-assisted digital therapeutics thus creates critical tension between technical efficiency and ethical responsibility.

AI technologies can increase accessibility, personalisation, and early intervention strategies; however, they need to be governed transparently, ethically safeguarded, and supported by strong data protection measures.

Furthermore, using technology alone as an intervention will not solve the social and structural issues surrounding digital addiction. A sustainable method of handling this situation can be achieved if the proper institutional policies are in place at the time of treatment, regulations are provided as guidelines by an organisation, individuals within the community are willing to adhere to the regulations, and there is a way to develop public awareness through public education programs.

5. COMMUNITY-BASED AND POLICY INTERVENTIONS

Digital addictions like excessive gaming, social media use, and compulsive smartphone use have quickly grown into a global public health problem that affects mental health, productivity, and social relationships (WHO, 2019; Kuss & Griffiths, 2017). While individual-level treatments, such as Cognitive-Behavioural Therapy (CBT) and AI-based digital therapeutics, are important, at the community and policy levels, how we respond to treatment in the wider social environment is important for prevention, early detection, and long-term recovery (Griffiths et al., 2016).

Community-level interventions seek to harness community resources (families, schools, organisations) to raise awareness, prevent substance use, and create pathways to accessible care. Policy-level interventions, on the other hand, establish regulatory structures that ensure ethical use of technology, safeguard vulnerable groups, and generate funding opportunities for prevention and treatment services (Li et al., 2022). Combining community and policy interventions leads to a multilevel approach to a public health problem. This approach considers both individuals' behavioural responses and the systemic societal factors that drive digital addiction.

6.1 Community-Based Interventions

Community-level efforts are essential for grassroots prevention and treatment, especially for adolescents and young adults, who are the most at-risk groups for digital addiction (Young, 2011). Community-based efforts can include schools, families, local organisations, and public messaging that help create an environment of digital well-being.

A. School-Based Digital Literacy and Prevention Programs

Schools play a crucial role in identifying and preventing harmful digital use by incorporating digital literacy into their curricula, thereby encouraging healthy digital behaviours and self-regulation (Kim, 2017). This could involve discussing issues related to cyberbullying and compulsive behaviours, while also developing better time management and offline practices. Additionally, using screening tools can help identify students at risk for problematic digital use (Kuss et al., 2014). For example, South Korea's "i-Seum" program offered classroom lessons and parent engagement to help children minimise screen time and become more socially successful and productive students (Kim, 2017).

B. Family-Centred Interventions

The family is an important influence on digital behaviours, especially in a child's early years and adolescence (Young, 2009). Community-based initiatives often involve parents, caregivers, and families in activities designed to improve communication and develop strategies to regulate technology use. Family-based strategies can include educating parents on non-punitive forms of screen-time regulation, family workshops focused on building problem-solving skills, and offering counselling to manage relational conflict stemming from technology overuse (Han & Renshaw, 2012). Studies show that when families are involved, treatment adherence improves, particularly when adolescents are engaged in video-gaming addiction, with failure to adhere negatively impacting recovery (King et al., 2019).

C. Digital Detox Camps and Retreats

Digital detox camps provide specialised environments where individuals can withdraw from digital devices and reevaluate their relationship with technology. Common elements of detox camps include outdoor activities, mindfulness courses, meditation, and group therapy aimed at achieving balance and wellness (Xanidis & Brignell, 2016). In South Korea, there are more than 200 government-sponsored detox camps that offer recreational and therapeutic programs targeted to at-risk adolescents who exhibit symptoms of digital addiction (Park et al., 2018). Moreover, in China, adolescents with significant gaming disorder may have to engage with an inpatient treatment centre (Li et al., 2022). It is essential to note that detox camps are sometimes included as part of a more extensive and comprehensive clinical program for treatment recovery from gaming disorder, and are for the purpose of immersing these adolescents in offline experiences and community support mechanisms to facilitate recovery.

D. Community-Based Peer Support Groups

Peer support groups represent a critical element of continuous social support and accountability for people recovering from digital addiction. Similar to 12-step addiction programs, peer groups provide an opportunity for individuals to share experiences, strategies for coping, and useful-life mechanisms for addressing problematic engagement with the digital world.. Examples of peer groups include Digital Wellness Clubs on college campuses, local community support groups organized by organizations like The Center for Humane Technology, and peer-support forums that are online and moderated for safety and constructive interaction (Montag et al.,

2021). These peer-practitioner networks provide a sense of belonging and empowerment that further support recovery (Montag et al., 2021).

6.2. Response to Policy

To address the environmental and structural issues associated with digital addiction, new governmental policies and laws will have to be put into place. Policymakers play a proven and essential role in establishing usage limits, ethical technology design, and funding research and treatment (Li et al., 2022).

A. Regulatory Interventions

Multiple nations have developed comprehensive policy plans to reduce unhealthy gaming and other screen time among children and youth. For example, in China, gaming is limited to only 3 hours per week under real-name registration designed to monitor gaming time (Li et al., 2022). In South Korea, the "Cinderella Law" bars youth under age 16 from gaming between midnight and 6:00 a.m. (Kim, 2017). The European Union's General Data Protection Regulation (GDPR) includes privacy protections to address harmful design practices while preventing manipulation through custom protocols based on individuals' data. In conclusion, the goals of these policy initiatives are to reduce gambling addiction, minimise risk, and enhance healthy digital engagement among children/young people through intervention and legislation of risky features of their online environment.

B. Designing policies that promote ethical technology

Policymakers are increasingly urging tech companies to prioritise user well-being over engagement through features such as time-limiting apps, transparency in algorithmic recommender systems (Torous et al., 2020), or banning tweets that engage in manipulative structures toward children. For example, Apple and Google are beginning to create digital well-being dashboards to help customers monitor and limit their screen time, due to public health considerations (Gao et al., 2020).

C. Funding & Financial Support for Research

Clinical trials, visibility initiatives, and treatment strategies can be funded through government sources. Funding can take the form of grants for research institutions, health organisations, or non-profits conducting epidemiology and efficacy research on the treatment of digital addiction (WHO, 2019). South Korea provides substantial funding to its National Information Society Agency (NIA) to run nationwide campaigns and treatment centres (Kim, 2017).

D. Global Concerns

Digital addiction is a global concern that requires all countries to work together on research, policies, and interventions. The World Health Organisation's decision in 2019 to include Gaming Disorder in the ICD-11 was not only important in the development of a global framework for diagnosing this addiction (WHO, 2019). Regional summits and initiatives supported by organisations such as the OECD and WHO encourage countries to share best practices for preventing and treating digital addiction (Montag et al., 2021).

7. CASE STUDIES OF SUCCESSFUL INTERVENTIONS

7.1 South Korea's National Digital Detox Program

7.1.1. Background and Rationale

With some of the highest rates of internet use and broadband connectivity in the world, South Korea is among the most digitally connected countries. The growth of technology has driven economic and social advancement, but has also increased rates of digital addiction, especially among youth and young adults (Koo, 2011).

When internet gaming addiction was recognised as a concern in the early 2000s, troubling accounts emerged showing the impact of excessive gaming on academic performance, family relationships, mental health, and instances of severely neglected care of children (Kim, 2017). By 2010, research suggested that 8% to 12% of Korean adolescents reported symptoms of internet addiction (Park et al., 2018). South Korea viewed the escalation of internet addiction as a public health crisis and, therefore, implemented a multi-tiered, nationwide strategy in response to the prevention and treatment of digital addictions. As part of the overall strategy, the government developed residential "digital detox" camps, digital citizenship education programs in schools, family counselling programs, and regulations on gaming behaviour (Young, 2009; Koo, 2011).

7.1.2. Program Components

Korea's National Digital Detox Program is overseen by the Ministry of Gender Equality and Family (MOGEF), National Information Society Agency (NIA), local government agencies, schools, and community organisations, with the overall objective of reducing digital device addiction, while utilising a holistic, multi-level, wrap-around approach (Kim, 2017). Digital addiction service delivery platforms generally comprise government-supported counselling centres that offer clinical evaluation, cognitive-behavioural therapy, and family therapy. The centres act as important nodes for early intervention (Han & Renshaw, 2012). When cases are much more severe, there are live-in residential digital detox programs (also called internet detox camps) that offer a structured, naturally social setting confined to a space without technology, while incorporating mindfulness training, outdoor experiences, and group therapy. These programs typically last two to four weeks, aiming to disrupt patterns of problematic behaviours and teach strategies to avoid harmful digital habits and discontent. By 2016, there were more than 200 camps funded by government support (Kim, 2017; Park et al., 2018; Xanidis & Brignell, 2016). Schools have considered incorporating digital literacy education, time management training, screening tools, and parental workshops as part of their i-Seum Program to combat technology-related addiction, especially among youth (Kim, 2017). South Korea has also taken several legislative measures to tackle technology-related addiction, such as the "Shutdown Law" introduced in 2011, banning minors under 16 years old from playing online games between midnight and 06:00, but this was abolished in 2021 in part due to the law being deemed unenforceable and largely ineffective (Li et al, 2022; Montag et al., 2021). Thus, the proactive stance of South Korea towards addressing digital addiction through a multi-dimensional approach to prevention, intervention, and regulation reflects a demonstrative interest in addressing digital addictions.

7.1.3. Implementation in Practice

The approach taken by the program entails a multi-system initiative:

- Early detection, which takes shape in school screenings and parent reporting;
- Outpatient therapy through community counselling centres for mild to moderate cases;
- Residential detox treatment centres for severe addiction cases;
- Post-treatment follow-up, including family therapy and community group meetings (King et al., 2019).

Residential camps highlight technology abstinence, physical activity, cognitive-behavioural therapy-based group sessions, and family involvement to support and reinforce behaviour changes (Han & Renshaw, 2012).

7.1.4. Evidence of Effectiveness

Research supports the notion that digital detox intervention programs in South Korea have produced short-term reductions in screen time and improved mental health indicators (i.e., anxiety and depression) (Park et al., 2018; Mohamed et al., 2022).

For example, Mohammed et al. (2022) reported that structured detox interventions significantly improved symptoms of adolescent electronic screen syndrome. In a separate context, King et al. (2019) reported that family involvement in therapy supported continued adherence to therapy and greater reductions in relapse.

However, in terms of sustainability, long-term reporting is problematic. Follow-up studies demonstrate that many participants returned to their old habits within months of their programs ending, without ongoing support from families and schools (Montag et al., 2021).

7.1.5 Challenges and Criticisms

Despite being historically viewed as an innovative solution, the program has received several criticisms:

- Sustainability: Detox camps are only short-term solutions; they lack structured follow-up measures for long-term outcomes (Park et al., 2018).
- Regulatory backlash: the Shutdown Law provoked public opposition, and frequently, a minor would utilise a parent's account (Li et al, 2022).
- Stigma and Rights: restraining therapy and enforcement could stigmatise the adolescent or infringe personal autonomy (Montag et al, 2021).
- Need for standardised metrics: different studies use different terms for digital addiction and different measures for analysis, which complicates the evaluation of treatments (Kuss et al., 2014).

7.1.6 Lessons for Global Policy and Practice

South Korea's experience provides some implications for countries experiencing digital addiction.

- Multi-level approach: Utilising both school-based prevention, family programs, and community-based family and clinical interventions is a much more complex and cohesive approach than singular strategies (Young, 2011).
- 2. Follow-up: detox programs need to have aftercare and relapse prevention in order to continue the benefits and gains (King et al, 2019).

- 3. Policy: regulation needs to establish evidence-based and respond to the changing technological and cultural paradigms (Li et al, 2022);
- 4. Evaluation- Considerations should be made about going forward for deriving consistent diagnostic and evaluative metrics internationally (WHO, 2019).

7.2 China's Gaming Restrictions Policy

7.2.1. Background and Rationale

As of 2021, China has one of the largest gaming markets in the world, with more than 668 million gamers, a large proportion of whom are children and adolescents (Li et al., 2022). While gaming has had a tremendous impact on China's digital economy, gaming addiction, otherwise known as "internet gaming disorder," has raised alarms over the last two decades (Montag et al., 2021).

Starting in the early 2010s, Chinese health authorities, as well as parents, became concerned with the adverse effects of excessive gaming, including reduced performance in school, sleep problems, mental health issues, and extreme cases in which there were severe bodily injuries as well (Kuss et al., 2014).

In 2019, the World Health Organisation (WHO) formally designated Gaming Disorder as a mental health condition within the ICD-11 classification (WHO, 2019). The designation enabled many to gain a global perspective, which in turn strengthened the need for specific policies to prevent and treat gaming-related conditions. Subsequently, the Chinese government started to enact rigorous regulatory policies to reduce the gaming hours for minors, restrict the potential for gaming design that motivates addiction, and protect the mental health of youth (Li et al., 2022).

7.2.2 Key Elements of the Policy

China's gaming restriction policy is a broad-based initiative aimed at combating digital addiction among minors, including playing time limits, real-name verification, content restrictions, and corporate responsibilities. Monitoring and enforcement of the policy are the responsibility of the National Press and Publication Administration (NPPA), alongside the Ministry of Education and the National Health Commission of the People's Republic of China. The strict rules of the policy are administered and enforced (Gao et al., 2020). Minors under 18 are permitted to play for three hours per week, one hour each day from Friday through Sunday, restricted to 8–9 PM, with additional playing time on national holidays. This policy represents a significant shift from the playing time regulations prior to 2019 (Li et al., 2022; Montag et al., 2021). Real-name verification, along with facial recognition, is a required measure to enforce playing time limits and to support companies' responsibilities for monitoring usage in real time (Li et al., 2022). The policies aim to reduce addictive aspects of video games by banning item systems, such as loot boxes and gameplay pay-to-win systems. The restrictions have also limited in-app purchases, removed inappropriate content from video games, and encouraged the development of educational or culturally valuable video games (Gao et al., 2020). Video game companies have a legal obligation to comply with regulations, and failure to do so may result in monetary fines or the revocation of their gaming license. Tencent and NetEase were fined for failing to comply with the regulations (Li et al., 2022; Montag et al., 2021).

7.2.3 Execution and Enforcement

The Chinese government employs technology-based enforcement mechanisms:

- A national database that links gamers' real names and data across gaming platforms.
- Facial recognition technology in government-issued identification cards is used to prevent minors from using adults' game accounts.
- Game applications would automatically shut down as soon as a daily or weekly specific time limit was reached.
- Parents and the community could call a hotline to report violations that would be made public.

This centralised enforcement method of the youth gaming laws represents one of the strongest attempts globally to regulate digital behaviours at the population level (Li et al., 2022).

7.2.4 Outcomes and Impacts

The restriction policy in China has swiftly displaced youth gaming in the short term, particularly with Tencent reporting a 92% reduction in time spent gaming among underage players in the first couple of months. Parents also reported that their youth regularly engaged more in their schoolwork and had better sleep patterns (Li et al., 2022). Notably, the policy disrupted the gaming industry, causing stock prices of major companies like Tencent and NetEase to drop and prompting game developers to pivot toward adult and international gaming markets to offset losses (Gao et al., 2020). In some cases, youth borrowed parents' accounts or used their own VPNs and/or accessed foreign locations to keep playing video games and engage in more offline gaming (Montag et al., 2021). As a result, the restrictions highlighted the difficulties with promoting full behavioural compliance.

7.2.5 Criticisms and Challenges

While China's gaming restriction policy is novel globally, it faces controversies and challenges. First, critics claim that it over-regulates minors and takes away any vestiges of freedom to choose their leisure activities (Montag et al., 2021). In addition, many minors find ways to circumvent the rules through account sharing and VPNs, raising concerns about the effectiveness of management, even with sophisticated monitoring systems (Li et al., 2022). Possible addictive consequences could appear, like binge game play during the designated hours, or even switching to another addiction, such as excessive use of smartphones or social media (Kuss et al., 2014). Lastly, from an economic perspective, the policy received some criticism for constraining creativity and innovation in the gaming industry, which may hinder China's ability to compete in the international market (Gao et al., 2020).

7.2.6 Implications for Global Strategy

China's experience provides valuable lessons for other countries wanting to regulate gaming:

- Technology can facilitate enforcement, but it will always be the cultural and social context that determines acceptance.
- In the short term, strict time limits are practical, but family involvement and education will determine long-term effectiveness (King et al., 2019).
- Moderation, established through parenting, education, and industry, will probably be the more sustainable approach compared to the more rigid structure of regulation or to no parenting or education at all.
- A collaborative approach among countries will be necessary to regulate cross-border gaming and digital addiction on a global scale (WHO, 2019).

7.3 Community-Based Interventions in the EU

7.3.1 Introduction

Digital addiction has been identified as a serious public health issue across the European Union (EU), in particular due to excessive use of social media, gaming, and other online platforms. Increasing numbers of adolescents and young adults have been diagnosed with internet use disorder (IUD) and gaming disorder (GD), all of which have raised considerable worry about mental health, academic outcomes, and social connections (Király et al., 2020; Rumpf et al., 2018).

In 2019, the World Health Organisation (WHO) recognised gaming disorder in its 11th Revision of the International Classification of Diseases (ICD-11), which influenced and encouraged policymakers in Europe to move to include preventive and treatment initiatives (WHO, 2019). Unlike countries such as China and South Korea, which have adopted heavily top-down regulatory approaches, EU member states focus on community-based and education-focused preventive approaches rather than regulatory initiatives (Sariyska et al., 2017).

7.3.2 A Framework for the EU Community-Based Interventions

The EU is adopting a public, public health, and community-centred approach to digital addiction, addressing issues related to awareness, prevention, and recovery, rather than over-regulation. Programs are implemented through schools, local health services, NGOs, and family support networks, and are effective (Stevens et al., 2021a).

Key principles:

Empower families and communities through various digital literacy programs.

- Screen for problematic use early in primary care and in schools.
- Integration of service into the local health care system.
- Cross-border work among EU member states to document best practices (Király et al., 2020).

7.3.3 Community-Based Interventions Types

In fact, Europe has prioritised digital literacy and education as part of a public health response to digital addiction, particularly for minors and their families. The European Commission's "Better Internet for Kids" (BIK) initiative provides information about internet safety, educational resources, and opportunities to connect with groups working on safe practices in their communities (Livingstone et al., 2019). In all EU member states, Safer Internet Centres (SICs) provide helplines and action lines regarding online risks and allow students, parents, and others to report harmful content. Schools and workshop settings may subsequently offer programming on digital citizenship (Stevens et al., 2021b), thereby shifting the conversation about healthy technology use from fear to education. With support in schools, you provide prevention initiatives that focus on early intervention; for example, the Digital Balance Program, developed in Finland, provides educators with training on problematic use of digital technologies and links individuals to resources if needed (Király et al., 2020). Additionally, Germany partners with educators, schools, and youth services with local mental health providers to screen and provide group support for students with internet and gaming use addiction (Rumpf et al., 2018). There are also peer-to-peer education options at partner schools in the Netherlands and Denmark that encourage students to engage with one another within their networks (Livingstone et al., 2019).

Community health and counselling services are another set of supports in addition to school initiatives. There are local addiction clinics that have specialised programs for gaming disorder. At the same time, community centres offer group therapy, family counselling, and workshops to help families find digital balance and harmony in their lives (Stevens et al., 2021b). In Italy and Spain, therapists are working with parents to develop digital detox plans that are feasible in parents' daily lives and accessible to families of varying income levels (Montag et al., 2021).

Support groups provide a non-judgmental way to share digital addiction experiences and strategies to reduce the addiction, as modelled on 12-step groups and programs as well (Király et al., 2020). Some groups combine online and in-person support during times such as the pandemic (Stevens et al., 2021b).

Similar to initiatives in EU member states, community programs can also be created to establish a uniform toolbox and share best practices. The EU Kids Online Network is researching how to use the digital risk and access research to reduce risks to the participants (Livingstone et al., 2019). The Pan European Game Information (PEGI) is a content rating system that provides guidelines for parents to check games for content (Stevens et al., 2021b). In addition, Horizon Europe is a funding program for research aimed at advancing digital well-being and preventing addiction, while facilitating cross-border collaboration and innovation.

7.3.4 Example in Action: "Safer Internet Day"

In practice, Safer Internet Day (SID) is an excellent example of a community initiative, which takes place annually as a member state activity throughout all EU Member States:

- Organised by the Insafe network, SID provides information about how to behave responsibly online via workshops, school activities, and social media (Livingstone et al., 2019).
- There are organisations, local communities, and technology companies that partner to raise awareness of digital addiction and online safety.
- In 2024, SID is expected to be viewed by over 180 million people worldwide, underscoring the importance of community engagement (Stevens et al., 2021a).

7.3.5 Results and Impact

The literature supports the idea that community initiatives in the EU have a positive impact on digital well-being:

- Király et al. (2020) found a significant decrease in adolescents' gaming disorder symptoms after an intervention, at school, and at the time, and again after 6 months.
- The Better Internet for Kids network found and reported a 30% increase in parental awareness of the risks associated with digital addiction from 2018 to 2022 (Livingstone et al., 2019).
- Rumpf and colleagues (2018) described the increased accessibility and reduced stigma associated with integrating gaming-based disease treatment into a local health service.

7.3.6 Challenges

There are some challenges:

- Limited funding or budget constraints in some parts of the EU.
- Inequitable access to services in rural vs urban areas.
- The pace of digital technology development is so rapid that programs and policies cannot keep up with the pace of change.

Table 5. Comparative International Policy Responses

Country	Strategy	Strength	Limitation
South Korea	Detox camps	Structured rehabilitation	Psychological pressure
China	Gaming restrictions	Reduced gaming time	Surveillance concerns
India	Awareness campaigns	Accessibility	Limited infrastructure

8. CHALLENGES IN TREATMENT DEVELOPMENT

A. Diagnostic and Conceptual Issues

Diagnostic woes and conceptual challenges majorly inhibit the development of effective treatments for digital addictions. Unlike gaming disorder, for which diagnoses were only recently inserted into ICD-11, there are still no widely recognised diagnostic criteria for the alternative types of digital addiction, coarsely defined as social media addiction, smartphone addiction, etc. (WHO, 2019). Inconsistencies in terminology continue to abound, as one model will posit internet addiction, another problematic internet use, and yet another screen dependency, thus confounding clinical assessment and research (Montag et al., 2021). In addition, given that depression, anxiety, ADHD, and substance abuse may co-occur with these alleged addictions, it is worth considering whether these could be secondary maladaptive behaviours rather than primary, thus complicating treatment strategies (King et al., 2019; Rumpf et al., 2018).

B. Technological Challenges

Technological challenges also slow down the development of treatment. The rapid pace of evolution in apps, online platforms, and digital games means that interventions may be outdated by the time they are implemented (Montag et al., 2021). Technology can also work in practical ways towards treatment through mobile apps, AI-assisted therapy, and online monitoring. However, these pose troubling concerns regarding privacy, security, and accessibility for the very vulnerable populations (Livingstone et al., 2019; Stevens et al., 2021b).

C. Cultural and Societal Barriers

Cultural and societal barriers make treatment even more challenging. The way we perceive digital addiction is profoundly shaped by our cultural norms, which can influence whether it is regarded as a serious clinical issue or merely a behavioural concern (Király et al., 2020). It is really sad that the stigma surrounding this issue, along with a general lack of public awareness, often prevents people from seeking the help they truly need. This can lead to delays in early intervention and make addiction worse, especially for young people (Montag et al., 2021).

D. Policy and Regulatory Challenges

On top of that, some serious policy and regulatory hurdles make things even more complicated. The lack of rules regarding addictive features on digital platforms—like loot boxes or algorithms designed to keep users engaged—puts individuals in a vulnerable position. Moreover, healthcare systems often fall short in providing adequate coverage for treatments related to digital addiction (King & Delfabbro, 2019a; Király et al., 2020). To make matters worse, the differences in how countries recognise digital addiction as a medical condition make it challenging to standardise treatment on a global scale.

E. Research Gaps and Ethical Concerns

Research gaps and ethical concerns can significantly hinder progress. It is important to recognise these issues as we move forward. Most studies are short-term or cross-sectional, with few randomised controlled trials to evaluate treatment efficacy over time (Stevens et al., 2021a; King et al., 2019). Ethical issues, including data privacy, informed consent, and balancing individual autonomy with public health objectives, must be addressed when deploying technology-based interventions (Livingstone et al., 2019; Montag et al., 2021

9. FUTURE DIRECTIONS

Digital addiction, which includes everything from internet browsing and online gaming to social media use and smartphone overuse, is becoming a significant public health issue around the world (Montag et al., 2021). To tackle this complex problem, future treatment approaches should focus on early detection, tailored care, innovative technology, community involvement, and integrating policies (Király et al., 2020; King et al., 2019).

Improving diagnostics is crucial. We need standardised criteria that are accepted globally for various types of digital addictions, not just gaming disorder. This will help us assess the situation accurately, conduct cross-cultural research, and plan effective interventions (WHO, 2019). Additionally, the combination of digital phenotyping and AI-driven monitoring offers exciting opportunities for early detection. By examining behavioural patterns, screen time, and app usage, we can craft personalised strategies to prevent issues before they arise (Montag et al., 2021).

Technological advancements are set to be a game-changer in treatment. With AI-driven interventions, gamified therapy programs, virtual reality (VR) exposure therapy, and mobile health (mHealth) apps, we now have scalable, adaptable, and engaging ways to approach treatment (Stevens et al., 2021a; King et al., 2019). These cutting-edge solutions enable ongoing monitoring, instant feedback, and tailored behaviour adjustments, which can significantly enhance adherence and outcomes. Additionally, working together with tech companies can help minimise exposure to addictive features on platforms (Livingstone et al., 2019; King & Delfabbro, 2019b). It is also vital to foster cross-cultural and international collaboration to ensure that interventions are culturally sensitive and effective globally.

When it comes to research priorities, we are looking at longitudinal studies, randomised controlled trials (RCTs), and standardised outcome measures to assess the effectiveness and sustainability of treatments (Stevens et al., 2021b; Király et al., 2020). Keeping ethical considerations in mind—such as data privacy, informed consent, and digital autonomy—is essential, especially as we begin to roll out AI, VR, and digital monitoring in treatment programs (Livingstone et al., 2019).

To sum it all up, the future of tackling digital addiction really depends on using integrated, flexible, and research-backed strategies. This involves combining technology with clinical support, engaging communities, and creating strong policy frameworks. Key factors such as early detection, tailored interventions, and global collaboration will be crucial to addressing the growing issue of digital addiction and promoting healthier digital habits worldwide.

10. CONCLUSION

Digital addiction has emerged as a significant concern in the 21st century, driven by the swift growth of internet technologies, social media, online gaming, and mobile apps. Its effects extend far beyond personal well-being, affecting mental health, academic success, relationships, and overall quality of life. Addressing this issue requires a mix of strategies that combine clinical methods, technology-driven solutions, community efforts, and regulatory actions (Király et al., 2020; Montag et al., 2021).

Diagnostic clarity is still a key element. While it was a positive move to include gaming disorder in the ICD-11, we still lack clear guidelines for other concerns like social media and smartphone addiction (WHO, 2019). Recent advancements, such as AI-driven monitoring and digital phenotyping, present exciting opportunities for early detection and tailored care. However, they also bring up important privacy and ethical issues (Montag et al., 2021). Technological innovations, including AI therapy, gamified treatments, and mobile health apps, are making it easier for young people to find support and stay engaged. Community-based strategies that involve schools, families, and peer networks are essential for building resilience and improving digital literacy (Livingstone et al., 2019).

We are facing ongoing challenges—such as the rapid pace of technological change, rising mental health concerns, and the lack of consistent global policies—that call for us to work together internationally and rely on evidence-based strategies. To foster healthy digital interactions and protect our society's well-being, we need a comprehensive, flexible, and ethical approach.

REFERENCES

American Psychiatric Association. (2013). *Diagnostic and statistical manual of mental disorders* (5th ed.). American Psychiatric Publishing., DOI: 10.1176/appi.books.9780890425596

Andreassen, C. S., Pallesen, S., & Griffiths, M. D. (2016). The relationship between addictive use of social media, narcissism, and self-esteem: Findings from a large national survey. *Addictive Behaviors*, *64*, 287–293. DOI: 10.1016/j.addbeh.2016.03.006 PMID: 27072491

Billieux, J., Maurage, P., Lopez-Fernandez, O., Kuss, D. J., & Griffiths, M. D. (2015). Can disordered mobile phone use be considered a behavioural addiction? An update on current evidence and a comprehensive model for future research. *Current Addiction Reports*, *2*(2), 156–162. DOI: 10.1007/s40429-015-0054-y

Brand, M., Young, K. S., Laier, C., Wölfling, K., & Potenza, M. N. (2019). Integrating psychological and neurobiological considerations regarding the development and maintenance of specific internet-use disorders: An Interaction of Person-Affect-Cognition-Execution (I-PACE) model. *Neuroscience and Biobehavioral Reviews*, *71*, 252–266. DOI: 10.1016/j.neubiorev.2016.08.033 PMID: 27590829

Davis, R. A. (2001). A cognitive-behavioural model of pathological internet use. *Computers in Human Behavior*, *17*(2), 187–195. DOI: 10.1016/S0747-5632(00)00041-8

Elhai, J. D., Levine, J. C., Dvorak, R. D., & Hall, B. J. (2017). Non-social features of smartphone use are most related to depression, anxiety, and problematic smartphone use. *Computers in Human Behavior*, *69*, 75–82. DOI: 10.1016/j.chb.2016.12.023

Fam, J. Y. (2018). Prevalence of internet gaming disorder in adolescents: A meta-analysis across three decades. *Scandinavian Journal of Psychology*, *59*(5), 524–531. DOI: 10.1111/sjop.12459 PMID: 30004118

Fitzpatrick, K. K., Darcy, A., & Vierhile, M. (2017). Delivering cognitive behaviour therapy to young adults with symptoms of depression and anxiety using a fully automated conversational agent (Woebot): A randomised controlled trial. *JMIR Mental Health*, *4*(2), e19. DOI: 10.2196/mental.7785 PMID: 28588005

Fulmer, R., Joerin, A., Gentile, B., Lakerink, L., & Rauws, M. (2018). Using psychological artificial intelligence (Tess) to relieve symptoms of depression and anxiety: Randomised controlled trial. *JMIR Mental Health*, *5*(4), e64. DOI: 10.2196/mental.9782 PMID: 30545815

Gao, L., Gan, Y., Zhang, Y., & Liu, R. (2020). Wearable devices for health monitoring in the Internet of Things: A survey. *Journal of Industrial Information Integration*, *17*, 100130. DOI: 10.1016/j.jii.2020.100130

Griffiths, M. D. (2016). Behavioural addiction in sport: The case of exercise addiction. *Journal of Behavioral Addictions*, *5*(2), 133–139. DOI: 10.1556/2006.5.2016.018

Griffiths, M. D., Kuss, D. J., & Demetrovics, Z. (2016). Social networking addiction: An overview of preliminary findings. In *Behavioural addictions* (pp. 119–141). Academic Press., DOI: 10.1016/B978-0-12-407724-9.00006-9

Gupta, A., Khan, A. M., & Gupta, A. (2021). Internet addiction and its correlates among Indian college students: A systematic review. *Indian Journal of Community Medicine : Official Publication of Indian Association of Preventive & Social Medicine*, *46*(3), 433–440. DOI: 10.4103/ijcm.IJCM_230_21

Han, D. H., & Renshaw, P. F. (2012). Bupropion in the treatment of problematic online game play in patients with major depressive disorder. *Journal of Psychopharmacology*, *26*(5), 689–696. DOI: 10.1177/0269881111400647 PMID: 21447539

Johnson, D., Deterding, S., Kuhn, K. A., Staneva, A., Stoyanov, S., & Hides, L. (2016). Gamification for health and wellbeing: A systematic review of the literature. *Internet Interventions : The Application of Information Technology in Mental and Behavioural Health*, *6*, 89–106. DOI: 10.1016/j.invent.2016.10.002 PMID: 30135818

Kim, J. (2017). South Korea's approach to combating gaming addiction. *Asia Pacific Journal of Social Work and Development*, *27*(2-3), 134–145. DOI: 10.1080/02185385.2017.1352170

King, D. L., & Delfabbro, P. H. (2019a). *Internet gaming disorder: Theory, assessment, treatment, and prevention*. Academic Press., DOI: 10.1016/C2017-0-02346-3

King, D. L., & Delfabbro, P. H. (2019b). Video game monetisation (e.g., 'loot boxes'): A blueprint for practical social responsibility measures. *International Journal of Mental Health and Addiction*, *17*(1), 166–179. DOI: 10.1007/s11469-018-0009-3

King, D. L., Delfabbro, P. H., Griffiths, M. D., & Gradisar, M. (2019). Cognitive-behavioural approaches to outpatient treatment of internet gaming disorder: A pilot study. *Journal of Clinical Psychology*, *73*(3), 301–309. DOI: 10.1002/jclp.22323

Király, O., Griffiths, M. D., King, D. L., Lee, H. K., Lee, S. Y., Bányai, F., Zsila, Á., Takács, Z. K., & Demetrovics, Z. (2020). Policy responses to problematic video game use: A systematic review of current measures and future possibilities. *Journal of Behavioral Addictions*, *9*(2), 257–271. DOI: 10.1556/2006.2020.00040 PMID: 28859487

Koo, C. (2011). Internet-addicted South Korean children and government efforts. *Journal of the American Medical Association, 306*(15), 1602–1603. DOI: 10.1001/jama.2011.1478

Kuss, D. J., & Griffiths, M. D. (2017). Social networking sites and addiction: Ten lessons learned. *International Journal of Environmental Research and Public Health, 14*(3), 311. DOI: 10.3390/ijerph14030311 PMID: 28304359

Kuss, D. J., Griffiths, M. D., Karila, L., & Billieux, J. (2014). Internet addiction: A systematic review of epidemiological research for the last decade. *Current Pharmaceutical Design, 20*(25), 4026–4052. DOI: 10.2174/13816128113199990617 PMID: 24001297

Kuss, D. J., Griffiths, M. D., Karila, L., & Billieux, J. (2019). Internet addiction: A systematic review of epidemiological research for the last decade. *Current Pharmaceutical Design, 25*(1), 6–18. DOI: 10.2174/1381612825666190115144101 PMID: 24001297

Kuss, D. J., & Lopez-Fernandez, O. (2016). Internet addiction and problematic internet use: A systematic review of clinical research. *World Journal of Psychiatry, 6*(1), 143–176. DOI: 10.5498/wjp.v6.i1.143 PMID: 27014605

Li, H., Wang, S., & Zhu, C. (2016). Effectiveness of a group-based cognitive behavioural therapy program for internet addiction among adolescents. *Addictive Behaviors, 55*, 65–71. DOI: 10.1016/j.addbeh.2016.01.010

Li, X., Wang, P., & Liu, H. (2022). Regulatory strategies for online gaming and digital addiction prevention in China. *Policy and Internet, 14*(3), 711–732. DOI: 10.1002/poi3.315

Lister, C., West, J. H., Cannon, B., Sax, T., & Brodegard, D. (2014). Just a fad? Gamification in health and fitness apps. *JMIR Serious Games, 2*(2), e9. DOI: 10.2196/games.3413 PMID: 25654660

Livingstone, S., Stoilova, M., & Nandagiri, R. (2019). Children's data and privacy online: Growing up in a digital age. An Evidence Review. London School of Economics. https://www.lse.ac.uk/media-and-communications

Meng, S. Q., Dong, F. L., & Wang, Z. L.. (2022). Global prevalence of digital addiction in the general population: A systematic review and meta-analysis. *Journal of Behavioral Addictions, 11*(2), 345–360. DOI: 10.1556/2006.2022.00032 PMID: 35150965

Miller, W. R., & Rollnick, S. (2013). *Motivational interviewing: Helping people change* (3rd ed.). Guilford Press.

Mohamed, S. M., Hamed, N. A., & Fahmy, A. M. (2022). Effect of digital detox program on electronic screen syndrome among preparatory school students. *Journal of Nursing Education and Practice, 12*(4), 20–30. DOI: 10.5430/jnep.v12n4p20 PMID: 36373487

Montag, C., Wegmann, E., Sariyska, R., Demetrovics, Z., & Brand, M. (2021). How to overcome taxonomical problems in the study of Internet use disorders and what to do with "smartphone addiction"? *Journal of Behavioral Addictions, 10*(1), 1–7. DOI: 10.1556/2006.8.2019.59 PMID: 31668089

Müller, K. W., Janikian, M., Dreier, M., Wölfling, K., Beutel, M. E., Tzavara, C., Richardson, C., & Tsitsika, A.Cross-national Epidemiology of Problematic Internet Use Study Group. (2015). Regular gaming behaviour and internet gaming disorder in European adolescents: Results from a cross-national representative survey of prevalence, predictors, and psychopathological correlates. *European Child & Adolescent Psychiatry, 24*(5), 565–574. DOI: 10.1007/s00787-014-0611-2 PMID: 25189795

Park, S., Kim, Y., & Cho, M. J. (2018). Prevalence of internet addiction and correlations with family factors among South Korean adolescents. *Adolescence, 53*(209), 469–478. DOI: 10.1080/01494929.2018.1440619 PMID: 19149152

Park, S., Lee, J. Y., Kim, J., & Han, D. H. (2022). Virtual reality-based intervention for gaming disorder: A randomised controlled trial. *Frontiers in Psychiatry, 13*, 837497. DOI: 10.3389/fpsyt.2022.837497

Peris, C., Pastor, J., & Martinez, V. (2020). Virtual reality in clinical psychology: Applications and possibilities. *Anales de Psicología, 36*(1), 1–13. DOI: 10.6018/analesps.337791

Petry, N. M., Rehbein, F., Ko, C. H., & O'Brien, C. P. (2018). Internet gaming disorder in the DSM-5. *Current Psychiatry Reports, 20*(2), 8. DOI: 10.1007/s11920-018-0877-6 PMID: 29504045

Rajpurohit, L., & Yadav, K. C. (2024). The impact of smartphone addiction on adolescents' quality of life: A systematic review. *Frontiers in Health Informatics, 13*(2), 45–58. DOI: 10.3389/fhi.2024.1053489

Rumpf, H. J., Achab, S., Billieux, J., Bowden-Jones, H., Carragher, N., Demetrovics, Z., Higuchi, S., King, D. L., Mann, K., Potenza, M. N., Saunders, J. B., Abbott, M., Ambekar, A., Aricak, O. T., Assanangkornchai, S., Bahar, N., Borges, G., Brand, M., & Campbell, M. (2018). Including gaming disorder in the ICD-11: The need to do so from a clinical and public health perspective. *Journal of Behavioral Addictions, 7*(3), 556–561. DOI: 10.1556/2006.7.2018.59 PMID: 30010410

Sariyska, R., Lachmann, B., Markett, S., & Montag, C. (2017). Internet use disorder: An overview of behavioural and neuroimaging findings. *Frontiers in Psychology, 8*, 61. DOI: 10.3389/fpsyg.2017.00061

Solankure, K., Sagare, S., & Bhoomika, B. J. (2025). Prevalence of smartphone addiction and its impact on sleep quality among school-going students: A cross-sectional study. *Journal of Ayurveda and Holistic Medicine, 13*(4), 3–11. DOI: 10.70066/jahm.v13i4.1835

Starcevic, V., Billieux, J., & Schimmenti, A. (2021). Selfitis, selfie addiction, Instagram addiction: A conceptual overview. *Current Opinion in Psychology, 39*, 49–54. DOI: 10.1016/j.copsyc.2020.08.014

Stevens, M. W., King, D. L., Dorstyn, D., & Delfabbro, P. H. (2021b). Cognitive-behavioural therapy for Internet gaming disorder: A systematic review and meta-analysis. *Clinical Psychology & Psychotherapy, 28*(3), 612–624. DOI: 10.1002/cpp.2539

Stevens, M. W. R., Dorstyn, D., Delfabbro, P. H., & King, D. L. (2021a). Global prevalence of gaming disorder: A systematic review and meta-analysis. *The Australian and New Zealand Journal of Psychiatry, 55*(6), 553–568. DOI: 10.1177/0004867420962851 PMID: 33028074

Torous, J., Myrick, K. J., Rauseo-Ricupero, N., & Firth, J. (2020). Digital mental health and COVID-19: Using technology today to accelerate the curve on access and quality tomorrow. *JMIR Mental Health, 7*(3), e18848. DOI: 10.2196/18848 PMID: 32213476

WHO. (2019). International Classification of Diseases for Mortality and Morbidity Statistics (11th Revision), World Health Organisation. https://icd.who.int/

Xanidis, N., & Brignell, C. M. (2016). The association between the use of social network sites, sleep quality, and cognitive function during the day. *Computers in Human Behaviour, 55*(Pt B), 121–126. DOI: 10.1016/j.chb.2015.09.004

Young, K. S. (1998). Internet addiction: The emergence of a new clinical disorder. *Cyberpsychology & Behavior, 1*(3), 237–244. DOI: 10.1089/cpb.1998.1.237

Young, K. S. (2009). Understanding online gaming addiction and treatment issues for adolescents. *The American Journal of Family Therapy, 37*(5), 355–372. DOI: 10.1080/01926180902942191

Young, K. S. (2011). CBT-IA: The first treatment model for internet addiction. *Journal of Cognitive Psychotherapy, 25*(4), 304–312. DOI: 10.1891/0889-8391.25.4.304

Compilation of References

Abbas, Z., Javied, U., & Pratt, S. (2023). Exploring the energy intensity – per capita income nexus: Evidence from middle-income and high-Income countries. *Journal of Environmental Economics and Policy*, *13*(1), 70–82. DOI: 10.1080/21606544.2023.2212367

Aboul-Yazeed, R. S., Darwish, A., & Hassanien, A. E. (2025). Flourish the mood: A systematic review on the impacts of metaverse on psychological and mental health. *Frontiers in Virtual Reality*, *6*, 1429038. DOI: 10.3389/frvir.2025.1429038

Ackerman, C. E. (2017). *Writing therapy: Using a pen and paper to enhance personal growth*. PositivePsychology.com. https://positivepsychology.com/writing-therapy/

Adamus, S., Bielski, K., Szatkowska, I., Gola, M., & Draps, M. (2025). Exploring the role of the amygdala in Compulsive Sexual Behavior Disorder via a parcellation pipeline based on Recurrence Quantification Analysis. *Journal of Behavioral Addictions*, *14*(1), 204–219. DOI: 10.1556/2006.2025.00014 PMID: 40063093

Adarsh, H., & Sahoo, S. (2023). Pornography and its impact on adolescent/teenage sexuality. *Journal of Psychosexual Health*, *5*(1), 35–39. DOI: 10.1177/26318318231153984

Áfra, E., Janszky, J., Perlaki, G., Orsi, G., Nagy, S., Arató, Á., & Darnai, G. (2023). Altered functional brain networks in problematic Internet use: resting-state fMRI study. *Research Square (Research Square)*. DOI: 10.21203/rs.3.rs-2718429/v1

Aftabi, P., & Bahramjerdi, S. F. N. (2023). Developing a decision-making framework within the management of historical cities: Towards integrated conservation and development of the Roudaki neighbourhood. *Land Use Policy*, *129*, 106653. Advance online publication. DOI: 10.1016/j.landusepol.2023.106653

Agasalim, A. A. (2024). Empirical Findings on the Relationship of Energy Consumption, Gross Domestic Product Per Capita and Carbon Dioxide (CO2) Emissions. *International Journal of Energy Economics and Policy*. DOI: 10.32479/ijeep.14062

Agbakoba, R., McGee-Lennon, M., Bouamrane, M.-M., Watson, N., & Mair, F. S. (2016). Implementation factors affecting the large-scale deployment of digital health and well-being technologies: A qualitative study of the initial phases of the 'Living-It-Up' programme. *Health Informatics Journal*, *22*(4), 867–877. DOI: 10.1177/1460458215594651 PMID: 26276795

Aghamiri, F. S., Luetz, J. M., & Hills, K. (2024). Why did God let this Happen? Assessing the Spiritual Impacts of Sexual Addiction on Intimate Female Partners: A Qualitative Investigation. *Sexuality & Culture*, *28*, 2113–2142. DOI: 10.1007/s12119-024-10221-3

Akbari, M., Seydavi, M., Sheikhi, S., & Spada, M. M. (2023). Problematic smartphone use and sleep disturbance: The roles of metacognitions, desire thinking, and emotion regulation. *Frontiers in Psychiatry*, *14*, 1137533. DOI: 10.3389/fpsyt.2023.1137533 PMID: 37593452

Akbar, Z., & Alamsyah, R. (2025). The impact of social media usage on student mental health: A study of social comparison and FOMO. *International Journal of Educational Studies*, *8*(1), 12–24.

Albayrak, R., & Özbek, Y. (2025). Determining the relationship of food neophobia, digital addiction, body image perception on social media with dietary inflammatory index among adolescents. *Frontiers in Public Health*, *13*, 1683764. Advance online publication. DOI: 10.3389/fpubh.2025.1683764 PMID: 41246100

Alimour, S. A., & Alrabeei, M. (2025). Redefining psychopathology in the context of digital overload: Emerging disorders in the age of information saturation. *Frontiers in Digital Health*, *7*, 1693287. DOI: 10.3389/fdgth.2025.1693287 PMID: 41312176

Aljomaa, S. S., Qudah, M. F. A., Albursan, I. S., Bakhiet, S. F., & Abduljabbar, A. S. (2016). Smartphone addiction among university students in the light of some variables. *Computers in Human Behavior*, *61*, 155–164. https://www.sciencedirect.com/science/article/pii/S0747563216302126. DOI: 10.1016/j.chb.2016.03.041

Allcott, H. (2020). *Digital Addiction*. AEA Randomized Controlled Trials., DOI: 10.1257/rct.5796-1.2000000000000002

Allen, M., Emmers, T., Gebhardt, L., & Giery, M. A. (1995). Exposure to pornography and acceptance of rape myths. *The Journal of Communication*, *45*(1), 5–26. DOI: 10.1111/j.1460-2466.1995.tb00711.x

Allison, K., Dawson, R. M., Messias, D. K. H., Culley, J. M., & Brown, N. (2023). Early adolescent online sexual risks on smartphones and social media: Parental awareness and protective practices. *The Journal of Early Adolescence, 44*(7), 882–908. DOI: 10.1177/02724316231212560

Al-Mansoori, R. S., Al-Thani, D., Ali, R., & Yan, Z. (2023). Designing for digital wellbeing: From theory to practice — a scoping review. *Human Behavior and Emerging Technologies, 9924029*, 1–24. Advance online publication. DOI: 10.1155/2023/9924029

Almourad, M. B., McAlaney, J., Skinner, T., Pleya, M., & Ali, R. (2020). Defining digital addiction: Key features from the literature. *Psihologija, 53*(3), 237–253. DOI: 10.2298/PSI191029017A

Alvarez-Segura, M., Fernández, I., El Kasmy, Y., Francisco, E., Gallo Martínez, S., Ortiz Jiménez, E. M., & Butjosa, A. (2025). Impact of pornography consumption on children and adolescents: A trauma-informed approach. *Frontiers in Child and Adolescent Psychiatry, 4*, 1567649. Advance online publication. DOI: 10.3389/frcha.2025.1567649 PMID: 41089467

Alzahrani, A. K. D., & Griffiths, M. D. (2025). Problematic gaming and students' academic performance: A systematic review. *International Journal of Mental Health and Addiction, 23*(5), 4062–4095. DOI: 10.1007/s11469-024-01338-5

AL-Zoubi., A. (2023, May). Digital technology and changes in media consumption: a case study of smartphone and app usage. In *International Conference on Business and Technology* (pp. 433-444). Cham: Springer Nature Switzerland.

American Psychiatric Association. (2013). *Diagnostic and statistical manual of mental disorders* (5th ed.). American Psychiatric Publishing.

American Psychological Association. (2023, May 9). *Health advisory on social media use in adolescence*. American Psychological Association. https://www.apa.org/topics/social-media-internet/health-advisory-adolescent-social-media-use

Amson, A., Bagnato, M., Remedios, L., Pritchard, M., Soulene, S., Gillis, G., & Kent, M. (2024). Beyond the Screen: Exploring the Dynamics of Social Media Influencers, Food Marketing, and Gendered Influences on Adolescent Diets. *Research Square (Research Square)*. DOI: 10.21203/rs.3.rs-3909431/v1

Anderson, E. L. (2018). Associations between early exposure to online pornography and problematic sexual behaviors in adolescence. *Journal of Adolescence, 63*, 84–95. https://doi.org/10.xxxx/j.adolescence.2018.xxxx

Anderson, E. L., Steen, E., & Stavropoulos, V. (2017). Internet use and problematic Internet use: A systematic review of longitudinal research trends in adolescence and emergent adulthood. *International Journal of Adolescence and Youth, 22*(4), 430–454. DOI: 10.1080/02673843.2016.1227716

Andrade, A. L. M. (Ed.). (2025). *Digital addictions: An interdisciplinary approach to behavioral addictions and digital media.* Springer Nature. DOI: 10.1007/978-3-031-87986-9

Andrade, L., & Viñán-Ludeña, M. (2025). Mapping research on ICT addiction: A comprehensive review of Internet, smartphone, social media, and gaming addictions. *Frontiers in Psychology, 16*, 1578457. Advance online publication. DOI: 10.3389/fpsyg.2025.1578457 PMID: 40443730

Andreassen, C. S., Billieux, J., Griffiths, M., Kuss, D., Demetrovics, Z., Mazzoni, E., & Pallesen, S. (2016). The relationship between addictive use of social media and video games and symptoms of psychiatric disorders: A large-scale cross-sectional study. *Psychology of Addictive Behaviors : Journal of the Society of Psychologists in Addictive Behaviors, 30*(2), 252–262. DOI: 10.1037/adb0000160 PMID: 26999354

Andreassen, C. S., Pallesen, S., & Griffiths, M. D. (2016). The relationship between addictive use of social media, narcissism, and self-esteem: Findings from a large national survey. *Addictive Behaviors, 64*, 287–293. DOI: 10.1016/j.addbeh.2016.03.006 PMID: 27072491

Anghel, O. (2025). INTERNET ADICTION AND ITS EFFECTS (FROM ARTS). *Review of Artistic Education.* DOI: 10.35218/rae-2025-0050

Antoniadou, N., Kokkinos, C. M., & Markos, A. (2016). Development, construct validation and measurement invariance of the Greek Cyber-Bullying/Victimization Experiences Questionnaire (CBVEQ-G). *Computers in Human Behavior, 65*, 380–390. DOI: 10.1016/j.chb.2016.08.032

An, Y., & Zhang, M. X. (2024). Relationship between problematic smartphone use and sleep problems: The roles of sleep-related compensatory health beliefs and bedtime procrastination. *Digital Health, 10*, 20552076241283338. DOI: 10.1177/20552076241283338 PMID: 39291154

Ardhanariswari, R., Azzahro, F., Fauzan, M., Pamuji, K., & Murniati, T. (2026). Digital Technology as a Tool for Fulfilling Women's Rights: A Legal Analysis of Online Gender-based Violence (OGBV) Within the Framework of SDG 5. *KnE Social Sciences, 11*(1), 213–234. DOI: 10.18502/kss.v11i1.20610

Arnett, J. J. (2000). Emerging adulthood: A theory of development from the late teens through the twenties. *The American Psychologist*, *55*(5), 469–480. DOI: 10.1037/0003-066X.55.5.469 PMID: 10842426

Ashata, G. P. (2024). Digital dynamics: Investigating the impact of social media on sexual behavior. *IDOSR Journal of Communication and English*, *9*(2), 1–6. DOI: 10.59298/IDOSR/JCE/92.16.202412

Astuti, S. A. T., & Winarti, Y. (2022). A scoping review: The impact of pornography addiction on adolescents. *Muhammadiyah International Public Health and Medicine Proceeding*, *2*(1), 366–381. DOI: 10.61811/miphmp.v1i2.265

Atalayer, D. (2017). Dürtüsellik ve Aşırı Yeme Arasındaki İlişki: Psikolojik ve Nörobiyolojik Yaklaşımlar. *Psikiyatride Guncel Yaklasimlar -. Psikiyatride Güncel Yaklaşımlar*, *10*(2), 1–1. DOI: 10.18863/pgy.358090

Atar, A. (2026). Neurobiological Consequences of High-Fat High-Sugar Diets on the Mesocorticolimbic System: A Narrative Review. *Current Nutrition Reports*, *15*(1), 6–6. DOI: 10.1007/s13668-026-00729-5 PMID: 41543783

Atkinson, G., Groom, B., Hanley, N., & Mourato, S. (2018). Environmental Valuation and Benefit-Cost Analysis in U.K. Policy. *Journal of Benefit-Cost Analysis*, *9*(1), 97–119. DOI: 10.1017/bca.2018.6

Attanasi, G., Maffioletti, A., Shalukhina, T., Bel, C., & Chérikh, F. (2021). Gender Differences in the Impact of COVID-19 Lockdown on Potentially Addictive Behaviors: An Emotion-Mediated Analysis. *Frontiers in Psychology*, *12*, 703897. Advance online publication. DOI: 10.3389/fpsyg.2021.703897 PMID: 34867588

Attwood, F. (2005). What do people do with porn? Qualitative research into the consumption, use, and experience of pornography and other sexually explicit media. *Sexuality & Culture*, *9*(2), 65–86. DOI: 10.1007/s12119-005-1008-7

Attwood, F., & Smith, C. (2014). Porn Studies: An introduction. *Porn Studies*, *1*(1-2), 1–6. DOI: 10.1080/23268743.2014.887308

Aydınlar, A., Mavi, A., Kütükçü, E., Kırımlı, E. E., Alış, D., Akın, A., & Altıntaş, L. (2024). Awareness and level of digital literacy among students receiving health-based education. *BMC Medical Education*, *24*(1), 38. DOI: 10.1186/s12909-024-05025-w PMID: 38191385

Aznar-Martínez, B., Lorente-De-Sanz, J., López-I-Martín, X., & Castillo-Garayoa, J. A. (2024). Pornography and gender-based violence: Two neglected topics in sexuality education. A systematic review. *Sex Education*, *25*(2), 256–272. DOI: 10.1080/14681811.2024.2316154

Bai, J., Zhu, H., Ran, X.-W., Qu, H., He, L., & Zhao, Y. (2025). The time-stamped effects of screen exposure on food intake in adults: A meta-analysis of experimental studies. *Appetite*, *206*, 107846–107846. DOI: 10.1016/j.appet.2024.107846 PMID: 39753153

Baikie, K. A., & Wilhelm, K. (2005). Emotional and physical health benefits of expressive writing. *Advances in Psychiatric Treatment*, *11*(5), 338–346. DOI: 10.1192/apt.11.5.338

Baker, Ö. E., & Bugay, A. (2011). Cyberbullying and loneliness: The mediating role of psychological symptoms. *Procedia: Social and Behavioral Sciences*, *30*, 276–280. DOI: 10.1016/j.sbspro.2011.10.253

Balakrishnan, V. (2018). Actions, emotional reactions and cyberbullying—From the lens of bullies, victims, bully-victims and bystanders among Malaysian young adults. *Telematics and Informatics*, *35*(4), 1190–1200. DOI: 10.1016/j.tele.2018.02.002

Ballester-Arnal, R., García-Barba, M., Castro-Calvo, J., Giménez-García, C., & Gil-Llario, M. D. (2022). Pornography consumption in people of different age groups: An analysis based on gender, contents, and consequences. *Sexuality Research & Social Policy*, *20*(2), 766–779. DOI: 10.1007/s13178-022-00720-z

Bandura, A. (1977). *Social learning theory*. Prentice Hall.

Bandura, A. (1986). *Social foundations of thought and action: A social cognitive theory*. Prentice-Hall.

Bandura, A. (2001). Social cognitive theory of mass communication. *Media Psychology*, *3*(3), 265–299. DOI: 10.1207/S1532785XMEP0303_03

Banet-Weiser, S. (2018). *Empowered: Popular feminism and popular misogyny*. Duke University Press.

Barbieri, V., Piccoliori, G., Engl, A., & Wiedermann, C. J. (2024). Impact of digital media, school problems, and lifestyle factors on youth psychosomatic health: A cross-sectional survey. *Children (Basel, Switzerland)*, *11*(7), 795. DOI: 10.3390/children11070795 PMID: 39062244

Barlett, C. P. (2015). Anonymously hurting others online: The effect of anonymity on cyberbullying frequency. *Psychology of Popular Media Culture*, *4*(2), 70–79. DOI: 10.1037/a0034335

Barlett, C. P. (2017). From theory to practice: Cyberbullying theory and its application to intervention. *Computers in Human Behavior*, *72*, 269–275. DOI: 10.1016/j.chb.2017.02.060

Barlett, C. P., Bennardi, C., Williams, S., & Zlupko, T. (2021). Theoretically predicting cyberbullying perpetration in youth with the BGCM: Unique challenges and promising research opportunities. *Frontiers in Psychology*, *12*, 708277. DOI: 10.3389/fpsyg.2021.708277 PMID: 34659022

Barlett, C. P., Kowalewski, D. A., Kramer, S. S., & Helmstetter, K. M. (2019). Testing the relationship between media violence exposure and cyberbullying perpetration. *Psychology of Popular Media Culture*, *8*(3), 280–286. DOI: 10.1037/ppm0000179

Barton, B. A., Adams, K. S., Browne, B. L., & Arrastia-Chisholm, M. C. (2018). The effects of social media usage on attention, motivation, and academic performance. *Active Learning in Higher Education*, *22*(1), 11–22. DOI: 10.1177/1469787418782817

Bateman, I., & Kling, C. (2020). Revealed Preference Methods for Nonmarket Valuation: An Introduction to Best Practices. *Review of Environmental Economics and Policy*, *14*(2), 240–259. DOI: 10.1093/reep/reaa009

Bava, S., & Tapert, S. F. (2010). Adolescent brain development and the risk for alcohol and other drug problems. *Neuropsychology Review*, *20*(4), 398–413. DOI: 10.1007/s11065-010-9146-6 PMID: 20953990

Beeson, D., Wolffsohn, J. S., Baigum, T., Qureshi, T., Gohil, S., Wahid, R., & Sheppard, A. L. (2024). Digital eye strain symptoms worsen during prolonged digital tasks, associated with a reduction in productivity. *Computers in Human Behavior Reports*, *16*, 100489. DOI: 10.1016/j.chbr.2024.100489

Benvegnù, G., Piva, A., Cadorin, C., Mannari, V., Girondini, M., Federico, A., Tamburin, S., & Chiamulera, C. (2023). The effects of virtual reality environmental enrichments on craving to food in healthy volunteers. *Psychopharmacology*, *241*(1), 49–60. DOI: 10.1007/s00213-023-06462-z PMID: 37697163

Bert, F., Giacometti, M., Gualano, M. R., & Siliquini, R. (2014). Smartphones and health promotion: A review of the evidence. *Journal of Medical Systems*, *38*(1), 9995. DOI: 10.1007/s10916-013-9995-7 PMID: 24346929

Berthon, P., Pitt, L., & Campbell, C. (2019). Addictive De-Vices: A Public Policy Analysis of Sources and Solutions to Digital Addiction. *Journal of Public Policy & Marketing*, *38*(4), 451–468. DOI: 10.1177/0743915619859852

Berthoud, H.-R. (2012). *The neurobiology of food intake in an obesogenic environment. 71(4), 478-487*. Cambridge University Press., DOI: 10.1017/S0029665112000602

Bhargava, V., & Velasquez, M. (2020). Ethics of the Attention Economy: The Problem of Social Media Addiction. *Business Ethics Quarterly*, *31*(3), 321–359. DOI: 10.1017/beq.2020.32

Bibi, K., Fatima, A., Amin, R., & Rowland, D. L. (2022). Understanding Serial Mediators of Problematic Pornography Use in Pakistani Men and Women. *International Journal of Environmental Research and Public Health, 19*(21), 14336. DOI: 10.3390/ijerph192114336 PMID: 36361229

Billieux, J., Maurage, P., Lopez-Fernandez, O., Kuss, D. J., & Griffiths, M. D. (2015). Can disordered mobile phone use be considered a behavioural addiction? An update on current evidence and a comprehensive model for future research. *Current Addiction Reports, 2*(2), 156–162. DOI: 10.1007/s40429-015-0054-y

Binford, W. (2018). Viewing pornography through a children's rights lens. *Sexual Addiction & Compulsivity, 25*(4), 415–444. DOI: 10.1080/10720162.2019.1578311

Błachnio, A., Przepiórka, A., & Gorbaniuk, O. (2024). Relationship between fear of missing out and adolescents' mental health. *Annals of Agricultural and Environmental Medicine : AAEM, 31*(2), 266–271.

Błachnio, A., Przepiorka, A., Gorbaniuk, O., Benvenuti, M., Ciobanu, A., Senol-Durak, E., Durak, M., Giannakos, M., Mazzoni, E., Pappas, I., Popa, C., Seidman, G., Wu, A., Yu, S., & Ben-Ezra, M. (2019). Cultural Correlates of Internet Addiction. *Cyberpsychology, Behavior and Social Networking, 22*(4), 258–263. DOI: 10.1089/cyber.2018.0667 PMID: 30958038

Blinka, L., Ševčíková, A., Dreier, M., Škařupová, K., & Wölfling, K. (2022). Online sex addiction: A qualitative analysis of symptoms in treatment-seeking men. *Frontiers in Psychiatry, 13*, 907549. DOI: 10.3389/fpsyt.2022.907549 PMID: 35873234

Bocci Benucci, S., Di Gesto, C., Ghinassi, S., Casale, S., & Fioravanti, G. (2024). Pornography use, problematic pornography use, impulsivity, and sensation seeking: A meta-analysis. *Journal of Sexual Medicine, 21*(10), 922–939. DOI: 10.1093/jsxmed/qdae101 PMID: 39183145

Boer, M., Stevens, G. W. J. M., Finkenauer, C., de Looze, M. E., & van den Eijnden, R. J. J. M. (2021). Social media use intensity, social media use problems, and mental health among adolescents. *Computers in Human Behavior, 116*, 106645. DOI: 10.1016/j.chb.2020.106645

Bond, E., & Phippen, A. (2020). Tackling teen sexting- policing challenges when society and technology outpace legislation. In *Advanced sciences and technologies for security applications* (pp. 157–177). https://doi.org/DOI: 10.1007/978-3-030-50613-1_7

Boniel-Nissim, M., Marino, C., Galeotti, T., Blinka, L., Ozoliņa, K., Craig, W., Lahti, H., Wong, S. L., Brown, J., Wilson, M., Inchley, J., & van den Eijnde, R. (Eds.). (2024). *A focus on adolescent social media use and gaming in Europe, Central Asia and Canada: Health Behaviour in School-aged Children international report from the 2021/2022 survey* (Vol. 6). World Health Organization Regional Office for Europe.

Bordoloi, M., Durkin, I., & Aggarwal, A. (2024). Effects of Pornography on Youth: A Review. *Missouri Medicine, 121*(3), 195–197. PMID: 38854615

Bossen, C., & Bertelsen, P. S. (2024). Digital health care and data work: Who are the data professionals? *The HIM Journal, 53*(3), 243–251. DOI: 10.1177/18333583231183083 PMID: 37491822

Bőthe, B., Koós, M., Tóth-Király, I., Orosz, G., & Demetrovics, Z. (2020a). Investigating the associations of pornography use frequency, problematic pornography use, and moral incongruence. *Journal of Sex Research, 57*(4), 442–456. DOI: 10.1080/00224499.2019.1654367

Bőthe, B., Tóth-Király, I., Orosz, G., Potenza, M. N., & Demetrovics, Z. (2020b). High-frequency pornography use may not always be problematic. *Journal of Sexual Medicine, 17*(4), 793–811. DOI: 10.1016/j.jsxm.2020.01.007 PMID: 32033863

Bőthe, B., Tóth-Király, I., Popova, N., Nagy, L., Koós, M., Demetrovics, Z., Potenza, M. N., Kraus, S. W., Ballester-Arnal, R., Batthyány, D., Bergeron, S., Billieux, J., Briken, P., Burkauskas, J., Cárdenas-López, G., Carvalho, J., Castro-Calvo, J., Chen, L., Ciocca, G., & Grubbs, J. B. (2025). Identification and comprehensive characterization of moral disapproval and behavioral dysregulation-based pornography-use profiles across 42 countries. *Journal of Behavioral Addictions, 14*(1), 131–154. DOI: 10.1556/2006.2024.00054 PMID: 39945767

Bőthe, B., Tóth-Király, I., Zsila, Á., Griffiths, M. D., Demetrovics, Z., & Orosz, G. (2018). The Development of the Problematic Pornography Consumption Scale (PPCS). *Journal of Sex Research, 55*(3), 395–406. DOI: 10.1080/00224499.2017.1291798 PMID: 28276929

Bouazza, S., Elkinany, S., Abbouyi, S., Rhazi, K., & Zarrouq, B. (2022). Association between problematic use of smartphones and mental health in the Middle East and North Africa (MENA) region: a systematic review. Research Square (United States). DOI: 10.21203/rs.3.rs-1662848/v1

Bowlby, J. (1988). *A secure base: Parent-child attachment and healthy human development*. Basic Books.

Boyd, D. (2014). *It's complicated: The social lives of networked teens*. Yale University Press., DOI: 10.5752/10054

Boyd, M. J., & Dobrow, J. (2011). Media literacy and positive youth development. *Advances in Child Development and Behavior*, *41*, 251–271. DOI: 10.1016/B978-0-12-386492-5.00010-5 PMID: 23259195

Boyland, E., Spanakis, P., O'Reilly, C., & Christiansen, P. (2024). Associations between everyday exposure to food marketing and hunger and food craving in adults: An ecological momentary assessment study. *Appetite*, *196*, 107241–107241. DOI: 10.1016/j.appet.2024.107241 PMID: 38307297

Bozzola, E. (2021). Media use during childhood and adolescence. *International Journal of Environmental Research and Public Health*, *18*(3), 967. DOI: 10.3390/ijerph18030967 PMID: 33499274

Brand, M., Antons, S., Bőthe, B., Demetrovics, Z., Fineberg, N., Jiménez-Múrcia, S., King, D. L., Mestre-Bach, G., Moretta, T., Müller, A., Wegmann, E., & Potenza, M. (2024). Current Advances in Behavioral Addictions: From Fundamental Research to Clinical Practice. *The American Journal of Psychiatry*, *182*(2), 155–163. DOI: 10.1176/appi.ajp.20240092 PMID: 39659159

Brand, M., Potenza, M. N., & Stark, R. (2022). Theoretical models of types of problematic usage of the Internet: When theorists meet therapists. *Current Opinion in Behavioral Sciences*, *45*, 101119. DOI: 10.1016/j.cobeha.2022.101119

Brand, M., Wegmann, E., Stark, R., Müller, A., Wölfling, K., Robbins, T. W., & Potenza, M. N. (2019). The Interaction of Person-Affect-Cognition-Execution (I-PACE) model for addictive behaviors: Update, generalization to addictive behaviors beyond internet-use disorders, and specification of the process character of addictive behaviors. *Neuroscience and Biobehavioral Reviews*, *104*, 1–10. DOI: 10.1016/j.neubiorev.2019.06.032 PMID: 31247240

Brand, M., Young, K. S., & Laier, C. (2014). Prefrontal control and Internet addiction: A theoretical model and review of neuropsychological and neuroimaging findings. *Frontiers in Human Neuroscience*, *8*, 375. Advance online publication. DOI: 10.3389/fnhum.2014.00375 PMID: 24904393

Brand, M., Young, K. S., Laier, C., Wölfling, K., & Potenza, M. N. (2016). Integrating psychological and neurobiological considerations regarding the development and maintenance of specific Internet-use disorders: An Interaction of Person-Affect-Cognition-Execution (I-PACE) model. *Neuroscience and Biobehavioral Reviews*, *71*, 252–266. DOI: 10.1016/j.neubiorev.2016.08.033 PMID: 27590829

Brem, M. J., Garner, A. R., Grigorian, H., Florimbio, A. R., Wolford-Clevenger, C., Shorey, R. C., & Stuart, G. L. (2018). Problematic pornography use and physical and sexual intimate partner violence perpetration among men in Batterer Intervention Programs. *Journal of Interpersonal Violence, 36*(11–12), NP6085–NP6105. Advance online publication. DOI: 10.1177/0886260518812806 PMID: 30461344

Brewer, G., & Kerslake, J. (2015). Cyberbullying, self-esteem, empathy and loneliness. *Computers in Human Behavior, 48*, 255–260. DOI: 10.1016/j.chb.2015.01.073

Browne, M. W., & Cudeck, R. (1993). Alternative ways of assessing model fit. In Bollen, K. A., & Long, J. S. (Eds.), *Testing structural equation models* (pp. 136–162). Sage Publications.

Bryant, C. (2009). *Adolescence, pornography and harm* (Trends & Issues in Crime and Criminal Justice No. 368). Australian Institute of Criminology.

Bucher, T. (2018). *If...Then: Algorithmic Power and Politics*. Oxford University Press. DOI: 10.1093/oso/9780190493028.001.0001

Bull, F. C., Al-Ansari, S. S., Biddle, S., Borodulin, K., Buman, M. P., Cardon, G., Carty, C., Chaput, J. P., Chastin, S., Chou, R., Dempsey, P. C., DiPietro, L., Ekelund, U., Firth, J., Friedenreich, C. M., Garcia, L., Gichu, M., Jago, R., Katzmarzyk, P. T., & Willumsen, J. F. (2020). World Health Organization 2020 guidelines on physical activity and sedentary behaviour. *British Journal of Sports Medicine, 54*(24), 1451–1462. DOI: 10.1136/bjsports-2020-102955 PMID: 33239350

Buragohain, D., Khichar, S., Deng, C., Meng, Y., & Chaudhary, S. (2025). Analyzing metaverse-based digital therapies, their effectiveness, and potential risks in mental healthcare. *Scientific Reports, 15*(1), 17066. DOI: 10.1038/s41598-025-00916-4 PMID: 40379748

Büsche, K., Stark, R., Brand, M., & Antons, S. (2022). Self-regulatory processes in problematic pornography use. *Current Addiction Reports, 9*(4), 344–352. DOI: 10.1007/s40429-022-00447-2

Byron, P. (2023). Porn literacy and young people's digital cultures. *Porn Studies, 11*(1), 32–39. DOI: 10.1080/23268743.2023.2174173

Byun, S., Ruffini, C., Mills, J. E., Douglas, A. C., Niang, M., Stepchenkova, S., Lee, S. K., Loutfi, J., Lee, J., Atallah, M., & Blanton, M. (2008). Internet addiction: Metasynthesis of 1996–2006 quantitative research. *Cyberpsychology & Behavior, 12*(2), 203–207. DOI: 10.1089/cpb.2008.0102 PMID: 19072075

Cacioppo, J. T., Hawkley, L. C., Ernst, J. M., Burleson, M., Berntson, G. G., Nouriani, B., & Spiegel, D. (2006). Loneliness within a nomological net: An evolutionary perspective. *Journal of Research in Personality*, *40*(6), 1054–1085. DOI: 10.1016/j.jrp.2005.11.007

Cahyani, A., Iskandarsyah, A., Cahyadi, S., & Srisayekti, W. (2023). Differences in the Model of Eating in the Absence of Hunger Before and During the COVID-19 Pandemic. *The Open Psychology Journal*, *16*(1), e18743501242291. Advance online publication. DOI: 10.2174/0118743501242291231024071127

Cain, L., Hernández-Cortés, D., Timmins, C., & Weber, P. (2024). Recent Findings and Methodologies in Economics Research in Environmental Justice. *Review of Environmental Economics and Policy*, *18*(1), 116–142. DOI: 10.1086/728100

Cain, N., & Gradisar, M. (2010). Electronic media use and sleep in school-aged children and adolescents: A Review. *Sleep Medicine*, *11*(8), 735–742. DOI: 10.1016/j.sleep.2010.02.006 PMID: 20673649

Campbell, C., & Cornish, F. (2010). Towards a "fourth generation" of approaches to HIV/AIDS management: Creating contexts for effective community mobilisation. *AIDS Care*, *22*(sup2, S2), 1569–1579. DOI: 10.1080/09540121.2010.525812 PMID: 21161761

Campbell, L., & Kohut, T. (2017). The use and effects of pornography in romantic relationships. *Current Opinion in Psychology*, *13*, 6–10. DOI: 10.1016/j.copsyc.2016.03.004 PMID: 28813295

Caninsti, R., & Rahayu, S. (2024). The Role of Smartphone Addiction on Bed Procrastination and Mindful Eating Behavior in Adolescents. *Indigenous Jurnal Ilmiah Psikologi*, *9*(1), 1–13. DOI: 10.23917/indigenous.v9i1.2804

Carbonell, X., Chamarro, A., Oberst, U., Rodrigo, B., & Prades, M. (2018). Problematic use of the Internet and smartphones in university students: 2006–2017. *International Journal of Environmental Research and Public Health*, *15*(3), 475. DOI: 10.3390/ijerph15030475 PMID: 29518050

Cardi, V., Meregalli, V., Rosa, E., Derrigo, R., Faustini, C., Keeler, J., & Lawrence, N. (2022). A community-based feasibility randomized controlled study to test food-specific inhibitory control training in people with disinhibited eating during COVID-19 in Italy. *Eating and Weight Disorders : EWD*, *27*(7), 2745–2757. DOI: 10.1007/s40519-022-01411-9 PMID: 35666376

Cardoso, J., Ramos, C., Brito, J., & Almeida, T. C. (2022, April). Predictors of Pornography Use: Difficulties in Emotion Regulation and Loneliness. *Journal of Sexual Medicine, 19*(4), 620–628. DOI: 10.1016/j.jsxm.2022.01.005 PMID: 35165051

Carnes, S., & Love, T. (2017). Separating Models Obscures the Scientific Underpinnings of Sex Addiction as a Disorder. *Archives of Sexual Behavior, 46*(8), 2253–2256. DOI: 10.1007/s10508-017-1072-8 PMID: 28948394

Carnevali, D., Cavazzana, L., Grimoldi, L., Magnoni, P., Principi, N., Pellai, A., Carnevali, D., Cavazzana, L., Grimoldi, L., Magnoni, P., Principi, N., & Pellai, A. (2022). The use of online pornography among minors: Epidemiological analysis of the phenomenon. *Minerva Pediatrics, 74*(5), 579–585. DOI: 10.23736/S2724-5276.19.05342-8 PMID: 35166482

Casale, S. (2020). Problematic social media use: Conceptualization, assessment and trends in scientific literature. *Addictive Behaviors Reports, 12*, 100281. DOI: 10.1016/j.abrep.2020.100281 PMID: 32426449

Castro-Calvo, J., Gil-Llario, M. D., Giménez-García, C., Gil-Juliá, B., & Ballester-Arnal, R. (2020). Occurrence and clinical characteristics of Compulsive Sexual Behavior Disorder (CSBD): A cluster analysis in two independent community samples. *Journal of Behavioral Addictions, 9*(2), 446–468. DOI: 10.1556/2006.2020.00025 PMID: 32554840

Celebic, G., & Rendulic, D. (2011). Basic concepts of information and communication technology. *Handbook [Electronic resourse].—URL:* http://www. itdesk. info/ handbook_basic_ ict_concepts. pdf *(дата обращения: 19.05. 2018).*

Cerniglia, L., & Cimino, S. (2022). Some Considerations about Pornography Watching in Early Adolescence. *International Journal of Environmental Research and Public Health, 19*(17), 108–118. DOI: 10.3390/ijerph191710818 PMID: 36078525

Ceylan, J. (2025). The moderating effects of gender and emotional eating on the relationship between social media addiction and hedonic hunger in university students. *Scientific Reports, 15*(1), 33469–33469. DOI: 10.1038/s41598-025-11668-6 PMID: 41022969

Challoumis, C. (2022). Conditions of the CM (Cycle of Money). In *Social and Economic Studies within the Framework of Emerging Global Developments, Volume -1, V. Kaya* (pp. 13–24). DOI: 10.3726/b19907

Challoumis, C. (2025a). QUANTIFICATION OF EVERYTHING METHOD IN ECONOMICS. *INDeCS, 23*(4), 323–339. https://www.indecs.eu/2025/indecs2025-pp323-339.pdf

Challoumis, C. (2025c). The impact factor of Tangibles and Intangibles of controlled transactions on economic performance. *Economic Alternatives, 31*(1), 64–76. https://www.unwe.bg/doi/eajournal/2025.1/EA.2025.1.04.pdf

Challoumis, C. (2025d). THE INFLATION ACCORDING TO THE CYCLE OF MONEY (C.M.). *Economic Alternatives, 2025*(2), 324–353. https://doi.org/https://doi.org/10.37075/EA.2025.2.03

Challoumis, C. (2019). The R.B.Q. (Rational, Behavioral and Quantified) Model. *Ekonomika (Niš), 98*(1), 6–18. DOI: 10.15388/Ekon.2019.1.1

Challoumis, C. (2023). FROM SAVINGS TO ESCAPE AND ENFORCEMENT SAVINGS. *Cógito (Salvador), XV*(4), 206–216.

Challoumis, C. (2024a). Approach on Arm's Length Principle and Fix Length Principle Mathematical Representations. In *Innovations and Contemporary Trends in Business & Economics* (pp. 25–44). Peter Lang., https://www.peterlang.com/search?searchstring=Approach+on+Arm's+Length+Principle+and+Fix+Length+Principle+Mathematical+Representations

Challoumis, C. (2024b). From Economics to Economic Engineering (The Cycle of Money): The case of Romania. *Cógito (Salvador), XVII*(2), 161–170.

Challoumis, C. (2024c). Integrating Money Cycle Dynamics and Economocracy for Optimal Resource Allocation and Economic Stability. *Journal of Risk and Financial Management, 17*(9), 1–25. DOI: 10.3390/jrfm17090422

Challoumis, C. (2024d). The Index of the Cycle of Money: The Case of Switzerland. *Journal of Risk and Financial Management, 17*(4), 1–24. https://doi.org/https://doi.org/10.3390/jrfm17040135. DOI: 10.3390/jrfm17040135

Challoumis, C. (2025b). The Economic Dimensions of Technology and Media in Digital Social Innovation. In *Examining the Intersection of Technology, Media, and Social Innovation*. IGI Global., https://www.igi-global.com/book/examining-intersection-technology-media-social/381810#table-of-contents DOI: 10.4018/979-8-3373-5307-4.ch013

Challoumis, C., & Eriotis, N. (2025). The Impact of Artificial Intelligence on the Greek Economy. *Journal of Open Innovation, 11*(3), 1–13. https://doi.org/https://doi.org/10.1016/j.joitmc.2025.100578. DOI: 10.1016/j.joitmc.2025.100578

Chatterjee, D., & Rai, R. (2023). Behind the screens: Proposing a mentalization-based theoretical model of problematic Internet use. *Cyberpsychology (Brno), 17*(5). Advance online publication. DOI: 10.5817/CP2023-5-6

Chatterjee, S., & Kar, S. K. (2023). Teen Pornography: An emerging mental health challenge. *Journal of Psychosexual Health, 5*(1), 30–34. DOI: 10.1177/26318318231154230

Chauhan, P., & Raj, T. (2025). *Optimizing Indian Tourism and Cultural Heritage: Bridging Policy Gaps through Integrated Governance, Agrotourism, and Regenerative Development.* International Journal For Multidisciplinary Research., DOI: 10.36948/ijfmr.2025.v07i04.54654

Chen, L., Jiang, X., Wang, Q., Bőthe, B., Potenza, M. N., & Wu, H. (2022). The Association between the Quantity and Severity of Pornography Use: A Meta-analysis. *Journal of Sex Research, 59*(6), 704–719. DOI: 10.1080/00224499.2021.1988500 PMID: 34723731

Chen, L., Wang, D., Wang, H., Zhang, Y., & Jiang, X. (2023). Moderating Role of Sexual Attitudes in the Association between Online Sexual Activity and Problematic Pornography Use: Evidence from the Chinese Community and Help-Seeking Men. *International Journal of Sexual Health : Official Journal of the World Association for Sexual Health, 35*(4), 555–572. DOI: 10.1080/19317611.2023.2257688 PMID: 38601807

Chen, R., Peng-Li, D., Turel, O., Sørensen, T., Bechara, A., Li, Y., & He, Q. (2018). Decision Making Deficits in Relation to Food Cues Influence Obesity: A Triadic Neural Model of Problematic Eating. *Frontiers in Psychiatry, 9*, 264. Advance online publication. DOI: 10.3389/fpsyt.2018.00264 PMID: 29962976

Chen, Y., Wang, Z., Zhao, J., Zhao, X., Zuo, S., & Liu, W. (2025). Paths to Policy Sustainability for Protecting Cultural Heritage: A Quantitative Analysis of Conservation Policies for the Great Wall Within the "Instrument–Objective–Stakeholder" Framework. *Sustainability (Basel), 17*(10), 4378. Advance online publication. DOI: 10.3390/su17104378

Chesney, R., & Citron, D. (2019). Deepfakes and the new disinformation war. *Foreign Affairs, 98*(1), 147–155.

Chew, H., Rajasegaran, N., & Chng, S. (2023). *Effectiveness of interactive technology-assisted interventions on promoting healthy food choices: a scoping review and meta-analysis. 130(7), 1250-1259.* Cambridge University Press., DOI: 10.1017/S0007114523000193

Chiu, M., & Chein, J. (2022). Digital Media and the Developing Brain. *Cambridge University Press eBooks* (s. 104-134). içinde Cambridge University Press. DOI: 10.1017/9781108976237.008

Cho, D.-J., Kim, H., Lee, J., & Park, S. (2018). Economic cost–benefit analysis of the addictive digital game industry. *Applied Economics Letters*, *25*(9), 638–642. DOI: 10.1080/13504851.2017.1355528

Choi, J.-S., King, D., & Jung, Y.-C. (2019). Editorial: Neurobiological Perspectives in Behavioral Addiction. *Frontiers in Psychiatry*, *10*, 3. Advance online publication. DOI: 10.3389/fpsyt.2019.00003 PMID: 30723426

Chou, C., & Hsiao, M. C. (2000). Internet addiction, usage, gratification, and pleasure experience: The Taiwan college students' case. *Computers & Education*, *35*(1), 65–80. DOI: 10.1016/S0360-1315(00)00019-1

Christensen, E., Albertella, L., Chamberlain, S. R., Suo, C., Brydevall, M., Grant, J. E., Yücel, M., & Lee, R. S. C. (2024). A comprehensive evaluation of the neurocognitive predictors of problematic alcohol use, eating, pornography, and internet use: A 6-month longitudinal study. *Journal of Behavioral Addictions*, *13*(3), 823–840. DOI: 10.1556/2006.2024.00041 PMID: 39141435

Christensen, E., Albertella, L., Chamberlain, S., Brydevall, M., Suo, C., Grant, J., Yücel, M., & Lee, R. (2023). The neurocognitive correlates of non-substance addictive behaviors. *Addictive Behaviors*, *150*, 107904–107904. DOI: 10.1016/j.addbeh.2023.107904 PMID: 37984220

Chun, J.-W., Choi, J., Cho, H., Choi, M.-R., Ahn, K., Choi, J.-S., & Kim, D.-J. (2018). Role of Frontostriatal Connectivity in Adolescents With Excessive Smartphone Use. *Frontiers in Psychiatry*, *9*, 437. Advance online publication. DOI: 10.3389/fpsyt.2018.00437 PMID: 30258373

Clare, B., Walter, E., & Harold, E. (2019). Free market for the environment. *Economic Policy*, *14*(1), 116–125. Advance online publication. DOI: 10.18288/1994-5124-2019-1-116-125

Clemente-Suárez, V. J., Beltrán-Velasco, A. I., Herrero-Roldán, S., Rodriguez-Besteiro, S., Martínez-Guardado, I., Martín-Rodríguez, A., & Tornero-Aguilera, J. F. (2024). Digital device usage and childhood cognitive development: Exploring effects on cognitive abilities. *Children (Basel, Switzerland)*, *11*(11), 1299. DOI: 10.3390/children11111299 PMID: 39594874

Cohen, D. (2008). Neurophysiological Pathways to Obesity: Below Awareness and Beyond Individual Control. *57(7)*, 1768-1773. American Diabetes Association. DOI: 10.2337/db08-0163

Cooper, A. (1998). Sexuality and the Internet: Surfing into the new millennium. *Cyberpsychology & Behavior*, *1*(2), 187–193. DOI: 10.1089/cpb.1998.1.187

Cooper, A., Delmonico, D. L., & Burg, R. (2000). Cybersex users, abusers, and compulsives: New findings and implications. *Sexual Addiction & Compulsivity, 7*(1-2), 5–29. DOI: 10.1080/10720160008400205

Coppola, I., & Pihkala, P. (2023). Complex dynamics of climate emotions among environmentally active Finnish and American young people. *Frontiers in Political Science, 4*, 1063741. Advance online publication. DOI: 10.3389/fpos.2022.1063741

Costa, F., Frecassetti, S., Rossini, M., & Portioli-Staudacher, A. (2023). Industry 4.0 digital technologies enhancing sustainability: Applications and barriers from the agricultural industry in an emerging economy. *Journal of Cleaner Production, 408*, 137208. DOI: 10.1016/j.jclepro.2023.137208

Couldry, N., & Mejias, U. A. (2019). *The costs of connection: How data is colonizing human life and appropriating it for capitalism.* Stanford University Press., DOI: 10.1515/9781503609754

Council of Europe. (2018). *Guidelines to respect, protect and fulfil the rights of the child in relation to the digital environment.* Council of Europe. https://rm.coe.int/guidelines-to-respect-protect-and-fulfil-the-rights-of-the-child-in-th/16808d881a

Courbet, D., Fourquet-Courbet, M.-P., & Amato, S. (2020). "Addictions" and Problematic Behaviors linked to Internet and Social Networks. *HAL (Le Centre pour la Communication Scientifique Directe).* https://hal-amu.archives-ouvertes.fr/hal-02616325 adresinden alındı

Coyle, K., Anderson, P., & Laris, B. A. (2015). Schools and sexuality education. In *Evidence-based approaches to sexuality education* (1st ed., pp. 23–45). Routledge.

Crabbe, M., & Flood, M. (2021). School-based education to address pornography's influence on young people: A proposed practice framework. *American Journal of Sexuality Education, 16*(1), 1–37. DOI: 10.1080/15546128.2020.1856744

Csereklyei, Z. (2020). Price and income elasticities of residential and industrial electricity demand in the European Union. *Energy Policy, 137*, 111079. DOI: 10.1016/j.enpol.2019.111079

Csibi, S., Griffiths, M. D., Cook, B., Demetrovics, Z., & Szabo, A. (2018). The Psychometric Properties of the Smartphone Application-Based Addiction Scale (SABAS). *International Journal of Mental Health and Addiction, 16*(2), 393–403. DOI: 10.1007/s11469-017-9787-2 PMID: 29670500

D'Angelo, J. D. (2020). Problematic and addictive technology use. In *Elsevier eBooks* (pp. 347–364). https://doi.org/DOI: 10.1016/B978-0-12-817319-0.00016-5

Dahl, D., & Bergmark, K. H. (2020). Problematic internet use: A scoping review – Longitudinal research on a contemporary social problem, 2006–2017. *Nordisk Alkohol- & Narkotikatidskrift : NAT*, *37*(6), 497–525. DOI: 10.1177/1455072520941997 PMID: 35308651

Dalbudak, E., Evren, C., Aldemir, S., & Evren, B. (2014). The severity of Internet addiction risk and its relationship with the severity of borderline personality features, childhood traumas, dissociative experiences, depression and anxiety symptoms among Turkish university students. *Psychiatry Research*, *219*(3), 577–582. DOI: 10.1016/j.psychres.2014.02.032 PMID: 25023365

Daneback, K., & Ross, M. W. (2011). The complexity of internet sexuality. *Advances in Psychosomatic Medicine*, *31*, 121–134. DOI: 10.1159/000328920 PMID: 22005208

Daneback, K., Ševčíková, A., & Ježek, S. (2018). Exposure to online sexual materials in adolescence and desensitization to sexual content. *Sexologies*, *27*(3), e71–e76. DOI: 10.1016/j.sexol.2018.04.001

Darvesh, N., Radhakrishnan, A., Lachance, C. C., Nincic, V., Sharpe, J. P., Ghassemi, M., Straus, S. E., & Tricco, A. C. (2020). Exploring the prevalence of gaming disorder and Internet gaming disorder: A rapid scoping review. *Systematic Reviews*, *9*(1), 68. DOI: 10.1186/s13643-020-01329-2 PMID: 32241295

David, I., Krutman, L., Fernández-Santaella, M., Andrade, J., Andrade, E., Oliveira, L., Pereira, M. G., Gomes, F. S., Gleiser, S., Oliveira, J. M., Araújo, R. L., Volchan, E., & Braga, F. (2017). Appetitive drives for ultra-processed food products and the ability of text warnings to counteract consumption predispositions. *Public Health Nutrition*, *21*(3), 543–557. DOI: 10.1017/S1368980017003263 PMID: 29173214

Davis, C., & Carter, J. (2014). If Certain Foods are Addictive, How Might this Change the Treatment of Compulsive Overeating and Obesity? *Current Addiction Reports*, *1*(2), 89–95. DOI: 10.1007/s40429-014-0013-z

Davis, R. A. (2001). A cognitive-behavioural model of pathological internet use. *Computers in Human Behavior*, *17*(2), 187–195. DOI: 10.1016/S0747-5632(00)00041-8

Dawson, K., Gabhainn, S. N., Friday, R., & MacNeela, P. (2024). Barriers and recommendations for parent–child conversations about pornography. *Frontiers in Sociology*, *9*, 1349549. DOI: 10.3389/fsoc.2024.1349549 PMID: 38726390

de Alarcón, R., de la Iglesia, J. I., Casado, N. M., & Montejo, A. L. (2019). Online Porn Addiction: What We Know and What We Don't-A Systematic Review. *Journal of Clinical Medicine*, *8*(1), 91. DOI: 10.3390/jcm8010091 PMID: 30650522

De Jesus Correa, J., Souza, J., & Da Silva, P. R. (2025). PSIQUIATRIA DA ADIÇÃO DIGITAL: IMPACTOS DO USO EXCESSIVO DE TECNOLOGIA NO SISTEMA DE RECOMPENSA. *Revista Ft*. DOI: 10.69849/revistaft/dt10202506041027

Deb, S., Strodl, E., & Sun, J. (2015). Academic stress, parental pressure, anxiety and mental health among Indian high school students. *International Journal of Psychology and Behavioral Sciences*, *5*(1), 26–34.

Dechezleprêtre, A., & Sato, M. (2017). The Impacts of Environmental Regulations on Competitiveness. *Review of Environmental Economics and Policy*, *11*(2), 183–206. DOI: 10.1093/reep/rex013

De, D., Alsharef, J., Aydemır, E., & Khera, A. (2025). Social Media Algorithms and Teen Addiction: Neurophysiological Impact and Ethical Considerations. *Cureus*, *17*(1). Advance online publication. DOI: 10.7759/cureus.77145 PMID: 39925596

Deleuze, J., Rochat, L., Romo, L., Van der Linden, M., Achab, S., Thorens, G., Khazaal, Y., Zullino, D., Maurage, P., Rothen, S., & Billieux, J. (2015). Prevalence and characteristics of addictive behaviors in a community sample: A latent class analysis. *Addictive Behaviors Reports*, *1*, 49–56. DOI: 10.1016/j.abrep.2015.04.001 PMID: 29531979

Dienlin, T., & Johannes, N. (2020). The impact of digital technology use on adolescent well-being. *Dialogues in Clinical Neuroscience*, *22*(2), 135–142. DOI: 10.31887/DCNS.2020.22.2/tdienlin PMID: 32699513

Dieris-Hirche, J., Bottel, L., Pape, M., Te Wildt, B. T., Wölfling, K., Henningsen, P., Timmesfeld, N., Neumann, A., Neusser, S., Beckers, R., & Herpertz, S.OMPRIS study group. (2021). Effects of an online-based motivational intervention to reduce problematic internet use and promote treatment motivation in internet gaming disorder and internet use disorder (OMPRIS): Study protocol for a randomised controlled trial. *BMJ Open*, *11*(8), e045840. DOI: 10.1136/bmjopen-2020-045840 PMID: 34344675

Dinçer, E. M., Durmuş, H., Demirgül, S. A., Kavla, Y., Kitapçıoğlu, S., Aktürk, İ., Bozdemir, T., Sandıkçı, T., Büyükçorak, M., & Barış, F. Y. (2025). A roadmap to online pornography use: Research, assessment, and treatment. *Addicta : The Turkish Journal on Addictions*, *12*(4), 498–514. DOI: 10.5152/ADDICTA.2025.25572

Ding, H., Cao, B., & Sun, Q. (2023). The association between problematic internet use and social anxiety within adolescents and young adults: A systematic review and meta-analysis. *Frontiers in Public Health*, *11*, 1275723. DOI: 10.3389/fpubh.2023.1275723 PMID: 37841708

Doane, A. N., Pearson, M. R., & Kelley, M. L. (2014). Predictors of cyberbullying perpetration among college students: An application of the theory of reasoned action. *Computers in Human Behavior*, *36*, 154–162. DOI: 10.1016/j.chb.2014.03.051

Dombrowski, S. C., Gischlar, K. L., & Durst, T. (2007). Safeguarding young people from cyber pornography and cyber sexual predation: A major dilemma of the internet. *Child Abuse Review*, *16*(3), 153–170. DOI: 10.1002/car.939

Domoff, S., Sutherland, E., Yokum, S., & Gearhardt, A. (2020). Adolescents' Addictive Phone Use: Associations with Eating Behaviors and Adiposity. *International Journal of Environmental Research and Public Health*, *17*(8), 2861–2861. DOI: 10.3390/ijerph17082861 PMID: 32326344

Dong, R., Yuan, D., Wei, X., Cai, J., Ai, Z., & Zhou, S. (2025). Exploring the relationship between social media dependence and internet addiction among college students from a bibliometric perspective. *Frontiers in Psychology*, *16*, 1463671. Advance online publication. DOI: 10.3389/fpsyg.2025.1463671 PMID: 40144033

Döring, N. M. (2009). The Internet's impact on sexuality: A critical review of 15 years of research. *Computers in Human Behavior*, *25*(5), 1089–1101. DOI: 10.1016/j.chb.2009.04.003

Draps, M., Kowalczyk-Grębska, N., Marchewka, A., Shi, F., & Gola, M. (2021). White matter microstructural and Compulsive Sexual Behaviors Disorder - Diffusion Tensor Imaging study. *Journal of Behavioral Addictions*, *10*(1), 55–64. DOI: 10.1556/2006.2021.00002 PMID: 33570504

Draps, M., Sescousse, G., Potenza, M. N., Marchewka, A., Duda, A., Lew-Starowicz, M., Kopera, M., Jakubczyk, A., Wojnar, M., & Gola, M. (2020). Gray Matter Volume Differences in Impulse Control and Addictive Disorders-An Evidence From a Sample of Heterosexual Males. *Journal of Sexual Medicine*, *17*(9), 1761–1769. DOI: 10.1016/j.jsxm.2020.05.007 PMID: 32690426

Dresp, B., & Hutt, A. (2022). Digital Addiction and Sleep. *International Journal of Environmental Research and Public Health*, *19*(11), 6910. Advance online publication. DOI: 10.3390/ijerph19116910 PMID: 35682491

Driessen, C., Chung, A., Martino, F., Cameron, A., Bhatti, A., Huse, O., & Backholer, K. (2025). Contemporary digital marketing techniques used in unhealthy food campaigns targeting young people. *Appetite*, *211*, 107989–107989. DOI: 10.1016/j.appet.2025.107989 PMID: 40185242

Duffy, A., Dawson, D. L., & das Nair, R. (2016). Pornography Addiction in Adults: A Systematic Review of Definitions and Reported Impact. *Journal of Sexual Medicine, 13*(5), 760–777. DOI: 10.1016/j.jsxm.2016.03.002 PMID: 27114191

Dumontheil, I. (2016). Adolescent brain development. *Current Opinion in Behavioral Sciences, 10*, 39–44. DOI: 10.1016/j.cobeha.2016.04.012

Durlak, J. A., Weissberg, R. P., Dymnicki, A. B., Taylor, R. D., & Schellinger, K. B. (2011). The impact of enhancing students' social and emotional learning: A meta-analysis. *Child Development, 82*(1), 405–432. DOI: 10.1111/j.1467-8624.2010.01564.x PMID: 21291449

Eke, D., & Stahl, B. (2024). Ethics in the governance of data and digital technology: An analysis of European data regulations and policies. *Digital Society : Ethics, Socio-Legal and Governance of Digital Technology, 3*(1), 11. DOI: 10.1007/s44206-024-00101-6

Ekhtiari, H., Sangchooli, A., Carmichael, O., Moeller, F., O'Donnell, P., Oquendo, M., Paulus, M. P., Pizzagalli, D. A., Ramey, T., Schacht, J. P., Zare-Bidoky, M., Childress, A. R., & Brady, K. (2024). Neuroimaging biomarkers of addiction. *Nature Mental Health, 2*(12), 1498–1517. DOI: 10.1038/s44220-024-00334-x PMID: 39281741

Elbaum, S., & Panter, J. (2025). Managing escalation in off-the-shelf large language models. *arXiv (Cornell University)*. https://doi.org//arxiv.2508.01056DOI: 10.48550

Elhai, J. D., Levine, J. C., Dvorak, R. D., & Hall, B. J. (2017). Non-social features of smartphone use are most related to depression, anxiety, and problematic smartphone use. *Computers in Human Behavior, 69*, 75–82. DOI: 10.1016/j.chb.2016.12.023

Elhai, J. D., Yang, H., & Montag, C. (2020). Fear of missing out (FoMO): Symptom associations with depression, anxiety, and problematic smartphone use. *Addictive Behaviors Reports, 11*, 100262.

Elliott, C., Truman, E., & Black, J. (2025). Food marketing to teenagers: Examining the digital palate of targeted appeals. *Appetite, 207*, 107912–107912. DOI: 10.1016/j.appet.2025.107912 PMID: 39956205

Ergün, N. (2023). Developing the online pornography addiction scale and examining its associations with psychosocial factors. *Behavioral Psychology/Psicología Conductual, 31*(2), 269–299. DOI: 10.51668/bp.8323203n

Eskandar, K. (2025). The digital trap: Unraveling the neuropsychological impact of technology addiction. *Neuropsychological Trends*, (37), 7–23. DOI: 10.7358/neur-2025-037-eska

Esposito, F., & Maciel Cathoud Ferreira, T. (2024). Addictive design as an unfair commercial practice: The case of hyper-engaging dark patterns. *European Journal of Risk Regulation, 15*(4), 999–1016. DOI: 10.1017/err.2024.8

European Commission. (2025). Digital Services Act. European Commission. https://digital-strategy.ec.europa.eu/en/policies/digital-services-act

European Parliament. (2024). *Digital markets and digital services: The Digital Services Act and the Digital Markets Act — Implementation and enforcement* (EPRS_ATA(2024)766256). European Parliamentary Research Service. https://www.europarl.europa.eu/thinktank/en/document/EPRS_ATA(2024)766256

European Union. (2016). Article 5: Principles relating to processing of personal data. In *Regulation (EU) 2016/679 (General Data Protection Regulation)*. European Union. https://gdpr-info.eu/art-5-gdpr/

Everitt, B. J., & Robbins, T. W. (2016). Drug Addiction: Updating Actions to Habits to Compulsions Ten Years On. *Annual Review of Psychology*, *67*(1), 23–50. DOI: 10.1146/annurev-psych-122414-033457 PMID: 26253543

Evren, C., Dalbudak, E., Topcu, M., Kutlu, N., Evren, B., & Pontes, H. M. (2018). Psychometric validation of the Turkish nine-item Internet Gaming Disorder Scale-Short Form (IGDS9-SF). *Psychiatry Research*, *265*, 349–354. DOI: 10.1016/j.psychres.2018.05.002 PMID: 29793049

Fahy, A. E., Stansfeld, S. A., Smuk, M., Smith, N. R., Cummins, S., & Clark, C. (2016). Longitudinal associations between cyberbullying involvement and adolescent mental health. *The Journal of Adolescent Health : Official Publication of the Society for Adolescent Medicine*, *59*(5), 502–509. DOI: 10.1016/j.jadohealth.2016.06.006 PMID: 27528471

Fam, J. Y. (2018). Prevalence of internet gaming disorder in adolescents: A meta-analysis across three decades. *Scandinavian Journal of Psychology*, *59*(5), 524–531. DOI: 10.1111/sjop.12459 PMID: 30004118

Fardouly, J., Magson, N. R., Rapee, R. M., Oar, E. L., Johnco, C. J., Richardson, C., & Freeman, J. (2022). Investigating longitudinal and bidirectional relationships between parental factors and time spent on social media during early adolescence. *New Media & Society*, *26*(3), 1610–1626. DOI: 10.1177/14614448221076155

Fattore, L., & Melis, M. (2016). Exploring gender and sex differences in behavioral dyscontrol: From drug addiction to impulse control disorders. *Frontiers in Psychiatry*, *7*, 19. DOI: 10.3389/fpsyt.2016.00019 PMID: 26941657

Fernandez, D. P., & Griffiths, M. D. (2021). Psychometric Instruments for Problematic Pornography Use: A Systematic Review. *Evaluation & the Health Professions, 44*(2), 111–141. DOI: 10.1177/0163278719861688 PMID: 31284745

Field, T. (2020). Adolescent pornography: A narrative review. *International Journal of Psychological Research and Reviews, 36*, 36. Advance online publication. DOI: 10.28933/ijprr-2020-03-0505

Filippone, L., Shankland, R., & Hallez, Q. (2022). The relationships between social media exposure, food craving, cognitive impulsivity and cognitive restraint. *Journal of Eating Disorders, 10*(1), 184. Advance online publication. DOI: 10.1186/s40337-022-00698-4 PMID: 36434703

Fisher, W. A., & Barak, A. (2001). Internet pornography: A social psychological perspective on internet sexuality. *Journal of Sex Research, 38*(4), 312–323. DOI: 10.1080/00224490109552102

Fitzpatrick, K. K., Darcy, A., & Vierhile, M. (2017). Delivering cognitive behaviour therapy to young adults with symptoms of depression and anxiety using a fully automated conversational agent (Woebot): A randomised controlled trial. *JMIR Mental Health, 4*(2), e19. DOI: 10.2196/mental.7785 PMID: 28588005

Flayelle, M., Brevers, D., King, D., Maurage, P., Perales, J., & Billieux, J. (2023). A taxonomy of technology design features that promote potentially addictive online behaviours. *Nature Reviews Psychology, 2*(3), 136–150. DOI: 10.1038/s44159-023-00153-4

Flood, M. (2009). The harms of pornography exposure among children and young people. *Child Abuse Review, 18*(6), 384–400. DOI: 10.1002/car.1092

Folkvord, F., Anschütz, D., Buijzen, M., & Valkenburg, P. (2012). The effect of playing advergames that promote energy-dense snacks or fruit on actual food intake among children. *The American Journal of Clinical Nutrition, 97*(2), 239–245. DOI: 10.3945/ajcn.112.047126 PMID: 23269821

Fortenberry, J. D. (2013). Sexual development in adolescents. In *Elsevier eBooks* (pp. 171-192). DOI: 10.1016/B978-0-12-387759-8.00007-6

Franjic, S. (2022). A few words about pornography. *International Journal of Social Science and Economics, 2*(1), 7. DOI: 10.22158/ijsse.v2n1p7

Frascella, J., Potenza, M., Brown, L., & Childress, A. (2010). Shared brain vulnerabilities open the way for nonsubstance addictions: Carving addiction at a new joint? *1187(1)*, 294-315. Wiley. DOI: 10.1111/j.1749-6632.2009.05420.x

Fretes, G., Véliz, P., Cerezo-Narváez, A., Williams, D., Sibille, R., Arts, M., & Leroy, J. (2025). Digital Marketing of Unhealthy Foods and Non-alcoholic Beverages to Children and Adolescents: A Narrative Review. *Current Developments in Nutrition*, *9*(2), 104545–104545. DOI: 10.1016/j.cdnut.2025.104545 PMID: 40046995

Fulmer, R., Joerin, A., Gentile, B., Lakerink, L., & Rauws, M. (2018). Using psychological artificial intelligence (Tess) to relieve symptoms of depression and anxiety: Randomised controlled trial. *JMIR Mental Health*, *5*(4), e64. DOI: 10.2196/mental.9782 PMID: 30545815

Galatzer-Levy, R. M. (2021). Adolescent boys and pornography: Notes on a complex system. *The Psychoanalytic Study of the Child*, *74*(1), 191–208. DOI: 10.1080/00797308.2020.1859279

Gao, L., Gan, Y., Zhang, Y., & Liu, R. (2020). Wearable devices for health monitoring in the Internet of Things: A survey. *Journal of Industrial Information Integration*, *17*, 100130. DOI: 10.1016/j.jii.2020.100130

Gearhardt, A., Bueno, N., DiFeliceantonio, A., Roberto, C., Jiménez-Múrcia, S., & Fernández-Aranda, F. (2023). Social, clinical, and policy implications of ultra-processed food addiction. *BMJ (Clinical Research Ed.)*, *383*, e075354. Advance online publication. DOI: 10.1136/bmj-2023-075354 PMID: 37813420

George, A. S., George, A. H., & Baskar, T. (2023). The death of analog: Assessing the Impacts of ubiquitous mobile technology. *Partners Universal Innovative Research Publication*, *1*(2), 15–33.

George, A., & Rupa, R. (2025). Swipe, click, regret: An opinion on persuasive e-commerce and consumer autonomy. *Frontiers in Artificial Intelligence*, *8*, 1684841–1684841. DOI: 10.3389/frai.2025.1684841 PMID: 41190037

Gerber, J. P. (2018). Social comparison on social media: A meta-analysis. *Social Psychology (Göttingen)*.

Gesser-Edelsburg, A., & Arabia, M. A. E. (2018). Discourse on exposure to pornography content online between Arab adolescents and parents: Qualitative study on its impact on sexual education and behavior. *Journal of Medical Internet Research*, *20*(10), e11667. DOI: 10.2196/11667 PMID: 30305264

Giansanti, D. (2025). Smartphone Addiction in Youth: A Narrative Review of Systematic Evidence and Emerging Strategies. *Psychiatry International*, *6*(4), 118–118. DOI: 10.3390/psychiatryint6040118

Gibbons, F. X., Kingsbury, J. H., Wills, T. A., Finneran, S. D., Cin, S. D., & Gerrard, M. (2016). Impulsivity moderates the effects of movie alcohol portrayals on adolescents' willingness to drink. *Psychology of Addictive Behaviors : Journal of the Society of Psychologists in Addictive Behaviors, 30*(3), 325–334. DOI: 10.1037/adb0000178 PMID: 27099959

Gillespie, T. (2018). *Custodians of the Internet: Platforms, Content Moderation, and the Hidden Decisions That Shape Social Media.* Yale University Press.

Gisbert-Pérez, J., Longobardi, C., Martí-Vilar, M., Mastrokoukou, S., & Badenes-Ribera, L. (2025). Prevalence of Internet gaming disorder in young adults: A systematic review and meta-analysis. *Addictive Behaviors, 174*, 108576. DOI: 10.1016/j.addbeh.2025.108576 PMID: 41317410

Gola, M., Lewczuk, K., Potenza, M. N., Kingston, D. A., Grubbs, J. B., Stark, R., & Reid, R. C. (2020). What should be included in the criteria for compulsive sexual behavior disorder? *Journal of Behavioral Addictions, 11*(2), 160–165. DOI: 10.1556/2006.2020.00090 PMID: 34329192

Gola, M., Wordecha, M., Sescousse, G., Lew-Starowicz, M., Kossowski, B., Wypych, M., Makeig, S., Potenza, M. N., & Marchewka, A. (2017). Can Pornography be Addictive? An fMRI Study of Men Seeking Treatment for Problematic Pornography Use. *Neuropsychopharmacology : Official Publication of the American College of Neuropsychopharmacology, 42*(10), 2021–2031. DOI: 10.1038/npp.2017.78 PMID: 28409565

Golden, S. D., McLeroy, K. R., Green, L. W., Earp, J. A., & Lieberman, L. D. (2015). Upending the social ecological model to guide health promotion efforts toward policy and environmental change. *Health Education & Behavior : The Official Publication of the Society for Public Health Education, 42*(1, Suppl), 8S–14S. DOI: 10.1177/1090198115575098 PMID: 25829123

Golec, K., Draps, M., Stark, R., Pluta, A., & Gola, M. (2021). Aberrant orbitofrontal cortex reactivity to erotic cues in compulsive sexual behavior disorder. *Journal of Behavioral Addictions, 10*(3), 646–656. Advance online publication. DOI: 10.1556/2006.2021.00051 PMID: 34437297

Gonçalves, L., Nardi, A., & King, A. (2023). Digital dependence in the past decade: A systematic review. *Journal of Addiction Research and Adolescent Behaviour, 6*(1), 1–18. DOI: 10.31579/2688-7517/059

Gonsalves, V. M., Hodges, H., & Scalora, M. J. (2015). Exploring the use of online sexually explicit material: What is the relationship to sexual coercion? *Sexual Addiction & Compulsivity, 22*(3), 207–221. DOI: 10.1080/10720162.2015.1039150

Görts, P., Savard, J., Görts-Öberg, K., Dhejne, C., Arver, S., Jokinen, J., Ingvar, M., & Abé, C. (2023). Structural brain differences related to compulsive sexual behavior disorder. *Journal of Behavioral Addictions*, *12*(1), 278–287. DOI: 10.1556/2006.2023.00008 PMID: 36943775

GOV.UK. (2024). *Online Safety Act: explainer*. https://www.gov.uk/government/publications/online-safety-act-explainer/online-safety-act-explainer#:~:text=The%20Act%20requires%20social%20media,are%20shielded%20from%20harmful%20content

Grant, J. E., Boutouis, S., Collins, M., & Chamberlain, S. R. (2025). Compulsive sexual behavior disorder: Rates and clinical correlates in a community sample. *Frontiers in Psychiatry*, *16*, 1561885. DOI: 10.3389/fpsyt.2025.1561885 PMID: 40475952

Green, L., Lumby, C., McKee, A., & Ólafsson, K. (2020). National contexts for the risk of harm being done to children by access to online sexual content. In Tsaliki, L., & Chronaki, D. (Eds.), *Discourses of anxiety over childhood and youth across cultures* (pp. xx–xx). Palgrave Macmillan., DOI: 10.1007/978-3-030-46436-3_11

Griffiths, M. D. (2016). Behavioural addiction in sport: The case of exercise addiction. *Journal of Behavioral Addictions*, *5*(2), 133–139. DOI: 10.1556/2006.5.2016.018

Griffiths, M. D., Kuss, D. J., & Demetrovics, Z. (2016). Social networking addiction: An overview of preliminary findings. In *Behavioural addictions* (pp. 119–141). Academic Press., DOI: 10.1016/B978-0-12-407724-9.00006-9

Grimland, M., Mori, Y., Lesinskiene, S., Li, L., Ong, S. H., Praharaj, S. K., Wiguna, T., Zamani, Z., Heinonen, E., Gilbert, S., Brunstein Klomek, A., & Sourander, A.EACMHS Study Group. (2025). Cyberbullying victimization and suicide attempt among adolescents: A cross-national comparison. *International Journal of Environmental Research and Public Health*, *22*(3), 385. DOI: 10.3390/ijerph22030385 PMID: 40238440

Gross, J. J. (1998). The emerging field of emotion regulation: An integrative review. *Review of General Psychology*, *2*(3), 271–299. DOI: 10.1037/1089-2680.2.3.271

Grubbs, J. B., Exline, J. J., Pargament, K. I., Hook, J. N., & Carlisle, R. D. (2015). Transgression as addiction: Religiosity and moral disapproval as predictors of perceived addiction to pornography. *Archives of Sexual Behavior*, *44*(1), 125–136. DOI: 10.1007/s10508-013-0257-z PMID: 24519108

Grubbs, J. B., & Kraus, S. W. (2021). Pornography use and psychological science: A call for consideration. *Current Directions in Psychological Science*, *30*(1), 68–75. DOI: 10.1177/0963721420979594

Grubbs, J. B., Kraus, S. W., Perry, S. L., Lewczuk, K., & Gola, M. (2020). Moral incongruence and compulsive sexual behavior: Results from cross-sectional interactions and parallel growth curve analyses. *Journal of Abnormal Psychology*, *129*(3), 266–278. DOI: 10.1037/abn0000501 PMID: 32027146

Grubbs, J. B., & Perry, S. L. (2019). Moral incongruence and pornography use: A critical review and integration. *Journal of Sex Research*, *56*(1), 29–37. DOI: 10.1080/00224499.2018.1427204 PMID: 29412013

Grubbs, J. B., Perry, S. L., Wilt, J. A., & Reid, R. C. (2019). Pornography Problems Due to Moral Incongruence: An Integrative Model with a Systematic Review and Meta-Analysis. *Archives of Sexual Behavior*, *48*(2), 397–415. DOI: 10.1007/s10508-018-1248-x PMID: 30076491

Grubbs, J. B., Volk, F., Exline, J. J., & Pargament, K. I. (2015). Internet pornography use: Perceived addiction, psychological distress, and the validation of a brief measure. *Journal of Sex & Marital Therapy*, *41*(1), 83–106. DOI: 10.1080/0092623X.2013.842192 PMID: 24341869

Grubbs, J. B., Wilt, J. A., Exline, J. J., Pargament, K. I., & Kraus, S. W. (2017). Moral disapproval and perceived addiction to internet pornography: A longitudinal examination. *Addiction (Abingdon, England)*, *113*(3), 496–506. DOI: 10.1111/add.14007 PMID: 28833800

Gualano, M. R., Bert, F., Martorana, M., Voglino, G., Andriolo, V., Thomas, R., Gramaglia, C., Zeppegno, P., & Siliquini, R. (2017). The long-term effects of bibliotherapy in depression treatment: Series of case reports. *BioMed Research International*, *2017*, 4306473.

Gujar, V. (2024). New age marketing: AI personalization strategies in digital world. *International Advanced Research Journal in Science. Engineering and Technology*, *11*(3), 288–296.

Gupta, A., Khan, A. M., & Gupta, A. (2021). Internet addiction and its correlates among Indian college students: A systematic review. *Indian Journal of Community Medicine : Official Publication of Indian Association of Preventive & Social Medicine*, *46*(3), 433–440. DOI: 10.4103/ijcm.IJCM_230_21

Gupta, S. (2024). Child pornography and internet subcultures in India - A legal perspective. *Journal of Law and Sustainable Development*, *12*(1), e2997. DOI: 10.55908/sdgs.v12i1.2997

Halloran, A., Rippin, H., Farrand, C., Wickramasinghe, K., Flore, R., Pires, S., . . . Granheim, S. (2021). *Slide to Order: A Food Systems Approach to Meal Delivery Apps: WHO European Office for the Prevention and Control of Noncommunicable Diseases.* Technical University of Denmark. https://local.forskningsportal.dk/local/dki-cgi/ws/cris-link?src=dtu&id=dtu-c652223c-b60d-4401-9b13-c333c62b730c&ti=Slide%20to%20Order%3A%20A%20Food%20Systems%20Approach%20to%20Meal%20Delivery%20Apps%3A%20WHO%20European%20Office%20for%20the%20Prevention%20and%20Control%20of%20Noncommunicable%20Diseases adresinden alındı

Han, D. H., & Renshaw, P. F. (2012). Bupropion in the treatment of problematic online game play in patients with major depressive disorder. *Journal of Psychopharmacology*, *26*(5), 689–696. DOI: 10.1177/0269881111400647 PMID: 21447539

Han, R., Todd, A., Wardak, S., Partridge, S., & Raeside, R. (2023). Feasibility and Acceptability of Chatbots for Nutrition and Physical Activity Health Promotion Among Adolescents: Systematic Scoping Review With Adolescent Consultation. *JMIR Human Factors*, *10*, e43227. Advance online publication. DOI: 10.2196/43227 PMID: 37145858

Hanseder, S., & Dantas, J. A. R. (2023). Males' Lived Experience with Self-Perceived Pornography Addiction: A Qualitative Study of Problematic Porn Use. *International Journal of Environmental Research and Public Health*, *20*(2), 1497. DOI: 10.3390/ijerph20021497 PMID: 36674250

Harris, J., & Taillie, L. (2023). More than a Nuisance: Implications of Food Marketing for Public Health Efforts to Curb Childhood Obesity. *Annual Review of Public Health*, *45*(1), 213–233. DOI: 10.1146/annurev-publhealth-090419-102616 PMID: 38109516

Harris, J., & Taillie, L. (2024). More than a Nuisance: Implications of Food Marketing for Public Health Efforts to Curb Childhood Obesity. *Carolina Digital Repository (University of North Carolina at Chapel Hill)*. DOI: 10.17615/whrd-4415

Harun, N. U., Jaafar, A. B., Razak, T. M. T. A., Rahman, N. A. A., & Musah, N. S. M. (2025). A Comprehensive Review of the Psychological, Societal, and Technological Dimensions of Pornography Use and Impact. *International Journal of Research and Innovation in Applied Science*, *9*(24), 977–984.

Hatef, E., Hudson Scholle, S., Buckley, B., Weiner, J. P., & Austin, J. M. (2024). Development of an evidence- and consensus-based digital healthcare equity framework. *JAMIA Open*, *7*(4), ooae136. Advance online publication. DOI: 10.1093/jamiaopen/ooae136 PMID: 39553827

Hawdon, J., Oksanen, A., & Räsänen, P. (2016). Exposure to online hate in four nations: A cross-national consideration. *Deviant Behavior*, *38*(3), 254–266. DOI: 10.1080/01639625.2016.1196985

Hawkley, L. C., & Cacioppo, J. T. (2010). Loneliness matters: A theoretical and empirical review. *Current Directions in Psychological Science*, *19*(2), 70–74. PMID: 20652462

Health in All Policies (HiAP) framework for country action. (2014). *Health promotion international, 29 Suppl 1*, i19–i28. https://doi.org/DOI: 10.1093/heapro/dau035

Healy-Cullen, S., Taylor, J. E., Ross, K., & Morison, T. (2021). Youth encounters with internet pornography: A survey of youth, caregiver, and educator perspectives. *Sexuality & Culture*, *26*(2), 491–513. DOI: 10.1007/s12119-021-09904-y

Healy-Cullen, S., Taylor, K., & Morison, T. (2024). Youth, pornography, and addiction: A Critical review. *Current Addiction Reports*, *11*(2), 265–274. DOI: 10.1007/s40429-024-00549-z

Hebebrand, J., Albayrak, Ö., Adan, R., Antel, J., Diéguez, C., Jong, J., & Dickson, S. (2014). "Eating addiction", rather than "food addiction", better captures addictive-like eating behavior. *Neuroscience and Biobehavioral Reviews*, *47*, 295–306. DOI: 10.1016/j.neubiorev.2014.08.016 PMID: 25205078

Heinrich, L. M., & Gullone, E. (2006). The clinical significance of loneliness: A literature review. *Clinical Psychology Review*, *26*(6), 695–718. DOI: 10.1016/j.cpr.2006.04.002 PMID: 16952717

He, J., Yu, S., & Zhang, J. (2025). Analysis and prediction of addiction among virtual reality users. *PLoS One*, *20*(3), e0318117. DOI: 10.1371/journal.pone.0318117 PMID: 40072966

Hellfeldt, K., López-Romero, L., & Andershed, H. (2020). Cyberbullying and psychological well-being in young adolescence: The potential protective mediation effects of social support from family, friends, and teachers. *International Journal of Environmental Research and Public Health*, *17*(1), 45. DOI: 10.3390/ijerph17010045 PMID: 31861641

He, Q., Turel, O., Brevers, D., & Bechara, A. (2017). Excess social media use in normal populations is associated with amygdala-striatal but not with prefrontal morphology. *Psychiatry Research. Neuroimaging*, *269*, 31–35. DOI: 10.1016/j.pscychresns.2017.09.003 PMID: 28918269

Hinduja, S., & Patchin, J. W. (2008). Cyberbullying: An exploratory analysis of factors related to offending and victimization. *Deviant Behavior*, *29*(2), 129–156. DOI: 10.1080/01639620701457816

Hinduja, S., & Patchin, J. W. (2015). *Bullying beyond the schoolyard: Preventing and responding to cyberbullying* (2nd ed.). Sage.

Holt-Lunstad, J. (2024). Social connection as a critical factor for mental and physical health: Evidence, trends, challenges, and future implications. *World Psychiatry; Official Journal of the World Psychiatric Association (WPA)*, *23*(3), 312–332. DOI: 10.1002/wps.21224 PMID: 39279411

Hossain, M. S., & Islam, M. S. (2025). Digital detox for young hearts: Bibliotherapy within a bio-psycho-social model embedding AETCOM in medical humanities for digital-age challenges.

Hough, K., Friuli, M., Avena, N., & Romano, A. (2026). The addicted brain: How processed foods hijack reward pathways. *Pharmacological Research*, *224*, 108097–108097. DOI: 10.1016/j.phrs.2026.108097 PMID: 41525853

Huesmann, L. R. (2007). The impact of electronic media violence: Scientific theory and research. *The Journal of Adolescent Health : Official Publication of the Society for Adolescent Medicine*, *41*(6), S6–S13. DOI: 10.1016/j.jadohealth.2007.09.005 PMID: 18047947

Hulme, K. (2018). *The effects of social media on self-esteem and emotional well-being* [Graduate Research Paper, University of Northern Iowa]. UNI ScholarWorks. https://scholarworks.uni.edu/grp/589/

Humphreys, G., Evans, R., Makin, H., Cooke, R., & Jones, A. (2020). Identification of Behavior Change Techniques From Successful Web-Based Interventions Targeting Alcohol Consumption, Binge Eating, and Gambling: Systematic Review. *23(2)*. JMIR Publications. DOI: 10.2196/22694

Hunt, L. (1996). *The invention of pornography: Obscenity and the origins of modernity, 1500–1800*. Zone Books.

Hutton, J., Piotrowski, J., Bagot, K., Blumberg, F., Canli, T., Chein, J., . . . Potenza, M. (2024). Digital Media and Developing Brains: Concerns and Opportunities. *11(2)*, 287-298. Springer Science+Business Media. DOI: 10.1007/s40429-024-00545-3

Ifland, J., & Brewerton, T. (2025). Binge-type eating disorders and ultra-processed food addiction: Phenomenology, pathophysiology and treatment implications. *Frontiers in Psychiatry, 16,* 1584891–1584891. DOI: 10.3389/fpsyt.2025.1584891 PMID: 40625723

Imataka, G., Izumi, S., Miyamoto, Y., & Maehashi, A. (2024). Gaming disorders: Navigating the fine line between entertainment and addiction—Gaming history, health risks, social consequences, and pathways to prevention. *Journal of Clinical Medicine, 13*(17), 5122. DOI: 10.3390/jcm13175122 PMID: 39274335

Ince, C., Antons, S., Ashton, S., Borgogna, N. C., Brand, M., Briken, P., Castro-Calvo, J., Chen, L., Coleman, E., Efrati, Y., Fernández, D. P., Fuss, J., Gleason, N., Gola, M., Jennings, T. L., Kowalewska, E., Kraus, S. W., Lewczuk, K., Grubbs, J. B., & Bőthe, B. (2026). Compulsive sexual behavior disorder (CSBD) and problematic pornography use (PPU): A comprehensive, interdisciplinary, and expert-informed narrative review with suggested future directions. *Journal of Behavioral Addictions, 15*(1), 32–98. DOI: 10.1556/2006.2025.00337 PMID: 41879870

Indonesia, C. N. N. (2022). *Studi: Sebanyak 2,45 juta remaja Indonesia kena gangguan jiwa* [Study: As many as 2.45 million Indonesian teenagers have mental disorders]. https://www.cnnindonesia.com/gaya-hidup/20221212142530-255-886337/studi-245-juta-remaja-indonesia-kena-gangguan-jiwa

Iyamu, I., Gómez-Ramírez, O., Xu, A. X., Chang, H. J., Watt, S., Mckee, G., & Gilbert, M. (2022). Challenges in the development of digital public health interventions and mapped solutions: Findings from a scoping review. *Digital Health, 8,* 20552076221102255. DOI: 10.1177/20552076221102255 PMID: 35656283

Jaiswal, N., Deshpande, S., Gokani, N., Sahore, A., & Gowande, T. (2025). Understanding Pornography Addiction in India: Insights from a Retrospective, Observational Study. *BJPsych Open, 11*(S1, Suppl 1), S46. DOI: 10.1192/bjo.2025.10153

James, S., Karthik, S., & Thomas, B. (2025). Chasing the digital high: Should hedonic consumption be viewed through the lens of behavioral addiction? *Frontiers in Psychiatry, 16,* 1681307. Advance online publication. DOI: 10.3389/fpsyt.2025.1681307 PMID: 41164096

Jaworska, D. (2025). Many faces of FoMO: A qualitative in-depth investigation of context-specific experiences, emotions, and coping strategies. *PLoS One, 20*(9), e0330978. DOI: 10.1371/journal.pone.0330978 PMID: 40892849

Jenaro, C., Flores, N., & Frías, C. P. (2018). Systematic review of empirical studies on cyberbullying in adults: What we know and what we should investigate. *Aggression and Violent Behavior, 38,* 113–122. DOI: 10.1016/j.avb.2017.12.003

Jenaro, C., Flores, N., & Frías, C. P. (2021). Anxiety and depression in cyberbullied college students: A retrospective study. *Journal of Interpersonal Violence*, *36*(1–2), 579–602. DOI: 10.1177/0886260517730030 PMID: 29294905

Jennings, T. L., Gleason, N., Pachankis, J. E., Bőthe, B., & Kraus, S. W. (2024). LGBQ-affirming clinical recommendations for compulsive sexual behavior disorder. *Journal of Behavioral Addictions*, *13*(2), 413–428. DOI: 10.1556/2006.2024.00012 PMID: 38592797

Jeong, H., Yim, H. W., Lee, S., Lee, H. K., Potenza, M. N., & Park, M. (2021). Joint effects of children's emotional problems and parental depressive symptoms on the occurrence of internet gaming disorder among children and adolescents: A longitudinal study. *Journal of Behavioral Addictions*, *10*(2), 244–252. DOI: 10.1556/2006.2021.00030 PMID: 34128830

Jha, A., & Banerjee, D. (2022). Neurobiology of sex and pornography addictions: A Primer. *Journal of Psychosexual Health*, *4*(4), 227–236. DOI: 10.1177/26318318221116042

Jiang, Q., & Li, Y. (2018). Factors affecting smartphone dependency among the young in China. *Asian Journal of Communication*, *28*(5), 508–525. DOI: 10.1080/01292986.2018.1431296

Jia, S., Todd, A., Vanderlee, L., Farrell, P., Allman-Farinelli, M., Sacks, G., Gibson, A. A., & Partridge, S. (2024). Offline to online: A systematic mapping review of evidence to inform nutrition-related policies applicable to online food delivery platforms. *BMC Medicine*, *22*(1), 542–542. DOI: 10.1186/s12916-024-03747-8 PMID: 39558372

Jia, Y., & Nkoulou Mvondo, G. F. (2025). Exploring the adverse effects of the metaverse on users' psychological well-being and self-esteem: A mixed-methods study. *Journal of Retailing and Consumer Services*, *86*, 104321. DOI: 10.1016/j.jretconser.2025.104321

Jin, J., Wei, H., Chai, Y., Wu, L., Chen, M., & Ding, K. (2026). The neurobiology of internet addiction: A scoping review of developmental and gender-specific mechanisms. *Frontiers in Psychology*, *17*, 1729470–1729470. DOI: 10.3389/fpsyg.2026.1729470 PMID: 41768176

Jin, Y., & Jiang, S. (2025). Theoretical perspectives on adolescent internet addiction: A comprehensive literature review. *Health & Social Care in the Community*, *2025*(1), 4875332. Advance online publication. DOI: 10.1155/hsc/4875332

Johnson, D., Deterding, S., Kuhn, K. A., Staneva, A., Stoyanov, S., & Hides, L. (2016). Gamification for health and wellbeing: A systematic review of the literature. *Internet Interventions : The Application of Information Technology in Mental and Behavioural Health, 6*, 89–106. DOI: 10.1016/j.invent.2016.10.002 PMID: 30135818

Joseph, R., Alonso-Alonso, M., Bond, D., Pascual-Leone, Á., & Blackburn, G. (2011). The neurocognitive connection between physical activity and eating behaviour. *12(10)*, 800-812. Wiley. DOI: 10.1111/j.1467-789X.2011.00893.x

Judge, A. C. D. E. (2008). *Sex education: Are schools teaching what teens need to know?* NEJM Journal Watch., DOI: 10.1056/WH200804030000006

Juul, F., Steele, E., Parekh, N., & Monteiro, C. (2025). The role of ultra-processed food in obesity. *Nature Reviews. Endocrinology, 21*(11), 672–685. DOI: 10.1038/s41574-025-01143-7 PMID: 40659796

Kaplan, M., Lazter, Y., Bőthe, B., & Gewirtz Meydan, A. (2025). The Sacred, the Sinful, and the Shamed: The Association Between Compulsive Sexual Behavior, Moral Disapproval, and Sexual Shame Among Jewish Religious Adolescents. *International Journal of Sexual Health : Official Journal of the World Association for Sexual Health, 37*(3), 486–502. DOI: 10.1080/19317611.2025.2530511 PMID: 40843156

Karaköse, T., Yıldırım, B., Tülübaş, T., & Kardas, A. (2023). *A comprehensive review on emerging trends in the dynamic evolution of digital addiction and depression. 14*. Frontiers Media., DOI: 10.3389/fpsyg.2023.1126815

Kardefelt-Winther, D. (2014). A conceptual and methodological critique of internet addiction research: Towards a model of compensatory internet use. *Computers in Human Behavior, 31*, 351–354. DOI: 10.1016/j.chb.2013.10.059

Karim, R., & Chaudhri, P. (2012). Behavioral addictions: An overview. *Journal of Psychoactive Drugs, 44*(1), 5–17. DOI: 10.1080/02791072.2012.662859 PMID: 22641961

Karyanta, N. A. (2012). *Terapi puisi: Dasar-dasar penggunaan puisi sebagai modalitas dalam psikoterapi* [Poetry therapy: Basics of using poetry as a modality in psychotherapy]. Universitas Sebelas Maret.

Kassa, P. (2025). Cognitive benefits and risks of digital technology engagement. *Discover Psychology, 6*(1), 10. Advance online publication. DOI: 10.1007/s44202-025-00527-0

Kató, S., Pintér-Eszenyei, Z. G., Rando Hurtado, M. A., Csinády, A. K., & Szemán-Nagy, A. (2024). Associations of sexual dysfunction with problematic pornography use and attachment styles: A cross-sectional study of Hungarian-Spanish samples. *European Psychiatry : The Journal of the Association of European Psychiatrists*, *67*(S1, Suppl 1), S49–S50. DOI: 10.1192/j.eurpsy.2024.153

Kaur, K., Gurnani, B., Nayak, S., Deori, N., Kaur, S., Jethani, J., & Mishra, D. (2022). Digital eye strain: A comprehensive review. *Ophthalmology and Therapy*, *11*(5), 1655–1680. DOI: 10.1007/s40123-022-00540-9 PMID: 35809192

Kaya, F. K., & Güllüpinar, F. (2025). The evolution of attention economy in the age of digital capitalism. *Journal of Consumer & Consumption Research*, *17*(1).

Kear, A., & Sasha, L. (2018). Digital Technology Disorder: Justification and a Proposed Model of Treatment. *International Journal of Advanced Computer Science and Applications*, *9*(8). Advance online publication. DOI: 10.14569/IJACSA.2018.090882

Keilty, P. (2015). Embodied engagements with online pornography. *The Information Society*, *32*(1), 64–73. DOI: 10.1080/01972243.2015.1107162

Kendrick, W. (1987). *The secret museum: Pornography in modern culture*. University of California Press.

Kessler, R. C., Barker, P. R., Colpe, L. J., Epstein, J. F., Gfroerer, J. C., Hiripi, E., Howes, M. J., Normand, S.-L. T., Manderscheid, R. W., Walters, E. E., & Zaslavsky, A. M. (2003). Screening for serious mental illness in the general population. *Archives of General Psychiatry*, *60*(2), 184–189. DOI: 10.1001/archpsyc.60.2.184 PMID: 12578436

Khedraki, R., Srivastava, A. V., & Bhavnani, S. P. (2022). Framework for digital health phenotypes in heart failure. *Heart Failure Clinics*, *18*(2), 223–244. DOI: 10.1016/j.hfc.2021.12.003 PMID: 35341537

Khemkhaeng, A. C., Pravat, P. N., Thiha, T., Hayma, T., & Zeya, Z. (2022). Enhancing adolescent well-being: The impact of comprehensive sex education on knowledge, consent, and sexual violence Prevention. *Jurnal Sosial Sains Terapan Dan Riset (Sosateris)*, *10*(2), 151–161. DOI: 10.35335/gze4k733

Kim, J. (2017). South Korea's approach to combating gaming addiction. *Asia Pacific Journal of Social Work and Development*, *27*(2-3), 134–145. DOI: 10.1080/02185385.2017.1352170

Kim, J., & Park, S. (2025). Empowering individual preferences in mobile notifications. *IEEE Access : Practical Innovations, Open Solutions*.

Kim, K. K., & Backonja, U. (2025). Digital health equity frameworks and key concepts: A scoping review. *Journal of the American Medical Informatics Association : JAMIA*, *32*(5), 932–944. DOI: 10.1093/jamia/ocaf017 PMID: 39936843

Kim, K., Lee, I., Kim, J., & Choi, J.-W. (2020). Dietary patterns and smartphone use in adolescents: A large-sample, cross-sectional study. *Research Square (Research Square)*. DOI: 10.21203/rs.3.rs-33267/v1

King, D. L., & Delfabbro, P. H. (2019a). *Internet gaming disorder: Theory, assessment, treatment, and prevention*. Academic Press., DOI: 10.1016/C2017-0-02346-3

King, D. L., & Delfabbro, P. H. (2019b). Video game monetisation (e.g., 'loot boxes'): A blueprint for practical social responsibility measures. *International Journal of Mental Health and Addiction*, *17*(1), 166–179. DOI: 10.1007/s11469-018-0009-3

King, D. L., Delfabbro, P. H., Griffiths, M. D., & Gradisar, M. (2019). Cognitive-behavioural approaches to outpatient treatment of internet gaming disorder: A pilot study. *Journal of Clinical Psychology*, *73*(3), 301–309. DOI: 10.1002/jclp.22323

Király, O., Griffiths, M. D., King, D. L., Lee, H. K., Lee, S. Y., Bányai, F., Zsila, Á., Takács, Z. K., & Demetrovics, Z. (2020). Policy responses to problematic video game use: A systematic review of current measures and future possibilities. *Journal of Behavioral Addictions*, *9*(2), 257–271. DOI: 10.1556/2006.2020.00040 PMID: 28859487

Klaassen, M. J. E., & Peter, J. (2014). Gender (In)equality in internet pornography: A content analysis of popular pornographic internet videos. *Journal of Sex Research*, *52*(7), 721–735. DOI: 10.1080/00224499.2014.976781 PMID: 25420868

Kohut, T., Fisher, W. A., & Campbell, L. (2017). Perceived Effects of Pornography on the Couple Relationship: Initial Findings of Open-Ended, Participant-Informed, "Bottom-Up" Research. *Archives of Sexual Behavior*, *46*(2), 585–602. DOI: 10.1007/s10508-016-0783-6 PMID: 27393037

Kolhe, D., & Naik, A. R. (2025). Digital detox as a means to enhance eudaimonic well-being. *Frontiers in Human Dynamics*, *7*, 1572587. DOI: 10.3389/fhumd.2025.1572587

Koob, G. F., & Volkow, N. D. (2016). Neurobiology of addiction: A neurocircuitry analysis. *The Lancet. Psychiatry*, *3*(8), 760–773. DOI: 10.1016/S2215-0366(16)00104-8 PMID: 27475769

Koo, C. (2011). Internet-addicted South Korean children and government efforts. *Journal of the American Medical Association*, *306*(15), 1602–1603. DOI: 10.1001/jama.2011.1478

Kor, A., Zilcha-Mano, S., Fogel, Y. A., Mikulincer, M., Reid, R. C., & Potenza, M. N. (2014). Psychometric development of the Problematic Pornography Use Scale. *Addictive Behaviors*, *39*(5), 861–868. DOI: 10.1016/j.addbeh.2014.01.027 PMID: 24583276

Kowalewska, E., Gola, M., Kraus, S. W., & Lew-Starowicz, M. (2020). Spotlight on Compulsive Sexual Behavior Disorder: A Systematic Review of Research on Women. *Neuropsychiatric Disease and Treatment*, *16*, 2025–2043. DOI: 10.2147/NDT.S221540 PMID: 32943868

Kowalski, R. M., Giumetti, G. W., Schroeder, A. N., & Lattanner, M. R. (2014). Bullying in the digital age: A critical review and meta-analysis of cyberbullying research among youth. *Psychological Bulletin*, *140*(4), 1073–1137. DOI: 10.1037/a0035618 PMID: 24512111

Kowalski, R. M., Limber, S. P., & Agatston, P. W. (2012). *Cyberbullying: Bullying in the digital age* (2nd ed.). Wiley-Blackwell.

Kraus, S. W., Krueger, R. B., Briken, P., First, M. B., Stein, D. J., Kaplan, M. S., Voon, V., Abdo, C. H. N., Grant, J. E., Atalla, E., & Reed, G. M. (2018). Compulsive sexual behaviour disorder in the ICD-11. *World Psychiatry; Official Journal of the World Psychiatric Association (WPA)*, *17*(1), 109–110. DOI: 10.1002/wps.20499 PMID: 29352554

Kraus, S. W., & Sweeney, P. J. (2019). Hitting the Target: Considerations for Differential Diagnosis When Treating Individuals for Problematic Use of Pornography. *Archives of Sexual Behavior*, *48*(2), 431–435. DOI: 10.1007/s10508-018-1301-9 PMID: 30229519

Kraus, S. W., Voon, V., & Potenza, M. N. (2016). Should compulsive sexual behavior be considered an addiction? *Addiction (Abingdon, England)*, *111*(12), 2097–2106. DOI: 10.1111/add.13297 PMID: 26893127

Kübler-Ross, E. (1969). *On death and dying*. Macmillan.

Kuhn, C. M., Wilson, W., & Swartzwelder, S. (2013). Enduring effects of adolescent drug exposure. *Biological Psychiatry*, *74*(7), 480–481. DOI: 10.1016/j.biopsych.2013.07.030 PMID: 24034365

Kühn, S., & Gallinat, J. (2014). Brain structure and functional connectivity associated with pornography consumption: The brain on porn. *JAMA Psychiatry*, *71*(7), 827–834. DOI: 10.1001/jamapsychiatry.2014.93 PMID: 24871202

Kumar, S., & Saxena, G. (2021). Child online pornography: Criminal methods and investigation. In *Combating the exploitation of children in cyberspace: Emerging research and opportunities* (pp. 117–145). IGI Global., DOI: 10.4018/978-1-7998-2360-5.ch006

Kuss, D. J., & Griffiths, M. D. (2017). Social networking sites and addiction: Ten lessons learned. *International Journal of Environmental Research and Public Health, 14*(3), 311. DOI: 10.3390/ijerph14030311 PMID: 28304359

Kuss, D. J., Griffiths, M. D., Karila, L., & Billieux, J. (2014). Internet addiction: A systematic review of epidemiological research for the last decade. *Current Pharmaceutical Design, 20*(25), 4026–4052. DOI: 10.2174/13816128113199990617 PMID: 24001297

Kuss, D. J., & Lopez-Fernandez, O. (2016). Internet addiction and problematic Internet use: A systematic review of clinical research. *World Journal of Psychiatry, 6*(1), 143–176. DOI: 10.5498/wjp.v6.i1.143 PMID: 27014605

Kwan, I., Dickson, K., Richardson, M., MacDowall, W., Burchett, H., & Stansfield, C. (2020). Cyberbullying and mental health: A systematic review. *The Journal of Adolescent Health : Official Publication of the Society for Adolescent Medicine, 66*(3), 231–242.

LaFata, E., Allison, K., Audrain-McGovern, J., & Forman, E. (2024). Ultra-Processed Food Addiction: A Research Update. *13(2)*, 214-223. Springer Science+Business Media. DOI: 10.1007/s13679-024-00569-w

LaFata, E., & Gearhardt, A. (2022). Ultra-Processed Food Addiction: An Epidemic? *Psychotherapy and Psychosomatics, 91*(6), 363–372. DOI: 10.1159/000527322 PMID: 36349805

Laier, C., Schulte, F. P., & Brand, M. (2013). Pornographic picture processing interferes with working memory performance. *Journal of Sex Research, 50*(7), 642–652. DOI: 10.1080/00224499.2012.716873 PMID: 23167900

Lakhan, S. (2025). Hijacked by the Feed: Social Media Neuroengineering-Induced Digital Anhedonia. *Cureus, 17*(4). Advance online publication. DOI: 10.7759/cureus.83256 PMID: 40309512

Landripet, I., & Štulhofer, A. (2021). Pornography use and sexual satisfaction: The role of sexual socialization. In Maggino, F. (Ed.), *Encyclopedia of quality of life and well-being research.* Springer., DOI: 10.1007/978-3-319-69909-7_4145-2

Layden, M. A. (2021). Pornified: Pornography's connection to long-term damage and violence. In Caffo, E. (Ed.), *Online child sexual exploitation: Treatment and prevention of abuse in a digital world* (pp. 57–74). Springer Nature Switzerland AG., DOI: 10.1007/978-3-030-66654-5_6

Lee, S., Yoon, J., Cho, Y., & Chun, J. (2024). A systematic review of chatbot-assisted interventions for substance use. *Frontiers in Psychiatry*, *15*, 1456689. DOI: 10.3389/fpsyt.2024.1456689 PMID: 39319358

Lemos, T., Coutinho, G., Silva, L., Stariolo, J., Campagnoli, R., Oliveira, L., Pereira, M. G., Mota, B. E. F., Souza, G. G. L., Canella, D. S., Khandpur, N., & David, I. (2022). Ultra-Processed Foods Elicit Higher Approach Motivation Than Unprocessed and Minimally Processed Foods. *Frontiers in Public Health*, *10*, 891546–891546. DOI: 10.3389/fpubh.2022.891546 PMID: 35801235

Leung, A. N. M., Wong, N., & Farver, J. M. (2018). Cyberbullying in Hong Kong Chinese students: Life satisfaction, and the moderating role of friendship qualities on cyberbullying victimisation and perpetration. *Personality and Individual Differences*, *133*, 7–12. DOI: 10.1016/j.paid.2017.07.016

Lewczuk, K., Wizła, M., Glica, A., & Dwulit, A. D. (2024). Compulsive Sexual Behavior Disorder and Problematic Pornography Use in Cisgender Sexual Minority Individuals: The Associations with Minority Stress, Social Support, and Sexualized Drug Use. *Journal of Sex Research*, *61*(8), 1246–1260. DOI: 10.1080/00224499.2023.2245399 PMID: 37676791

Li, H., Wang, S., & Zhu, C. (2016). Effectiveness of a group-based cognitive behavioural therapy program for internet addiction among adolescents. *Addictive Behaviors*, *55*, 65–71. DOI: 10.1016/j.addbeh.2016.01.010

Linardon, J. (2020). Can Acceptance, Mindfulness, and Self-Compassion Be Learned by Smartphone Apps? A Systematic and Meta-Analytic Review of Randomized Controlled Trials. *Behavior Therapy*, *51*(4), 646–658. DOI: 10.1016/j.beth.2019.10.002 PMID: 32586436

Linardon, J., & Fuller-Tyszkiewicz, M. (2020). Attrition and adherence in smartphone-delivered interventions for mental health problems: A systematic and meta-analytic review. *Journal of Consulting and Clinical Psychology*, *88*(1), 1–13. DOI: 10.1037/ccp0000459 PMID: 31697093

Lin, C. Y., Broström, A., Nilsen, P., Griffiths, M. D., & Pakpour, A. H. (2017). Psychometric validation of the Persian Bergen Social Media Addiction Scale using classic test theory and Rasch models. *Journal of Behavioral Addictions*, *6*(4), 620–629. DOI: 10.1556/2006.6.2017.071 PMID: 29130330

Lin, C.-Y., Imani, V., Griffiths, M., & Pakpour, A. (2020). Validity of the Yale Food Addiction Scale for Children (YFAS-C): Classical test theory and item response theory of the Persian YFAS-C. *Eating and Weight Disorders : EWD*, *26*(5), 1457–1466. DOI: 10.1007/s40519-020-00956-x PMID: 32676845

Lin, Y.-H., Chiang, C., Lin, P.-H., Chang, L.-R., Ko, C.-H., Lee, Y.-H., & Lin, S.-H. (2016). Proposed Diagnostic Criteria for Smartphone Addiction. *PLoS One*, *11*(11), e0163010. Advance online publication. DOI: 10.1371/journal.pone.0163010 PMID: 27846211

Lister, C., West, J. H., Cannon, B., Sax, T., & Brodegard, D. (2014). Just a fad? Gamification in health and fitness apps. *JMIR Serious Games*, *2*(2), e9. DOI: 10.2196/games.3413 PMID: 25654660

Liu, J., & Ellis, D. (2021). Editorial: Eating in the Age of Smartphones: The Good, the Bad, and the Neutral. *Frontiers in Psychology*, *12*, 796899. Advance online publication. DOI: 10.3389/fpsyg.2021.796899 PMID: 34938246

Liu, Y., Li, L., Wang, Y., Ghahremani, D., Chen, J., Okita, K., Guo, W., & Liao, Y. (2021). Editorial: Neurobiological Biomarkers for Developing Novel Treatments of Substance and Non-substance Addiction. *Frontiers in Psychiatry*, *12*, 811032. Advance online publication. DOI: 10.3389/fpsyt.2021.811032 PMID: 34987436

Livingstone, S., Stoilova, M., & Nandagiri, R. (2019). Children's data and privacy online: Growing up in a digital age. An Evidence Review. London School of Economics. https://www.lse.ac.uk/media-and-communications

Livingstone, S., & Helsper, E. (2010). Balancing opportunities and risks in teenagers' use of the Internet. *New Media & Society*, *12*(2), 309–329. DOI: 10.1177/1461444809342697

Li, W. (2023). Gender stereotyping in media - Bias and discrimination. *Lecture Notes in Education Psychology and Public Media*, *29*(1), 237–241. DOI: 10.54254/2753-7048/29/20231518

Li, X., Wang, P., & Liu, H. (2022). Regulatory strategies for online gaming and digital addiction prevention in China. *Policy and Internet*, *14*(3), 711–732. DOI: 10.1002/poi3.315

Li, Y., & Wang, X. (2025). The relationship between fear of missing out and problematic social media use: A moderated mediation model. *Scientific Reports*, *15*, 2468.

Lochner, C., van den Berg, G., Chamberlain, S. R., Marincowitz, C., & Coetzee, B. (2024). Family functioning and problematic usage of the internet in youth: A cross-sectional investigation. *Journal of Psychiatric Research, 173*, 239–244. DOI: 10.1016/j.jpsychires.2024.03.038 PMID: 38554619

Lopez-Fernandez, O. (2020). Considering existing classic and contemporary proposals for preventing online addiction problems: Some old recipes for new problems. *Journal of Behavioral Addictions*, *9*(4), 903–907. DOI: 10.1556/2006.2020.00084 PMID: 33242026

Love, T., Laier, C., Brand, M., Hatch, L., & Hajela, R. (2015). Neuroscience of Internet Pornography Addiction: A Review and Update. *Behavioral Sciences (Basel, Switzerland)*, *5*(3), 388–433. DOI: 10.3390/bs5030388 PMID: 26393658

Luo, T., Wang, M., & Wu, L. (2025). Fear of missing out and problematic social media use: A moderated mediation model of social comparison and self-control. *International Journal of Mental Health and Addiction*, *23*(1).

Lustig, R. (2020). Ultraprocessed Food: Addictive, Toxic, and Ready for Regulation. *Nutrients*, *12*(11), 3401–3401. DOI: 10.3390/nu12113401 PMID: 33167515

Lu, Z. (2025). Mapping adolescent problematic social media use patterns across 41 countries/regions: A multilevel latent class analysis with social determinants. *Addictive Behaviors*, *172*, 108523. DOI: 10.1016/j.addbeh.2025.108523 PMID: 41110245

Maas, M. K., Wright, P. J., Rothman, E. F., Nelson, K. M., Weigle, P., & Herbenick, D. (2025). Pornography use during adolescence: The current state of knowledge and recommendations. In Christakis, D. A., & Hale, L. (Eds.), *Handbook of children and screens* (pp. 341–347). Springer., DOI: 10.1007/978-3-031-69362-5_47

Mabonga, B. (2024). *Impact of social media use (Instagram) on body image and self-esteem: The role of social comparison and FOMO* [Tesis Master, Bournemouth University]. Bournemouth University Institutional Repository. https://eprints.bournemouth.ac.id/40501/

Ma, C., Wang, Z., Li, C., Lu, J., Long, J., Li, R., Wu, Q., Jiang, H., Du, J., Li, R., Wang, P., Ma, L., Li, H., Hui, S., Zhao, W., Zhong, N., & Zhao, M. (2021). The clinical consistency and utility of ICD-11 diagnostic guidelines for gaming disorder: A field study among the Chinese population. *Frontiers in Psychiatry*, *12*, 781992. DOI: 10.3389/fpsyt.2021.781992 PMID: 35002801

MacIntyre, C. R., Chen, X., Kunasekaran, M., Quigley, A., Lim, S., Stone, H., & Gurdasani, D. (2023). Artificial intelligence in public health. *The Journal of International Medical Research, 51*(3), 03000605231159335. DOI: 10.1177/03000605231159335 PMID: 36967669

Madsen, K. R., Damsgaard, M. T., Petersen, K. J., Qualter, P., & Holstein, B. E. (2024). Bullying at school, cyberbullying, and loneliness: National representative study of adolescents in Denmark. *International Journal of Environmental Research and Public Health, 21*(4), 414. DOI: 10.3390/ijerph21040414 PMID: 38673326

Maes, C., Vandenbosch, L., & Wright, P. J. (2024). The impact of online pornography consumption on youth. In Rich, G. J., Kumar, V. K., & Farley, F. H. (Eds.), *Handbook of media psychology: The science and the practice* (pp. 101–111). Springer Nature Switzerland AG., DOI: 10.1007/978-3-031-56537-3_8

Magis-Weinberg, L., Suleiman, A. B., & Dahl, R. E. (2021). Context, development, and digital media: Implications for very young adolescents in LMICs. *Frontiers in Psychology, 12*, 632713. DOI: 10.3389/fpsyg.2021.632713 PMID: 33967899

Maksi, S., Keller, K., Dardis, F., Vecchi, M., Freeman, J., Evans, R., Boyland, E., & Masterson, T. (2024). The food and beverage cues in digital marketing model: Special considerations of social media, gaming, and livestreaming environments for food marketing and eating behavior research. *Frontiers in Nutrition, 10*, 1325265. Advance online publication. DOI: 10.3389/fnut.2023.1325265 PMID: 38384857

Maldonado-Devincci, A. M., Badanich, K. A., & Kirstein, C. L. (2010). Alcohol during adolescence selectively alters immediate and long-term behavior and neurochemistry. *Alcohol (Fayetteville, N.Y.), 44*(1), 57–66. DOI: 10.1016/j.alcohol.2009.09.035 PMID: 20113874

Mancini, C., Reckdenwald, A., & Beauregard, E. (2012). Pornographic exposure over the life course and the severity of sexual offenses: Imitation and cathartic effects. *Journal of Criminal Justice, 40*(1), 21–30. DOI: 10.1016/j.jcrimjus.2011.11.004

Maqsood, S., Ahmed, F., Arshad, M., Ikram, A., & Abdullahi, M. (2025). Comparative Analysis of Food Addiction and Obesity. *Critical Reviews in Food Science and Nutrition, 13*(8), e70799. Advance online publication. DOI: 10.1002/fsn3.70799 PMID: 40822524

Marchetti, I. (2023). The Structure of Compulsive Sexual Behavior: A Network Analysis Study. *Archives of Sexual Behavior, 52*(3), 1271–1284. DOI: 10.1007/s10508-023-02549-y PMID: 36735169

Marciano, L., Camerini, A.-L., & Morese, R. (2021). *The Developing Brain in the Digital Era: A Scoping Review of Structural and Functional Correlates of Screen Time in Adolescence. 12*. Frontiers Media., DOI: 10.3389/fpsyg.2021.671817

Marciano, L., Schulz, P. J., & Camerini, A.-L. (2020). Cyberbullying perpetration and victimization in youth: A meta-analysis of longitudinal studies. *Journal of Computer-Mediated Communication, 25*(2), 163–181. DOI: 10.1093/jcmc/zmz031

Marinucci, M., Pancani, L., Aureli, N., & Riva, P. (2022). Online social connections as surrogates of face-to-face interactions. *Computers in Human Behavior, 128*, 107102. DOI: 10.1016/j.chb.2021.107102

Martin, K., Shilton, K., & Smith, J. (2019). Business and the Ethical Implications of Technology: Introduction to the Symposium. *Journal of Business Ethics, 160*(2), 307–317. DOI: 10.1007/s10551-019-04213-9

Masri-Zada, T., Martirosyan, S., Abdou, A., Barbar, R., Kades, S., Makki, H., . . . Agrawal, D. (2025). The Impact of Social Media & Technology on Child and Adolescent Mental Health. *PubMed, 9*(2), 111-130. https://pubmed.ncbi.nlm.nih.gov/40520349 adresinden alındı

Massey, K., Burns, J., & Franz, A. (2020). Young people, sexuality and the age of pornography. *Sexuality & Culture, 25*(1), 318–336. DOI: 10.1007/s12119-020-09771-z

Mastrobattista, L., Pérez, L., Gallimberti, L., Genetti, B., Andreotti, A., Fassinato, D., & Mortali, C. (2024). Psychosocial risk and protective factors for youth problem behavior are associated with food addiction in the Generation Z. *Frontiers in Public Health, 12*, 1414110. Advance online publication. DOI: 10.3389/fpubh.2024.1414110 PMID: 38859893

Mattuck, R., Blanchet, R., & Wait, A. D. (2005). Data representativeness for risk assessment. *Environmental Forensics, 6*(1), 65–70. DOI: 10.1080/15275920590913886

Maurya, C., Muhammad, T., Dhillon, P., & Maurya, P. (2022). The effects of cyberbullying victimization on depression and suicidal ideation among adolescents and young adults: A three- year cohort study from India. *BMC Psychiatry, 22*(1), 599. Advance online publication. DOI: 10.1186/s12888-022-04238-x PMID: 36085004

Maza, M., Fox, K., Kwon, S.-J., Flannery, J., Lindquist, K., Prinstein, M., & Telzer, E. (2023). Association of Habitual Checking Behaviors on Social Media With Longitudinal Functional Brain Development. *JAMA Pediatrics, 177*(2), 160–160. DOI: 10.1001/jamapediatrics.2022.4924 PMID: 36595277

McArthur, J., Stewart, S., & Al-Hamdani, M. (2024). Vaping frequency in young users: The role of gender and age among regular users. *Substance Use & Misuse, 59*(12), 1778–1784. DOI: 10.1080/10826084.2024.2374975 PMID: 39028136

McCausland, H., Gearhardt, A., Peralta, J., & LaFata, E. (2025). A Critical Evaluation of the Terms Used To Describe Foods Implicated in Addictive-Like Eating. *Current Addiction Reports, 12*(1), 71. Advance online publication. DOI: 10.1007/s40429-025-00689-w

McGloin, A., & Eslami, S. (2014). *Digital and social media opportunities for dietary behaviour change. 74(2), 139-148.* Cambridge University Press., DOI: 10.1017/S0029665114001505

McGlynn, C., & Rackley, E. (2017). Image-based sexual abuse. *Oxford Journal of Legal Studies, 37*(3), 534–561. DOI: 10.1093/ojls/gqw033

McLeroy, K. R., Bibeau, D., Steckler, A., & Glanz, K. (1988). An ecological perspective on health promotion programs. *Health Education Quarterly, 15*(4), 351–377. DOI: 10.1177/109019818801500401 PMID: 3068205

Méndez, M., Padrón, I., Fumero, A., & Marrero, R. (2024). Effects of internet and smartphone addiction on cognitive control in adolescents and young adults: A systematic review of fMRI studies. *Neuroscience and Biobehavioral Reviews, 159*, 105572–105572. DOI: 10.1016/j.neubiorev.2024.105572 PMID: 38320657

Meng, S. Q., Dong, F. L., & Wang, Z. L.. (2022). Global prevalence of digital addiction in the general population: A systematic review and meta-analysis. *Journal of Behavioral Addictions, 11*(2), 345–360. DOI: 10.1556/2006.2022.00032 PMID: 35150965

Merdeka.com. (2022). *Mahasiswa Unhas bunuh diri karena tugas, Dekan: Tidak ada hubungannya* [Unhas student commits suicide due to assignments, Dean: No connection]. https://www.merdeka.com/peristiwa/mahasiswa-unhas-gantung-diri-diduga-karena-tugas-kuliah-dekan-tidak-ada-hubungannya.html

Meule, A., & Gearhardt, A. (2014). Food Addiction in the Light of DSM-5. *Nutrients, 6*(9), 3653–3671. DOI: 10.3390/nu6093653 PMID: 25230209

Miller, W. R., & Rollnick, S. (2013). *Motivational interviewing: Helping people change* (4th ed.). Guilford Press.

Minkler, M., & Wallerstein, N. (2008). *Community-based participatory research for health: From process to outcomes* (2nd ed.). Jossey-Bass.

Moghimi, E., Davis, C., Bonder, R., Knyahnytska, Y., & Quilty, L. (2021). Exploring women's experiences of treatment for binge eating disorder: Methylphenidate vs. cognitive behavioural therapy. *Progress in Neuro-Psychopharmacology & Biological Psychiatry, 114*, 110492–110492. DOI: 10.1016/j.pnpbp.2021.110492 PMID: 34863926

Mohamed, S. M., Hamed, N. A., & Fahmy, A. M. (2022). Effect of digital detox program on electronic screen syndrome among preparatory school students. *Journal of Nursing Education and Practice, 12*(4), 20–30. DOI: 10.5430/jnep.v12n4p20 PMID: 36373487

Molle, R., Fatemi, H., Dagher, A., Levitan, R., Silveira, P., & Dubé, L. (2016). *Gene and environment interaction: Is the differential susceptibility hypothesis relevant for obesity? 73, 326-339*. Elsevier BV., DOI: 10.1016/j.neubiorev.2016.12.028

Monacis, L., Palo, V., Griffiths, M. D., & Sinatra, M. (2016). Validation of the Internet Gaming Disorder Scale - Short-Form (IGDS9-SF) in an Italian-speaking sample. *Journal of Behavioral Addictions, 5*(4), 683–690. DOI: 10.1556/2006.5.2016.083 PMID: 27876422

Montag, C., Lachmann, B., Herrlich, M., & Zweig, K. (2019). Addictive features of social media/messenger platforms and freemium games against the background of psychological and economic theories. *International Journal of Environmental Research and Public Health, 16*(14), 2612. DOI: 10.3390/ijerph16142612 PMID: 31340426

Montag, C., & Walla, P. (2016). Carpe diem instead of losing your social mind: Beyond digital addiction and why we all suffer from digital overuse. *Cogent Psychology, 3*(1), 1157281. DOI: 10.1080/23311908.2016.1157281

Montag, C., Wegmann, E., Sariyska, R., Demetrovics, Z., & Brand, M. (2021). How to overcome taxonomical problems in the study of Internet use disorders and what to do with "smartphone addiction"? *Journal of Behavioral Addictions, 10*(1), 1–7. DOI: 10.1556/2006.8.2019.59 PMID: 31668089

Moreno, M. A., & Radesky, J. S. (2024). Benefits and harms of proposed social media legislation. *JAMA Pediatrics, 178*(9), 857. DOI: 10.1001/jamapediatrics.2024.2380 PMID: 39037793

Moreno, M., Riddle, K., Jenkins, M. C., Singh, A. P., Zhao, Q., & Eickhoff, J. (2022). Measuring problematic internet use. *JMIR Public Health and Surveillance, 8*(1), e27719. DOI: 10.2196/27719 PMID: 34081596

Moreno-Padilla, M., Alacreu-Crespo, A., Guillaume, S., & Paso, G. (2022). The outcome-representation learning model: Impairments in decision-making in adolescents with excess weight. *Current Psychology*, *42*(26), 22404–22414. DOI: 10.1007/s12144-022-03299-1

Morgan, C., & Klein, C. (2024). How online data informs forensic mental health evaluations of sexual behavior: An overview. *Behavioral Sciences & the Law*, *42*(3), 186–204. DOI: 10.1002/bsl.2650 PMID: 38459739

Morin, J.-P., Rodríguez-Durán, L., Guzmán-Ramos, K., Perez-Cruz, C., Ferreira, G., Díaz-Cintra, S., & Pacheco-López, G. (2017). *Palatable Hyper-Caloric Foods Impact on Neuronal Plasticity. 11*. Frontiers Media., DOI: 10.3389/fnbeh.2017.00019

Mortier, P., Auerbach, R. P., Alonso, J., Bantjes, J., Benjet, C., Cuijpers, P., Ebert, D. D., Green, J. G., Hasking, P., Nock, M. K., O'Neill, S., Pinder-Amaker, S., Sampson, N. A., Vilagut, G., Zaslavsky, A. M., Bruffaerts, R., Kessler, R. C., Boyes, M., Kiekens, G., & Vives, M.WHO WMH-ICS Collaborators. (2018). Suicidal thoughts and behaviors among first-year college students: Results from the WMH-ICS project. *Journal of the American Academy of Child and Adolescent Psychiatry*, *57*(4), 263–273. DOI: 10.1016/j.jaac.2018.01.018 PMID: 29588052

Mujica, A., Crowell, C., Villano, M., & Uddin, K. (2022). ADDICTION BY DESIGN: Some Dimensions and Challenges of Excessive Social Media Use. *Medical Research Archives*, *10*(2). Advance online publication. DOI: 10.18103/mra.v10i2.2677

Müller, K. W., Janikian, M., Dreier, M., Wölfling, K., Beutel, M. E., Tzavara, C., Richardson, C., & Tsitsika, A.Cross-national Epidemiology of Problematic Internet Use Study Group. (2015). Regular gaming behaviour and internet gaming disorder in European adolescents: Results from a cross-national representative survey of prevalence, predictors, and psychopathological correlates. *European Child & Adolescent Psychiatry*, *24*(5), 565–574. DOI: 10.1007/s00787-014-0611-2 PMID: 25189795

Mullis, M. D. (2022). Parent-child communication about sex. *The International Encyclopedia of Health Communication*, 1-4. https://doi.org/DOI: 10.1002/9781119678816.iehc0887

Ndayambaje, E., & Okereke, P. U. (2025). The Psychopathology of Problematic Smartphone Use (PSU): A Narrative Review of Burden, Mediating Factors, and Prevention. *Health Science Reports*, *8*(5), e70843. DOI: 10.1002/hsr2.70843 PMID: 40415982

Nesi, J. (2022). The facts about pornography use in teens. *Brown University Child and Adolescent Behavior Letter*, *38*(12), 8. DOI: 10.1002/cbl.30677

Nesi, J., Subrahmanyam, K., Valkenburg, P., Morita, H., Ehrenreich, S., Chiu, M., & Weinstein, E. (2022). *Handbook of Adolescent Digital Media Use and Mental Health*. Cambridge University Press., DOI: 10.1017/9781108976237

Ng, W. (2015). Learners in a digital society: Digital practices of young people and their teaching implications. In *New digital technology in education* (pp. 51–71). Springer., DOI: 10.1007/978-3-319-05822-1_3

Nikken, P., & Schols, M. (2015). How and why parents guide the media use of young children. *Journal of Child and Family Studies*, *24*(11), 3423–3435. DOI: 10.1007/s10826-015-0144-4 PMID: 26472932

Núñez-Rodríguez, S., Burgos-González, D., Mínguez-Mínguez, L. A., Menéndez-Vega, F., Antoñanzas-Laborda, J. L., González-Bernal, J. J., & González-Santos, J. (2025). Effectiveness of therapeutic interventions in the treatment of internet gaming disorder: A systematic review. *European Journal of Investigation in Health, Psychology and Education*, *15*(4), 49. DOI: 10.3390/ejihpe15040049 PMID: 40277866

Odgers, C. L., & Jensen, M. R. (2020). Annual research review: Adolescent mental health in the digital age. *Journal of Child Psychology and Psychiatry, and Allied Disciplines*, *61*(3), 336–348. DOI: 10.1111/jcpp.13190 PMID: 31951670

Odgers, C. L., Schueller, S. M., & Ito, M. (2020). Screen time, social media use, and adolescent development. *Annual Review of Developmental Psychology*, *2*(1), 485–502. DOI: 10.1146/annurev-devpsych-121318-084815

Odlaug, B. L., Lust, K., Schreiber, L. R., Christenson, G., Derbyshire, K., Harvanko, A., Golden, D., & Grant, J. E. (2013). Compulsive sexual behavior in young adults. *Annals of Clinical Psychiatry*, *25*(3), 193–200. DOI: 10.1177/104012371302500305 PMID: 23926574

OECD. (2021). *21st-century readers: Developing literacy skills in a digital world.* OECD Publishing. https://www.oecd.org/content/dam/oecd/en/publications/reports/2021/05/21st-century-readers_26f2b462/a83d84cb-en.pdf

Office of the Surgeon General (OSG). (2023). *Social Media and Youth Mental Health: The U.S. Surgeon General's Advisory*. US Department of Health and Human Services. https://www.hhs.gov/sites/default/files/sg-youth-mental-health-social-media-advisory.pdf

Ojala, M. (2022). How do young people deal with border tensions when making climate-friendly food choices? On the importance of critical emotional awareness for learning for social change. *Climate (Basel)*, *10*(1), 8. DOI: 10.3390/cli10010008

Ong, R. H. S., Sim, H. S., Bergman, M. M., How, C. H., Png, C. A. L., Lim, C. S., Peh, L. H., & Oh, H. C. (2024). Prevalence and associations of problematic smartphone use with smartphone activities, psychological well-being, and sleep quality in a household survey of Singapore adults. *PLoS One*, *19*(12), e0315364. DOI: 10.1371/journal.pone.0315364 PMID: 39693321

Openshaw, L. L. (2011). School-based support groups for traumatized students. *School Psychology International*, *32*(2), 163–178. DOI: 10.1177/0143034311400830

Ophir, Y., Rosenberg, H., Lipshits-Braziler, Y., & Amichai-Hamburger, Y. (2020). "Digital adolescence": The effects of smartphones and social networking technologies on adolescents' well-being. In N. Van Zalk & C. P. Monks (Eds.), *Online peer engagement in adolescence: Positive and negative aspects of online social interaction* (pp. 122-139). Routledge/Taylor & Francis Group. https://doi.org/DOI: 10.4324/9780429468360-8

Organisation for Economic Co-operation and Development. (2025). Children in the digital environment. OECD. https://www.oecd.org/en/topics/children-in-the-digital-environment.html

Paasonen, S. (2011). Revisiting cyberfeminism. *Communications*, *36*(3), 335–352. DOI: 10.1515/comm.2011.017

Pala, S. Ç., Ünsal, A., Emiral, G. Ö., & Demirtaş, Z.. (2021). Cyberbullying and multidimensional perceived social support among high school students in Turkey. *Journal of Istanbul Faculty of Medicine*, *84*(1), 104–112. DOI: 10.26650/IUITFD.2019.0106

Palazzolo, F. (2023). Internet pornography use disorder: In search of a non-pathologizing description of an evolving clinical issue. *Sexual Health & Compulsivity*, *30*(4), 328–341. DOI: 10.1080/26929953.2023.2254785

Panagiotidi, M., & Overton, P. G. (2018). The relationship between internet addiction, attention deficit hyperactivity disorder symptoms and online activities. *Comprehensive Psychiatry*, *87*, 7–11. DOI: 10.1016/j.comppsych.2018.08.004 PMID: 30176388

Paquette, M. M., Bergeron, S., Bigras, N., Koós, M., Nagy, L., Kraus, S. W., Demetrovics, Z., Potenza, M. N., Ballester-Arnal, R., Batthyány, D., Billieux, J., Briken, P., Burkauskas, J., Cárdenas-López, G., Carvalho, J., Castro-Calvo, J., Chen, L., Ciocca, G., Corazza, O., & Bőthe, B. (2025). Sexual satisfaction across cultures, genders, languages, and sexual orientations: Validation of the Global Measure of Sexual Satisfaction. *Psychology of Sexual Orientation and Gender Diversity*. Advance online publication. DOI: 10.1037/sgd0000774

Parasuraman, S., Sam, A. T., Yee, S. W. K., Chuon, B. L. C., & Ren, L. Y. (2017). Smartphone usage and increased risk of mobile phone addiction: A concurrent study. *International Journal of Pharmaceutical Investigation*, *7*(3), 125. https://pmc.ncbi.nlm.nih.gov/articles/PMC5680647/. DOI: 10.4103/jphi.JPHI_56_17 PMID: 29184824

Pardhan, S., Parkin, J., Trott, M., & Driscoll, R. (2022). Risks of digital screen time in children and adolescents. *The Journal of School Health*, *92*(8), 765–773. DOI: 10.1111/josh.13170 PMID: 35253225

Park, B. Y., Wilson, G., Berger, J., Christman, M., Reina, B., Bishop, F., Klam, W. P., & Doan, A. P. (2016). Is Internet pornography causing sexual dysfunctions? A review with clinical reports. *Behavioral Sciences (Basel, Switzerland)*, *6*(3), 17. DOI: 10.3390/bs6030017 PMID: 27527226

Park, S., Kim, Y., & Cho, M. J. (2018). Prevalence of internet addiction and correlations with family factors among South Korean adolescents. *Adolescence*, *53*(209), 469–478. DOI: 10.1080/01494929.2018.1440619 PMID: 19149152

Park, S., Lee, J. Y., Kim, J., & Han, D. H. (2022). Virtual reality-based intervention for gaming disorder: A randomised controlled trial. *Frontiers in Psychiatry*, *13*, 837497. DOI: 10.3389/fpsyt.2022.837497

Pasquale, L., Zippo, P., Curley, C., O'Neill, B., & Mongiello, M. (2020). Digital age of Consent and age verification: Can they protect children? *IEEE Software*, *39*(3), 50–57. DOI: 10.1109/MS.2020.3044872

Patel, D. G., Kshatri, A. H. S., Kommuru, S., & Javvaji, C. K. (2025). A narrative review of digital addiction and health. *Cureus*, *17*(12). PMID: 41625856

Patel, D., Kshatri, A., Kommuru, S., & Javvaji, C. (2025). A Narrative Review of Digital Addiction and Health: A New Challenge for Modern Medicine. *Cureus*, *17*(12). Advance online publication. DOI: 10.7759/cureus.100491 PMID: 41625856

Paterna, A., Alcaraz-Ibáñez, M., Aguilar-Parra, J. M., Salavera, C., Demetrovics, Z., & Griffiths, M. D. (2024). Problematic smartphone use and academic achievement: A systematic review and meta-analysis. *Journal of Behavioral Addictions*, *13*(2), 313–326. DOI: 10.1556/2006.2024.00014 PMID: 38669081

Patwardhan, V., Mallya, J., Kaliappan, S., & Kumar, D. (2024). Influence of social media on young adults' food consumption behavior: Scale development. *Cogent Social Sciences*, *10*(1), 2391016. Advance online publication. DOI: 10.1080/23311886.2024.2391016

Paul, M., Maglaras, L., Ferrag, M. A., & Almomani, I. (2023). Digitization of healthcare sector: A study on privacy and security concerns. *ICT Express*, *9*(4), 571–588. DOI: 10.1016/j.icte.2023.02.007

Paulus, F. W., Nouri, F., Ohmann, S., Möhler, E., & Popow, C. (2024). The impact of internet pornography on children and adolescents: A systematic review. *L'Encéphale*, *50*(6), 649–662. DOI: 10.1016/j.encep.2023.12.004 PMID: 38519310

Paulus, F. W., Ohmann, S., von Gontard, A., & Popow, C. (2018). Internet gaming disorder in children and adolescents: A systematic review. *Developmental Medicine and Child Neurology*, *60*(7), 645–659. DOI: 10.1111/dmcn.13754 PMID: 29633243

Peñafiel Mora, V. F., Granda, M. F., & Parra, O. (2025). Technology-based interventions to address internet addictive behaviors: Systematic review. *Discover Mental Health*, *5*(1), 167. DOI: 10.1007/s44192-025-00187-5 PMID: 41171525

Peng, P., Chen, Z., Ren, S., Liu, Y., He, R., Liang, Y., Tan, Y., Tang, J., Chen, X., & Liao, Y. (2023). Determination of the cutoff point for Smartphone Application-Based Addiction Scale for adolescents: A latent profile analysis. *BMC Psychiatry*, *23*(1), 675. DOI: 10.1186/s12888-023-05170-4 PMID: 37716941

Peng, Z., Jia, Q., Mao, J., Luo, X., Huang, A., Zheng, H., Jiang, S., Ma, Q., Ma, C., & Yi, Q. (2025). Neurotransmitters crosstalk and regulation in the reward circuit of subjects with behavioral addiction. *Frontiers in Psychiatry*, *15*, 1439727. DOI: 10.3389/fpsyt.2024.1439727 PMID: 39876994

Peris, C., Pastor, J., & Martinez, V. (2020). Virtual reality in clinical psychology: Applications and possibilities. *Anales de Psicología*, *36*(1), 1–13. DOI: 10.6018/analesps.337791

Perlman, D., & Peplau, L. A. (1982). Theoretical approaches to loneliness. In Peplau, L. A., & Perlman, D. (Eds.), *Loneliness: A sourcebook of current theory, research and therapy* (pp. 123–134). Wiley-Interscience.

Peter, J., & Valkenburg, P. M. (2016). Adolescents and Pornography: A Review of 20 Years of Research. *Journal of Sex Research*, *53*(4-5), 509–531. DOI: 10.1080/00224499.2016.1143441 PMID: 27105446

Petry, N. M., Rehbein, F., Ko, C. H., & O'Brien, C. P. (2018). Internet gaming disorder in the DSM-5. *Current Psychiatry Reports*, *20*(2), 8. DOI: 10.1007/s11920-018-0877-6 PMID: 29504045

Pew Research Center. (2022). *Teens, social media and technology 2022*. Pew Research Center.

Potenza, M. N. (2018). Pornography in the current digital technology environment: An overview of a special issue on pornography. *Sexual Addiction & Compulsivity, 25*(4), 241–247. DOI: 10.1080/10720162.2019.1567411

Powell, A., & Henry, N. (2014). Blurred Lines? Responding to 'Sexting' and Gender-based Violence among Young People. *Children Australia, 39*(2), 119–124. DOI: 10.1017/cha.2014.9

Prasad, S., & Kumar, R. (2025). *From detection to detox: A hybrid model of machine learning and bibliotherapy in digital dementia care*. ResearchGate.

Prause, N. (2019). Porn is for masturbation. *Archives of Sexual Behavior, 48*(8), 2271–2277. DOI: 10.1007/s10508-019-1397-6 PMID: 30847758

Pretlow, R., Stock, C., Allison, S., & Roeger, L. (2015). Treatment of Child/Adolescent Obesity Using the Addiction Model: A Smartphone App Pilot Study. *Childhood Obesity, 11*(3), 248–259. DOI: 10.1089/chi.2014.0124 PMID: 25760813

Privara, M., & Bob, P. (2023). Pornography consumption and cognitive-affective distress. *The Journal of Nervous and Mental Disease, 211*(8), 641–646. DOI: 10.1097/NMD.0000000000001669 PMID: 37505898

Przybylski, A. K., Murayama, K., DeHaan, C. R., & Gladwell, V. (2013). Motivational, emotional, and behavioral correlates of fear of missing out. *Computers in Human Behavior, 29*(4), 1841–1848. DOI: 10.1016/j.chb.2013.02.014

Przybylski, A. K., & Nash, V. (2018). Internet filtering and adolescent exposure to online sexual material. *Cyberpsychology, Behavior and Social Networking, 21*(7), 405–410. DOI: 10.1089/cyber.2017.0466 PMID: 29995533

Pursey, K., Yokum, S., Brain, K., & Burrows, T. (2024). Neural Responses in Addictive Eating: a Systematic Review. *11(2)*, 173-190. Springer Science+Business Media. DOI: 10.1007/s40429-023-00538-8

Pursey, K., Babicola, L., Ventura, R., & Segni, M. (2024). Editorial: Dysfunctional motivation in eating behaviors: a complex gene x environment interplay. *Frontiers in Behavioral Neuroscience, 18*, 1367256. Advance online publication. DOI: 10.3389/fnbeh.2024.1367256 PMID: 38405038

Qualter, P., Vanhalst, J., Harris, R., Van Roekel, E., Lodder, G., Bangee, M., Maes, M., & Verhagen, M. (2015). Loneliness across the life span. *Perspectives on Psychological Science : A Journal of the Association for Psychological Science, 10*(2), 250–264. DOI: 10.1177/1745691615568999 PMID: 25910393

Rainwater, L. (1974). The effects of pornography. In *Deviance and liberty* (pp. 8–25). Routledge., DOI: 10.4324/9780203793343-16

Raj, G., Sharma, A. K., & Arora, Y. (2024). Analyzing the effect of digital technology on mental health. In *Strategies for E-Commerce Data Security* (pp. 54–82). IGI Global. DOI: 10.4018/979-8-3693-6557-1.ch003

Rajpurohit, L., & Yadav, K. C. (2024). The impact of smartphone addiction on adolescents' quality of life: A systematic review. *Frontiers in Health Informatics, 13*(2), 45–58. DOI: 10.3389/fhi.2024.1053489

Ramadhan, R. N., Rampengan, D. D., Yumnanisha, D. A., Setiono, S. B., Tjandra, K. C., Ariyanto, M. V., Idrisov, B., & Empitu, M. A. (2024). Impacts of digital social media detox for mental health: A systematic review and meta-analysis. *Narra J, 4*(2), e786. DOI: 10.52225/narra.v4i2.786 PMID: 39280291

Ramsey, N., Obeidallah, M., & Abraham, A. (2023). Impact of covid-19 on adolescent health and use of social media. *Current Opinion in Pediatrics, 35*(3), 362–367. DOI: 10.1097/MOP.0000000000001248 PMID: 37036294

Rank, M. R. (2023). *Talking to children about pornography.* https://doi.org/DOI: 10.4324/9781003189787-10

Reangsing, C., Wongchan, W., Trakooltorwong, P., Thaibandit, J., & Oerther, S. (2025). Effects of cognitive behavioral therapy (CBT) on addictive symptoms in individuals with internet gaming disorders: A systematic review and meta-analysis. *Psychiatry Research, 348,* 116425. DOI: 10.1016/j.psychres.2025.116425 PMID: 40054044

Rebello, C., & Greenway, F. (2016). Reward-Induced Eating: Therapeutic Approaches to Addressing Food Cravings. *33(11)*, 1853-1866. Adis, Springer Healthcare. DOI: 10.1007/s12325-016-0414-6

Rector, N. A., & Roger, D. (1996). Cognitive style and symptom presentation in depression. *Journal of Affective Disorders, 39*(2), 79–87.

Reed, K. P., Cooper, R. L., Nugent, W. R., & Russell, K. (2016). Cyberbullying: A literature review of its relationship to adolescent depression and current intervention strategies. *Journal of Human Behavior in the Social Environment, 26*(1), 37–45. DOI: 10.1080/10911359.2015.1059165

Rehm, J., Fischer, B., Graham, K., Haydon, E., Mann, R. E., & Room, R. (2004). The importance of environmental modifiers of the relationship between substance use and harm. *Addiction (Abingdon, England), 99*(6), 663–666. DOI: 10.1111/j.1360-0443.2004.00719.x PMID: 15139864

Robb, M. B., & Lauricella, A. R. (2014). Connecting child development and technology: What we know and what it means. In *Technology and digital media in the early years* (1st ed., pp. 16–32). Routledge., DOI: 10.4324/9781315856575-18

Roberto, C. A. (2023). An inconvenient truth: Difficult problems rarely have easy solutions. *The Behavioral and Brain Sciences*, *46*, e173. DOI: 10.1017/S0140525X23000882 PMID: 37646295

Robinson, L., Cotten, S. R., Ono, H., Quan-Haase, A., Mesch, G., Chen, W., Schulz, J., Hale, T. M., & Stern, M. J. (2015). Digital inequalities and why they matter. *Information Communication and Society*, *18*(5), 569–582. DOI: 10.1080/1369118X.2015.1012532

Robinson, T. E., & Berridge, K. C. (2008). Incentive sensitization theory. *Philosophical Transactions of the Royal Society of London. Series B, Biological Sciences*, *363*(1507), 3137–3146. DOI: 10.1098/rstb.2008.0093 PMID: 18640920

Robinson, T. E., & Berridge, K. C. (2025). The Incentive-Sensitization Theory of Addiction 30 Years On. *Annual Review of Psychology*, *76*(1), 29–58. DOI: 10.1146/annurev-psych-011624-024031 PMID: 39094061

Rojas-Estrada, E., Vizcaíno-Verdú, A., & Bonilla-Del-Río, M. (2024). Sexual (Mis) information. In *Advances in educational technologies and instructional design book series* (pp. 265-284). https://doi.org/DOI: 10.4018/979-8-3693-2053-2.ch015

Romer, D. (2016). Introduction to the issue "adolescents in the digital age: Effects on health and development.". *Media and Communication*, *4*(3), 1–3. DOI: 10.17645/mac.v4i3.658

Romero-Rodríguez, J., Berral-Ortiz, B., Martínez-Domingo, J., & Victoria-Maldonado, J. (2024). Online protection measures to prevent sexting among minors. In *Advances in educational technologies and instructional design book series* (pp. 246-264). https://doi.org/DOI: 10.4018/979-8-3693-2053-2.ch014

Rumpf, H. J., Achab, S., Billieux, J., Bowden-Jones, H., Carragher, N., Demetrovics, Z., Higuchi, S., King, D. L., Mann, K., Potenza, M. N., Saunders, J. B., Abbott, M., Ambekar, A., Aricak, O. T., Assanangkornchai, S., Bahar, N., Borges, G., Brand, M., & Campbell, M. (2018). Including gaming disorder in the ICD-11: The need to do so from a clinical and public health perspective. *Journal of Behavioral Addictions*, *7*(3), 556–561. DOI: 10.1556/2006.7.2018.59 PMID: 30010410

Russell, D. W. (1996). UCLA Loneliness Scale (Version 3): Reliability, validity, and factor structure. *Journal of Personality Assessment*, *66*(1), 20–40. DOI: 10.1207/s15327752jpa6601_2 PMID: 8576833

Ru, Y., Norlizah, H. C., Burhanuddin, N. A. N., Liu, H., & Dong, J. (2025). The correlation between mindfulness and problematic smartphone use: A meta-analysis. *Addictive Behaviors, 164*, 108272. DOI: 10.1016/j.addbeh.2025.108272 PMID: 39923383

Sabet, A. G., & Gountas, S. (2019). Social comparison on Instagram and its relationship with self-esteem. *The International Journal of Health, Wellness & Society, 9*(3), 33–47.

Sabina, C., Wolak, J., & Finkelhor, D. (2008). The nature and dynamics of internet pornography exposure for youth. *Cyberpsychology & Behavior, 11*(6), 691–693. DOI: 10.1089/cpb.2007.0179 PMID: 18771400

Sadeeq, M., & Kumar, V. (2021). Inferring social relationships: Interrelated impact of personological factors and cyber bullying [Doctoral dissertation, Lovely Professional University]. Shodhganga. https://shodhganga.inflibnet.ac.in/handle/10603/123456

Sahin, M. (2012). The relationship between the cyberbullying/cybervictimization and loneliness among adolescents. *Children and Youth Services Review, 34*(4), 834–837. DOI: 10.1016/j.childyouth.2012.01.010

Salimian, P. K., Chunara, R., & Weitzman, E. R. (2014). Averting the perfect storm: Addressing youth substance use risk from social media use. *Pediatric Annals, 43*(10), 411. DOI: 10.3928/00904481-20140924-08 PMID: 25290130

Samala, A. D., Rawas, S., Criollo-C, S., Fortuna, A., Feng, X., Prasetya, F., & Hidayat, R. (2024). Social media in education. *Asian Journal of University Education, 20*(3), 524–539. DOI: 10.24191/ajue.v20i3.27869

Samsudin, E. Z., Yaacob, S. S., Wee, C. X., Ruzlin, A. N. M., Azzani, M., Jamil, A. T., & Mohamad, M. (2023). Prevalence of cyberbullying victimisation and its association with family dysfunction, health behaviour and psychological distress among young adults in urban Selangor, Malaysia: A cross-sectional study. *BMJ Open, 13*(11), e072801. DOI: 10.1136/bmjopen-2023-072801 PMID: 37967999

Samsudin, S.. (2024). Cyberbullying victimization, loneliness and well-being among adolescents. *Children and Youth Services Review, 148*, 106896.

Sancho-Cantus, D. (2024). Pornography addiction: Conceptual and methodological approaches in the post-pandemic era. Mini-Review. *Global Journal of Addiction & Rehabilitation Medicine, 7*(4). Advance online publication. DOI: 10.19080/GJARM.2024.07.555718

Sariyska, R., Lachmann, B., Markett, S., & Montag, C. (2017). Internet use disorder: An overview of behavioural and neuroimaging findings. *Frontiers in Psychology*, *8*, 61. DOI: 10.3389/fpsyg.2017.00061

Saruco, E., & Pleger, B. (2021). A Systematic Review of Obesity and Binge Eating Associated Impairment of the Cognitive Inhibition System. *Frontiers in Nutrition*, *8*, 609012–609012. DOI: 10.3389/fnut.2021.609012 PMID: 33996871

Schepis, T. S., Marlowe, D. B., & Forman, R. F. (2008). The availability and portrayal of stimulants over the internet. *The Journal of Adolescent Health : Official Publication of the Society for Adolescent Medicine*, *42*(5), 458–465. DOI: 10.1016/j.jadohealth.2007.11.140 PMID: 18407040

Schiebener, J., Laier, C., & Brand, M. (2015). Getting stuck with pornography? Overuse or neglect of cybersex cues in a multitasking situation is related to symptoms of cybersex addiction. *Journal of Behavioral Addictions*, *4*(1), 14–21. DOI: 10.1556/JBA.4.2015.1.5 PMID: 25786495

Schimmenti, A. (2023). Beyond Addiction: Rethinking Problematic Internet use from a Motivational Framework. *Clinical Neuropsychiatry*, *20*(6), 471–478. DOI: 10.36131/cnfioritieditore20230601 PMID: 38344462

Schmidt, C., Morris, L. S., Kvamme, T. L., Hall, P., Birchard, T., & Voon, V. (2017). Compulsive sexual behavior: Prefrontal and limbic volume and interactions. *Human Brain Mapping*, *38*(3), 1182–1190. DOI: 10.1002/hbm.23447 PMID: 27787929

Schmitt, K. L., & Woolf, K. D. (2018). Cognitive development in digital contexts. *Journal of Children and Media*, *1-3*, 1–3. Advance online publication. DOI: 10.1080/17482798.2018.1522116

Schneider, J. P., O'Donnell, L., & Smith, E. (2012). The impact of cybersex addiction on the family: Results of a survey. *Sexual Addiction & Compulsivity*, *19*(1–2), 123–146. DOI: 10.1080/10720162.2012.658344

Servidio, R., Soraci, P., Griffiths, M. D., Boca, S., & Demetrovics, Z. (2024). Fear of missing out and problematic social media use: A serial mediation model of social comparison and self-esteem. *Addictive Behaviors Reports*, *19*, 100536. DOI: 10.1016/j.abrep.2024.100536 PMID: 38495391

Seto, M. C. (2015). *Internet sexual offending: Theory, practice, and policy*. American Psychological Association., DOI: 10.1037/14644-000

Setty, E. (2022). Digital media and relationships, sex, and health education in the classroom. *Pastoral Care in Education*, *41*(3), 289–305. DOI: 10.1080/02643944.2022.2095418

Setyawati, R., Hartini, N., & Suryanto, S. (2020). The Psychological Impacts of Internet Pornography Addiction on Adolescents. Humaniora. *Journal of Indonesian Culture and Society, 11*(3), 235–244. DOI: 10.21512/humaniora.v11i3.6682

Shafly, M. S. N., Ahadiah, H. R., Syadza, L., Algristian, H., & Setyorini, D. (2025). Compulsive Sexual Behavior as a Maladaptive Coping Mechanism in Bipolar Affective Disorder: A Case Report. *Sinergi International Journal of Psychology, 3*(3), 137–147. DOI: 10.61194/psychology.v3i3.785

Shanmugasundaram, M., & Tamilarasu, A. (2023). *The impact of digital technology, social media, and artificial intelligence on cognitive functions: a review. 2*. Frontiers Media., DOI: 10.3389/fcogn.2023.1203077

Shannon, H., Bush, K., Villeneuve, P. J., Hellemans, K. G., & Guimond, S. (2022). Problematic Social Media Use in Adolescents and Young Adults: Systematic Review and Meta-analysis. *JMIR Mental Health, 9*(4), e33450. DOI: 10.2196/33450 PMID: 35436240

Sharma, R. (2020). Vital need for sex education in Indian youth and adolescents. *Indian Journal of Pediatrics, 87*(4), 255. DOI: 10.1007/s12098-020-03240-z PMID: 32048223

Shulman, E. P., Smith, A. R., Silva, K., Icenogle, G., Duell, N., Chein, J., & Steinberg, L. (2016). The Dual Systems Model: Review, reappraisal, and reaffirmation. *Developmental Cognitive Neuroscience, 17*, 103–117. DOI: 10.1016/j.dcn.2015.12.010 PMID: 26774291

Simon, L., & Daneback, K. (2013). Adolescents' use of the internet for sex education: A thematic and critical review of the literature. *International Journal of Sexual Health : Official Journal of the World Association for Sexual Health, 25*(4), 305–319. DOI: 10.1080/19317611.2013.823899

Singh, R. (2024). Cyber pornography and its control mechanisms: An evaluation. *Research Review, 9*(12), 73–78.

Sinha, R. (2017). *Role of addiction and stress neurobiology on food intake and obesity. 131, 5-13*. Elsevier BV., DOI: 10.1016/j.biopsycho.2017.05.001

Smaniotto, B., Bigot, J. L., & Camps, F. (2021). "Pornography addiction": Elements for discussion of a case report. *Archives of Sexual Behavior, 51*(2), 1375–1381. DOI: 10.1007/s10508-021-02133-2 PMID: 34786657

Smits, M., Kim, C. M., Van Goor, H., & Ludden, G. D. (2022). From digital health to digital well-being. *Journal of Medical Internet Research, 24*(4), e33787. DOI: 10.2196/33787 PMID: 35377328

Solankure, K., Sagare, S., & Bhoomika, B. J. (2025). Prevalence of smartphone addiction and its impact on sleep quality among school-going students: A cross-sectional study. *Journal of Ayurveda and Holistic Medicine*, *13*(4), 3–11. DOI: 10.70066/jahm.v13i4.1835

Soler, I., Sánchez, C., & Quiles-Soler, M. (2021). Nomophobia in teenagers: Digital lifestyle, social networking and smartphone abuse. *Communicatio Socialis*, *34*(4), 17–32. DOI: 10.15581/003.34.4.17-32

Solly, J., Hook, R., Grant, J., Cortese, S., & Chamberlain, S. (2021). Structural gray matter differences in Problematic Usage of the Internet: a systematic review and meta-analysis. *27(2)*, 1000-1009. Springer Nature. DOI: 10.1038/s41380-021-01315-7

Spada, M. M. (2014). An overview of problematic Internet use. *Addictive Behaviors*, *39*(1), 3–6. DOI: 10.1016/j.addbeh.2013.09.007 PMID: 24126206

Spence, C., Okajima, K., Cheok, A., Petit, O., & Michel, C. (2015). Eating with our eyes: From visual hunger to digital satiation. *Brain and Cognition*, *110*, 53–63. DOI: 10.1016/j.bandc.2015.08.006 PMID: 26432045

Srnicek, N. (2017). *Platform capitalism*. Polity Press.

Starcevic, V., Billieux, J., & Schimmenti, A. (2021). Selfitis, selfie addiction, Instagram addiction: A conceptual overview. *Current Opinion in Psychology*, *39*, 49–54. DOI: 10.1016/j.copsyc.2020.08.014

Stark, R., & Klucken, T. (2017). Neuroscientific approaches to (online) pornography addiction. In *Studies in neuroscience, psychology and behavioral economics* (pp. 109-124). https://doi.org/DOI: 10.1007/978-3-319-46276-9_7

Stark, R., Markert, C., Kruse, O., Walter, B., Strahler, J., & Klein, S. (2022). Individual cortisol response to acute stress influences neural processing of sexual cues. *Journal of Behavioral Addictions*, *11*(2), 506–519. DOI: 10.1556/2006.2022.00037 PMID: 35895611

Statista. (2024). Canada: experiences with cyberbullying, 2024. Statista. https://www.statista.com/statistics/1498106/canada-experienced-witnessed-cyberbullying/

Statista. (2024). *Cyberbullying – Statistics & facts*. https://www.statista.com/topics/1809/cyber-bullying/

Statista. (2025). *UK girls on upsetting online experiences 2016–2023*. https://www.statista.com/statistics/1448496/uk-girls-on-upsetting-online-experiences/

Steel, C. M. (2015). Web-based child pornography: The global impact of deterrence efforts and its consumption on mobile platforms. *Child Abuse & Neglect*, *44*, 150–158. DOI: 10.1016/j.chiabu.2014.12.009 PMID: 25605590

Steele, V. R., Staley, C., Fong, T., & Prause, N. (2013). Sexual desire, not hypersexuality, is related to neurophysiological responses elicited by sexual images. *Socio-affective Neuroscience & Psychology*, *3*(1), 20770. DOI: 10.3402/snp.v3i0.20770 PMID: 24693355

Steinberg, L. (2008). A social neuroscience perspective on adolescent risk-taking. *Developmental Review*, *28*(1), 78–106. DOI: 10.1016/j.dr.2007.08.002 PMID: 18509515

Steinberg, L. (2014). *Age of opportunity: Lessons from the new science of adolescence*. Houghton Mifflin Harcourt.

Steinfeld, N. (2020). Parental mediation of adolescent Internet use: Combining strategies to promote awareness, autonomy and self-regulation in preparing youth for life on the web. *Education and Information Technologies*, *26*(2), 1897–1920. DOI: 10.1007/s10639-020-10342-w

Stevens, M. W. R., Dorstyn, D., Delfabbro, P. H., & King, D. L. (2021a). Global prevalence of gaming disorder: A systematic review and meta-analysis. *The Australian and New Zealand Journal of Psychiatry*, *55*(6), 553–568. DOI: 10.1177/0004867420962851 PMID: 33028074

Stevens, M. W. R., King, D. L., Dorstyn, D., & Delfabbro, P. H. (2019). Cognitive-behavioral therapy for Internet gaming disorder: A systematic review and meta-analysis. *Clinical Psychology & Psychotherapy*, *26*(2), 191–203. DOI: 10.1002/cpp.2341 PMID: 30341981

Stevens, M. W., King, D. L., Dorstyn, D., & Delfabbro, P. H. (2021b). Cognitive-behavioural therapy for Internet gaming disorder: A systematic review and meta-analysis. *Clinical Psychology & Psychotherapy*, *28*(3), 612–624. DOI: 10.1002/cpp.2539

Steward, T., & Wierenga, C. (2022). Foreword to the special issue on the neuroscience of obesity and related disorders. *23(4)*, 679-681. Springer Science+Business Media. DOI: 10.1007/s11154-022-09739-4

Steyer, I. (2014). Gender representations in children's media and their influence. *Campus-Wide Information Systems*, *31*(2/3), 171–180. DOI: 10.1108/CWIS-11-2013-0065

Stone, R. (2026). *Women targeted by AI-generated sexual imagery describe lasting harm*. Rolling Stone.

Strasburger, V. C. (2010). Sexuality, contraception, and the media. *Pediatrics, 126*(3), 576–582. DOI: 10.1542/peds.2010-1544 PMID: 20805150

Štulhofer, A., Kohut, T., & Koletić, G. (2022). Pornography use in adolescence and young adulthood. In *Focus on sexuality research* (pp. 385-421). https://doi.org/DOI: 10.1007/978-3-030-84273-4_14

Sunday, O. J., Adesope, O. O., & Maarhuis, P. L. (2021). The effects of smartphone addiction on learning: A meta-analysis. *Computers in Human Behavior Reports, 4*, 100114. DOI: 10.1016/j.chbr.2021.100114

Tabish, S. (2025). From evolution to obsession: Understanding digital addiction among youth in the modern age. *American Journal of Health Research, 13*(4), 248–258. DOI: 10.11648/j.ajhr.20251304.17

Talan, M. İ., Bostan, G., & Öztürk, Y. (2021). Investigation of the relationship between high school students' cyberbullying and cyber victimization situations and their perceptions of loneliness. *Journal of Research in Education and Society, 8*(2), 378–398. DOI: 10.51725/etad.905167

Tao, T. J., Lim, T. K., Yeung, E. T. F., Liu, H., Shris, P. B., Ma, L. K. Y., & Hou, W. K. (2023). Internet-based cognitive behavioral therapy. npj. *Digital Medicine, 6*(1), 80. PMID: 37117458

Teo, E., Goh, D., Vijayakumar, K., & Liu, J. (2018). To Message or Browse? Exploring the Impact of Phone Use Patterns on Male Adolescents' Consumption of Palatable Snacks. *Frontiers in Psychology, 8*, 2298. Advance online publication. DOI: 10.3389/fpsyg.2017.02298 PMID: 29358925

Tereshchenko, S. (2023). Neurobiological risk factors for problematic social media use as a specific form of Internet addiction: A narrative review. *World Journal of Psychiatry, 13*(5), 160–173. DOI: 10.5498/wjp.v13.i5.160 PMID: 37303928

Termann, S. (2025). The dopamine collapse hypothesis. *SSRN*.

Teymur, Z., & ÖNEY, B. (2024). HEDONİK AÇLIK VE OBEZİTE. *DergiPark (Istanbul University)*. https://dergipark.org.tr/tr/pub/arsagbil/issue/86259/1460606 adresinden alındı

Thorneycroft, R., Smith, E., & Nicholas, L. (2024). Whose concerns? Young adults discussing (their) concerns with pornography. *Sex Education, 25*(4), 465–480. DOI: 10.1080/14681811.2024.2356635

Timotheou, S., Miliou, O., Dimitriadis, Y., Sobrino, S. V., Giannoutsou, N., Cachia, R., & Ioannou, A. (2023). Impacts of digital technologies on education. *Education and Information Technologies, 28*(6), 6695–6726. DOI: 10.1007/s10639-022-11431-8 PMID: 36465416

Tokunaga, R. S. (2017). A meta-analysis of the relationships between psychosocial problems and internet habits: Synthesizing internet addiction, problematic internet use, and deficient self-regulation research. *Communication Monographs, 84*(4), 423–446. DOI: 10.1080/03637751.2017.1332419

Tomei, A., Studer, J., & Gmel, G. (2021). Prosocialness in young males with substance and behavioral addictions. *Journal of Behavioral Addictions, 10*(2), 327–337. DOI: 10.1556/2006.2021.00035 PMID: 34191744

Torous, J., Myrick, K. J., Rauseo-Ricupero, N., & Firth, J. (2020). Digital mental health and COVID-19: Using technology today to accelerate the curve on access and quality tomorrow. *JMIR Mental Health, 7*(3), e18848. DOI: 10.2196/18848 PMID: 32213476

Torraco, R. J. (2016). Writing integrative literature reviews: Using the past and present to explore the future. *Human Resource Development Review, 15*(4), 404–428. DOI: 10.1177/1534484316671606

Tse, N., Siu, A., & Tsang, S.. (2024). Group motivational interviewing for adolescents at risk of internet gaming disorder: A mixed-methods preliminary evaluation. *Clinical Social Work Journal.* Advance online publication. DOI: 10.1007/s10615-024-00968-5

Tsochantaridou, A., Sergentanis, T., Grammatikopoulou, M., Merakou, K., Vassilakou, T., & Kornarou, E. (2023). Food Advertisement and Dietary Choices in Adolescents: An Overview of Recent Studies. *Children (Basel, Switzerland), 10*(3), 442–442. DOI: 10.3390/children10030442 PMID: 36980000

Tunney, C., & Rooney, B. (2023). Using theoretical models of problematic internet use to inform psychological formulation: A systematic scoping review. *Clinical Child Psychology and Psychiatry, 28*(2), 810–830. DOI: 10.1177/13591045221104569 PMID: 36916053

Turner, K. H., Jolls, T., Hagerman, M. S., O'Byrne, W., Hicks, T., Eisenstock, B., & Pytash, K. E. (2017). Developing digital and media literacies in children and adolescents. *Pediatrics, 140*(Supplement_2), S122–S126. DOI: 10.1542/peds.2016-1758P PMID: 29093046

Twenge, J. M., & Campbell, W. K. (2018). Associations between screen time and lower psychological well-being among children and adolescents. *Preventive Medicine Reports*, *12*, 271–283. DOI: 10.1016/j.pmedr.2018.10.003 PMID: 30406005

Tymofiyeva, O., Yuan, J., Kidambi, R., Huang, C.-Y., Henje, E., Rubinstein, M., Jariwala, N., Max, J. E., Yang, T. T., & Xu, D. (2020). Neural Correlates of Smartphone Dependence in Adolescents. *Frontiers in Human Neuroscience*, *14*, 564629. Advance online publication. DOI: 10.3389/fnhum.2020.564629 PMID: 33132878

U.S. Department of Health and Human Services & Office of the Surgeon General. (2023). *Surgeon General's advisory on youth mental health and social media*. U.S. Department of Health and Human Services. https://www.hhs.gov/sites/default/files/sg-youth-mental-health-social-media-advisory.pdf

Uclés-Torrents, M., Ruiz-Gamarra, G., & Aparicio-Martinez, P. (2026). Social Media Use, Affect, and Dietary Choices Across Age Groups—Insights from the Special Issue "The Impact of Social Media on Eating Behavior". *Nutrients*, *18*(2), 335–335. DOI: 10.3390/nu18020335 PMID: 41599948

Ukabuiro, I. K., & Agomah, S. A. (2025). A digital persuasive system to mitigate health risks. *European Journal of Innovative Studies and Sustainability*, *1*(3), 28–45. DOI: 10.59324/ejiss.2025.1(3).04

Uludag, K. (2023). Personalized video recommendation system and its potential role as a trigger of addiction. *Scientific Studios on Social and Political Psychology*, *29*(2), 44–46. DOI: 10.61727/sssppj/2.2023.44

Uma, P., Buzana, T., & Iluzija, B. (2014). PSIHOLOGIJA, https://citeseerx.ist.psu.edu/viewdoc/summary?doi=10.1.1.461.8490 adresinden alındı

UNESCO. (2018). *Global framework of reference on digital literacy skills*. UNESCO. https://unesdoc.unesco.org/ark:/48223/pf0000265403

UNICEF. (2021). *The state of the world's children 2021: On my mind*. UNICEF. https://www.unicef.org/reports/state-worlds-children-2021

UNICEF. (2023). [*For every child, digital*. UNICEF.]. *The State of the World's Children*, •••, 2023.

UNICEF. (2025). *Keeping children safe online: trends in online platform regulation and emerging lessons*. UNICEF. https://www.unicef.org/media/177636/file/FINAL_Policy%20brief_online%20platform%20regulation.pdf.pdf

Upadhyaya, H. (2024). *Digital education and economic transformation*. Meadow Publication.

Valkenburg, P. M., & Peter, J. (2013). The differential susceptibility to media effects model. *The Journal of Communication, 63*(2), 221–243. DOI: 10.1111/jcom.12024

van den Eijnden, R. J. J. M., Lemmens, J. S., & Valkenburg, P. M. (2016). The Social Media Disorder Scale: Validity and psychometric properties. *Computers in Human Behavior, 61*, 478–487. DOI: 10.1016/j.chb.2016.03.038

van Deursen, A. J. A. M., & Helsper, E. J. (2015). The third-level digital divide: Who benefits most from being online? *Communication and Information Technologies Annual, 10*, 29–52. DOI: 10.1108/S2050-206020150000010002

van Dijck, J., Poell, T., & de Waal, M. (2018). *The platform society: Public values in a connective world.* Oxford University Press. DOI: 10.1093/oso/9780190889760.001.0001

VanderBroek-Stice, L., Stojek, M., Beach, S., vanDellen, M., & MacKillop, J. (2017). Multidimensional assessment of impulsivity in relation to obesity and food addiction. *Appetite, 112*, 59–68. DOI: 10.1016/j.appet.2017.01.009 PMID: 28087369

Varela, J. J., Hernández, C., Ramos Miranda, R., Barlett, C. P., & Rodríguez-Rivas, M. E. (2022). Victims of cyberbullying: Feeling loneliness and depression among youth and adult Chileans during the pandemic. *International Journal of Environmental Research and Public Health, 19*(10), 5886. DOI: 10.3390/ijerph19105886 PMID: 35627423

Vasiliu, O. (2023). An integrative model as a step toward increasing the awareness of eating disorders in the general population. *Frontiers in Psychiatry, 14*, 1184932. Advance online publication. DOI: 10.3389/fpsyt.2023.1184932 PMID: 37205977

Vaterlaus, J. M., Beckert, T. E., & Bird, C. V. (2015). At a certain age it's not appropriate to monitor one's child. *Emerging Adulthood, 3*(5), 353–358. DOI: 10.1177/2167696815581277

Vera-Gray, F., McGlynn, C., Kureshi, I., & Butterby, K. (2021). Sexual violence as a sexual script in mainstream online pornography. *British Journal of Criminology, 61*(5), 1243–1260. DOI: 10.1093/bjc/azab035

Vertongen, R., Chamberlain, K., & Van Ommen, C. (2022). Pornography and adolescents: Unravelling dominant research assumptions. *Porn Studies, 9*(4), 430–444. DOI: 10.1080/23268743.2022.2114532

Vertongen, R., Van Ommen, C., & Chamberlain, K. (2022). Adolescent dilemmas about viewing pornography and their efforts to resolve them. *Journal of Adolescent Research, 40*(1), 226–254. DOI: 10.1177/07435584221133307

Vicens, A., & Satter, R. (2026). Investigation reveals misuse of AI image generation for sexualized content. *Reuters*. https://www.reuters.com/world/us/rise-ai-generated-child-sexual-imagery-reports-2026-02-20/

Vieira, C., & Griffiths, M. D. (2024). Problematic pornography use and mental health: A systematic review. *Sexual Health & Compulsivity*, *31*(3), 207–247. DOI: 10.1080/26929953.2024.2348624

Vinnakota, D., Arafat, S. M. Y., Kar, S. K., Sivasubramanian, M., Hossain, S. R., Parsa, A. D., & Kabir, R. (2021). Pornography and sexual violence against women in India: A scoping review. *Journal of Psychosexual Health*, *3*(3), 216–221. DOI: 10.1177/26318318211023935

Vladimiros, P. (2025). The Edible Interface: How Mass-Market Foods Became Sophisticated Delivery Systems for Biological Influence. Zenodo *(CERN European Organization for Nuclear Research)*. DOI: 10.5281/zenodo.17815936

Volkow, N. D., Koob, G. F., & McLellan, A. T. (2016). Neurobiologic Advances from the Brain Disease Model of Addiction. *The New England Journal of Medicine*, *374*(4), 363–371. DOI: 10.1056/NEJMra1511480 PMID: 26816013

Volkow, N. D., Wang, G. J., Fowler, J. S., Tomasi, D., Telang, F., & Baler, R. (2010). Addiction: Decreased reward sensitivity and increased expectation sensitivity conspire to overwhelm the brain's control circuit. *BioEssays : News and Reviews in Molecular, Cellular and Developmental Biology*, *32*(9), 748–755. DOI: 10.1002/bies.201000042 PMID: 20730946

Voon, V., Mole, T. B., Banca, P., Porter, L., Morris, L., Mitchell, S., Lapa, T. R., Karr, J., Harrison, N. A., Potenza, M. N., & Irvine, M. (2014). Neural correlates of sexual cue reactivity in individuals with and without compulsive sexual behaviours. *PLoS One*, *9*(7), e102419. DOI: 10.1371/journal.pone.0102419 PMID: 25013940

Vu, H., François, K. K., Hung, N. X., Trung, N. V., & Hieu, N. L. (2024). Potential of digital health solutions. In *Digitalization of Medicine in LMICs* (pp. 51–68). Springer.

Wang, J., & Zhao, Y. (2024). Social comparison on social media and its influence on subjective well-being: A systematic review. *International Journal of Environmental Research and Public Health*, *21*(3), 345. PMID: 38541344

Wattick, R., Olfert, M., Claydon, E., Hagedorn, R., Barr, M., & Brode, C. (2023). Early life influences on the development of food addiction in college attending young adults. *Eating and Weight Disorders : EWD*, *28*(1), 14. Advance online publication. DOI: 10.1007/s40519-023-01546-3 PMID: 36807705

Watts, L. K., Wagner, J., Velasquez, B., & Behrens, P. I. (2017). Cyberbullying in higher education: A literature review. *Computers in Human Behavior*, *69*, 268–274. DOI: 10.1016/j.chb.2016.12.038

Wdowiak, K., Maciocha, A., & Wąż, J. (2025). Pornography through the lens of the 21st century and its impact on society. *Journal of Psychiatry & Clinical Psychology/Psychiatria i Psychologia Kliniczna, 25*(2). https://doi.org/DOI: 10.15557/PiPK.2025.0018

Weber, M., Quiring, O., & Daschmann, G. (2012). Peers, parents and pornography: Exploring adolescents' exposure to sexually explicit material and its developmental correlates. *Sexuality & Culture*, *16*(4), 408–427. DOI: 10.1007/s12119-012-9132-7

Wegmann, E., Antons, S., Schmidt, L. D., Klein, L., Montag, C., Rumpf, H. J., Müller, S. M., & Brand, M. (2025). Feels good, and less bad: Problematic use of the Internet is associated with heightened experiences of both gratification and compensation. *Journal of Behavioral Addictions*, *14*(1), 263–275. DOI: 10.1556/2006.2024.00067 PMID: 39786377

Weill Cornell Medicine. (2025). *Study finds addictive screen use, not total screen time, linked to youth suicide risk.* https://news.weill.cornell.edu/news/2025/06/study-finds-addictive-screen-use-not-total-screen-time-linked-to-youth-suicide-risk

Wéry, A., & Billieux, J. (2017). Problematic cybersex: Conceptualization, assessment, and treatment. *Addictive Behaviors*, *64*, 238–246. DOI: 10.1016/j.addbeh.2015.11.007 PMID: 26646983

Wéry, A., Deleuze, J., Canale, N., & Billieux, J. (2018). Emotionally laden impulsivity interacts with affect in predicting addictive use of online sexual activity in men. *Comprehensive Psychiatry*, *80*, 192–201. DOI: 10.1016/j.comppsych.2017.10.004 PMID: 29128857

Whatnall, M., Skinner, J., Leary, M., & Burrows, T. (2022). Food Addiction: A Deep Dive into 'Loss of Control' and 'Craving'. *Current Addiction Reports*, *9*(4), 318–325. DOI: 10.1007/s40429-022-00431-w

Whitehand, J. (2022). The problem of separate worlds. *Urban Morphology*, *14*(2). Advance online publication. DOI: 10.51347/jum.v14i2.5150

WHO. (2019). International Classification of Diseases for Mortality and Morbidity Statistics (11th Revision), World Health Organisation. https://icd.who.int/

Wilcox, H. C., & Wyman, P. A. (2004). Self-esteem, perceived social support, and suicidal ideation and behavior among African American public housing residents. *Archives of Suicide Research : Official Journal of the International Academy for Suicide Research*, *8*(3), 239–252. PMID: 16081390

Williams, L. (1989). *Hard core: Power, pleasure, and the frenzy of the visible.* University of California Press.

Willie, M., Maqbool, M., & Qadir, A. (2024). From click to calories: Navigating the impact of food delivery apps on obesity. *Open Health*, *5*(1), 20230022. Advance online publication. DOI: 10.1515/ohe-2023-0022

Willis, M., Bridges, A. J., & Sun, C. (2022). Pornography use, gender, and sexual objectification: A multinational study. *Sexuality & Culture*, *26*(4), 1298–1313. DOI: 10.1007/s12119-022-09943-z

Willoughby, B. J., Busby, D. M., & Young-Petersen, B. (2018). Understanding associations between personal definitions of pornography, using pornography, and depression. *Sexuality Research & Social Policy*, *16*(3), 342–356. DOI: 10.1007/s13178-018-0345-x

Willoughby, B. J., Carroll, J. S., Busby, D. M., & Brown, C. C. (2016). Differences in Pornography Use Among Couples: Associations with Satisfaction, Stability, and Relationship Processes. *Archives of Sexual Behavior*, *45*(1), 145–158. DOI: 10.1007/s10508-015-0562-9 PMID: 26228990

Wizła, M., & Lewczuk, K. (2024). The Associations Between Attachment Insecurity and Compulsive Sexual Behavior Disorder or Problematic Pornography Use: The Mediating Role of Emotion Regulation Difficulties. *Archives of Sexual Behavior*, *53*(9), 3419–3436. DOI: 10.1007/s10508-024-02904-7 PMID: 38898361

Wojciechowski, J., Draps, M., Kublik, E., Dubiejko, P., Wolak, T., & Gola, M. (2025). Enhanced conditioning and disrupted extinction processes in men struggling with compulsive sexual behaviors. *Journal of Behavioral Addictions*, *14*(1), 191–203. DOI: 10.1556/2006.2025.00012 PMID: 40014056

Wolf, N., Henemann, G., Schmitgen, M., Koenig, J., Bach, P., & Wolf, R. (2025). Screens and brains: Multimodal neuroimaging insights into mechanisms of problematic smartphone use. *Progress in Neuro-Psychopharmacology & Biological Psychiatry*, *142*, 111531–111531. DOI: 10.1016/j.pnpbp.2025.111531 PMID: 41120086

World Health Organization & International HBSC Network. (2023). *Problematic social media use. HBSC Data Browser.* World Health Organization. https://data-browser.hbsc.org/measure/problematic-social-media-use/

World Health Organization. (1986). *Ottawa Charter for Health Promotion.* World Health Organization. https://www.who.int/teams/health-promotion/enhanced-wellbeing/first-global-conference

World Health Organization. (2014). *Preventing suicide: A global imperative* (community-based approaches section). World Health Organization. https://www.who.int/publications/i/item/9789241564779

World Health Organization. (2018). *International classification of diseases (11th revision).*

World Health Organization. (2020). *Addictive behaviours: Gaming disorder.* https://www.who.int/news-room/questions-and-answers/item/addictive-behaviours-gaming-disorder

World Health Organization. (2022). *Guidelines on mental health at work.* World Health Organization. https://www.who.int/publications/i/item/9789240053052

World Health Organization. (2022). *International classification of diseases for mortality and morbidity statistics* (11th ed.).

World Health Organization. (2023). *Commercial determinants of health.* World Health Organization. https://www.who.int/news-room/fact-sheets/detail/commercial-determinants-of-health

World Health Organization. (2024). *Global brief for World Mental Health Day 2024: Mental health is a universal human right.* World Health Organization. https://www.who.int/publications/i/item/9789240029200

World Health Organization. (2025). *Ethics and governance of artificial intelligence for health: Guidance on large multi-modal models.* World Health Organization. https://iris.who.int/server/api/core/bitstreams/e9e62c65-6045-481e-bd04-20e206bc5039/content

Wright, A. J. (2018). Comprehensive assessment of substance abuse and addiction risk in adolescence. In T. MacMillan & A. Sisselman-Borgia (Eds.), *New directions in treatment, education, and outreach for mental health and addiction* (pp. 25–55). Springer International Publishing/Springer Nature. https://doi.org/DOI: 10.1007/978-3-319-72778-3_3

Wright, P. J. (2011). Mass media effects on youth sexual behavior. *Annals of the International Communication Association*, *35*(1), 343–385. DOI: 10.1080/23808985.2011.11679121

Wright, P. J., Tokunaga, R. S., & Herbenick, D. (2025). Pornography Use, Moral Incongruence, Psychological Distress, and Sexual Satisfaction. *Archives of Sexual Behavior*, *54*(1), 7–17. DOI: 10.1007/s10508-024-03055-5 PMID: 39718733

Wuersch, L., Neher, A., & Peter, M. K. (2023). Digital internal communication. *International Journal of Management Reviews*, *25*(3), 614–639. DOI: 10.1111/ijmr.12323

Wylie, K. (2010). Sex education and the influence on sexual wellbeing. *Procedia: Social and Behavioral Sciences*, *5*, 440–444. DOI: 10.1016/j.sbspro.2010.07.119

Xanidis, N., & Brignell, C. M. (2016). The association between the use of social network sites, sleep quality, and cognitive function during the day. *Computers in Human Behaviour, 55*(Pt B), 121–126. DOI: 10.1016/j.chb.2015.09.004

Xiao, Y., Meng, Y., Brown, T. T., Keyes, K. M., & Mann, J. J. (2025). Addictive use of social media and mobile phones, but not total time, kopingis associated with future suicidal behavior. *International Journal of Environmental Research and Public Health*, *22*(1), 57. PMID: 39857510

Xiong, J., Liu, C., Zhao, Y., & Chen, L. (2025). Longitudinal associations between problematic pornography use and adolescent mental health: Mediating roles of sleep disturbance and shame. *Journal of Behavioral Addictions*, *14*(1), 45–60.

Yang, J., Fu, X., Liao, X., & Li, Y. (2020). Association of problematic smartphone use with poor sleep quality, depression, and anxiety: A systematic review and meta-analysis. *Psychiatry Research*, *284*, 112686. DOI: 10.1016/j.psychres.2019.112686 PMID: 31757638

Yang, Y., Wu, Q., & Morys, F. (2021). Brain Responses to High-Calorie Visual Food Cues in Individuals with Normal-Weight or Obesity: An Activation Likelihood Estimation Meta-Analysis. *Brain Sciences*, *11*(12), 1587–1587. DOI: 10.3390/brainsci11121587 PMID: 34942889

Ybarra, M. L., & Mitchell, K. J. (2005). Exposure to internet pornography among children and adolescents: A national survey. *Cyberpsychology & Behavior*, *8*(5), 473–486. DOI: 10.1089/cpb.2005.8.473 PMID: 16232040

Ye, X. (2025). Dark patterns and addictive designs. *Weizenbaum Journal of the Digital Society*, *5*(3), Article 2.

Young, K. S. (1998). Internet addiction: The emergence of a new clinical disorder. *Cyberpsychology & Behavior*, *1*(3), 237–244. DOI: 10.1089/cpb.1998.1.237

Young, K. S. (2009). Understanding online gaming addiction and treatment issues for adolescents. *The American Journal of Family Therapy*, *37*(5), 355–372. DOI: 10.1080/01926180902942191

Young, K. S. (2011). CBT-IA: The first treatment model for internet addiction. *Journal of Cognitive Psychotherapy*, *25*(4), 304–312. DOI: 10.1891/0889-8391.25.4.304

Yue, Z. (2022). Sexual media and behaviors. In *Elsevier eBooks* (pp. 239-247). https://doi.org/DOI: 10.1016/B978-0-12-818872-9.00189-8

Yu, J. J., Kim, H., & Hay, I. (2013). Understanding adolescents' problematic Internet use from a social/cognitive and addiction research framework. *Computers in Human Behavior*, *29*(6), 2682–2689. DOI: 10.1016/j.chb.2013.06.045

Yu, S., & Sussman, S. (2020). Does Smartphone Addiction Fall on a Continuum of Addictive Behaviors? *International Journal of Environmental Research and Public Health*, *17*(2), 422–422. DOI: 10.3390/ijerph17020422 PMID: 31936316

Zalaquett, C. P., & Chatters, S. J. (2014). Cyberbullying in College. *SAGE Open*, *4*(1), 215824401452672. DOI: 10.1177/2158244014526721

Zaman, S. B., Khan, R. K., Evans, R. G., Thrift, A. G., Maddison, R., & Islam, S. M. S. (2022). ICT adoption for older adults. *JMIR Aging*, *5*(1), e25251. DOI: 10.2196/25251 PMID: 34994695

Zarate, D., Hobson, B. A., March, E., Griffiths, M. D., & Stavropoulos, V. (2022). Psychometric properties of the Bergen Social Media Addiction Scale: An analysis using item response theory. *Addictive Behaviors Reports*, *17*, 100473. DOI: 10.1016/j.abrep.2022.100473 PMID: 36536822

Zen, M., Hendriks, J., & Burns, S. (2024). Sexually explicit media literacy education: A scoping review of parental perspectives and relevant resources. *Sex Education*, *25*(3), 359–375. DOI: 10.1080/14681811.2024.2338275

Zhai, B., & Fang, G. (2025). The relationship between social media use intensity and life satisfaction: A moderated mediation model. *Frontiers in Psychology*, *16*, 1463671.

Zhang, D., Huebner, E. S., & Tian, L. (2020). Longitudinal associations among neuroticism, depression, and cyberbullying in early adolescents. *Computers in Human Behavior*, *112*, 106475. DOI: 10.1016/j.chb.2020.106475

Zhang, H.-B., Zheng, H., Zhang, Y., & Zhao, D. (2020). *Commentary: Compulsive drug use is associated with imbalance of orbitofrontal- and prelimbic-striatal circuits in punishment-resistant individuals. 14, 49-49.* Frontiers Media., DOI: 10.3389/fncir.2020.00049

Zhou, R., Morita, N., Ogai, Y., Saito, T., Zhang, X., Yang, W., & Yang, F. (2024). Meta-Analysis of Internet Gaming Disorder Prevalence: Assessing the Impacts of DSM-5 and ICD-11 Diagnostic Criteria. *International Journal of Environmental Research and Public Health*, *21*(6), 700. DOI: 10.3390/ijerph21060700 PMID: 38928946

Zhu, L., & Lan, J. (2024). The Influence of Negative Emotion and Self-Acceptance on Suicidal Ideation of Disabled College Students: The Mediating Effect of Hopelessness. *Iranian Journal of Public Health*, *53*(12), 2759–2767. DOI: 10.18502/ijph.v53i12.17319 PMID: 39759216

Zuboff, S. (2019). *The age of surveillance capitalism*. PublicAffairs.

Zurcher, J. D. (2017). Exploring descriptive norms of parent-child communication about pornography among parents of middle-schoolers in the US. *Journal of Children and Media*, *11*(4), 381–398. DOI: 10.1080/17482798.2017.1312471

About the Contributors

Özgün Arda Kus graduated from Maltepe University, Department of Public Relations and Advertising, with a full scholarship, and also pursued a double major in Psychology. He completed his first Master's degree in the Department of Sales and Marketing at Okan University, Business Administration Department. His second Master's degree is in Department of Addiction and Rehabilitation, Institute of Health Sciences. He completed his Ph.D. education in the Department of Public Relations and Advertising at Istanbul University with a thesis titled "Digital Games as an Interactive Communication Space; A study on the effects of playing motivations on digital game addiction." He is currently continuing his academic studies as an Assistant Professor at the Department of Public Relations and Advertising at Usküdar University Faculty of Communication. He has participated in various international and national certificate programs in the fields of marketing and psychology. He has authored the internationally published books "The Concept of Mobile Marketing, A Study for Istanbul and Generation Y," and "Relationships Among Game, Digital Game, Addiction, and Motivation Concepts," and has served as co-editor for the compilation books "Digital Forms of Games 1,2 and 3". He is also co-editor of "Critical Perspectives on Digital Culture and Gaming" and "Advancements in Digital Broadcasting and Content Platforms" published by IGI Global. He has also presented papers at international scientific conferences and contributed chapters and articles to various books. The areas of research and interest for Ozgün Arda Kus include: digital games, alienation, self, mobile marketing, consumer behaviors and generations, mood disorders, and behavioral addictions. He is a full member of the Turkish Psychological Association.

***

P. C. Ahamed is a Rehabilitation Council of India–registered Clinical Psychologist (RCI No. A42422) with extensive training and experience across premier mental health and academic institutions in India. He holds advanced qualifications including an M.Phil. in Clinical Psychology from the Central Institute of Psychiatry, Ranchi, an M.Phil. in Cognitive Science from the University of Hyderabad, and a Fellowship in Psychiatric Rehabilitation from the National Institute of Mental Health and Neuro Sciences (NIMHANS), Bengaluru. His professional experience spans roles as Clinical Psychologist at NIMHANS, Assistant Professor and Clinical Psychologist at Rajagiri College of Social Sciences, Resident Psychologist at IIT Palakkad, and Counsellor at IIT Roorkee, where he has worked extensively with university students and young adults. A UGC-NET–qualified professional and University Second Rank holder in M.A. Psychology, he is also an author and editor of books and book chapters, with multiple national and international research publications and invited talks in India and abroad. His areas of expertise include anxiety and mood disorders, adolescent mental health, substance use and behavioural addictions (including internet and gaming addiction), psychological assessment, Cognitive Behaviour Therapy, Motivational Interviewing, psychiatric rehabilitation, and tele-counselling. He is an active member of several national and international professional associations.

Constantinos Challoumis is a Visiting Professor at the National and Kapodistrian University of Athens (NKUA), at AUEB, and at CNAM University (France) via Descartes College, and an Assistant Professor in IT, Law, and Management at Philips University. He holds a PhD in Economics (NKUA), is a Postdoc cand. (NKUA), and has 7 BScs (1 of which is a cand.) and 8 MScs (1 of which is a cand.). His research spans economics, accounting, law, technology, and quantitative modeling.

Ruchika Dwivedi serves as Assistant Professor II in the Department of Forensic Science at JECRC University, Jaipur. Her research expertise encompasses fingerprints, forensic biology, and questioned documents. She has authored research papers, delivered conference presentations, contributed poster presentations, and served as co-guide for paper presentations, actively advancing forensic science scholarship.

Zeba Jinwala is a Clinical Psychologist associated with the Wellness Centre at Indian Institute of Technology Roorkee, India. She holds an M.Phil. in Clinical Psychology and works extensively with university students, providing psychological assessment and evidence-based therapeutic interventions. Her clinical approach integrates Cognitive-Behavioral Therapy, mindfulness-based interventions, and solution-focused therapy, and she practices from a queer-affirmative and inclusive framework. Her research interests include cognitive biases, obsessive–compulsive disorder, sleep behaviour, and psychological wellbeing among young adults. In addition to her institutional role, she maintains an independent freelance clinical practice, offering counselling and psychotherapy to diverse clients while advocating for accessible and stigma-free mental health care.

Elif Kurtulus Anarat is working as an assistant professor in the department of Psychology (English), Elif Kurtuluş Anarat graduated from Boğaziçi University, Guidance and Psychological Counseling Department in 2011. In 2012, with Dr. Feyza Bayraktar and Prof. Dr. Fatoş Erkman, she conducted research for the Turkish adaptation study of the Yale Food Addiction Scale. In 2019, she completed her master's degree in Üsküdar University, Department of Clinical Psychology, with her thesis titled "Examination of The Mediating Role of Perceived Father Acceptance and Rejection in the Relationship of Eating Attitudes with Loneliness and Belongingness". She completed the Doğuş University Clinical Psychology Ph.D. Program in July 2022 with her dissertation titled "Examination of the Mediator Role of Uncertainty Intolerance and Impulsivity Levels in the Relationship between Eating Behavior and Personality Traits of University Students".

Raghu N. is an Associate Professor at Jain (Deemed-to-be University), recognized for his commitment to fostering a dynamic and engaging learning environment that inspires students to explore their capabilities and achieve academic excellence, with a strong passion for teaching and mentoring, He consistently strives to cultivate critical thinking, innovation, and lifelong learning among his students. His research contributions span across reputed journals, book chapters, and international conference proceedings, reflecting both depth and diversity in his academic pursuits. Dr. Raghu N also holds patents that highlight his technical expertise and his dedication to leveraging technology for societal benefit. His work emphasizes practical innovation aimed at addressing real-world challenges. He is actively involved in community service as a National Service Scheme (NSS) Programme Officer. Over the past five years, he has played a pivotal role in organizing and leading numerous outreach initiatives focused on social awareness, environmental sustainability, and community development. His efforts demonstrate a strong commitment to nurturing socially responsible citizens. Dr. Raghu N is also an active member of several esteemed professional bodies, including the International Association of Engineers (IAENG), the International Association of Computer Science and Information Technology (IACSIT), the Institute for Engineering Research and Publication (IFERP), the Indian Academicians and Researchers Association, the Optical Society of India, and the Asia-Pacific Chemical, Biological & Environmental Engineering Society (APCBEES). His involvement in these organizations reflects his dedication to continuous professional growth and collaboration within the global research community.

Tawheed Nabi is an Associate Professor of Economics at the Mittal School of Business, Lovely Professional University, India.

Srinivasan Nagaraj is currently working in Chitanya Bharathi Institute of Technology, Proddatur as Professor in Computer Science and Engineering Department. He completed his M.Tech(CSE) from Acharya Nagarjuna University and was awarded with Ph.D. from Annamalai University in 2023. He published more than 20 research papers in National and International journals, he published 5 patents to his credit and also participated in 15 National and International Conferences. He taught all Computer science and Machine Learning subjects for Undergraduate and Post graduate students. He has a stint of 24 years of experience in various reputed colleges and universities at various academic and administrative positions.

Kadriye Olğaç Ak is a Research Assistant in the Department of Nursing, Faculty of Health Sciences at Mardin Artuklu University. She completed her Master's degree in Public Health Nursing at Dicle University and is currently pursuing her PhD in Public Health Nursing at Atatürk University. Her research interests include public health nursing, health promotion, disease prevention, women's health, cultural health beliefs, health education, digital health, technology addictions, behavioral health, and community-based nursing interventions. She has participated in various national and international scientific projects and has authored studies in the fields of public health and nursing. Through her research and professional activities, she aims to contribute to evidence-based practices that promote health, well-being, and culturally sensitive nursing care in an increasingly digital society.

Pawan Pant is working as an Assistant Professor of Management at the University School of Business, Chandigarh University, Mohali, Punjab. He has published two research papers, one national and one international journal. He has 10 years of teaching experience and worked as an Assistant Manager (Purchase) at Pacific Industries Ltd., Udaipur (Rajasthan) for one year. His area of specialization is Economics.

K. Shyam Sunder Reddy is a Professor in the Department of Computer Science and Engineering with over 137years of teaching and research experience. He obtained his Ph.D. in Computer Science and Engineering from JNTUA and specializes in Artificial Intelligence, Machine Learning, Data Analytics, and Database Management Systems. He has published several research papers in reputed Scopus and SCIE indexed journals, authored a textbook on Database

Management Systems, and contributed actively to academic research, conferences, and professional organizations.

Ratan Sarkar is an Assistant Professor in the Department of Education, Tezpur University (A Central University), Assam, India. Previously, he served nearly seven years as Assistant Professor in the Department of Teachers' Training (B.Ed.), Prabhat Kumar College, Contai (Vidyasagar University), and as Guest Faculty at National Institute for Empowerment of Persons with Intellectual Disabilities, Regional Centre, Kolkata. He holds a Ph.D. in Education from Pondicherry University, an M.Ed. and M.Phil. in Special Education from Ramakrishna Mission Vivekananda Educational and Research Institute, Belur Math, and an M.A. in Education and Technology from Tata Institute of Social Sciences, Mumbai. He began his academic journey with a B.Ed. in Special Education (Jadavpur University) and a B.A. in English (Hons) from Siliguri College (University of North Bengal), Darjeeling. Dr. Sarkar has published extensively in leading journals (SAGE, Springer, Routledge, Wiley), authored books, chapters, and reviews, and led projects under the Ministry of Education, Govt. of India. His works on inclusive education, EdTech, disability studies, policy advocacy to advance equitable learning ecosystems.

Geetika Saxena is an Assistant Professor of Forensic Science at JECRC University, Jaipur, Rajasthan. Dr. Saxena dual master in Forensic Science and Clinical Psychology are unique and valuable, allowing her to approach juvenile delinquency from both a scientific and psychological perspective. Her primary research area of juvenile delinquency is crucial for understanding the motivations and behaviours of young offenders, and her work in this field can contribute to developing effective prevention and intervention strategies.

Richa Saxena serves as an Assistant Professor in the Department of Psychology at Kanad Assistant Professor, Haridwar. Holding degrees in both Psychology and English along with a Ph.D. and SLET, she is a seasoned psychologist excelling in clinical and counseling practices extended across Manishav, Samadhan, and online platforms. Her research prowess is evidenced by participation in numerous national and international conferences, earning prestigious best paper awards, while her 14 years of experience shine through engaging radio programs, public speaking, and master training for personality development programs. Through dynamic workshops and a pivotal role in women's empowerment via skill development initiatives, she continues to make significant contributions to mental health and community upliftment.

S Deborah Sharon is currently studying MSc Forensic Psychology under Lovely Professional University, Punjab. ORCID ID: 0009-0002-7834-8560.

Sujatha Somesula is currently working as an Assistant Professor in the Department of Computer Science and Engineering at Chaitanya Bharathi Institute of Technology in Proddatur. She completed her M.Tech in CSE from JNTUA in Ananthapuram. Her research includes two patents and two book chapters published with a well-known academic publisher. She has also participated in national and international conferences. With over six years of teaching experience, she has held academic positions at various colleges and universities. She has taught subjects such as Cloud Computing, Computer Networks, Internet of Things (IoT), Database Management Systems (DBMS), Computer Science, and Machine Learning to both undergraduate and postgraduate students. Her area of interests is Neural Networks in Deep Learning, Artificial Intelligence and Machine Learning, particularly in intelligent systems and data-driven modeling.

Mohammad Amin Wani is an Assistant Professor of Psychology with a strong background in teaching, research, and mentorship. He has demonstrated proficiency in implementing engaging teaching strategies that enhance student learning experiences and improve performance. His expertise in research is evident through his mentorship of students in research projects, fostering critical thinking and academic excellence.

Index

A

B

C

D

E

F

H

www.ingramcontent.com/pod-product-compliance
Lightning Source LLC
LaVergne TN
LVHW062337300926
849161LV00007B/1731